A B O U T   T H E   A U T H O R

J. Susan Milton is professor of statistics at Radford University. Dr. Milton received a B.S. from Western Carolina University, an M.A. from the University of North Carolina at Chapel Hill, and a Ph.D. in statistics from Virginia Polytechnic Institute and State University. She is a Danforth Associate and is a recipient of the Radford University Foundation Award for Excellence in Teaching. Dr. Milton is the author of *Introduction to Probability and Statistics: Principles and Applications for Engineering and the Computing Sciences,* as well as *Introduction to Statistics, Probability with the Essential Analysis, Applied Statistics with Probability,* and *A First Course in the Theory of Linear Statistical Models.*

To my family:

Joan and Tom Savage
Enid Milton
Stephanie and David Savage
Deborah Savage and Tim Woolf

STATISTICAL
METHODS IN THE
BIOLOGICAL
AND HEALTH SCIENCES

Third Edition

J. Susan Milton
Radford University

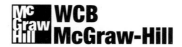

Boston   Burr Ridge, IL   Dubuque, IA   Madison, WI   New York   San Francisco
St. Louis   Bangkok   Bogotá   Caracas   Lisbon   London   Madrid
Mexico City   Milan   New Delhi   Seoul   Singapore   Sydney   Taipei   Toronto

WCB/McGraw-Hill

A Division of the McGraw-Hill Companies

STATISTICAL METHODS IN THE BIOLOGICAL AND HEALTH SCIENCE,
THIRD EDITION

This book is printed on acid-free paper.

6 7 8 9 0 QPF/QPF 0 7 6 5

ISBN 0–07–290148–9

Vice president and editorial director: *Kevin T. Kane*
Publisher: *John-Paul Lenney*
Sponsoring editor: *William K. Barter*
Marketing Manager: *Mary K. Kittell*
Project Manager: *Cathy Ford Smith*
Production Supervisor: *Laura Fuller*
Freelance design coordinator: *Mary I. Christianson*
Supplement coordinator: *Rita Hingtgen*
Compositor: *Interactive Composition Corporation*
Typeface: *10.5/12 Times Roman*
Printer: *Quebecor Printing Book Group/Fairfield, P.4*

p. 131: excerpt from Mark Stevens, *Three Mile Island*, © 1980. Reprinted with permission from Random House, Inc.

Library of Congress Cataloging-in-Publication Data

Milton J. Susan (Janet Susan)
   Statistical methods in the biological and health sciences / J.
Susan Milton. — 3rd ed.
       p.   cm.
   Includes bibliographical references and index.
   ISBN 0–07–290148–9
   J. Life sciences—Statistical methods.   J. Title.
QH323.5.M54   1999
519.5–dc21   **98   18214**
                                                    CIP

www.mhhe.com

CONTENTS

It has become increasingly evident that the interpretation of much of the research in the biological and health sciences depends to a large extent on statistical methods. For this reason, it is essential that students in these fields be exposed to statistical reasoning early in their careers. This text is intended for a first course in statistical methods for undergraduate students in the biological and health sciences. However, it can also be used to advantage by graduate students with little or no prior experience with statistical methods.

This text is not a statistical cookbook, nor is it a manual for researchers. We attempt to find a middle road—to give the student an understanding of the logic behind statistical techniques as well as practice in using them. Knowledge of calculus is not assumed, and readers with an adequate background in high school algebra should be able to follow the arguments presented.

We chose the examples and exercises specifically for the student of biological and health sciences. These are drawn from genetics, general biology, ecology, and medicine, and, except where indicated otherwise, data are simulated. However, the simulation is done with care so that the results of the analysis are consistent with recently reported research. In this way, the student will gain some insight into the types of problems that interest current workers in the biological sciences. Many exercises are open-ended to stimulate some classroom discussion.

It is assumed that the student has access to some type of electronic calculator. Many such calculators are on the market, and most have some built-in statistical capability. Use of these calculators is encouraged, for it allows the student to concentrate on the interpretation of the analysis rather than on the arithmetic computations. Instruction in the use of the TI83 graphing calculator is given in the text. This calculator, which is relatively new on the market, will perform most of the statistical tests presented in the text. It will also derive many of the confidence intervals described and has available most of the statistical tables discussed in the manuscript.

We should point out that most of the data sets presented are rather small so that the student will not be overwhelmed by the computational aspects of statistical analysis. This does not imply that very small samples are acceptable in biological research. In fact, most major research projects involve a tremendous investment in time and money and result in a large body of data. Such data lend themselves to analysis via the electronic computer. For this reason, we include some instruction in the interpretation of computer output. The package chosen for illustrative purposes is SAS (Statistical Analysis System: SAS Institute, Inc., Raleigh, North Carolina). This was done because of its widespread availability and ease of use. We do not intend to imply that it is superior to other well-known packages such as SPSSX (Statistical Package for the Social Sciences), BMD (Biomedical Computer Programs, University of California Press), or

MINITAB (Duxbury Press). An introduction to SAS together with the computer code required to generate the output is given in an optional Technology Tools section at chapter end.

This is a substantial revision of the second edition of the text. Reviewers' comments have been incorporated into the text to strengthen the discussions in many places. New exercises have been added throughout the text. A Technology Tools section introducing SAS programming and the TI83 graphing calculator has been added at the end of many chapters. New discussions include those of back-to-back stem-and-leaf plots, a simplified discussion of variance comparisons, and an expanded T table. The text continues to place a heavy emphasis on the finding and interpretation of P values.

A number of different courses can be taught from this book. They can vary in length from one semester to one year. It is difficult to determine exactly what material can be covered in a given time, since this is a function of class size, academic maturity of the students, and the inclination of the instructor. However, we do offer some guidelines for the use of this text in the chapter summaries below.

Chapter 1   This is an introduction to descriptive statistics. The notion of population versus sample is introduced early and stressed. The exploratory data analysis (EDA) topics of stem-and-leaf diagrams and box plots have been expanded. The importance of assessing shape, location, and variability is emphasized.

Chapter 2   This chapter introduces probability from an intuitive point of view. Tree diagrams are introduced and their use in solving genetics problems is emphasized. Counting techniques are given and tied to the problem of calculating probabilities via the classical method. If time does not permit coverage of the entire chapter, we suggest that Sections 2.1 and 2.2 be covered.

Chapter 3   This chapter covers the axioms of probability and the theorems that follow from the axioms. The topics of independence, conditional probability, and Bayes' Theorem are found here. A section entitled "Diagnostic Tests and Relative Risk" is included, presenting applications of conditional probability that are of special interest to students in the medical fields. This chapter can be skipped if time does not permit its coverage.

Chapter 4   This chapter covers discrete random variables only, introducing the notions of density, cumulative distribution, and expectation.

Chapter 5   This chapter parallels the ideas presented in Chapter 4 but applies them to continuous random variables. A subsection on the normal probability rule and its application to the construction of medical charts is given.

Chapter 6   In Chapter 6 we discuss point and interval estimation of the mean as well as hypothesis testing on the value of this parameter. A section on random sampling and randomization is included. The use of the P value is explained and emphasized throughout this chapter and the remainder of the text. A section on the effect of sample size on the length of confidence intervals and on the power of a test is given.

Chapter 7   This chapter is a short chapter on inferences concerning the variance and the standard deviation of a random variable. The discussion of variance comparisons has been simplified to include a rule-of-thumb check for equality. The formal F test is still included in the text.

Chapter 8   In Chapter 8 we discuss inferences on a proportion and the comparison of two proportions, with the Central Limit Theorem used to justify the techniques given.

Chapter 9   In Chapter 9 we compare two means via point and interval estimation and hypothesis tests. Preliminary *F* tests for comparing variances are discussed. Both the pooled and the Smith-Satterthwaite procedures for comparing means based on independent samples are explained. Discussion of how to use SAS for these tests is included. The chapter ends with a section about paired data.

Chapter 10   Chapter 10 introduces techniques used to compare the means of more than two populations, including discussions of the one-way classification model, randomized blocks, and the two-way classification model. The material includes a discussion of the effectiveness of blocking and Bonferroni *T* tests for conducting paired comparisons. Notes on computing are given throughout the chapter.

Chapter 11   This chapter presents a thorough discussion of simple linear regression and correlation. A section on multiple regression has been added.

Chapter 12   Categorical data problems are considered here, with an emphasis on tests of independence and tests of homogeneity in 2×2 and $r \times c$ tables.

Chapter 13   In this chapter, distribution-free alternatives to the classical procedures given in earlier chapters are presented. The material includes sections on the Lilliefors test for normality, Bartlett's tests for equal variances, and a small sample binomial test on proportions.

Many courses on this level are one semester in length, and it would be difficult to cover the entire text in that time. Sections that can be omitted with little loss of continuity are labeled as optional.

Thanks are due to Maggie Rogers, Bill Barter, and Cathy Smith for their encouragement and direction during the revision of this text and to Joann Fisher for the typing of the manuscript. My appreciation goes to Tonya Porter for her help in the preparation of the solutions manual. I also wish to recognize Joan Savage and Charlene Lutes for their help as biological consultants. Special thanks are offered to the following reviewers for their helpful suggestions: Charles M. Biles, Ph.D., Humboldt State University; John E. Boyer, Jr., Kansas State University; Annette Bucher, Colorado State University; Christiana Drake, University of California; Dr. R. K. Elswick, Jr., Medical College of Virginia, Virginia Commonwealth University; Thomas J. Glover, Hobart and William Smith Colleges; Golde I. Holtzman, Virginia Tech (VPI); Mark Krailo, University of Southern California; Benny Lo, NW Polytechnic University; Christopher Morrell, Loyola College; Lisa Sullivan, Boston University; Andrew Jay Tierman, Saginaw Valley State University; Mark S. West, Auburn University; and Robert F. Woolson, Ph.D., The University of Iowa.

J. Susan Milton

Descriptive Methods

Statistics has become an indispensable tool for most scientists. What is statistics and how can statistical techniques be used to answer the practical questions posed by scientists?

Statistics has been defined as the art of decision making in the face of uncertainty. We begin by describing a typical problem that calls for a statistical solution. We use this example to introduce some of the language underlying the field of statistics. The terms are used here on an intuitive level. They are defined in a more technical sense later, as the need arises.

A researcher studying heart disease in persons 18 years old or older has identified four factors as being potentially associated with the development of the disease: age, weight, number of cigarettes smoked per day, and family history of heart disease. The researcher wants to gather evidence that either confirms these factors as contributing to the development of the disease or shows them to be unimportant. How should she or he proceed?

This is inherently a statistical problem. What characteristics identify it as such? Simply these:

1. Associated with the problem is a large group of objects (in this case, people) about which inferences are to be made. This group of objects is called the *population.*
2. Certain characteristics of the members of the population are of particular interest. The value of each of these characteristics may change from object to object within the population. They are called *random variables:* variables because they change in value; random because their behavior depends on chance and is somewhat unpredictable.
3. The population is too large to study in its entirety. So we must make inferences about the population based on what is observed by studying only a portion, or *sample,* of objects from the population.

In the study of factors affecting heart disease, the population is the set of all persons suffering from the disease. The random variables of interest are the patient's age and weight, number of cigarettes smoked per day, and family history. It is impossible to identify and study every person with heart disease. Thus any conclusions that are reached must be based on studying only a portion, or a sample, of these people.

Random variables fall into two broad categories: continuous and discrete. A *continuous random variable* is a variable that prior to the experiment being conducted can assume any value in some interval or continuous span of real numbers. Measurements of things such as time, length, height, age, weight, speed, temperature, and pressure are usually assumed to be continuous. The variable age in the study of heart disease is continuous, as is the variable weight. The age of a person in the study conceivably can lie anywhere between 18 and, say, 110 years, a continuous time span. The person's weight may lie anywhere from perhaps 90 to 600 pounds! A *discrete random variable* is a variable that assumes its values at isolated points. Thus the set of possible values is either finite or countably infinite. Discrete random variables often arise in practice in connection with count variables. The number of cigarettes smoked per day is discrete. If we count a portion of a cigarette smoked as being a cigarette smoked, then the set of possible values is {0, 1, 2, 3, 4, 5, . . .}, a countably infinite collection. If family history is studied by recording the number of natural parents and grandparents who experienced heart disease, then this variable also is discrete. Its set of possible values is {0, 1, 2, 3, 4, 5, 6}, a finite collection. Random variables are usually denoted by capital letters.

A descriptive measure associated with a random variable when the variable is considered over the entire population is called a *parameter*. Parameters are usually denoted by Greek letters. To remember that parameters describe populations, just remember that both of these words begin with the letter *p*. One commonly encountered parameter is the population average value, or the population mean. This parameter is denoted by the Greek letter μ. For example, in the study of heart disease, the researcher would be interested in determining the average number of cigarettes smoked per day by members of the population. The exact value of this parameter cannot be obtained unless every member of the population is surveyed. Since this cannot be done, the exact value of μ will remain unknown even after our study is complete. However, we will be able to use statistical methods to approximate its value based on data obtained from a sample of patients drawn from the population.

A descriptive measure associated with a random variable when the variable is considered only over a sample is called a *statistic*. This is easy to remember because the words *statistic* and *sample* both begin with the letter *s*. Statistics serve two purposes. They describe the sample at hand, and they serve as approximations for corresponding population parameters. For example, the average number of cigarettes smoked per day by members of a sample of heart disease patients is a statistic. It is called a sample average or sample mean. Its value for a given sample probably will not equal the population mean μ exactly. However, it is hoped that it is at least close in value to μ.

A statistician or user of statistics is always working in two worlds. The ideal world is at the population level and is theoretical in nature. It is the world that we would like to see. The world of reality is the sample world. This is the level at which we really operate. We hope that the characteristics of our sample reflect well the characteristics of the population. That is, we treat our sample as a microcosm that mirrors the population. The idea is illustrated in Figure 1.1.

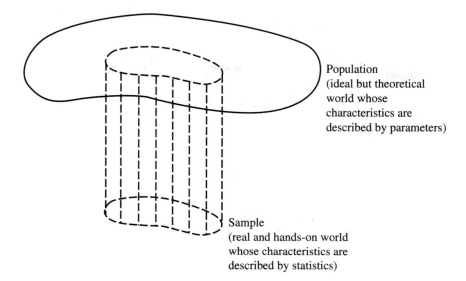

Population
(ideal but theoretical
world whose
characteristics are
described by parameters)

Sample
(real and hands-on world
whose characteristics are
described by statistics)

FIGURE 1.1

The sample is viewed as a miniature population. We hope that the behavior of
the random variable under study over the sample gives an accurate picture of its
behavior in the population.

We shall be interested primarily in three questions concerning the behavior of a
random variable. These are:

1. What is the location of the variable? That is, about what value does the variable
   fluctuate?
2. How much variation is involved? That is, do the observed values of the variable
   tend to cluster closely together or are they widely spread?
3. What is the shape of the distribution? That is, do the values tend to fall into a bell-
   shaped, flat, u-shaped, or some other distinctive pattern?

In this chapter we introduce some graphical and some analytical techniques that can be
used to answer these questions.

1.1
DISTRIBUTION TABLES: DISCRETE DATA

Recall that a discrete random variable is a random variable that can assume at most
either a finite or a countably infinite number of possible values. Discrete random variables arise frequently in survey data. For example, we might want to compare the opinion of females concerning the issue of abortion to that of males. Hence one variable in
the study is "sex." This variable is discrete since it assumes only the two naturally occurring values "male" or "female." We might ask the question, Do you favor legalized
abortion on demand during the first trimester of pregnancy? Since the answer to this

question varies from respondent to respondent, we are dealing with a random variable. The researcher could decide to record each response as "yes," "no," "undecided," or "refuses to answer." In this way a discrete random variable with four possible values is created. To understand and summarize such data, it is helpful to display the data in table or graphical form. These tables or graphs usually display the possible values of the random variable along with information on the number of times each value occurs. These counts are called *frequency counts* or simply *frequencies*. Example 1.1.1 illustrates the idea.

EXAMPLE 1.1.1. A comparative study of two adult homes in western Virginia is conducted. The purpose of the study is to determine the type of patients being served and to ascertain where patients go upon discharge from the home. Four discrete random variables are involved. They are sex (coded by the researcher as F = female or M = male), diagnosis (coded as MR = mentally retarded, MI = mentally ill, PI = physically ill), age, and destination after leaving the home (coded as 1 = died, 2 = home of relative, 3 = hospital, 4 = street, 5 = another home for adults, 6 = nursing home, 7 = not discharged at present). (Data presented are for one home and are taken from a larger study conducted by the statistical laboratory and Debbie Thompson, Department of Social Work, Radford University, 1990.)

Sex	Diagnosis	Age	Destination	Sex	Diagnosis	Age	Destination
M	MI	29	2	F	MI	72	6
M	MR	35	7	M	MI	52	7
F	PI	34	7	F	PI	31	7
M	MI	36	7	M	PI	35	7
F	MR	25	7	M	PI	42	7
F	MI	20	7	F	MI	29	2
F	PI	31	7	F	MR	61	7
F	PI	89	1	F	MI	18	3
M	MR	42	7	F	MR	64	7
M	MI	41	7	M	PI	51	7
F	PI	47	7	F	PI	30	7
M	PI	41	2	F	MR	35	7
M	MI	87	7	M	PI	40	6
F	MR	56	1	M	MR	76	3
F	MR	50	7	M	PI	59	7
F	PI	28	7	F	MI	71	6
M	MR	35	7	F	MI	62	7
F	PI	23	7	F	MI	65	3
F	MR	39	3	M	MR	51	7
M	PI	42	7	F	MR	18	7

The frequencies for the variable *diagnosis* are shown in Table 1.1. Notice that this table lists the category into which the response falls along with the number of observations per category.

In most studies frequency counts are obtained, and they do give valuable insight into the behavior of the random variable under study. However, frequency counts alone can be misleading. For example, suppose that we hear that 10 new cases of acquired immunodeficiency syndrome (AIDS) were diagnosed at a particular hospital during

TABLE 1.1

Frequency distribution for the variable *diagnosis* of Example 1.1.1

Category	Frequency
MI (mentally ill)	12
MR (mentally retarded)	13
PI (physically ill)	15

the month of June. Is this cause for alarm? Maybe—maybe not. It depends, of course, on the number of persons screened for the disease. Ten cases discovered among 20 persons tested certainly paints an entirely different picture than does 10 cases found among 1000 persons tested. To put a frequency count into perspective we report the count relative to the total, thus forming a *relative frequency*. Table 1.2 gives the frequencies and relative frequencies for the variable *diagnosis* of Example 1.1.1. Relative frequencies can be multiplied by 100 to yield the percentage of observations falling into each category. This information is useful since percentages are readily understood by everyone. Table 1.3 gives the complete summary of the variable *diagnosis*.

Table 1.4 is a summary table of the data as produced by SAS. SAS, which stands for Statistical Analysis System, is a statistical computing package that is in widespread use among data analysts, statisticians, and researchers. Some key SAS basics will be explained in the Technology Tools sections of this text. Notice that SAS has automatically listed the diagnosis values in alphabetical order. It has also included a column called "cumulative frequency" and one called "cumulative percent." The word *cumulative* means to accumulate or sum the values. Thus the cumulative frequency 25 is obtained by adding the number of mentally retarded patients (13) found in the second row to the number of mentally ill patients (12) found in the first row; the

TABLE 1.2

Frequency and relative frequency distributions for the variable *diagnosis* of Example 1.1.1

Category	Frequency	Relative frequency
MI (mentally ill)	12	12/40 = .300

TABLE 1.3

Complete summary table for the variable *diagnosis* of Example 1.1.1

Category	Frequency	Relative frequency	Percentage
MI (mentally ill)	12	12/40 = .300	30.0
MR (mentally retarded)	13	13/40 = .325	32.5
PI (physically ill)	15	15/40 = .375	37.5

■ **TABLE 1.4**

Frequencies and percentages for the variable diagnosis of
Example 1.1.1

Diagnose	Frequency	Percent	Cumulative frequency	Cumulative percent
MI	12	30.0	12	30.0
MR	13	32.5	25	62.5
PI	15	37.5	40	100.0

cumulative frequency 40 is the sum of all of the counts listed in the frequency column
(40 = 12 + 13 + 15). Note that if the data are entered correctly the last number in the
cumulative frequency column should be the sample size.

The cumulative percent column is obtained by summing the percent column; its
last entry should always be 100%. However, in some tables the percentages might not
add to 100% exactly due to rounding differences. We should point out that when the
variable values are nonnumeric or have no natural linear order, the cumulative distribution might not be meaningful. However, it does give a verification that all the data in
the sample have been included. The SAS code used to produce this table is given in the
Technology Tools section at the end of this chapter.

Bar Graphs

A vertical bar graph can be used to convey information visually. Each category is represented by a vertical bar with each bar being of the same width. The heights of the
bars are dependent upon the number of observations per category. The vertical scale
of the graph can represent frequencies, relative frequencies, or percentages. Each type
of graph is informative, with the latter two having the advantage that their vertical
scales are not data dependent. They range from 0 to 1 in the case of a relative frequency bar graph and from 0 to 100% in the case of a percentage bar graph. Figure 1.2
shows each of these graphs for the variable *diagnosis* of Example 1.1.1. Bars can be
constructed horizontally if so desired. In fact, horizontal bar charts are sometimes
preferable in report writing as they tend to require less space than do vertical bar
charts. Figure 1.3 shows the horizontal bar graph for the variable *diagnosis* as produced by SAS. Notice that this graph also automatically gives the summary information contained in Table 1.4.

Bivariate Data: Two-Way Tables

Sometimes we want to study two discrete random variables simultaneously. For example, we might want to use the data of Example 1.1.1 to investigate a possible association between the sex of a patient and the diagnosis given. To begin such a study, we
construct a two-way table. Such a table contains r rows, where r is the number of possible responses for the first variable, and c columns, where c is the number of responses

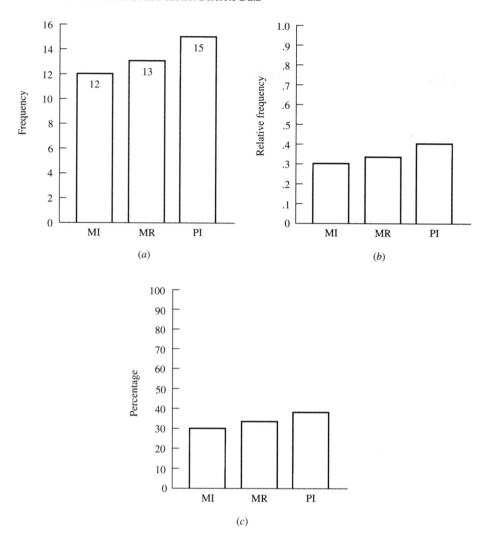

FIGURE 1.2

(a) Frequency bar graph for the variable *diagnosis,* of Example 1.1.1; (b) relative frequency bar graph for the variable *diagnosis;* (c) percentage bar graph for the variable *diagnosis.*

associated with the second variable. Thus a two-way table has $r \cdot c$ categories or cells. Information concerning frequencies, relative frequencies, and percentages is commonly included in the table. It also includes the distribution for each variable individually along the margins of the table.

EXAMPLE 1.1.2. Consider the data of Example 1.1.1. The random variable *sex* has two possible responses. If we use this variable to form the rows of our table, then $r = 2$. The

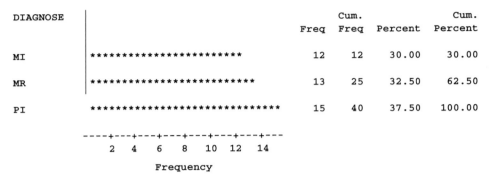

A Horizontal Bar Graph:
Variable Diagnosis

FIGURE 1.3

A horizontal bar graph for the variable *diagnosis* of Example 1.1.1 as produced by SAS.

TABLE 1.5

Two-way distribution table for the study of Example 1.1.1 with $r = 2$, $c = 3$, and $r \cdot c = 6$ cells

Sex	Diagnosis		
	MI	**MR**	**PI**
F	Females who are mentally ill	Females who are mentally retarded	Females who are physically ill
M	Males who are mentally ill	Males who are mentally retarded	Males who are physically ill

random variable *diagnosis* has three responses, and hence the table has $c = 3$ columns. This results in a two-way table with $r \cdot c = 2 \cdot 3 = 6$ cells. These cells are shown in Table 1.5. The distribution of the 40 patients among the 6 cells is shown in Table 1.6.

Two-way tables can be formed that allow a quick comparison of one group of individuals within a sample to another. For instance, in the study of Example 1.1.1 it would be of interest to compare the diagnosis of males to that of females. Since the frequencies, relative frequencies, and percentages reported in Table 1.6 refer to cells, some additional computations are required to make the comparison. Notice that there are 17 males in the sample. Of these, 5 are mentally ill, 5 are mentally retarded, and 7 are physically ill. This information can be used to obtain the distribution of the variable *diagnosis* for the males within the sample. This distribution is shown in Table 1.7a. The distribution of the variable *diagnosis* for the 23 females in the sample is included in Table 1.7b. Notice that there are some differences in distribution between the two groups, the most notable being that, at the present time, the percentage of physically ill males (41.18%) is somewhat larger than the percentage of physically ill females (34.78%).

TABLE 1.6

Two-way distribution table of *sex* by *diagnosis* for the data of Example 1.1.1*

Sex	Diagnosis			Distribution of *sex*
	MI	MR	PI	
F	7	8	8	23
	.175	.200	.200	.575
	17.5%	20.0%	20.0%	57.5%
M	7	5	7	17
	.125	.125	.175	.425
	12.5%	12.5%	17.5%	42.5%
Distribution of *diagnosis*	12	13	15	40
	.300	.325	.375	
	30.0%	32.5%	37.5%	

*The first number in each cell gives the cell frequency followed by the cell relative frequency and cell percentage.

TABLE 1.7a

Distribution of the variable *diagnosis* for the males of Example 1.1.1

Sex	Diagnosis			
	MI	MR	PI	
F				
M	5	5	7	17
	$\frac{5}{17} = .2941$	$\frac{5}{17} = .2941$	$\frac{7}{17} = .4118$	
	29.41%	29.41%	41.18%	

TABLE 1.7b

Distribution of the variable *diagnosis* for both males and females

Sex	Diagnosis			
	MI	MR	PI	
F	7	8	8	23
	$\frac{7}{23} = .3043$	$\frac{8}{23} = .3478$	$\frac{8}{23} = .3478$	
	30.43%	34.78%	34.78%	
M	5	5	7	17
	$\frac{5}{17} = .2941$	$\frac{5}{17} = .2941$	$\frac{7}{17} = .4118$	
	29.41%	29.41%	41.18%	

▨   **TABLE 1.8**

Two-way table used to investigate the association between
sex and _diagnosis,_ for the data of Example 1.1.1, as
produced by SAS

```
Two-Way Table Used to Investigate
The Relationship Between Sex and Diagnosis


                   |  Table of sex by DIAGNOSE

     Sex           |  DIAGNOSE

     Frequency|           |           |           |
     Percent  |           |           |           |
     Row Pct  |           |           |           |
     Col Pct  |  MI       |  MR       |  PI       |   Total
     ---------+-----------+-----------+--------+
     F        |        7  |        8  |        8  |     23
              |    17.50  |    20.00  |    20.00  |   57.50
              |    30.43  |    34.78  |    34.78  |
              |    58.33  |    61.54  |    53.33  |

     ---------+-----------+-----------+--------+
     M        |        5  |        5  |        7  |     17
              |    12.50  |    12.50  |    17.50  |   42.50
              |    29.41  |    29.41  |    41.18  |
              |    41.67  |    38.46  |    46.67  |

     ---------+-----------+-----------+--------+
     Total           12         13         15         40
                   30.00      32.50      37.50     100.00
```

SAS includes a procedure for producing two-way tables quickly. Table 1.8 is the SAS version of the two-way table for the data of Example 1.1.1. Notice that SAS automatically lists row and column headings in alphabetical order. The upper left-hand corner of the SAS printout explains the numbers contained in each cell of the table. The first number is the cell frequency. For example, from the table we can see that there were 7 mentally ill females in the sample. The second number gives the cell percentage. We can see that the 7 mentally ill females make up 17.5% of the entire sample. The third number gives the row percentage. In the example, we can now see that of the _females_ in the sample, 30.43% were mentally ill. Notice that the row percentages match those found by hand and given in Table 1.7b. Table 1.8 lets us see that of the patients who were mentally ill, 58.33% were female. Notice that the distribution of _sex_ is found as row totals and percentages in SAS, which match the values found in Table 1.6; the distribution of _diagnosis_ is shown as column totals and percentages, which also match the values found in Table 1.6. The SAS code for producing two-way tables is found in the Technology Tools section at the end of this chapter.

Remember that all we have done in the examples in this section is describe a sample of patients from a particular adult home. Techniques for drawing conclusions about the population of patients served by this home from the sample will be presented in chapters to come.

■ EXERCISES 1.1

1. The following data are from a second adult home taken from the study described in
   Example 1.1.1.

Sex	Diagnosis	Age	Destination	Sex	Diagnosis	Age	Destination
F	MI	67	6	M	MR	80	7
M	PI	71	7	M	MI	83	2
F	PI	54	1	M	PI	49	3
F	MI	63	7	F	PI	78	6
F	MI	48	7	M	MI	57	7
M	MI	56	7	M	MR	69	3
M	PI	62	3	F	MI	83	7
F	MR	57	2	F	PI	92	1
F	PI	81	7	F	PI	55	3
F	PI	36	7	F	PI	63	6
F	PI	72	3	F	PI	64	4
F	PI	65	3	M	PI	89	7

   (a) Construct a summary table for the variable *diagnosis*.
   (b) Construct a percentage bar graph for the variable *diagnosis*. Comment on any
       differences that you observe between this graph and that given in Figure 1.2c.
2. (a) See the data of Example 1.1.1 and Exercise 1 to construct frequency bar
       graphs for the variable *destination* for the two homes. Why is a comparison
       of this variable for the two samples based on these graphs alone not appro-
       priate?
   (b) Construct relative frequency bar graphs for the variable *destination* for each
       home. Comment on any apparent differences observed.
   (c) Construct a two-way table of *sex* versus *destination* for each group.
   (d) Construct a two-way table of *diagnosis* versus *destination* for each group.
3. Construct a two-way table of *sex* versus *diagnosis* for the data of Exercise 1. Compare this table to that given in Table 1.6. Comment on any apparent differences that
   you observe.
4. Construct a two-way table of *sex* versus *diagnosis* that displays the distribution of
   the variable *diagnosis* for each sex for the data of Exercise 1. Comment on any notable differences between males and females for this sample.
5. A study is conducted to investigate the association between diet and the development
   of headaches. Two groups of chronic headache sufferers are identified. These are
   coded as V = vascular headaches and T = tension headaches. A control group
   consisting of persons who claim to have headaches infrequently was also included
   in the study. These persons are coded as C. Each individual is also identified by
   sex. The study group is as follows: (Based on a study reported in Patricia
   Guarnieri, Cynthia Radnitz, and Edward Blanchard, "Assessment of Dietary Risk
   Factors in Chronic Headache," *Biofeedback and Self-Regulation,* vol. 15, March
   1990, pp. 15–25.)

Sex	Diagnosis	Sex	Diagnosis	Sex	Diagnosis	Sex	Diagnosis
M	V	F	V	M	V	M	V
F	V	F	T	M	V	F	T
F	V	M	C	M	V	M	V
M	T	F	V	M	C	F	C
F	T	M	V	F	V	M	T
M	V	M	C	F	T	M	V
M	V	F	C	F	V	M	T
M	C	F	V	F	V	M	C
F	C	F	V	F	V	F	V
F	V	F	C	F	V	F	V
F	C	M	V	F	V	F	V
M	V	F	T	F	V	F	T
F	C	F	C	F	T	F	V
F	C	F	C	F	T	F	T
M	V	F	V	F	C	F	V
F	C	F	C	F	V	F	C
F	V	F	C	F	T	F	T
M	V	M	V	M	C	F	V
F	C	F	T	F	T	M	C
F	C	F	C	M	C	M	T
F	T	M	V	F	V	F	C
M	V	F	T	M	C	F	T
M	T	F	C	M	T	F	V
F	V	M	C	F	V	F	V
M	T	F	T	F	C	F	T
F	V	F	V	F	V	M	T
F	V	F	T	F	C	F	V
F	V	F	V	F	C	F	V
F	T	F	V	F	V	F	V
F	V	F	V	F	C	F	C
F	T	F	V	F	T	F	V
F	V	F	C	F	V	M	T
F	V	F	V	M	C	M	T
F	T	F	V	M	T	M	C
F	C	F	C	M	T	F	C
F	V	M	T	F	V	F	C
M	C	F	V	F	C	M	T
M	T	M	T	F	T	F	V
F	T	F	V	F	V	F	C
F	V	F	T	F	T	F	T
F	V	M	C	F	C	F	C
F	V	F	V	F	V	F	V
F	V	F	C				

(*a*) Construct a two-way distribution table of *sex* versus *diagnosis*.

(*b*) Construct a two-way table that allows one to compare the diagnosis for males to that for females.

6. In many disciplines, questions are asked to determine the strength of the opinion held by a group of people concerning a given topic. Responses are scored on what

is called a "Likert" scale. A typical Likert scale will label responses as follows:

1 = strongly disagree
2 = somewhat disagree
3 = neutral
4 = somewhat agree
5 = strongly agree
6 = not applicable

In a study of student opinion this statement was made: "The Health Center at R.U. has hours that are convenient for students." A sample of 246 students was obtained and each student was classified according to his or her gender and his or her response to this statement on the Likert scale. Use the SAS printout given in Table 1.9 to answer these questions.

(a) There are only 245 student responses accounted for in the table. There are several reasons for obtaining a missing response. List some of these reasons.
(b) How many students in the sample were female and strongly agreed with the statement?
(c) What percentage of the sample was female and strongly agreed with the statement?
(d) What percentage of the females strongly agreed with the statement?
(e) What percentage of the males strongly agreed with the statement?
(f) Of those that strongly agreed, what percentage was female?

TABLE 1.9
Two-way summary table for the variables gender and health center hours

Table of Gender by Q2

```
Gender    Q2

Frequency|
Percent  |
Row Pct  |strongly|somewhat|neutral|somewhat|strongly|  not    |
Col Pct  |disagree|disagree|       | agree  | agree  |applicable| Total
---------+--------+--------+-------+--------+--------+----------+
f        |     18 |     20 |    23 |     45 |     20 |       16 |  142
         |   7.35 |   8.16 |  9.39 |  18.37 |   8.16 |     6.53 | 57.96
         |  12.68 |  14.08 | 16.20 |  31.69 |  14.08 |    11.27 |
         |  78.26 |  50.00 | 47.92 |  61.64 |  68.97 |    50.00 |
---------+--------+--------+-------+--------+--------+----------+
m        |      5 |     20 |    25 |     28 |      9 |       16 |  103
         |   2.04 |   8.16 | 10.20 |  11.43 |   3.67 |     6.53 | 42.04
         |   4.85 |  19.42 | 24.27 |  27.18 |   8.74 |    15.53 |
         |  21.74 |  50.00 | 52.08 |  38.36 |  31.03 |    50.00 |
---------+--------+--------+-------+--------+--------+----------+
Total         23       40      48       73       29        32     245
            9.39    16.33   19.59    29.80    11.84     13.06  100.00

Frequency missing = 1
```

TABLE 1.10

**Two-way table for the variables species
and presence of grooming**

```
           Table of species by response

Species       Response

Frequency|
Percent
Row Pct
Col Pct  | no      |yes      |  Total
---------+--------+---------+
       1 |    40  |     25  |     65
         |  30.77 |   19.23 |  50.00
         |  61.54 |   38.46 |
         |  53.33 |   45.45 |
---------+--------+---------+
       2 |    35  |     30  |     65
         |  26.92 |   23.08 |  50.00
         |  53.85 |   46.15 |
         |  46.67 |   54.55 |
---------+--------+---------+
Total         75        55       130
            57.69     42.31    100.00
```

(g) From an intuitive standpoint, does it appear that males and females probably differ substantially in their opinion toward health center hours? Explain your reasoning.

(h) Give some reasons why a student might check "not applicable" as a response to the statement.

(Based on data gathered at Radford University, March 1997.)

7. A study is conducted to investigate the association between spider species and various activities that spiders perform. Use the data of Table 1.10 to answer these questions.

(a) Which species had the highest percentage of its members participating in the grooming activity?

(b) What percentages of the entire sample of 130 spiders participated in grooming?

(c) Based on these data, do you think that there might be a substantial difference in grooming habits between these two species? Explain your answer.

(Based on an experiment conducted by Travis Alderman, Department of Biology, Radford University, Spring 1997.)

1.2

A QUICK LOOK AT DISTRIBUTION: STEM AND LEAF

Before beginning to analyze a data set it is important to realize what the data represent. In particular, it is important to realize that each number in a data set is an observed value of some random variable. Sometimes we have data for the entire population; usually we do not. When the data available are population data, any pertinent question can be answered by direct observation. There is no uncertainty concerning the characteristics of the population. However, if the data represent only a sample of observations drawn from the population, then statistical methods are needed to ascertain the nature of the population.

Consider a discrete quantitative random variable with a large number of possible values or a continuous random variable. Our first task is to get some idea of the distribution of the random variable. That is, we want to determine where the values are centered, whether they are widely spread, and whether or not they fall into a distinctive pattern. To do so, we shall employ some of the tools of exploratory data analysis (EDA). In the words of John W. Tukey, a well-known data analyst and the author of many EDA techniques [16]

> We will be exploring numbers. We need to handle them easily and look at them effectively. Techniques for handling and looking—whether graphical, arithmetic, or intermediate—will be important. The simpler we can make these techniques the better—so long as they work—and work well.

A technique for looking at distribution that has been found to work well is the stem-and-leaf diagram. It is easy to construct, and the construction can be done quickly. As you shall see, the data set is essentially reproduced in the stem-and-leaf diagram. Thus we create a diagram in which data points are grouped in such a way that we can see the shape of the distribution while retaining the individuality of the data points. A stem-and-leaf diagram consists of a series of horizontal rows of numbers. The number used to label a row is called its *stem,* and the remaining numbers in the row are called *leaves.* The stem is the major portion of the number. For example, if we look at the numbers 3.1, 3.2, 3.7, and 3.5, what first catches the eye is the fact that all these numbers are in the "threes." The stem of each number is 3. The leaf of each number gives secondary information about the number. In our example the leaf of each number is the number after the decimal place. It gives more specific information about these numbers that are all in the "threes." There are no hard-and-fast rules about how to construct a stem-and-leaf diagram. Roughly, the steps are as follows:

Constructing a Simple Stem-and-Leaf Diagram

1. Choose some convenient numbers to serve as stems. To be useful in ascertaining shape at least five stems are needed. The stems chosen are usually the first one or two digits of the numbers in the data set.
2. Label the rows via the chosen stems.
3. Reproduce the data graphically by recording the digit following the stem as a leaf on the appropriate stem.
4. Turn the graph on its side to see how the numbers are distributed. In particular, try to answer such questions as
   a. Do the data tend to cluster near a particular stem or stems or do they spread rather evenly across the diagram?
   b. Do the data tend to taper toward one end or the other of the diagram?
   c. If a smooth curve is sketched across the top of the diagram, does it form a rough bell? Is it flat? Is it symmetric?

An example should clarify the idea.

1		1	0 2		1	0 2 4 0 9 2 1 1 4 3 5		1	0 2 4 0 9 2 1 1 4 3 5
2		2	0		2	0 2 7 2 3 4 1 1		2	0 2 7 2 3 4 1 1
3		3	3		3	3 1 0		3	3 1 0
4		4			4	1 0 1		4	1 0 1
5		5			5	0 1		5	0 1
6		6			6	3		6	3
7		7			7	7		7	7
8		8			8	3		8	3
(a)		(b)			(c)			(d)	

FIGURE 1.4

Stem-and-leaf display for the magnitude of a sample of California earthquakes as measured on the Richter scale: (a) choosing stems, (b) recording the first four data points, (c) the entire data set displayed and (d) looking for shape.

EXAMPLE 1.2.1. Consider these observations on the random variable X, the magnitude of a California earthquake as measured on the Richter scale:

1.0	8.3	3.1	1.1	5.1
1.2	1.0	4.1	1.1	4.0
2.0	1.9	6.3	1.4	1.3
3.3	2.2	2.3	2.1	2.1
1.4	2.7	2.4	3.0	4.1
5.0	2.2	1.2	7.7	1.5

The first digits of these numbers are 1, 2, 3, 4, 5, 6, 7, 8. These digits will serve as stems and row labels. See Figure 1.4a. We next represent the data graphically by recording the number appearing after the decimal point as a leaf on the appropriate stem. The first four data points are shown in Figure 1.4b. The entire data set is displayed in Figure 1.4c. To get an idea of shape, turn the book on its side and look at the smooth curve that has been drawn in Figure 1.4d. From this, it can be seen that these data cluster at the lower end of the scale; most quakes were rather mild. If this sample is an accurate indication of the severity of California earthquakes, then it would seem rather unusual to see a very severe quake. Notice also that the display is not symmetric. Rather, there is a long tail or tapering toward the upper or right end of the display. Data such as these are said to be skewed right. If the long tail were to the left, we would say that the data are skewed left. (Based on data found in Robert Iacopi, *Earthquake Country,* Lane Books, Menlo Park, Calif., 1971.)

Sometimes using the first one or two digits of the data points as stems does not provide enough stems to allow us to detect the shape. One way to overcome this problem is to use double stems. That is, use each stem twice—once to graph the low leaves 0, 1, 2, 3, 4 and then again to graph the high leaves 5, 6, 7, 8, 9. Example 1.2.2 illustrates a double-stem diagram.

EXAMPLE 1.2.2. In a study of growth in males these observations are obtained on X, the circumference in centimeters of a child's head at birth.

33.1	34.6	34.2	36.1	34.2	35.6
34.5	35.8	34.5	34.2	34.3	35.2
33.7	36.0	34.2	34.7	34.6	34.3
33.4	34.9	33.8	33.6	35.2	34.6
33.7	34.8	33.9	34.7	35.1	34.2
36.5	34.1	34.0	35.1	35.3	

```
33 | 1 4
33 | 7 7 8 9 6
34 | 1 2 2 0 2 2 3 3 2
34 | 5 6 9 8 5 7 7 6 6
35 | 1 2 1 3 2
35 | 8 6
36 | 0 1
36 | 5
```

FIGURE 1.5

A double stem-and-leaf display giving the circumference in centimeters of a child's head at birth based on the data of Example 1.2.2.

If we use the first two digits as stems, we will only have four stems, 33, 34, 35, 36. Since this is not enough to allow us to detect shape, we will use each of these twice and form a double-stem display. The display is shown in Figure 1.5. Notice that in each case the low leaves 0, 1, 2, 3, 4 are graphed on the first stem with the high leaves 5, 6, 7, 8, 9 following. From this we can see that the data tend to cluster in the 34-centimeter area. Although there is not perfect symmetry, these data are more nearly symmetric than the earthquake data of Example 1.2.1.

Stem-and-leaf diagrams are useful for comparing two data sets of a similar nature. For example, we might want to compare cholesterol levels for males and females; we might want to display the results of two different weight loss programs side by side; or we might want a visual representation of the growth over time of a species of tree at two different elevations. Comparisons of this sort can be made via what is called a "back-to-back" stem-and-leaf diagram. Example 1.2.3 illustrates this technique.

EXAMPLE 1.2.3. A study is conducted to compare the growth over 10 years in red oak trees at elevations of 975 meters and 675 meters. The variable measured is the length of the core sample covering the last 10 years of growth rings in centimeters. See Figure 1.6. These data are obtained:

975 m			675 m		
3.8	2.8	6.0	1.8	2.3	1.0
1.3	3.8	1.7	2.3	1.1	2.9
2.6	1.5	1.9	2.0	1.1	0.8
2.2	4.0	2.5	2.2	2.6	1.6
2.0	1.7	0.7	2.4	2.1	1.7

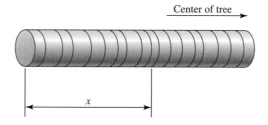

Center of tree

x

FIGURE 1.6

A typical core sample. Each ring represents one year of growth. The variable X is the length in centimeters of the last 10 rings.

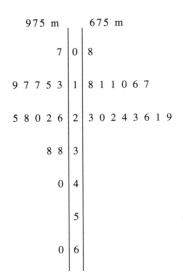

975 m   675 m

7	0	8
9 7 7 5 3	1	8 1 1 0 6 7
5 8 0 2 6	2	3 0 2 4 3 6 1 9
8 8	3	
0	4	
	5	
0	6	

FIGURE 1.7

A back-to-back stem-and-leaf diagram for the variable *X*, the growth over 10 years of red oak trees at two different elevations.

We could construct a stem-and-leaf diagram for each data set separately. However, since the purpose of the study is comparison and there is some overlap of stems, both data sets can be represented conveniently on the same set of stems. To do so, we let the leading digit of each number be its stem; the second digit of each will form the leaf. The stems are placed in the center of the diagram. The leaves for 975-meter elevation are shown on the left of the stems; those for the 675-meter elevation are on the right. Figure 1.7 shows the back-to-back stem-and-leaf diagram. There are several things to notice here. First, even though there were no observations with a stem of 5, this stem was included in the diagram. This was done so that the eye gets the proper perspective with respect to spread or dispersion at the 675-meter elevation. Second, it appears that there is a difference in the distribution of the variable growth at these two elevations. The values at 975 meters are more widely spread than those at 675 meters as evidenced by four data points that are larger than any seen at the 675-meter elevation. It also seems that the center of the data at 675 meters is below that at 975 meters because the former data set contains no values larger than 2.9, whereas the latter has several values that exceed that value. Keep in mind that these statements are only tentative observations based on a picture. In later chapters you will learn how to compare locations and variability analytically. (Based on data obtained by Allison Field, Department of Biology, Radford University, Fall 1996.)

Many of the statistical procedures presented later are developed under the assumption that the random variable studied has at least an approximate bell-shaped distribution. The stem-and-leaf diagram is an aid in determining whether or not this assumption is reasonable. For example, it would be surprising to hear that the random variable *X*, the magnitude of a California earthquake as measured on the Richter scale, has a bell-shaped distribution. The stem-and-leaf diagram of Figure 1.4*d* does not look at all like a bell. On the other hand, the diagram of Figure 1.5, although not perfectly symmetric, does tend to have a rough bell shape. It would not be surprising to hear a claim that *X*, the circumference of a male child's head at birth, has a bell-shaped distribution.

■ **EXERCISES 1.2**

1. One important variable used to measure the development stage of AIDS in infected patients is the ratio of T helper to T suppressor lymphocytes. The normal range for this random variable is 1.0 to 2.9. These data are obtained on a sample of randomly selected AIDS patients: (Based on information found in Interpretive Data Guide, ARUP Laboratories, 1996.)

.45	.52	.98	.62	.62
.40	.78	.53	.71	.71
.66	.71	.68	.70	.51
.79	.61	.67	.81	.84
.82	.91	.90	1.00	1.10

(a) Construct a stem-and-leaf diagram for these data using stems 4, 5, 6, 7, 8, 9, 10, and 11. Graph the point 1.00 as 10/0 and the point 1.10 as 11/0. (Remember that the decimal point itself does not appear as part of the stem.)

(b) Comment on the pattern or shape suggested by these data.

(c) Does it appear that the ratio of T helper to T suppressor lymphocytes for AIDS patients is probably lower than that for persons without AIDS? Explain.

2. A long runout landslide is a landslide in which the debris has traveled many times
   ∴ drop height over flat or gently sloping ground. A study of the reach (distance
      ∍led by the debris) of such landslides is conducted. These data are obtained:
        ∍d on data reported in Charles Campbell, "Self-Lubrication for Long Runout
        lides," *Journal of Geology,* November 1989, pp. 653–665.)

Re.... , км					
1.4	9.8	3.2	7.1	7.9	8.6
6.1	10.3	4.0	8.6	6.7	6.6
6.2	6.8	7.2	11.5	3.4	5.8
2.7	5.6	8.3	9.3	5.8	6.8

(a) Construct a stem-and-leaf diagram for these data. Use the integer part of each number as the stem and the first digit after the decimal as the leaf.

(b) Do you think that it would be unusual in the future to see a long runout landslide with a reach of 10 or more kilometers? Explain.

(c) By inspection, give a rough approximation of the average reach of these landslides.

3. A new vaccine is being developed to innoculate children against diphtheria. The standard protective level attained by older vaccines is 1 μg/ml 1 month after immunization. These data are obtained on the protective level of the new vaccine after 1 month: (Based on a report in the *Journal of Family Practice,* January 1990, pp. 27–30.)

12.5	13.8	13.0	13.5	13.2
12.2	13.4	14.0	13.6	13.3
13.3	14.1	14.6	13.1	12.1
13.7	13.4	12.8	12.6	12.7

(a) Form a double stem-and-leaf diagram for these data.

(b) Would you be surprised to hear a claim that X, the protective level after 1 month for the new vaccine, follows a bell-shaped distribution?

(c) By inspection of the stem-and-leaf diagram, approximate the average protection level using the new vaccine. Would you be surprised to hear a claim that the new vaccine tends to give a higher level of protection than the standard?

4. A study of male cardiac clinic patients is conducted. The purpose of the study is to pinpoint variables that contribute to stress in these patients. Stress is measured by means of the Hamilton anxiety score. These scores fall on a scale from 1 to 25 with 18 denoting moderate stress and 25 denoting severe stress. Two groups of patients are to be compared. These data are obtained: (Based on data reported in Earl Burch, Jr., and Jeffery Brandenburg, "Variables Contributing to Distress in Male Cardiac Patients," *Journal of Family Practice,* January 1990, pp. 43–47.)

Living alone				Living with others			
8.6	9.0	9.3	9.6	13.2	15.4	17.5	18.5
9.3	13.5	9.5	8.3	14.7	16.9	14.0	13.3
10.1	11.0	10.3	8.1	14.2	16.0	13.6	14.6
9.4	8.7	10.7	9.4	15.6	17.3	18.1	15.2
14.2	8.2	12.9	11.6	18.0	16.1	17.4	17.2

(a) Construct stem-and-leaf diagrams for each group.

(b) Does either distribution appear to be bell-shaped?

(c) Does either distribution appears to be skewed? If so, in what direction?

(d) Construct a back-to-back stem-and-leaf diagram for these data.

(e) Which group tends to have a lower average stress score?

(f) Based on these data, can we conclude that the average stress score for all male cardiac patients living alone falls below that of all male cardiac patients living with others? Explain.

5. Tethered locusts (acridid grasshoppers) are used in an experiment to study in-flight steering. Interest centers on the reaction of the locust to an acoustic stimulus and to a visual stimulus. In each case the variable of interest is the latency, the time that elapses between receipt of the stimulus and the head movement made by the locust that results in a course alteration. These data are obtained: (Based on data found in C. H. F. Rowell, "Descending Interneurones of the Locust Reporting Deviation from Flight Course: What Is Their Role in Steering?" *Journal of Experimental Biology,* vol. 146, September 1989, pp. 177–194.)

Latency, ms					
Acoustic			**Visual**		
86	106	117	72	95	73
102	109	120	99	71	90
103	113	101	102	97	71
99	114	126	75	80	70
108	107	109	100	104	81
100	107	106	103	101	103
115			77	78	89

(a) Construct a double stem-and-leaf diagram for each data set. Use the first two digits of each number as the stem. The stem for a two-digit number such as 86 is 08.

(b) Would you be surprised to hear a claim that latency is symmetrically distributed in both cases?

(c) Would you be surprised to hear a claim that latency follows a bell-shaped distribution in both cases?

(d) Under which stimulus is latency more widely dispersed?

6. Trace elements of zinc and copper are present in foods under normal circumstances. These elements can be toxic and can cause problems by competing with each other and thus impeding absorption by the body. A study of the levels of these elements in infant formulas is conducted. Each data point represents the average level in milligrams per liter for samples of equal size selected from among the top 16 brands on the market. (Based on data found in B. Lonnerdal, "Trace Element Absorption in Infants as a Foundation to Setting Upper Limits for Trace Elements in Infant Formulas," *Journal of Nutrition,* December 1989, pp. 1839–1844.)

Zinc			
3.0	5.8	5.6	4.8
5.1	3.6	5.5	4.7
5.7	5.0	5.9	5.7
4.4	5.4	4.2	5.3

Copper			
.40	.51	.47	.55
.56	.41	.60	.46
.60	.61	.48	.63
.50	.45	.62	.57

(a) Construct a double stem-and-leaf diagram for each data set.

(b) Does either data set exhibit a skew? If so, in which direction?

(c) A new formula is produced and its average copper level is estimated to be .53. Does this figure seem to be excessively high compared to formulas currently on the market? Explain.

(d) Would it be unusual to observe an estimated average zinc level less than 4.0 for the new formula? Explain.

7. Construct stem-and-leaf diagrams for the variable *age* of Example 1.1.1 and Exercise 1 of Section 1.1. Do the age distributions of the two homes appear to be similar in shape and location? Explain.

8. A study is conducted to help understand the effect of smoking on sleep patterns. The random variable considered is X, the time in minutes that it takes to fall asleep. Samples of smokers and nonsmokers yield these observations on X:

Nonsmokers					
17.2	19.7	18.1	15.1	18.3	17.6
16.2	19.9	19.8	23.6	24.9	20.1
19.8	22.6	20.0	24.1	25.0	21.4
21.2	18.9	22.1	20.6	23.3	20.2
21.1	16.9	23.0	20.1	17.5	21.3
21.8	22.1	21.1	20.5	20.4	20.7
19.5	18.8	19.2	22.4	19.3	17.4

Smokers					
15.1	20.5	17.7	21.3	16.0	24.8
16.8	21.2	18.1	22.1	15.9	25.2
22.8	22.4	19.4	25.2	18.3	25.0
25.8	24.1	15.0	24.1	21.6	16.3
24.3	25.7	15.2	18.0	23.8	17.9
23.2	25.1	16.1	17.2	24.9	19.9
15.7	15.3	19.9	23.1	23.0	25.1

(a) Construct a back-to-back stem-and-leaf diagram for these data. Use the integers from 15 to 25 inclusive as stems.

(b) Would you be surprised to hear someone claim that there is no difference in the distribution of X for the two groups? Explain.

9. Burning of vegetation in grass, shrub, and forest land is a common occurrence. Some burns are accidental, whereas others are planned burns for the purpose of creating post-fire habitat for the benefit of plants and animals. However, soil that has been exposed to high heat can become sterile. A study is conducted to study the effect of soil sterilization on the growth of plants. Radish plants were used in the study. The variable measured was the dry weight of the plant at the end of 4 weeks. These data were obtained: (Based on a study conducted by Joy Burcham, Department of Biology, Radford University, Fall 1996.)

Sterile soil (dry weight in grams)			Nonsterile Soil (dry weight in grams)		
9	28	26	16	19	13
10	18	17	15	14	2
10	28	10	7	11	6
30	30	11	9	6	3
25	35	34	18	14	11
9	15		20		

(a) Construct a double stem-and-leaf diagram for each of these data sets. Does either diagram appear to be roughly bell-shaped? Which seems to be more widely dispersed? Which seems to have the lower center of location?

(b) Construct a back-to-back double stem-and-leaf diagram for these data. Comment on what these data seem to say about the ability of radishes to grow in sterile soil.

■ 1.3
FREQUENCY DISTRIBUTIONS: HISTOGRAMS

In Section 1.2 we introduced the stem-and-leaf diagram, a quick graphical technique for organizing numerical data sets in which the number of distinct values is large. The stem-and-leaf diagram gives us a rough idea of the shape of a distribution as well as its location. The technique works well for data sets that are not widely dispersed. However, if the data points cover a wide range of values, it is difficult to pick appropriate stems. In this case, we need an alternative way to group data so that shape can be ascertained. The diagrams constructed to detect shape in this case are called *histograms*. Three types of histograms (frequency, relative frequency, and percentage) will be demonstrated. The technique has been in use for many years, with the origin of the term *histogram* credited to Karl Pearson in 1895.

A frequency histogram is a vertical or horizontal bar graph. It depicts the distribution of values in such a way that the area of each bar is proportional to the number of objects in the category or class represented by the bar. Thus a histogram for continuous data serves the same purpose as the bar graphs presented in Section 1.1. Since a data set with a large number of different numeric values has no obvious natural classes, we must devise a scheme for defining them. We want to define equal-sized classes in such a way that each observation clearly falls into exactly one of them. Many such schemes have been devised over the years. The technique illustrated here is one that works well. These rules for creating classes will be used. They will be illustrated step by step in Example 1.3.1.

Rules for Breaking Data into Classes

1. Decide on the number of classes wanted. The number chosen depends on the number of observations available. Table 1.11 gives suggested guidelines for the number of classes to be used as a function of sample size. It is based on Sturges' rule, a formula developed by H. A. Sturges in 1926. This rule states that k, the number of classes, is given by $k = 1 + 3.322 \log_{10} n$ where n is the sample size. This formula was used to derive the class numbers given in Table 1.11. You can verify some of these values for yourself. (H. A. Sturges, "The Choice of a Class Interval," *Journal of the American Statistical Association,* vol. 21, 1926, pp. 65–66.)

2. Locate the largest observation and the smallest observation. Find the difference between these two observations. Subtract in the order of largest minus smallest. This difference is called the *range* of the data.

3. Find the minimum class size required to cover this range by dividing the range by the number of classes desired. This value is the minimum size required to cover the range if the lower boundary for the first category is taken to be the smallest data point. However, to ensure that no data point falls on a boundary, we will define boundaries in such a way that they involve one more decimal place than the data. Hence we will start the first class slightly *below* the first data point. By doing this, the minimum width required to cover the range is not long enough to trap the largest

TABLE 1.11

Suggested number of classes to be used in subdividing numeric data as a function of sample size

Sample size	Number of classes
Less than 16	Not enough data
16–31	5
32–63	6
64–127	7
128–255	8
256–511	9
512–1023	10
1024–2047	11
2048–4095	12
4096–8190	13

■ **TABLE 1.12**

Units and half units for data reported to the stated degree of accuracy

Data reported to nearest	Unit	$\frac{1}{2}$ unit
Whole number	1	.5
Tenth (1 decimal place)	.1	.05
Hundredth (2 decimal places)	.01	.005
Thousandth (3 decimal places)	.001	.0005
Ten thousandth (4 decimal places)	.0001	.00005

data point in the last class. For this reason the actual class width used must be a little longer than minimum. The actual class width is found by rounding the minimum width *up* to the same number of decimal places as the data itself. If the minimum width by chance already has the same number of decimal places as the data, we still round up one unit. For example, if we have data reported to one decimal place accuracy and the minimum width required to cover the range is found to be 1.7, we bump this up to 1.8 to obtain the actual class width to be used.

4. The lower boundary for the first class lies $\frac{1}{2}$ unit below the smallest observation. Table 1.12 gives units and half units for various types of data sets. The remaining class boundaries are found by adding the class width to the preceding boundary value.

EXAMPLE 1.3.1. A study of ultrasonic calling in young Mongolian gerbils was conducted. Each animal was isolated for 1 minute on each of the first 14 days of its life, and the sounds that the animal produced were recorded. One variable of interest was the number of calls emitted. There was some concern that the daily handling of the experimental animals might have influenced their behavior. To detect this possible source of error, a group of control animals, animals that had not been handled at all, was studied on the fifth day. The data for this day for the two groups are as follows:

	Number of calls per animal				
Experimental			**Control**		
135	149	130 (smallest)	123	112	112
137	151	151	109	105	121
148	143	139	118	106	100
152	154	151	116	115	115
144	146	137	96	120	112
138	145	156 (largest)	88	112	122
142	136	138	102	123	128
145	150	144	117	110	124
147	151	142	119	98	109
147	138	155	101	111	90

Consider first the data for the experimental animals. Our task is to separate these data into classes. Notice that there are 30 data points. The guidelines given in Table 1.11 suggest that we divide the data into five classes. Now we locate the largest data point (156) and the smallest (130). These are used to find the width of the interval containing all the data

TABLE 1.13

Experimental animals: Frequency distribution

Class	Boundaries	Frequency
1	129.5 to 135.5	2
2	135.5 to 141.5	7
3	141.5 to 147.5	10
4	147.5 to 153.5	8
5	153.5 to 159.5	3

points. In this case, the data are covered by an interval of width $156 - 130 = 26$ units. To find the minimum width required for each class this number is divided by the number of classes desired. Here the minimum class width is $26/5 = 5.2$ units. To find the *actual* class width to be used in splitting the data, we round the minimum width *up* to the same number of decimal places as the data. Here the data are reported in whole numbers. Thus we round the minimum width, 5.2, up to the nearest whole number, 6. The classes actually used will be of width 6. The first class starts $\frac{1}{2}$ unit below the smallest observation. Since the data here are whole numbers, we see from Table 1.12 that a unit is 1 and a half unit is .5. We will start the first class .5 below the smallest observation. That is, the lower boundary for the first class is $130 - .5 = 129.5$. The remaining class boundaries are found by successively adding the actual class width (6) to the preceding boundary value until all data points are covered. In this manner we obtain the following five classes for the experimental animals: 129.5 to 135.5, 135.5 to 141.5, 141.5 to 147.5, 147.5 to 153.5, 153.5 to 159.5. Note that since the boundaries have one more decimal place than the data, no data point can fall on a boundary; each data point must fall into one and only one class. Now the data can be summarized in table form by counting the number of observations in each class (see column 3 of Table 1.13).

The graph of the frequency distribution is shown in Figure 1.8. This graph is called a frequency *histogram.* Notice that since the bars are of the same width by design, the area of each bar is directly proportional to its height. Since its height is equal to the number of observations in the class represented by the bar, the area of each bar is also directly proportional to the number of observations in its respective class as desired. This property of a histogram is

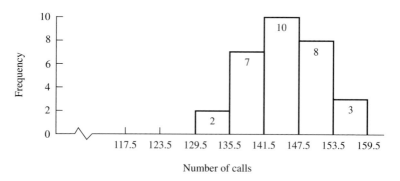

FIGURE 1.8

Frequency histogram (experimental).

TABLE 1.14

Control animals: Frequency distribution

Class	Boundaries	Frequency
1	87.5 to 96.5	3
2	96.5 to 105.5	5
3	105.5 to 114.5	9
4	114.5 to 123.5	11
5	123.5 to 132.5	2

useful since it is fairly easy to visually compare areas. Histograms paint a visual picture of the frequency distribution of the numbers in a data set.

For the control animals, the smallest observation is 88, the largest is 128, and the range is 40. The minimum class width needed to divide the data into five classes is 8. Notice that even though this is a whole number already, we still bump it up one unit to 9 to obtain the actual class width. This is to account for the fact that the lower boundary for the first class lies slightly below the smallest data point. In this case this boundary is 87.5. Table 1.14 gives the frequency table for the control animals, and Figure 1.9 gives the corresponding frequency histogram. Note that the histogram for the controls is somewhat different in shape from that of the experimental animals. The histograms are also located at different places along the horizontal axis. This implies that there might, in fact, be some basic differences in the behavior of the two groups of animals.

Figure 1.10 gives the SAS version of the histogram shown in Figure 1.8. Notice that the bars in SAS are labeled via the class midpoints rather than the class boundaries. For example, the boundaries for the first class are 129.5 and 135.5. The class midpoint is $(129.5 + 135.5)/2 = 132.5$. The SAS code used to produce this histogram is found in the Technology Tools section at the end of this chapter.

As mentioned in Section 1.1, frequency counts are important, but they do not tell the complete story concerning the distribution of a random variable. To put a frequency into perspective we also report the count relative to the total thus forming the relative frequency distribution of the variable. When the relative frequency is multiplied by 100, we obtain the percentage distribution. Tables 1.15 and 1.16 summarize what is known thus far

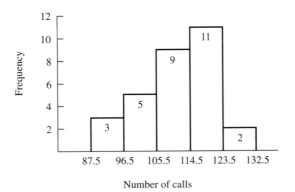

FIGURE 1.9

Frequency histogram (controls).

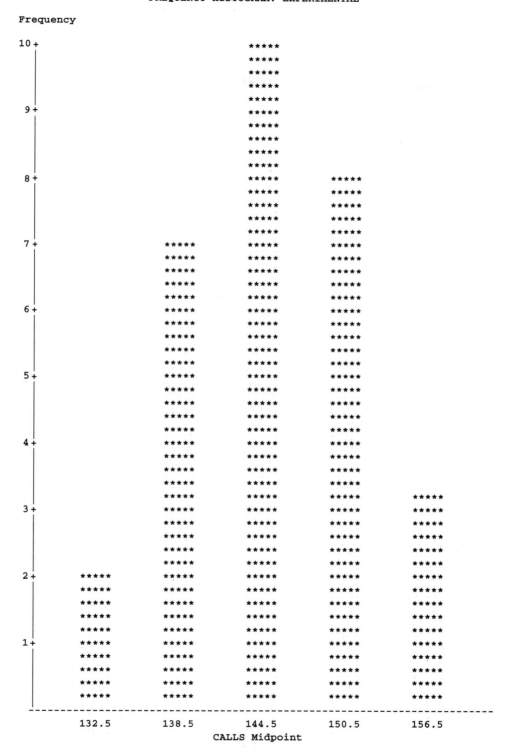

FIGURE 1.10

SAS version of the histogram for the experimental animals of Example 1.3.1.

TABLE 1.15

Experimental animals

Class	Boundaries	Frequency	Relative frequency	Percentage
1	129.5 to 135.5	2	.0667	6.67
2	135.5 to 141.5	7	.2333	23.33
3	141.5 to 147.5	10	.3333	33.33
4	147.5 to 153.5	8	.2667	26.67
5	153.5 to 159.5	2	.1000	10.00

TABLE 1.16

Control animals

Class	Boundaries	Frequency	Relative frequency	Percentage
1	87.5 to 96.5	3	.1000	10.00
2	96.5 to 105.5	5	.1667	16.67
3	105.5 to 114.5	9	.3000	30.00
4	114.5 to 123.5	11	.3667	36.67
5	123.5 to 132.5	2	.0667	6.67

concerning the distribution of the random variable *number of calls* for the experimental and control groups, respectively.

One further point should be noted. The procedure presented here for constructing a histogram works well if the data set does not have any values that are extremely out of line with the rest of the data. For example, suppose that the data set for experimental animals in Example 1.3.1 contains the value 201. This number is much bigger than the rest of the data. It will have a large impact on the value of the range; in fact, the range changes from 26 to 71. This, in turn, changes the class width from 5.2 to 14.2. What effect does this have on the histogram? To see, consider Figure 1.11. The most important thing to notice is that by expanding the class width, the bulk of the data falls into two very large classes. We lose all sense of the shape of the data. It is evident that when a data set contains unusual values, the textbook procedure should be modified. Exercise 10 (of Section 1.3) outlines two solutions to this problem.

Cumulative Distributions

In addition to the frequency, relative frequency, and percentage distributions among classes it is of interest to consider the cumulative frequency, relative cumulative frequency, and cumulative percentage distributions for numeric variables. Recall from our discussion in the discrete case that cumulative values are obtained by adding. Thus the cumulative frequency for a given class is the number of observations falling in that class or in any class below it; the relative cumulative frequency is the fraction of observations falling in or below the class; and the cumulative percentage is the percentage of observations falling in or below the class. These distributions for the data of Example 1.3.1 are given in Tables 1.17 and 1.18.

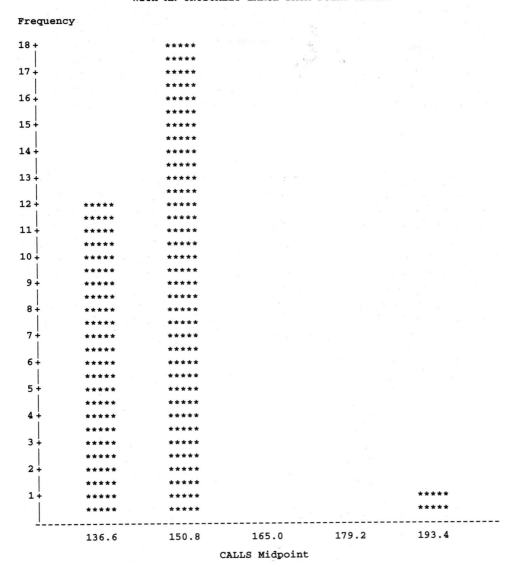

FIGURE 1.11

Figure 1.12 shows a horizontal histogram for the data on experimental animals given in Example 1.3.1. Notice that the figure also includes the information on frequencies, percentages, cumulative frequencies, and cumulative percentages shown in Table 1.17.

Example 1.3.2. illustrates the breakdown of a data set in which data are not whole-number data.

TABLE 1.17

Experimental animals: Cumulative distributions

Class	Boundaries	Cumulative frequency	Relative cumulative frequency	Cumulative percentage
1	129.5 to 135.5	2	$2/30 = .0667$	6.67
2	135.5 to 141.5	9	$9/30 = .3000$	30.00
3	141.5 to 147.5	19	$19/30 = .6333$	63.33
4	147.5 to 153.5	27	$27/30 = .900$	90.00
5	153.5 to 159.5	30	$30/30 = 1.000$	100.00

TABLE 1.18

Control animals: Cumulative distributions

Class	Boundaries	Cumulative frequency	Relative cumulative frequency	Cumulative percentage
1	87.5 to 96.5	3	$3/30 = .1000$	10.00
2	96.5 to 105.5	8	$8/30 = .2667$	26.67
3	105.5 to 114.5	17	$17/30 = .5667$	56.67
4	114.5 to 123.5	28	$28/30 = .9334$	93.34
5	123.5 to 132.5	30	$30/30 = 1.0000$	100.00

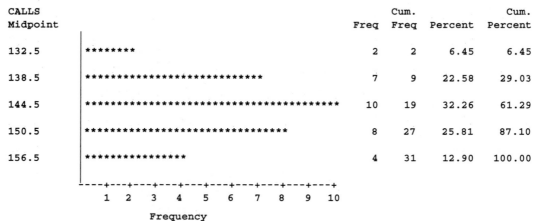

```
                  SUMMARY TABLE AND HORIZONTAL HISTOGRAM:
                               EXPERIMENTAL

CALLS                                                      Cum.              Cum.
Midpoint                                        Freq       Freq   Percent    Percent

132.5    *******                                  2         2      6.45       6.45

138.5    **************************               7         9     22.58      29.03

144.5    ***************************************  10        19     32.26      61.29

150.5    *********************************         8        27     25.81      87.10

156.5    ****************                          4        31     12.90     100.00

         ---+---+---+---+---+---+---+---+---+
          1   2   3   4   5   6   7   8   9   10
               Frequency
```

FIGURE 1.12

A horizontal histogram showing frequency, percentage, cumulative frequency, and cumulative percentage distribution for the data on experimental animals of Example 1.3.1.

TABLE 1.19

Distribution of time to onset of reaction

Class	Boundaries	Frequency	Relative frequency	Percentage	Cumulative frequency	Relative cumulative frequency	Cumulative percentage
1	3.75 to 5.95	2	2/40 = .050	5	2	2/40 = .050	5
2	5.95 to 8.15	4	4/40 = .100	10	6	6/40 = .150	15
3	8.15 to 10.35	10	10/40 = .250	25	16	16/40 = .400	40
4	10.35 to 12.55	16	16/40 = .400	40	32	32/40 = .800	80
5	12.55 to 14.75	6	6/40 = .150	15	38	38/40 = .950	95
6	14.75 to 16.95	2	2/40 = .050	5	2	40/40 = 1.000	100

EXAMPLE 1.3.2. Many people experience systemic allergic reactions to insect stings. These reactions differ from patient to patient not only in severity but also in time to onset of the reaction. The following data represent the time to onset of the reaction in 40 patients who experienced a systemic reaction to a bee sting.

(Data are in minutes.)

10.5	11.2	9.9	15.0	11.4	12.7	16.5	10.1
12.7	11.4	11.6	6.2	7.9	8.3	10.9	8.1
3.8	10.5	11.7	8.4	12.5	11.2	9.1	10.4
9.1	13.4	12.3	5.9	11.4	8.8	7.4	8.6
13.6	14.7	11.5	11.5	10.9	9.8	12.9	9.9

From Table 1.11 we see that it is appropriate to divide these data into six categories. The largest observation is 16.5, the smallest is 3.8, and the range is 12.7. The minimum category width required to cover the range is $12.7/6 = 2.12$. Since the data are reported to one decimal place accuracy, we round 2.12 up to 2.2 to obtain the actual category width. From Table 1.12 we see that $\frac{1}{2}$ unit for one decimal place data is .05. The lower boundary for the first category is .05 below the smallest observation, or $3.80 - .05 = 3.75$. The complete frequency and cumulative frequency breakdown for the data is shown in Table 1.19.

EXERCISES 1.3

1. One variable of interest in a study of the Xanthid crab, a small crab found near Gloucester Point, Virginia, is the number of eggs spawned per individual. The following observations were obtained for 45 crabs:

1,959	4,534	7,020	6,725	6,964	7,428	9,359	9,166
2,802	2,462	4,000	3,378	7,343	4,189	8,973	4,327
2,412	7,624	1,548	4,801	737	5,321	849	5,749
6,837	8,639	7,417	6,082	10,241	962	3,894	1,801
5,099	6,627	4,484	5,633	4,148	6,588	5,847	4,632
6,472	8,372	8,225	6,142	12,130			

(*a*) Find the largest and smallest observations.
(*b*) Find the range.
(*c*) If the guidelines of Table 1.11 are used, how many classes are needed to subdivide these data?

(d) What minimum class width is needed to cover the range if six classes are used?

(e) Find the actual class width to be used in partitioning the data set.

(f) Find the lower boundary for the first class.

(g) Determine the summary table for the data set and construct a relative frequency histogram.

(h) Would you be surprised to hear someone claim that the random variable *number of eggs spawned* exhibits a bell-shaped distribution? Explain.

2. In studying growth patterns in children, one important variable is the age of the child when the adolescent growth spurt begins. The following observations were obtained in a study of 35 boys and 40 girls (age is in years):

Boys							Girls							
16.0	14.9	14.1	14.8	14.4	14.0	14.6	12.2	13.7	13.3	12.3	12.5	12.9	11.9	11.6
15.2	14.7	13.6	14.6	16.1	13.2	13.2	13.4	12.4	12.6	13.5	12.5	13.4	11.7	13.5
14.9	14.1	15.4	15.3	14.4	14.8	14.8	13.7	12.1	14.1	11.8	12.8	12.9	11.6	14.3
13.5	15.1	13.5	15.0	14.6	15.4	15.9	13.1	13.3	13.5	14.7	12.3	11.6	13.1	12.6
13.7	15.9	14.7	14.5	14.4	13.8	15.3	12.7	12.7	12.0	11.4	13.5	12.4	12.1	12.1

(a) Break each data set into the number of classes suggested in Table 1.11, using the method demonstrated in this section.

(b) Construct relative frequency histograms for each data set. Comment on any apparent similarities or differences in the histograms.

3. In patients with Duchenne muscular dystrophy, serum levels of creatine kinase are dramatically elevated over the normal value of less than 50 units/liter. The following data are serum creatine kinase activities measured in 24 young Duchenne patients (in units per liter):

3720	3796	3340	5600	3802	3580
5500	2000	1571	2360	1500	1840
3723	3790	3345	3805	5595	3577
1995	5504	2055	1573	1835	1505

(a) Break the data set into the number of classes suggested in Table 1.11.

(b) Find the summary table for the data set.

(c) Construct a percentage histogram for the data and describe its shape and location.

4. *Relative cumulative frequency ogive.* If the random variable under study is continuous, then a line graph of the cumulative distribution can be used to obtain valuable information. The graph is obtained by plotting the upper boundary of each class on the horizontal axis and the relative cumulative frequency on the vertical axis. The points obtained are then joined by line segments. The graph is completed by extending a line segment to pass through the point 0 at the lower boundary of the first class. Such a graph is called a relative cumulative frequency ogive. For example, consider the data of Example 1.3.2. The variable *time to onset of reaction* to an insect sting is continuous. The relative cumulative frequency ogive is constructed from the information found in Table 1.19 and is shown in Figure 1.13. We now ask two questions:

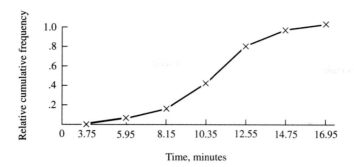

FIGURE 1.13
Relative cumulative frequency ogive.

1. About what proportion of patients have experienced a reaction within 10 minutes?
2. By what time has a reaction occurred in half of the patients?

The first question can be answered graphically by locating 10 on the horizontal axis, projecting a vertical line up to the ogive, and then projecting a horizontal line over to the vertical axis (see Figure 1.14). The desired proportion is seen to be approximately .37. The second question is answered by locating .5 on the vertical axis and then reversing the process. The answer is seen to be approximately 11 minutes. (See Figure 1.14.)

(*a*) For each data set of Exercise 2 construct a relative cumulative frequency ogive. Use the ogive to approximate the age by which 50% of the boys have begun the adolescent growth spurt; do the same for the girls. Does there appear to be much difference between the two values?

(*b*) By age 12, approximately what proportion of the girls had experienced the beginning of the growth spurt? By age 14, approximately what proportion of the boys had experienced the beginning of the growth spurt?

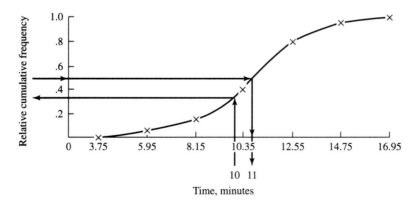

FIGURE 1.14
Projection method for estimating percentages.

5. (*a*) Plot a relative cumulative frequency ogive for the data set of Exercise 3.
   (*b*) Based on these data, what proportion of Duchenne patients have serum creatine kinase levels of at least 50 times the normal value?

6. In a study designed to correlate seasonal change in plasma testosterone with the reproductive cycle in lizards, the following data were obtained from a sample of 33 lizards of a particular species captured in the month of August. (Testosterone levels are in nanograms per milliliter.)

7.5	7.2	3.0	12.1	15.1	12.1	11.5	11.8	7.2	13.2	13.6
8.2	9.5	8.4	13.3	12.5	12.4	2.1	10.7	9.4	6.7	6.8
6.1	8.3	7.9	6.0	7.6	13.2	4.5	9.3	8.1	3.5	9.0

In October a sample of 40 lizards of the same species had the following plasma testosterone levels:

43.7	37.2	29.0	31.6	47.5	48.3	38.3	29.7
32.5	45.2	36.1	30.5	37.2	50.5	36.9	44.5
35.9	28.7	37.5	30.2	36.9	43.2	27.0	26.2
41.8	26.4	34.3	28.6	35.9	22.0	45.4	30.3
29.8	46.1	42.7	31.5	37.4	25.1	27.2	45.0

   (*a*) Find the summary table for each data set using the number of classes suggested in Table 1.11.
   (*b*) Construct relative frequency histograms for both data sets.
   (*c*) Compare the histograms in light of the additional observation that secondary sex characteristics develop in young lizards in the winter and mating takes place in summer.

7. Some efforts are currently being made to make textile fibers out of peat fibers. This would provide a source of cheap feedstock for the textile and paper industries. One variable being studied is *X*, the percentage of ash content of a particular variety of peat moss. Assume that a random sample of 50 mosses yields these observations: (Based on data found in "Peat Fibre: Is There Scope in Textiles?" *Textile Horizons,* vol. 2, no. 10, October 1982, p. 24.)

.5	1.8	4.0	1.0	2.0
1.1	1.6	2.3	3.5	2.2
2.0	3.8	3.0	2.3	1.8
3.6	2.4	.8	3.4	1.4
1.9	2.3	1.2	1.9	2.3
2.6	3.1	2.5	1.7	5.0
1.3	3.0	2.7	1.2	1.5
3.2	2.4	2.5	1.9	3.1
2.4	2.8	2.7	4.5	2.1
1.5	.7	3.7	1.8	1.7

   (*a*) Construct a stem-and-leaf diagram for these data. Use the numbers 0, 1, 2, 3, 4, 5 as stems.
   (*b*) Is there any reason to suspect that *X* does not follow a bell-shaped distribution?
   (*c*) Use the method outlined in this section to subdivide these data. Use Table 1.11 to determine the appropriate number of classes.
   (*d*) Construct a summary table for these data.

8. Acute exposure to cadmium produces respiratory distress and kidney and liver damage and may result in death. For this reason, the level of airborne cadmium dust and cadmium oxide fume in the air is monitored. This level is measured in milligrams of cadmium per cubic meter of air. A sample of 35 readings yield these data: (Based on a report in *Environmental Management,* September 1981, p. 414.)

.044	.030	.052	.044	.046
.020	.066	.052	.049	.030
.040	.045	.039	.039	.039
.057	.050	.056	.061	.042
.055	.037	.062	.062	.070
.061	.061	.058	.053	.060
.047	.051	.054	.042	.051

(a) Construct a stem-and-lead diagram for these data. Use the numbers 02, 03, 04, 05, 06, 07 as stems.

(b) Would you be surprised to hear someone claim that the random variable X, the cadmium level in the air, follows a bell-shaped distribution?

(c) Use the method outlined in this section to break these data into six classes.

(d) Construct a summary table for these data.

(e) Construct a relative frequency histogram for these data. Does the histogram exhibit a bell shape?

(f) Construct a relative cumulative frequency ogive for these data. Use the ogive to approximate that point above which 50% of the readings should fall.

9. A study is conducted to compare the diversity of the plants found in a burned and an unburned portion of a national forest. For each site, the variable recorded is the Sequential Comparison Index (SCI) for the site. A high SCI value indicates that many different species were found at the site; a low SCI indicates the presence of only a few species. These data were obtained for samples of 35 burned and 35 unburned sites.

Burned				
0.155	1.317	0.196	1.753	0.503
0.303	1.564	1.795	2.017	0.901
1.686	0.591	2.527	0.733	1.555
1.055	0.109	1.000	2.377	0.729
1.214	1.523	0.459	1.192	1.377
0.713	1.269	1.418	1.368	1.469
2.067	2.479	1.423	2.179	0.141

Unburned				
1.856	0.892	1.662	0.804	0.998
1.518	1.507	2.122	0.380	1.234
0.382	1.187	2.203	0.648	0.517
0.498	0.029	0.383	0.489	0.010
1.044	0.935	0.374	0.423	1.483
1.624	0.559	0.939	0.171	0.805
1.282	0.544	1.505	0.635	0.777

(Based on information gathered by Jackie Cummings, Department of Biology, Radford University, Fall 1996.)

(*a*) A SAS version of a horizontal histogram and summary table for each group is shown in Figure 1.15. We let SAS choose its own classes to construct these charts. That is, we did not feed SAS the midpoints that the text procedure identifies. Is SAS, by default, using the text algorithm to determine class numbers, class boundaries, and class midpoints? Explain your answer.

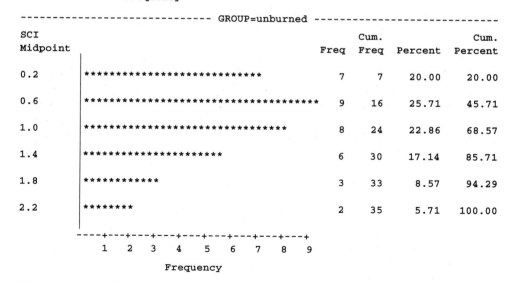

```
                              SAS DOES ITS THING

---------------------------- GROUP=burned ----------------------------
SCI                                      Cum.                Cum.
Midpoint                        Freq     Freq    Percent    Percent

  0.2    |*********                 5      5     14.29      14.29

  0.6    |***********               6     11     17.14      31.43

  1.0    |********                  4     15     11.43      42.86

  1.4    |********************      11     26     31.43      74.29

  1.8    |******                    3     29      8.57      82.86

  2.2    |********                  4     33     11.43      94.29

  2.6    |****                      2     35      5.71     100.00

         ----+---+---+---+---+--
             2   4   6   8  10
               Frequency

---------------------------- GROUP=unburned ----------------------------
SCI                                      Cum.                Cum.
Midpoint                        Freq     Freq    Percent    Percent

  0.2    |**************************       7      7     20.00      20.00

  0.6    |*************************************   9     16     25.71      45.71

  1.0    |*******************************  8     24     22.86      68.57

  1.4    |********************      6     30     17.14      85.71

  1.8    |************              3     33      8.57      94.29

  2.2    |********                  2     35      5.71     100.00

         ----+---+---+---+---+---+---+---+---+
             1   2   3   4   5   6   7   8   9
               Frequency
```

FIGURE 1.15

SAS analysis of the data of Exercise 9.

(b) What class width is SAS using in each case?

(c) What is the upper class boundary for SAS's first class? Does any data point actually fall on this boundary? Could a future data point with three-decimal-place accuracy fall on this boundary?

(d) If we use the text algorithm for finding boundaries, what are the boundaries for the first class in each case? Could a future data point with three-decimal-place accuracy fall on this boundary?

(e) If SAS is available, redraw the histograms using the text algorithm and compare the results to those shown here.

(f) If SAS is available, change the data point .459 in the data for burned sites to .400. Rerun the chart and see how SAS handles a data point that falls on the current boundary.

10. *Histogram: unusual values.* Consider the experimental data of Example 1.3.1 with the extra point 201 added. We present here two solutions for representing the data via a histogram. In each case the area of the bar for a class is proportional to the number of observations in the class.

   Adding an extended class. We keep the class boundaries for the bulk of the data as outlined in the text. We add one more class to cover the unusual point. By necessity, the class width of this added class will be larger than the others. So that the area of the bar will be proportional to the number of observations in the class, the height of the bar no longer equals the number of observations in the class.

(a) Define the extended class boundaries to be 159.5 to 201.5. What is the class width?

(b) What is the total area of the frequency histogram for the bulk of the data? Each observation is represented by how much area?

(c) What should be the area of the bar representing the extended class?

(d) What should be the height of the extended class bar so that its area will be that found in part c?

   Adding more classes. Keep the class boundaries for the bulk of the data as outlined in the text. Add more classes of the same class width until the unusual value is covered. Usually this will result in some empty classes and some gaps in the histogram, but it will preserve the idea that classes are of the same width and that the height of the bar for a frequency histogram is the class frequency.

(e) Consider the SAS output shown in Figure 1.16. How many classes were added to cover the point 201?

(f) If the point 185 were added to the control data of Example 1.3.1, how many additional classes would be needed to cover this point? How many would be empty?

11. Consider the data of Example 1.3.1. Construct a back-to-back double stem-and-leaf diagram for these data. That is, graph both the experimental and control data on the same stem-and-leaf diagram using stems of 08, 08, 09, 09, 10, 10, 11, 11, 12, 12, 13, 13, 14, 14, 15, 15. This diagram points out clearly one major difference in these two data sets. What is this major difference? Which technique, stem-and-leaf diagrams, or histograms, gives the better impression of potential shape in the population?

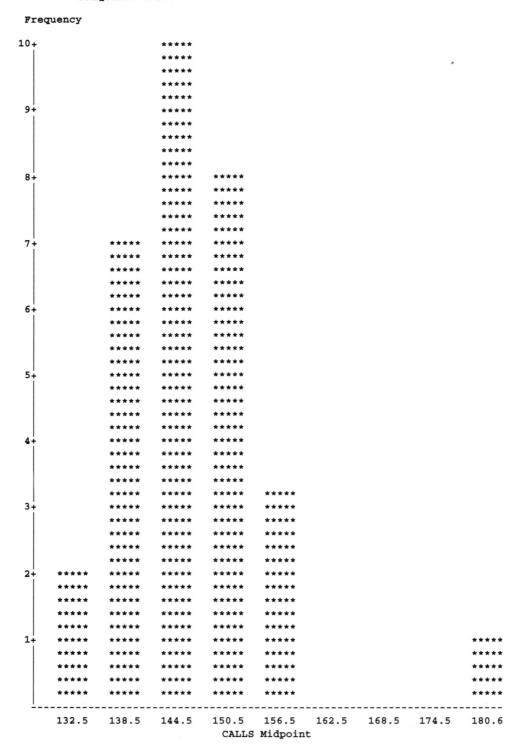

FIGURE 1.16

Adding extra classes to cover unusual data points.

▩ 1.4

MEASURES OF LOCATION OR CENTRAL TENDENCY

Recall that the primary purpose of statistics is to draw conclusions about a population based on information obtained from a sample. We have already seen two techniques, the stem-and-leaf diagram and histogram, that can be used to ascertain shape. These diagrams also give a rough idea of location or central tendency. In this section we consider two measures of location, the mean and the median. The population mean is the average value of the random variable over the population. Its value is denoted by μ. The population median is the point M with the property and approximately 50% of the population values fall-on or below M with the rest falling above M. Both μ and M are parameters. Their values are not known and cannot be found from a sample. However, it is possible to approximate or estimate them from a sample via the sample mean and the sample median. These statistics, which we shall define in this section, are denoted by $\bar{x}$ and $\tilde{x}$, respectively. Figure 1.17 illustrates the idea.

Sample Mean

The most common measure of location is the average or mean value. The mean of a sample is the arithmetic average of the observations. Definition 1.4.1 states this using summation notation. In this notation, the capital Greek sigma Σ is used to indicate addition. For example, Σx means to add the data points. If you are unfamiliar with this notation, see Appendix A.

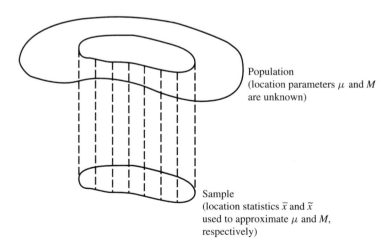

Population
(location parameters μ and M are unknown)

Sample
(location statistics $\bar{x}$ and $\tilde{x}$ used to approximate μ and M, respectively)

▩ **FIGURE 1.17**

The statistics $\bar{x}$ and $\tilde{x}$ are used to describe location in the sample and to approximate the values of μ and M, respectively.

DEFINITION 1.4.1. SAMPLE MEAN. Let $x_1, x_2, \ldots, x_n$ be a set of n observations on a variable X. The arithmetic average of these values is called the *sample mean* and is denoted by $\bar{x}$ (pronounced "x bar"). That is,

$$\text{Sample mean} = \bar{x} = \frac{x_1 + x_2 + \cdots + x_n}{n} = \frac{\sum x}{n}$$

Whenever a computation is done, the question arises, How many decimal places should be reported in the final answer? This is especially true now that most computations are done on handheld calculators or by prewritten computer programs. These typically report results to as high as eight-decimal-place accuracy. Unless the data themselves are reported to this degree of accuracy, it is not necessary or desirable to report all these values. There are no rigid rules concerning how many decimal places to retain. We shall use the convention that when computing means, the result will be reported to one more decimal place than the data. The last decimal place will be found by rounding rather than by truncation. For example, if we average the values 23.72, 89.10, and 112.56 on a standard scientific calculator, we see 75.12666667. This average will be reported as 75.127. An exception to this convention will be made if $\bar{x}$ has a finite decimal expansion. For example, if we average 1, 2, 5, and 1 we shall report the mean as $9/4 = 2.25$. *Warning:* When doing a series of arithmetic operations, do not round until the final result has been calculated. Otherwise, rounding error will be compounded.

EXAMPLE 1.4.1. In a study of water pollution, samples of mussels were taken from two localities in Sweden. The variables of interest are X and Y, the lead concentration (milligrams per gram dry weight) from the Smygehuk and Falsterbo Kanal areas, respectively. The following data were obtained:

Smygehuk	Falsterbo Kanal
106.3	113.0
209.3	140.5
246.5	163.3
252.3	185.7
294.4	202.5
	207.2

Since we are sampling from two distinct populations, two sample means $\bar{x}$ and $\bar{y}$ are involved. Here

$$\bar{x} = \frac{106.3 + 209.3 + \cdots + 294.4}{5} = 221.76$$

$$\bar{y} = \frac{113.0 + 140.5 + \cdots + 207.2}{6} = 168.70$$

Can we conclude from these statistics that, without a doubt, the average lead concentration found in mussels at Smygehuk, μ_X, exceeds the average at Falsterbo Kanal, μ_Y? The answer to this question is no. We do not have population data; we have only small samples drawn from these populations. The sample means differ greatly, which leads us to strongly suspect that $\mu_X \neq \mu_Y$. However, we cannot make this claim with 100% certainty.

Notice that $\bar{X}$ is a random variable. Its value will vary from sample to sample. For example, if we took 10 samples each of size 5 from the population of mussels at Smygehuk and computed the sample mean for each sample, we would not expect to obtain the same value is each case. The $\bar{x}$ values should differ from one another because of chance factors involved in the sampling process. The distribution of $\bar{X}$ is considered in Chapter 7.

Most scientific calculators and all calculators with statistical capability will calculate $\bar{x}$ automatically as data are entered in the "statistics" mode. Since the steps required to find $\bar{x}$ differ from calculator to calculator we cannot give specific calculator instructions here. You are urged to learn how to use your calculator to find the sample mean. The steps required for the TI83 are given in the Technology Tools section at the end of this chapter.

Sample Median

The second measure of location is the median. Roughly speaking, the median is the number located in the "middle" of the ordered data set.

DEFINITION 1.4.2. Let $x_1, x_2, \ldots, x_n$ be a sample of observations arranged in order from smallest to largest. The sample median is the middle observation if n is odd. If n is even, it is the average of the two middle observations. We shall denote the sample median by $\tilde{x}$ (pronounced "x tilde").

If n is small, it is easy to spot the middle of the data set. However, if n is large, it is useful to have a formula that pinpoints the location of the middle observation or observations. The formula is given below, and its use is illustrated in Example 1.4.2.

$$\text{Median location} = \frac{n+1}{2}$$

EXAMPLE 1.4.2. Consider the data of Example 1.4.1 which has already been ordered. Since $n = 5$ for the Smygehuk sample, the median location is $(n+1)/2 = 6/2 = 3$. The sample median is the third observation. That is, $\tilde{x} = 246.5$. For the Falsterbo Kanal data, $n = 6$ and $(n+1)/2 = 7/2 = 3.5$. We interpret this to mean that the median is the average of the third and fourth observations. Here

$$\tilde{y} = \frac{163.3 + 185.7}{2} = 174.5$$

In summarizing data, it is useful to report both the sample mean and the sample median. They both measure location but in a slightly different way.

The sample median has one advantage over the sample mean as a measure of location. In particular, it is *resistant*. This means that its value changes only slightly when a small part of the data is deleted or replaced by new numbers that might be very different from the original ones. This property is desirable when a data set contains a number that is far removed from the rest of the data points. A number of this sort is called an *outlier* or a "wild" number. Its presence can drastically affect the value of the sample mean; it has little or no effect on the value of the sample median. Outliers arise for two reasons: (1) They are legitimate observations whose values are simply unusually large or small, or (2) they are the result of an error in measurement, poor experimental technique, or a mistake in recording the data. In the first case it is suggested that the presence of the outlier be reported and that sample statistics be reported both with and without the outlier. In the second case, the data point can be corrected if possible or else dropped from the data set. A graphical method for detecting outliers is given in Section 1.6.

■ EXERCISES 1.4

1. Consider the following data sets:

Data set I			Data set II			
2	4	0	1	1	5	7
1	4	3	3	4	6	
3	1	1	2	1	5	

   For each data set find the sample mean and sample median.

2. In a study of parasites, the distribution of the tick *Ixodes trianguliceps* in field mice was considered. The following observations were obtained on the number of ticks found on 44 mice.

0	2	0	0	2	2	0	0	1
1	3	0	0	1	0	0	1	0
1	4	0	0	1	4	2	0	0
1	0	0	2	2	1	1	0	6
0	5	1	3	0	1	0	1	

   (*a*) Construct a frequency bar graph for these data and estimate the sample mean by inspection.
   (*b*) Calculate the sample mean and compare this value to your estimate from part *a*.
   (*c*) Find the sample median.

3. *Outliers.* Often studies of birds are conducted by capturing, banding, and releasing the birds so that their movements can be followed. One variable studied was the flight distance from the point of release of a bird just banded to its first perch. The following data were obtained on two types of birds, the robin and the mourning dove (distance is given in feet):

Robin (I)			Mourning dove (II)			
128.8	57.2	48.2	40.0	381.7	358.9	1200.0*
160.0	65.2	69.2	80.0	266.8	13.9	
192.1	68.9	117.3	313.9	162.7	165.5	
163.4	24.7	36.5	175.7	76.0	317.2	
186.4	37.4	140.8	55.5	22.1	300.6	
156.2	99.7	59.3	44.7	170.0	197.7	
70.0	265.0	71.3	166.7	263.7	288.1	
10.0	78.7	105.3	83.4	369.7	102.0	

(a) Find the sample mean and median for each data set. Do they seem similar with respect to either of these measures?

(b) Note that the starred observation in the data set for mourning doves is very different from the others. It is an *outlier*. To see the effect of this outlier, drop it from the data set and calculate the mean and median for the remaining 24 observations. Which measure is least affected by the presence of the outlier? Do you see why it is desirable to report both the mean and the median of a data set? Does there appear to be an outlier in data set I?

4. Find the sample mean and median for each of the data sets of Exercise 9 of Section 1.3

5. Find the sample mean and median for the data of Exercise 1 of Section 1.2.

6. Find the sample mean and median for the data of Exercise 8 of Section 1.3.

7. Count data are something reported in scientific journals in table form. For example, a study of the number of species found on slides of water taken from a river near a source of pollution might yield these data:

Number of species x	Number of slides f
0	1
1	3
2	2
4	8
5	2

The complete data set actually consists of these data:

```
0   2   4   4
1   2   4   4
1   4   4   5
1   4   4   5
```

The mean for this sample can be calculated in the usual way. In this case $\bar{x} = 3.1$ This mean can be found more quickly by multiplying each value of x listed by its corresponding frequency, adding these terms, and then dividing by the sum of the frequencies. For these data,

$$\bar{x} = \frac{0(1) + 1(3) + 2(2) + 4(8) + 5(2)}{16}$$

Use this technique and the frequency bar graph found in Exercise 2 to verify your answer to part *b* of Exercise 2.

1.5

MEASURES OF VARIABILITY OR DISPERSION

Recall that the behavior of a random variable is determined by chance. Hence the observed values of a random variable differ from one another to some extent. In some cases the differences are slight; in others they are pronounced. Since we hope that the

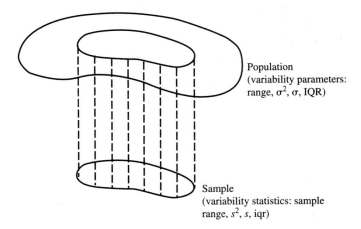

Population
(variability parameters:
range, σ^2, σ, IQR)

Sample
(variability statistics: sample
range, s^2, s, iqr)

FIGURE 1.18
The statistics sample range, s^2, s, and iqr are used to describe
variability in the sample and to approximate the population
variability parameters.

characteristics of our sample reflect well the corresponding population characteristics,
we measure variability in the sample to understand the extent of the variation that exists in the population. In this section we consider four measures of variation: the sample range, sample variance s^2, sample standard deviation s, and interquartile range iqr.
These statistics describe variability in the sample and are used to approximate the population range, population variance σ^2, population standard deviation σ, and population
interquartile range IQR, respectively. See Figure 1.18. An example will demonstrate
the need for these measures in addition to the measures of location introduced in the
last section.

EXAMPLE 1.5.1. In a study of scholastic sports injuries, 25 school districts within a state
were selected and polled. The following data were obtained on the number of serious injuries incurred by male athletes while participating in basketball and football:

Basketball					Football				
1	2	4	4	7	1	7	7	6	1
3	3	2	4	5	2	6	1	7	2
2	4	3	5	3	1	3	2	7	5
4	4	3	6	5	6	1	7	4	1
5	6	4	6	5	5	7	6	3	2

Table 1.20 is the frequency table for these data. The relative frequency histogram for each
data set is shown in Figure 1.19. It is evident that even though both histograms are centered
at 4, their shapes are quite different. Let X denote the number of basketball injuries reported
per district, and Y the number of football injuries. A quick calculation will show that
$\bar{x} = \bar{y} = 4$. Notice that the sample medians are identical to the sample means. If we used
only location to compare the two data sets, we would erroneously conclude that there was
no difference between them.

TABLE 1.20

Frequency distributions of scholastic sports injuries

Basketball injuries			Football injuries		
Number of cases	Frequency	Relative frequency	Number of cases	Frequency	Relative frequency
1	1	.040	1	6	.240
2	3	.120	2	4	.160
3	5	.200	3	2	.080
4	7	.280	4	1	.040
5	5	.200	5	2	.080
6	3	.120	6	4	.160
7	1	.040	7	6	.240

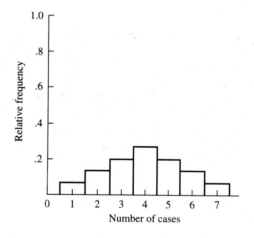

(a)

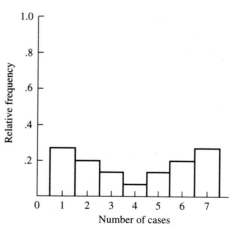

(b)

FIGURE 1.19

Relative frequency histograms:
(a) basketball and
(b) football.

The characteristic that is not being detected analytically by the sample mean or the sample median is *variability*. There is some fluctuation in the observations. They are not all the same. Some lie close to the mean; others do not. We need a measure that detects the extent of this variability. We want a statistic with the property that when data points are clustered near the mean, its value will be small; when data points are more widely dispersed with many lying quite far from the mean, its value will be large. Figure 1.20 illustrates the idea. Several such statistics have been proposed. Perhaps the most logical way to begin to measure variability about the mean is to find the distance of each data point from the mean and sum these distances. Each distance is found by subtracting the mean from the data point. That is, they are found by forming the difference $x - \bar{x}$ for each observation. A quick example will show that although this proposal is appealing, it will not work!

EXAMPLE 1.5.2. Consider the following set of observations:

$$x_1 = 2 \quad x_3 = 1 \quad x_5 = 4$$
$$x_2 = 5 \quad x_4 = 3$$

The sample mean for this data set is

$$\bar{x} = \frac{\sum x}{5} = \frac{2 + 5 + 1 + 3 + 4}{5} = 3$$

The sum of the differences between the observations and the sample mean is

$$(2 - 3) + (5 - 3) + (1 - 3) + (3 - 3) + (4 - 3) = (-1) + 2 + (-2) + 0 + 1 = 0$$

The proposed method of measuring variability makes it appear that there is no fluctuation in the data. The problem is evident. We are allowing negative differences associated with the data points that lie below $\bar{x}$ to cancel positive ones that arise when a data point lies above $\bar{x}$.

This problem must be corrected to obtain a satisfactory measure of variability about the mean.

Sample Variance

There are two ways to avoid the problem of allowing negative differences to cancel positive ones. We could just ignore the negative signs and work with the magnitude of the differences involved, or we could square the differences. The latter procedure is the

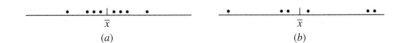

(a)   *(b)*

FIGURE 1.20

(a) Data points are clustered near the sample mean. Variability about the mean is small.
(b) Data points are more widely dispersed. Our statistic measuring variability should be larger in case *(b)* than in case *(a)*.

technique usually employed. Hence our measure of variability will make use of the sum of the squares of the differences between the data points and the sample mean $\sum (x - \bar{x})^2$. Is this sum sufficient to do the job? To answer this question, consider two samples each drawn from the same population. Assume that one sample is of size 5 and the other of size 5000. Which will have a larger value for the statistic $\sum (x - \bar{x})^2$? The second one will, naturally, because of sample size difference alone. To make sure that differences in sample size do not influence our measure of variability, we work not with the sum of the squared differences but with the average squared difference. Hence a logical measure of variability about the mean is the arithmetic average of these squared differences,

$$\frac{\sum (x - \bar{x})^2}{n}$$

This measure is acceptable and is preferred by many. However, it can be shown that this estimator on the average tends to underestimate the population variance σ^2. That is, if we draw many samples each of the same size and calculate

$$\sum \frac{(x - \bar{x})^2}{n}$$

for each, these values when plotted on a number line will form a pattern similar to that shown in Figure 1.21. This situation can be remedied by dividing the sum of the squared differences by $n - 1$ instead of n. The resulting statistic is called the *sample variance*. The pattern of values expected when σ^2 is estimated by

$$\frac{\sum (x - \bar{x})^2}{n - 1}$$

is shown in Figure 1.22. The definition of sample variance is formalized here.

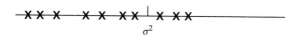

FIGURE 1.21
When using $\sum (x - \bar{x})^2/n$ to estimate σ^2, most estimates will fall below σ^2. That is, this statistic tends to underestimate σ^2.

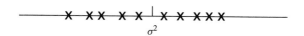

FIGURE 1.22
When using $\sum (x - \bar{x})^2/(n - 1)$ to estimate σ^2, the values vary about σ^2 as an average.

DEFINITION 1.5.1. Sample variance. Let $x_1, x_2, \ldots, x_n$ be a set of n observations on a variable X with sample mean $\bar{x}$. The *sample variance* is denoted by s^2 and is given by

$$s^2 = \frac{\sum (x - \bar{x})^2}{n - 1}$$

We shall report sample variances to two decimal places beyond the data.

EXAMPLE 1.5.3. The data set

2   1   4
5   3

has a sample mean of 3. Its sample variance is given by

$$
\begin{aligned}
s^2 &= \frac{\sum (x - \bar{x})^2}{n - 1} \\
&= \frac{(2 - 3)^2 + (5 - 3)^2 + (1 - 3)^2 + (3 - 3)^2 + (4 - 3)^2}{4} \\
&= \frac{(-1)^2 + 2^2 + (-2)^2 + 0^2 + 1^2}{4} \\
&= \frac{1 + 4 + 4 + 0 + 1}{4} = \frac{10}{4} = 2.50
\end{aligned}
$$

The formula for the sample variance given in Definition 1.5.1 does involve a fair amount of computation, especially if the data set is large. Calculators with statistical capability have the formula for s^2 programmed internally. You should use this feature of your calculator to find s^2 rather than the definition.

Keep in mind the practical interpretation of s^2. The measure is defined in such a way that it cannot be negative. Furthermore, if most of the observations lie close to the mean, the variance will be small. However, if the data points exhibit a fair amount of variability in the sense that values quite frequently lie far from the mean, then the variance will be large.

We are now in a position to investigate further the differences that exist between the two data sets of Example 1.5.1.

EXAMPLE 1.5.4. Consider the histograms of Figure 1.19. Most of the observations obtained on basketball injuries lie close to the mean value of 4, as evidenced by the bulge in the center of histogram a. However, very few of the observations obtained on football injuries lie near 4. This is apparent from the dip in the center of histogram b. Intuitively, then, we would expect the sample variance for the data on basketball injuries to be smaller than that for the data on football injuries. To verify this, we compute s^2 for each data set and report its value to two decimal places. The calculation is done on a TI83 calculator. You should verify the values given below.

Basketball	Football
$\bar{x} = 4$	$\bar{y} = 4$
$\tilde{x} = 4$	$\tilde{y} = 4$
$s_X^2 = 2.17$	$s_Y^2 = 6.00$

(Notice that we have rounded $s^2 = 2.166666$ to 2.17 so that s^2 is reported to two more decimal places than the data.) As expected, $s_X^2 < s_Y^2$.

Sample Standard Deviation

A second measure of variability is the sample standard deviation. We define this measure now.

> **DEFINITION 1.5.2. Sample standard deviation.** Let $x_1, x_2, \ldots, x_n$ be a set of n observations on a variable X with sample variance s^2. The *sample standard deviation* is denoted by s and is defined by

$$s = \sqrt{s^2}$$

Standard deviations will be reported to one decimal place beyond that of the data.

Note that the sample standard deviation is simply the nonnegative square root of the sample variance. Since these two measures of variability are so closely related, the natural question to ask is, Why bother with both of them? There is one very practical reason for wanting to measure variability by using the standard deviation of the data set. Consider the data on the number of football and basketball injuries reported in 25 school districts. The unit associated with each data point and with each sample mean is an "injury." When the sample variance is calculated, the differences between the observed values and the sample mean are *squared*. The unit associated with the sample variance is therefore a "squared injury"! This does not make any sense. However, since the sample standard deviation is the square root of the sample variance, the unit associated with s is again an "injury." It often happens that the original unit is meaningless when squared. For this reason, usually no unit is attached to a variance. However, the unit associated with a standard deviation will always be the same as that associated with the original data and so will always be physically meaningful.

> **EXAMPLE 1.5.5.** The sample variance for the number of basketball-related injuries is 2.17 (see Example 1.5.4). The sample standard deviation is $s = \sqrt{s^2} = \sqrt{2.166666} = 1.5$. Notice that when finding the standard deviation we do not round the variance before taking the square root.

Sample Range

The next measure of variability to be considered is the sample range. This measure is the easiest to compute, and we define it here.

> **DEFINITION 1.5.3. Sample range.** Let $x_1, x_2, \ldots, x_n$ be a set of n observations on a variable X. The *sample range* is the difference between the largest and smallest observations with subtraction being in the order of largest minus smallest.

This measure of variability was used in Section 1.3 in constructing histograms. A large range implies that the data are spread over a large interval; a small range guarantees that the data are concentrated in a small segment of the number line.

Interquartile Range

The variance, standard deviation, and range are the measures of variability most often encountered. However, they are all rather seriously affected by outliers. Thus, a single wild number can inflate their value and give a somewhat misleading impression of the variation that exists among the bulk of the data. It is useful to have a measure of variability that is resistant to outliers. Our fourth measure of variation, the interquartile range, is such a measure. The sample interquartile range, iqr, represents the length of the interval that contains roughly the middle 50% of the data. If the iqr is small, then much of the data lies close to the center of the distribution; if it is large, the data tend to be widely dispersed. These steps are used to calculate the iqr.

Finding the Sample Interquartile Range

1. Find the median location, $(n + 1)/2$, where n is the sample size. If the sample size is an odd number then this location will be an integer. Otherwise, it will be a number halfway between two integers. For example, if $n = 17$ then the median location is $(17 + 1)/2 = 9$, an integer. If $n = 18$ then the median location is $(18 + 1)/2 = 9.5$, the number halfway between the integers 9 and 10.
2. If necessary, truncate the median location by ignoring the .5. For example, if the median location is 9.5, then the truncated location is 9. If the location is already an integer then no truncation is necessary.
3. Find the quartile location q by

$$q = \frac{\text{truncated median location} + 1}{2}$$

4. Find q_1 by counting up from the smallest data point to location q. If q is an integer, then q_1 is the data point in position q. If q is not an integer, then q_1 is the average of the data points in positions $q - .5$ and $q + .5$. Approximately 25% of the data will fall on or below q_1.
5. Find q_3 by counting down from the largest data point to position q as in part 4. Approximately 75% of the data will fall on or below q_3.
6. Define iqr by iqr $= q_3 - q_1$.

> **EXAMPLE 1.5.6.** A study of the type of sediment found at two different deep-sea drilling sites is conducted. The random variable of interest is the percentage by volume of cement found in core samples. By cement we mean dissolved and reprecipitated carbonate material. These data are obtained: (Based on information found in Andreas Wetzel, "Influence of Heat Flow on Ooze/Chalk Cementation: Quantification from Consolidation Parameters in DSDP Site 504 and 505 Sediments," *Journal of Sedimentary Petrology,* July 1989, pp. 539–547.)

Site I, % cement				Site II, % cement		
10	21	12	12	1	10	14
20	13	24	36	9	21	19
31	18	17	16	15	17	13
37	16	32	13	25	22	20
14	49	25	19	24	12	23
13	32	27		15	20	18

The double stem-and-leaf diagram for the data of site I is shown in Figure 1.23. The sample is size $n = 23$. The median location is $(n + 1)/2 = 12$. The quartile location is $q = (12 + 1)/2 = 6.5$. To find q_1 we use the stem-and-leaf diagram to locate the sixth and

```
1 | 0  4  3  3  2  2  3
1 | 8  6  7  6  9
2 | 0  1  4
2 | 5  7
3 | 1  2  2
3 | 7  6
4 |
4 | 9
```

FIGURE 1.23

Double stem-and-leaf diagram for the percentage by volume of cement in core samples taken at deep-sea drilling site I.

seventh data points counting from the smaller numbers up. These values are 13 and 14, respectively. Hence $q_1 = (13 + 14)/2 = 13.5$. To find q_3 we find the sixth and seventh data points counting from the higher numbers down. These points are 31 and 27, respectively, yielding $q_3 = (31 + 27)/2 = 29$. The sample interquartile range is $q_3 - q_1 = 29 - 13.5 = 15.5$.

Multiple Data Sets (Optional)

Measures of the central tendency, the variability, and the range provide valuable information about a data set. Often, however, we are concerned with not just a single data set, but the way in which a particular set of measurements behaves as a function of time, or dose of drug, or some other variable. At each time point, drug dose, and so on, a different data set is obtained. This may involve a very large number of data points, so a convenient way of graphing the data that provides maximum information is desirable. One such method is illustrated in Example 1.5.7.

EXAMPLE 1.5.7. The concentration of lactate in arterial blood was measured in a sample of six young men before and at several times during controlled exercise and in the recovery period following. The data in Table 1.21 were obtained. The mean and standard deviation for the data set at each time point may be computed and are given in Table 1.22. Then

TABLE 1.21

Arterial concentrations of lactate (millimoles/liter)

Rest, minutes	Exercise, minutes				Recovery, minutes			
	5	10	20	30	5	20	35	65
.93	7.60	8.25	6.70	6.49	4.35	2.05	1.35	.85
.55	3.95	4.31	8.85	4.38	6.22	2.98	2.02	.58
.87	6.54	6.52	4.56	8.75	2.45	1.17	.76	.95
.62	4.27	5.15	7.29	6.72	3.57	2.71	1.21	1.10
.72	5.85	7.31	5.88	4.88	3.81	1.84	1.58	.62
.79	5.41	6.30	6.96	7.70	5.62	2.36	1.29	.79

TABLE 1.22

Lactate concentration

Rest, minutes		Exercise, minutes				Recovery, minutes			
		5	10	20	30	2	20	35	65
$\bar{x}$	.747	5.603	6.307	6.707	6.487	4.337	2.185	1.368	.815
s	.146	1.377	1.425	1.435	1.653	1.387	.649	.417	.197

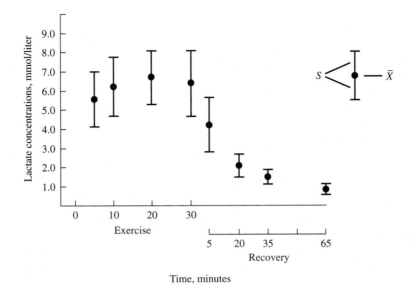

FIGURE 1.24

Lactate concentration over time.

a graph can be constructed in which the mean lactate concentration in millimoles per liter is plotted as a function of time. The standard deviation of each time point in the data set is shown as a set of brackets extending above and below the mean value points, as shown in Figure 1.24. Just a glance at this graph gives an idea of the change in blood lactate during exercise and recovery and allows a quick assessment of the variability at different time points.

You should be warned of one thing. Many graphs of the sort described in Example 1.5.7 appear in the literature. Other graphs of a similar appearance are used also. In these graphs, however, a measure of variability known as the *standard error of the mean* (SE) is used to determine the length of the brackets extending above and below the mean. The concept of standard error is introduced in Chapter 6. Graphs of either sort should be clearly marked to indicate which measure of variability is being used.

There are other statistical measures to describe data sets. We presented here the most commonly encountered ones. Several others are mentioned in the exercises for reference purposes. The sample mean, variance, and standard deviation are used extensively throughout this text; the sample median plays an important role in our discussion of distribution-free methods in Chapter 13.

▨ EXERCISES 1.5

1. Find the sample range, s^2, and s for the data of Exercise 1 of Section 1.4.
2. Find the sample range, s^2, and s for the data of Exercise 2 of Section 1.4.
3. (*a*) Find s^2 and s for each of the data sets of Exercise 3 of Section 1.4.
   (*b*) Drop the outlier from the data on mourning doves and recompute s^2 and s. Are these measures of variability resistant to the outlier?

(c) Find iqr for each of the data sets of Exercise 3 of Section 1.4.

(d) Drop the outlier from the data on mourning doves and recompute iqr. Is this measure of variability resistant to the outlier?

(e) Find the range for each of the data sets of Exercise 3 of Section 1.4.

(f) Drop the outlier from the data on mourning doves and recompute the range. Is this measure of variability resistant to the outlier?

4. Based on the histograms for the data of Exercise 6 of Section 1.3, which data set do you think has the larger variance? Compute s^2 for each group of verify your answer. What physical unit of measurement is associated with s?

5. Find s^2, s, the sample range, and iqr for the data of Exercise 7 of Section 1.3.

6. Find s^2, s, the sample range, and iqr for the data of Exercise 8 of Section 1.3. What physical unit of measurement is associated with s?

7. (a) Construct a double stem-and-leaf diagram for the site II data of Example 1.5.6. Compare the shape of this distribution to that of site I.

(b) Find the sample mean and median for each sample.

(c) Find s^2 and s for each sample.

8. Consider the data of Exercise 1 of Section 1.2.

(a) Find $\bar{x}$, $\tilde{x}$, s, s^2, range, and iqr for these data.

(b) Suppose that an additional observation of .72 is obtained. Will any of the statistics of part a be affected much by the addition of this point? Explain.

(c) Now add the observation 2.8 to the original data set. Will this point have a big impact on the value of any of the statistics of part a? If so, which ones are affected? Check your answer by calculating $\bar{x}$, $\tilde{x}$, s, s^2, range, and iqr for the expanded data set.

9. Consider the data of Exercise 9 of Section 1.3.

(a) Give an example of an additional SCI reading that would change the range for the unburned data rather dramatically. Would it change the value of the median to any large extent?

(b) Give an example of an additional SCI reading that would have little effect on the sample mean, standard deviation, and variance for the burned data.

10. *Coefficient of Variation.* The coefficient of variation is a measure used to compare the variability in one data set with that in another in situations in which a direct comparison of standard deviations is not convenient or realistic. For example, in a study of milk consumption in the United States, it is reported that the mean number of gallons of milk consumed per family unit per week is 8 with a sample standard deviation of 3 gallons. A similar study in Canada reports the mean consumption to be 12 liters with a sample standard deviation of 4 liters. It makes no sense to compare these standard deviations directly because they are reported in different units. A quick way to compare variability is with the *coefficient of variation* (CV), given by

$$CV = \frac{s}{\bar{x}}(100)$$

The coefficients of variation for the two samples are $(3/8)100 = 37.5$ and $(4/12)100 = 33.3$, respectively. The data from the United States exhibit more variability than do the Canadian data.

(a) An experiment is conducted to investigate the effect of a new dog food on weight gain in pups during the first 8 weeks of their lives. It is reported that the mean weight gain in a group of Great Dane pups is 30 pounds with a standard deviation of 10 pounds; the mean weight gain in a group of Chihuahua pups is 3 pounds with a standard deviation of 1.5 pounds. Calculate the coefficient of variation for each group. Which group exhibits the greater variability? Why is a direct comparison of standard deviations misleading here?

(b) A study of weights of 2-year-old girls in Great Britain yielded a sample mean of 12.74 kilograms with a sample standard deviation of 1.60 kilograms. A similar study in the United States resulted in a sample mean of 29.2 pounds with a sample standard deviation of 2 pounds. Find the coefficient of variation for each group. Which group exhibits greater variability?

11. Verify the values given in Table 1.22.

12. A study of two anesthetics is conducted using conscious, freely moving rats. The measured response is the percentage change in pressure of CO_2 in arterial blood after administration of identical doses of the drug. These data are obtained: (Based on information found in Linas V. Kudzma et al., "A Novel Class of Analgesic and Anesthetic Agents," *Journal of Medicinal Chemistry,* December 1989, pp. 2534–2542.)

Percent change, mmHg				
Compound I		**Compound II**		
27.2	31.7	55.1	65.8	63.6
30.1	32.0	56.3	58.3	64.0
30.5	28.6	60.0	57.1	65.3
28.4	29.2	63.5	55.4	62.8
30.7	33.0	64.9	56.5	59.5
31.3	31.7	62.7	55.1	
30.5	32.6	60.5	57.0	
30.1	28.2	59.2	59.3	
29.6	29.1	63.7	60.7	
30.2	30.7	64.1	62.1	

(a) Construct a stem-and-leaf diagram for each data set. Which data set appears to be more widely dispersed?

(b) Calculate the sample mean and median for each data set.

(c) Calculate the sample variance and sample standard deviation for each data set. Verify your answer to part a. What unit of measurement is associated with the sample standard deviation?

(d) Calculate the sample range and sample interquartile range for each data set.

(e) Based on the characteristics that you have observed in these samples, would you be surprised to hear a claim that there is no difference in the way that rats react to these compounds? Explain.

(f) Construct a diagram similar to that given in Figure 1.24 to compare the two data sets.

13. The technique illustrated in Exercise 7 of Section 1.4 can be used to compute s^2 from data reported in frequency table form. To do so we use a computational

shortcut for s^2. This shortcut states that

$$s^2 = \frac{n \sum x^2 - \left(\sum x \right)^2}{n(n-1)}$$

To use this shortcut, we multiply each value of x by its corresponding frequency and sum these values to obtain $\sum x$; we multiply the square of each x by the corresponding frequency to obtain $\sum x^2$. These values are then substituted into the shortcut formula to obtain s^2. For the data of Exercise 7 of Section 1.4,

$$\sum x = 0(1) + 1(3) + 2(2) + 4(8) + 5(2) = 49$$

$$\sum x^2 = 0^2(1) + 1^2(3) + 2^2(2) + 4^2(8) + 5^2(2) = 189$$

The sample variance for these data is

$$s^2 = \frac{16(189) - (49)^2}{16(15)} = 2.60$$

(a) Use this technique to verify the values given in Example 1.5.4 and Table 1.20.

(b) Use this technique to find the sample variance for the data of Exercise 2 of Section 1.4.

1.6

BOX PLOTS (OPTIONAL)

The box plot is a graphical representation of a data set that gives a visual impression of location, spread, and the degree and direction of skewness. It also allows for the identification of outliers. It is especially useful when one wants to compare two or more data sets. The method of construction demonstrated here is that given by Lambert H. Koopmans [7].

Constructing a Box Plot

1. A horizontal or vertical reference scale is constructed.
2. Find the sample median, q_1, q_3, and iqr as explained in Section 1.5.
3. Find two points f_1 and f_3, called "inner fences," by

$$f_1 = q_1 - 1.5(\text{iqr})$$

$$f_3 = q_3 + 1.5(\text{iqr})$$

Points that fall below f_1 or above f_3 are considered to be outliers.

4. Find two points a_1 and a_3, called "adjacent values." The point a_1 is the smallest data point that does not qualify as an outlier; a_3 is the largest data point that does not qualify as an outlier.

5. Find two points F_1 and F_3, called "outer fences," by

$$F_1 = q_1 - 2(1.5)(\text{iqr})$$

$$F_3 = q_3 + 2(1.5)(\text{iqr})$$

6. Locate the points found thus far on the horizontal or vertical scale. Their relative positions are shown in Figure 1.25a.
7. Construct a box with ends at q_1 and q_3 with an interior line drawn at the median as shown in Figure 1.25b.
8. Indicate adjacent values by x and connect them to the box with dashed lines. The dashed lines are called "whiskers." Locate any data points falling between the inner and outer fences and denote these by open circles. These points are considered to be mild outliers. Indicate data points that fall on or beyond the outer fences with asterisks. These points are considered to be extreme outliers (see Figure 1.25c).

The location of the midline of the box is an indication of the shape of the distribution. If the line is badly off center, then we know that the distribution is skewed in the direction of the longer end of the box.

Before we illustrate this technique, the notion of fences needs to be clarified. It can be shown that when sampling from a normal distribution, a symmetric bell-shaped distribution that will be studied in detail in Chapter 5, only about 7 values in every 1000 fall beyond the inner fences. Since these values are very unusual, they are deemed to be outliers. Outliers must be treated with care since, as you have seen, their presence can have a dramatic impact on $\bar{x}$, s^2, s, and the range, the usual measures of location and variation. When an outlier is found, one should consider its source. Is it a legitimate data point whose value is simply unusually large or small? Is it a misrecorded value? Is it the result of some error or accident in experimentation? In the last two instances the point can be deleted from the data set and the analysis completed on the remaining data. In the first case, we suggest that the presence of the outlier be made known and that statistics be reported both with and without the outlier. In this way, the

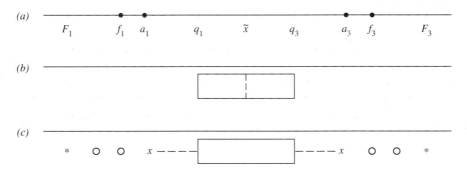

FIGURE 1.25

(a) Relative positions of median ($\tilde{x}$), quartiles (q_1) and q_3, adjacent values (a_1 and a_3), inner fences (f_1 and f_3), and outer fences (F_1 and F_3). (b) A box is drawn with ends at q_1 and q_3 and interior line at $\tilde{x}$. (c) Adjacent values are indicated by x; mild outliers are indicated by open circles; extreme outliers are shown as asterisks.

decision of whether or not to include the outlier in future analyses can be made by the researcher who is the subject matter expert.

EXAMPLE 1.6.1. A study of posttraumatic amnesia after a closed head injury is conducted. One variable studied is the length of hospitalization in days. The stem-and-leaf diagram for the data is shown in Figure 1.26. (Based on information found in Jerry Mysia et al., "Prospective Assessment of Posttraumatic Amnesia: A Comparison of GOAT and the OGMS," *Journal of Head Trauma Rehabilitation,* March 1990, pp. 65–77.) For these data the median location is $(n + 1)/2 = 11$ and the median is 40 days. The quartile location is $q =$ (truncated median location $+ 1)/2 = 6$. The points q_1 and q_3 are 32 and 47, respectively. The interquartile range is iqr $= q_3 - q_1 = 15$. The inner fences are

$$f_1 = q_1 - 1.5(\text{iqr}) \quad f_3 = q_3 + 1.5(\text{iqr})$$

$$= 32 - 22.5 \qquad = 47 + 22.5$$

$$= 9.5 \qquad = 69.5$$

The adjacent values are $a_1 = 12$ and $a_3 = 61$. The outer fences are

$$F_1 = q_1 - 2(1.5)(\text{iqr}) \quad F_3 = q_3 + 2(1.5)(\text{iqr})$$

$$= 32 - 45 \qquad = 47 + 45$$

$$= -13 \qquad = 92$$

The data set contains two points, 8 and 89, that qualify as mild outliers. The point 108 qualifies as an extreme outlier. Notice that since F_1 is negative, it is physically impossible to see an extreme outlier on the lower end of the scale. The box plot is shown in Figure 1.27. Notice that the midline of the box is near its center, indicating a nearly symmetric distribution. Are the outliers real observations that must be taken into account or are they the result of errors in data collection? In this case, it would be easy to check patient records to find the answer, and this should be done before proceeding with any further analysis of the data.

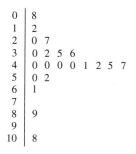

0	8
1	2
2	0 7
3	0 2 5 6
4	0 0 0 0 1 2 5 7
5	0 2
6	1
7	
8	9
9	
10	8

FIGURE 1.26

Stem-and-leaf diagram for the data of Example 1.6.1. Data represent length of hospitalization in days of posttraumatic amnesia patients ($n = 21$).

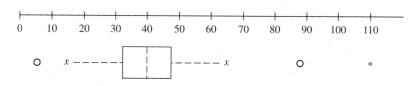

FIGURE 1.27

Box plot for the data of Example 1.6.1.

One further point should be made. This outlier test is based on the assumption that sampling is from a normal distribution. If the distribution is skewed, it is likely that the values that define the long tail of the skew will be identified as outliers. Are they really unusual values? Possibly not. The outlier test should be used in conjunction with a stem-and-leaf plot or a histogram.

▣ EXERCISES 1.6

1. In the study of Example 1.6.1 the variable X, the length of coma in days of patients suffering a closed head injury, was also considered. These data were collected:

2	8	9	14	16
6	10	8	7	
13	12	11	11	
11	13	15	10	
11	15	12	20	

   (a) Construct a stem-and-leaf diagram for these data. Do these data appear to be symmetrically distributed?
   (b) Construct a box plot for the data. Does the box plot give the same impression of symmetry as you received from the stem-and-leaf diagram?
   (c) Are there any data points that qualify as outliers?

2. Construct box plots for each of the data sets given in Example 1.5.6. Use these plots to compare these data sets with respect to location and variability. Which is more nearly symmetric? Does either data set contain outliers?

3. These data are obtained on the average density of the planets that comprise our solar system and our moon: (Based on Nigel Henbert, "Rocky Dwarfs and Gassy Giants," *New Scientist*, February 10, 1990, pp. 1–4.)

Mercury	5.42	Mars	3.94
Earth	5.52	Jupiter	1.32
Saturn	0.69	Uranus	1.26
Venus	5.25	Neptune	1.64
Moon	3.34	Pluto	2.10

   Do any of these values qualify as outliers?

4. Ozone levels around Los Angeles have been measured as high as 220 parts per billion (ppb). Concentrations this high can cause the eyes to burn and are a hazard to both plant and animal life. These data are obtained on the ozone level in a forested area near Seattle, Washington: (Based on information found in "Twigs," *American Forests*, April 1990, p. 71.)

160	176	160	180	167	164
165	163	162	168	173	179
170	196	185	163	162	163
172	162	167	161	169	178
161					

(a) Construct a double stem-and-leaf diagram for these data. Do these data appear to be skewed? If so, in which direction?

(b) Construct a box plot for these data and identify the outlier that exists.

(c) Assume that the outlier is a legitimate reading. In this case, which measure of location is least affected by the outlier? Which measure of variability is least affected by the outlier?

5. Two drugs, amantadine (A) and rimantadine (R), are being studied for use in combating the influenza virus. A single 100-mg dose is administered orally to healthly adults. The variable studied is T_{max}, the time in minutes required to reach maximum plasma concentration. These data are obtained: (Based on information found in Gordon Douglas, Jr., "Drug Therapy," *New England Journal of Medicine,* vol. 322, February 1990, pp. 443–449.)

T_{max} (A)			T_{max} (R)		
105	123	12.4	221	227	280
126	108	134	261	264	238
120	112	130	250	236	240
119	132	130	230	246	283
133	136	142	253	273	516
145	156	170	256	271	
200					

(a) Construct a box plot for each data set and identify outliers.

(b) Calculate $\bar{x}$ and s^2 for the data of set A.

(c) Assume that the outlier of set A is the result of a misplaced decimal point. Correct the error by deleting the decimal and see what changes this makes in your box plot. Recompute $\bar{x}$ and s^2, using the correct data point, and compare your results to those of part b.

(d) Is there an outlier in set R? If so, is there an obvious legitimate reason to delete it from the data set?

6. Consider the data of Exercise 3 of Section 1.4.

(a) Construct a histogram for each data set. Be careful to handle the outlier in the mourning dove data set as suggested in Section 1.3. Comment on the suggested shape of each distribution.

(b) Construct a box plot for each data set. Does the outlier test seem appropriate in each case? Explain.

7. Hydroponics is the science of growing plants in a nutrient solution alone. A study was conducted to compare this method of growing Echinacea (coneflower) to the traditional method of growing in soil. One variable measured at the end of the study is the height of each plant. The box plots shown in Figure 1.28 summarize the data gathered. In the plots, group 1 is the hydroponic group.

(a) Approximate the median for each group.

(b) Which group is more nearly symmetric?

(c) Which group has the larger inner quartile range?

(d) Which group has a data point that is possibly an extreme outlier? Can you say for certain that the point in question is an outlier? Explain.

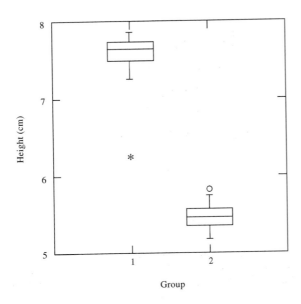

Box plot of Echinacea plant heights.

(e) Based on these plots do you think that hydroponics tends to produce taller plants than growing in soil? Explain.
(Based on a study by Mary Cappuccio, Department of Biology, Radford University, 1996.)

■ 1.7
HANDLING GROUPED DATA (OPTIONAL)

In some instances in the literature, data are presented in table or category form. Neither the raw data nor summary measures are given. When this occurs, it is helpful to be able to extract from the table at least a rough approximation of various summary measures for the underlying data set. Methods for doing so are given in the following examples.

EXAMPLE 1.7.1. In a study of Down's syndrome, 180 children who had the disorder were examined. Table 1.23 gives the frequency distribution for the variable X, the child's IQ. To use this table to approximate the mean IQ, first we determine the midpoint of each category or class. The *midpoint* is the arithmetic average of the lower and upper class boundaries. Thus the midpoint for the first class, which we denote by m_1, is

$$m_1 = \frac{10.5 + 20.5}{2} = 15.5$$

Successive class midpoints $m_2, m_3, \ldots, m_9$ are given in Table 1.23.

As long as the classes are not excessively wide, the midpoint of each class serves as a good approximation for each of the values in the class. Thus in approximating the sample

■ **TABLE 1.23**
Frequency distribution of IQ

Class	Class boundaries	Class midpoint m_i	Frequency f_i
1	10.5 to 20.5	15.5	4
2	20.5 to 30.5	25.5	34
3	30.5 to 40.5	35.5	0
4	40.5 to 50.5	45.5	70
5	50.5 to 60.5	55.5	43
6	60.5 to 70.5	65.5	19
7	70.5 to 80.5	75.5	7
8	80.5 to 90.5	85.5	2
9	90.5 to 100.5	95.5	1

mean, each of the four observations in class 1, whose actual values are unknown to us, is replaced by the number 15.5; each of the 34 observations in class 2 is replaced by the number 25.5; this procedure is continued for the other classes until finally the one observation in class 9 is replaced by the value 95.5. To approximate $\bar{x}$, we add these values and divide by 180, the total number of children in the study. Thus

$$\bar{x} \doteq \frac{4(15.5) + 34(25.5) + 0(35.5) + \cdots + 2(85.5) + 1(95.5)}{180}$$

$$= 47.4$$

where the symbol $\doteq$ means "approximately equal to." The mean IQ for this group of children is approximately 47.4.

A similar procedure can be used to approximate the sample variance for grouped data. Once again, the method is based on the assumption that the class midpoint provides a good approximation for each of the observations in the class. It also utilizes the shortcut formula for s^2 given in Exercise 1.5.13.

DEFINITION 1.7.1. $\bar{x}$ and s^2, grouped data. Let $x_1, x_2, x_3, \ldots, x_n$ be a set of n observations on a variable X categorized into k classes. Let m_i and f_i $(i = 1, 2, 3, \ldots, k)$ denote the class midpoint and class frequency, respectively, for each class. Then

$$\bar{x} \doteq \sum_{i=1}^{k} \frac{f_i m_i}{n}$$

and

$$s^2 \doteq \frac{n \sum_{i=1}^{k} f_i m_i^2 - \left(\sum_{i=1}^{k} f_i m_i \right)^2}{n(n-1)}$$

EXAMPLE 1.7.2. The approximate value of s^2 for the grouped data for Example 1.7.1 is given by

$$s^2 \doteq \frac{n \sum_{i=1}^{k} f_i m_i^2 - \left(\sum_{i=1}^{k} f_i m_i \right)^2}{n(n-1)}$$

$$= \frac{180 \sum_{i=1}^{9} f_i m_i^2 - \left(\sum_{i=1}^{9} f_i m_i \right)^2}{180(179)}$$

For these data

$$\sum_{i=1}^{9} f_i m_i^2 = 4(15.5)^2 + 34(25.5)^2 + \cdots + 2(85.5)^2 + 1(95.5)^2$$

$$= 445{,}595$$

and

$$\sum_{i=1}^{9} f_i m_i = 4(15.5) + 34(25.5) + \cdots + 2(85.5) + 1(95.5)$$

$$= 8540$$

Thus

$$s^2 \doteq \frac{180(445{,}595) - 8540^2}{180(179)} = 225.81$$

and

$$s \doteq \sqrt{225.81} \doteq 15.0$$

We outline here a method that can be used to approximate any specified observation in a data set from grouped data. When the point of interest is the "middle" of the data set, the method can be applied to obtain an approximation for the sample median.

Assume that $x_1, x_2, x_3, \ldots, x_n$ is a linearly ordered set of observations on a variable X. Let x_j denote any one of these observations. To approximate x_j from grouped data, the following steps are used:

1. Locate the class in which x_j falls; denote the class frequency for this class by f.
2. Find the lower and upper class boundaries for this class; denote them by l and u, respectively.
3. Find the difference between j and the cumulative frequency for the class immediately preceding the one in which x_j falls; denote this difference by d.
4. The approximate value of x_j is

$$x_j \doteq l + \frac{d}{f}(u - l)$$

This procedure is easy to apply. Consider Example 1.7.3.

EXAMPLE 1.7.3. A study is conducted to assess the effect of alcohol on serum cholesterol levels. One variable of interest is X, the amount of alcohol consumed per week per subject. The data for the 923 subjects who participated in the study are given in Table 1.24.

TABLE 1.24

Frequency distribution of alcohol consumption (in ounces)

Class	Class boundaries	Frequency f	Cumulative frequency	Relative cumulative frequency
1	0 to .5	201	201	.218
2	.5 to 3.5	372	573*	.621
3	3.5 to 9.5	260	833	.903
4	9.5 to 19.5	80	913	.989
5	≥ 19.5	10	923	1.000

The total number of observations is $n = 923$. Since this number is odd, the median location is $(n + 1)/2 = 462$ and the sample median is $\tilde{x} = x_{462}$. Thus we are trying to approximate $x_j = x_{462}$. From the cumulative frequency distribution it can be seen that the 462d observation lies in the second class (denoted*). The class frequency for this class is $f = 372$. Its lower class boundary is $l = .5$; its upper boundary is $u = 3.5$. The difference between j and the cumulative frequency for class 1 is $d = 462 - 201 = 261$. Thus

$$\tilde{x} = x_{462} \doteq l + \frac{d}{f}(u - l)$$

$$= .5 + \frac{261}{372}(3.5 - .5)$$

$$= 2.6$$

(The symbol $\doteq$ means "approximately equal to.") The approximate median alcohol consumption is 2.6 ounces per week.

EXERCISES 1.7

1. Consider Table 1.25.
   (a) Complete Table 1.25 by finding the midpoint and cumulative frequency for each class.
   (b) Approximate the sample mean, variance, standard deviation, and median.

TABLE 1.25

Frequency distribution

Class	Class boundaries	Class midpoint	Frequency	Cumulative frequency
1	4.5 to 9.5		1	
2	9.5 to 14.5		2	
3	14.5 to 19.5		5	
4	19.5 to 24.5		3	

2. A study is conducted on the age of women using oral contraceptives. The grouped data in Table 1.26 are reported.
   (a) Complete Table 1.26 by finding the class midpoint and cumulative frequency for each class.
   (b) Approximate the sample mean, variance, standard deviation, and median.
3. A study of Hodgkin's disease was conducted. The study was restricted to patients under age 40. One purpose of the study was to compare the distribution of cases by age in men to that in women. The grouped data shown in Table 1.27 were reported.
   (a) Complete Table 1.27 by finding the midpoint and cumulative frequency for each class.
   (b) For each group, approximate the sample mean, variance, standard deviation, and median. Point out the similarities and differences in the two groups.

TABLE 1.26

Frequency distribution of age (in years)

Class	Class boundaries	Class midpoint	Frequency	Cumulative frequency
1	14.5 to 19.5		171	
2	19.5 to 24.5		785	
3	24.5 to 29.5		837	
4	29.5 to 34.5		554	
5	34.5 to 39.5		382	
6	39.5 to 44.5		432	
7	44.5 to 49.5		562	
8	49.5 to 54.5		610	
9	54.5 to 59.5		490	
10	59.5 to 64.5		258	
11	64.5 to 69.5		153	
12	69.5 to 74.5		60	

TABLE 1.27

Distribution of cases by age

		Men		
Class	Class boundaries	Class midpoint	Frequency	Cumulative frequency
1	4.5 to 9.5		1	
2	9.5 to 14.5		4	
3	14.5 to 19.5		7	
4	19.5 to 24.5		23	
5	24.5 to 29.5		16	
6	29.5 to 34.5		7	
7	34.5 to 39.5		10	

		Women		
Class	Class boundaries	Class midpoint	Frequency	Cumulative frequency
1	4.5 to 9.5		0	
2	9.5 to 14.5		2	
3	14.5 to 19.5		10	
4	19.5 to 24.5		7	
5	24.5 to 29.5		3	
6	29.5 to 34.5		5	
7	34.5 to 39.5		2	

TECHNOLOGY TOOLS

The calculations necessary to summarize or display data from even a small data set can be tedious and time-consuming. There are many handheld calculators on the market that are programmed to do statistical calculations. Several computer packages exist whose primary purpose is statistical analysis. In the Technology Tools sections of this text (found at the end of most chapters) we discuss one computer package and one specific calculator. If you have access to these particular tools, then the instructions given can be followed exactly. If you are using a different calculator or program, the steps must be modified. The calculator chosen for this text is the TI83; the computer package to be used is SAS.

TI83 Graphics Calculator

The TI83 graphics calculator provides a powerful tool for aiding in the analysis of statistical data. It is easy to use. The instructions that we give will allow you to perform many of the operations presented in this text, and we will use data from the text to illustrate the use of the calculator. If you own one of these calculators, you are urged to study your user's guide. You will find that the calculator can do far more than we can explain in this text.

I. Reset/Clear

We begin by considering how to reset the TI83 to its factory setting. In these instructions we state the keystroke and the purpose of the keystroke. You should watch what appears on your screen. Many of the steps are self-explanatory and you will soon be able to perform the steps without having to memorize the routines given in the text.

	TI83 Keystroke	Purpose
1.	2ND	1. Resets to factory settings
	$+$	
	5	
	1	
	2	
2.	2ND	2. Darkens screen (if necessary)
	$\triangle$ (hold)	
3.	CLEAR	3. Clears screen

Note: 2ND $\triangledown$ (hold) lightens the screen if necessary.

This reset process erases all stored data, settings, and programs. If you are not saving anything this routine can be used to clear the calculator before beginning each new problem.

If you want to clear old data from the calculator without changing anything else, the following keystrokes can be used.

TI83 Keystroke	Purpose
STAT	Clears the stat data editor;
4	returns to blank screen
2ND	
1	
ENTER	
CLEAR	

Note: These instructions clear data from column L1. To clear columns L1 and

L2, add

, (comma)
2ND
2
just before ENTER.

II. Histograms

The TI83 calculator can be used to construct histograms. To use it to do so, you must know the lower boundary of the first class, the upper boundary of the last class, and the class width. We illustrate by constructing the histogram shown in Figure 1.8. The data used are that of Example 1.3.1. It is assumed that the calculator has been cleared.

TI83 Keystroke	**Purpose**
1. STAT 1	1. Accesses the stat data editor
2. 135 ENTER	2. Enters data (be sure to enter each data point; dots indicate that we have not shown all of the data here)
137 ENTER ⋮ 155 ENTER	
3. WINDOW	3. Accesses window to set class boundaries and class width
4. 129.5 ENTER	4. Sets xmin to 129.5
159.5 ENTER	Sets xmax to 159.5
6 ENTER	Sets class width to 6
(−)5 ENTER	Sets ymin to − 5 to provide some room below the histogram
20 ENTER ENTER	Allows for a maximum class frequency of 20
5. 2ND Y = ENTER cursor to ON ENTER ▽ ▷ ▷ ENTER GRAPH	5. Draws histogram

| 6. | TRACE | 6. | Determines frequencies and boundaries by moving cursor to right or left |

III. Finding $\bar{x}$, s, s^2, q_1, q_3, and the median

The TI83 calculator will compute most of the statistics described in this book. We demonstrate how this is done for a single data set using the site I data of Example 1.5.6. Note that the calculator does not estimate q_1 and q_3 as was done in the text. Rather, if the median location is an integer, then the quartile location is taken to be the median location divided by 2; if the median location is not an integer, then the quartile location will agree with those in the book. It is assumed that the calculator has been cleared.

TI83 Keystroke		**Purpose**
1.	STAT 1	1. Accesses the stat data editor
2.	10 ENTER 20 ENTER $\vdots$ 19 ENTER	2. Enters data
3.	STAT $\triangleright$ 1 ENTER (use $\triangledown$ to view others)	3. Calculates basic statistics
4.	VARS 5 3 X^2 ENTER	4. Calculates s^2

Note that since the median location is 12, an integer, the TI83 takes the quartile location to be the median location divided by 2. In this case the quartile location is 6. This yields $q_1 = 13$ and $q_3 = 31$. These values differ a little from those given in the text. The next section, Sorting, shows you how to get the textbook quartiles easily.

IV. Sorting

If you want to find q_1 and q_3 as was done in this book, the sorting feature is useful. We illustrate this procedure via the site I data of Example 1.5.6. It is assumed that the calculator has been cleared.

TI83 Keystroke	**Purpose**
1. STAT 1	1. Accesses the stat data editor

2.	10	2. Enters data (be sure to enter
	ENTER	each data point; dots indicate
	20	that we have not shown all
	ENTER	of the data here)
	⋮	
	19	
	ENTER	
3.	STAT	3. Sorts data and displays the
	2	sorted list
	2ND	
	1	
	ENTER	
	STAT	
	1	

Note that from the textbook example, the quartile location is 6.5. To find q_1, all we have to do is find the 6th and 7th data points in the now-sorted list and average them. In this case the 6th value is 13 and the 7th is 14. The average and therefore the value of q_1 is 13.5. The quartile q_3 can be found by finding the 6th and 7th points counting from the largest values back.

V. Box Plots

The TI83 will construct two types of box plots. One uses the maximum and minimum values of x to define the whiskers. The other defines the whiskers via the adjacent values as was done in the text. The latter plot will show and flag outliers. We demonstrate the construction of a box plot using the data of Example 1.6.1.

TI83 Keystroke				**Purpose**
Max/Min		**Outliers**		
1.	STAT	1.	STAT	1. Accesses the stat data
	1		1	editor
2.	8	2.	8	2. Enters data (be sure to enter
	ENTER		ENTER	each data point; dots indicate
	12		12	that we have not shown all of
				the data here)
	ENTER		ENTER	
	⋮		⋮	
	108		108	
3.	WINDOW	3.	WINDOW	3. Sets the x scale below
	0		0	xmin and above
	▽		▽	xmax; provides room under
	110		110	box plot
	▽		▽	
4.	2ND	4.	2ND	4. Draws the box plot
	$Y=$		$Y=$	
	ENTER		ENTER	

cursor to ON	cursor to ON	
ENTER	ENTER	
$\triangledown$	$\triangledown$	
$\triangleright$	$\triangleright$	
$\triangleright$	$\triangleright$	
$\triangleright$	$\triangleright$	
$\triangleright$		
ENTER	ENTER	
GRAPH	GRAPH	
5. TRACE	5. TRACE	5. Reads values of median, q_1, q_3, max x, min x (or a_1, a_3, and outliers)

The SAS Statistical Software Package

There are many statistical software packages on the market. Among the systems in widespread use are SPSS (Statistical Package for the Social Sciences, McGraw-Hill), BMD (Biomedical Computer Programs, University of California Press), MINITAB (Pennsylvania State University), and SAS (Statistical Analysis System, SAS Institute, Inc.). To use any such system to do simple analyses one needs little background in computer science.

We present here a very brief introduction to SAS programming to give you some experience with statistical packages. Once this experience has been gained, it is not difficult to adjust to other packages as they are similar. We introduce SAS by presenting some sample programs that can be modified to analyze the data sets presented in this chapter. You should consult the appropriate expert at your own installation to determine how to access SAS, save and run programs, and obtain output at your site.

I. One-way frequency tables

We begin by presenting the program used to produce Table 1.4 of the text. Data are from Example 1.1.1.

Each SAS program in this text consists of three parts: the data step, the data input step, and the data analysis step. The purpose of the data step is to name the data set, name the variables, set printing options, and create new variables if necessary. The first line of code that we shall use is

OPTIONS LS = 80   PS = 60   NODATE;

The words OPTIONS is a SAS keyword. It must be spelled correctly. This line indicates that output should be printed 80 characters to a line and 60 lines to a page. This sets the printing format to print on typewriter or notebook-size paper rather than oversized computer paper. The option NODATE suppresses the printing of the day's data on the output. Notice that this SAS command ends in a semicolon. *SAS commands can begin in any column and always end with a semicolon.* The next line is

DATA HOME;

In this line we are naming the data set HOME because the data is from a home for adults. Data set names can be at most eight letters and should reflect the context of the study. The word DATA is a SAS keyword. We next name the variables via an INPUT statement. Variable names like data set names can be at most eight letters and should reflect the variables under study. In this case we write

INPUT   SEX $ DIAGNOSE $ AGE   DEST;

This line tells SAS that each line of data will contain the value of each of four variables. These are the sex of the patient, the diagnosis, the patient's age, and the destination after leaving the home. The $ after SEX and DIAGNOSE indicates that the values of these variables will be letters rather than numbers. The next line of the program is

LINES;

This line of code tells SAS that the data follows immediately and ends the data step for this program.

The data input step now begins. In this step we enter the data as shown in Example 1.1.1. The data lines look like

```
M    MI    29   2  ⎫
M    MR    35   7  ⎬  first 3 lines of data
F    PI    34   7  ⎭
⋮

F    MR    18   7  }  last line of data
```

Note that the dots indicate that we have not shown all of the data here even though all of it would be entered into the computer. Notice that there are no semicolons at the end of data lines. To signal the end of the data lines, a line with only a semicolon is used. This line is

;

This completes the data input step.

SAS uses a series of procedures, or PROCS, to analyze the data. Throughout this text a number of commonly used procedures will be introduced. The procedure that was used to produce Table 1.4 was PROC FREQ. The SAS keyword PROC stands for the word *procedure;* the procedure desired is one that produces frequency counts, cumulative frequency counts, and percentages. Its name naturally is PROC FREQ. To tell SAS what is wanted, we write

PROC   FREQ;   TABLES   DIAGNOSE;

The word TABLES is a SAS keyword. We are asking for a table of frequencies for the variable DIAGNOSE, which is one of the four variables in our data set. This completes the data analysis step for our first program.

Titles can be added after a PROC step if desired. In this case, let us entitle our table

Frequencies and Percentages:
Variable Diagnosis

To accomplish this we write

```
TITLE    'Frequencies and Percentages:';
TITLE2   'Variable Diagnosis';
```

Notice that the first TITLE statement produces the first line of the title; it does not have to be numbered. The second line produces the second line of the title; it must be numbered. Also notice that titles are enclosed in single quotes and end with a semicolon. In this discussion and those to come we shall write SAS code in capital letters for ease of reading. However, *the code does not have to be entered into the computer in capital letters.*

Our first program looks like this.

```
OPTIONS   LS = 80   PS = 60   NODATE;
DATA HOME;
INPUT   SEX $   DIAGNOSE $   AGE   DEST;
LINES;
M   MI   29   2
M   MR   35   7
F   PI   34   7
⋮
F   MR   18   7
;
PROC FREQ; TABLES DIAGNOSE;
TITLE   'Frequencies and Percentages:';
TITLE2 'Variable Diagnosis';
```

This program can be adjusted to handle other data by changing the name of the data set, the variable names, and the title.

II. Horizontal bar graph: discrete data

We now present the code required to produce a horizontal bar graph. The data used are that of Example 1.1.1. The code below produced the graph shown in Figure 1.3. We shall give the SAS code and a brief explanation of the code. In the following there is a space between the command lines. This is done to leave room for the explanation of the code. When you type the program into the computer file do not leave blank lines in the program.

SAS Code	Purpose
OPTIONS LS = 80 PS = 60 NODATE;	Sets printing specifications
DATA HOME;	Names the data set
INPUT SEX $ DIAGNOSE $ AGE DEST;	Names the variables
LINES;	Signals that the data follows immediately
M MI 29 2	
M MR 35 7	Data lines
F PI 34 7	
⋮	

SAS Code	Purpose
F MR 18 7	
;	Signals the end of the data
PROC CHART;	Calls for the procedure used to create bar graphs
HBAR DIAGNOSE/DISCRETE;	Asks for a horizontal bar graph for the variable DIAGNOSE; lets SAS know that the variable DIAGNOSE is discrete
TITLE 'A Horizontal Bar Graph:';	Titles the first line
TITLE2 'Variable Diagnosis';	Titles the second line

Note that vertical bar graphs can be formed. To do so, change the code HBAR to VBAR.

III. Two-way tables

Two-way tables can be formed via PROC FREQ. We present here the code used to create Table 1.8. It is based on the raw data given in Example 1.1.1.

SAS Code	Purpose
OPTIONS LS = 80 PS = 60 NODATE;	Sets printing specifications
DATA HOME;	Names the data set
INPUT SEX $ DIAGNOSE $ AGE DEST;	Names the variables
LINES;	Signals that the data follows immediately
M MI 29 2	
M MR 35 7	Data line
F PI 34 7	
:	
F MR 18 7	
;	Signals the end of the data
PROC FREQ;	Calls for the frequency procedure
TABLES SEX*DIAGNOSE;	Asks for a two-way table to be formed; the row variable, SEX, is named first, followed by the column variable, DIAGNOSE
TITLE 'Two-Way Table Used to Investigate';	Titles the first line
TITLE2 'The Relationship Between Sex and Diagnosis';	Titles the second line

IV. Histograms: vertical and horizontal

We illustrate the SAS procedure for drawing a vertical histogram using the data of Example 1.3.1. The following code was used to create the histograms given in Figures 1.10 and 1.12.

SAS Code	Purpose
OPTIONS LS = 80 PS = 60 NODATE;	Sets printing specifications
DATA GERBILS;	Names data set
INPUT GROUP $ @; DO I = 1 to 30;	Inputs data; allows the data
INPUT CALLS @ @; OUTPUT;	to be input by only entering
	the group identifier once
LINES;	Signals that the data
	follows immediately
e 135 137 148 152 . . . 155	Enters data for the experimental
	group
c 123 109 118 116 . . . 90	Enters data for the control group
;	Signals the end of the data
DATA EXP; SET GERBILS;	Forms a new data set that
IF GROUP = 'e';	contains only the data for
	the experimental animals
PROC CHART; VBAR CALLS/	Asks for a vertical
MIDPOINTS = 132.5 138.5 144.5	histogram for the variable
150.5 156.5;	CALLS; specifies that SAS
	uses the same midpoints as
	those in the text;
	reproduces Figure 1.10
TITLE 'FREQUENCY HISTOGRAM:	Titles output
EXPERIMENTAL';	
PROC CHART; HBAR CALLS/	Asks for a horizontal
MIDPOINTS = 132.5 138.5 144.5	histogram for the variable
150.5 156.6;	CALLS; specifies
	midpoints; reproduces
	Figure 1.12
TITLE 'SUMMARY TABLE AND	Titles first line of output
HORIZONTAL HISTOGRAM'	
TITLL2 'EXPERIMENTAL';	Titles second line of output

V. Summary statistics/stem-and-leaf/box plots

The data of Example 1.6.1 are used to illustrate the procedure PROC UNIVARIATE. This procedure will compute all of the statistics discussed in this chapter and will also construct a stem-and-leaf diagram and a box plot for the data.

SAS Code	Purpose
OPTIONS LS = 80 PS = 60 NODATE;	Sets printing specifications
DATA AMNESIA;	Names data set
INPUT DAYS @ @;	Names variables; @ @
	allows us to put more than
	one data point per line;
	there must be at least one
	space between each data value

LINES;					Signals that the data follows immediately
					Data lines
8	12	20	27	30	
32	35	36	40	40	
40	40	41	42	45	
47	50	52	61	89	
108					
;					Signals the end of the data
PROC UNIVARIATE PLOT;					Calls for basic statistics to be evaluated and plots to be drawn

TITLE 'BASIC STATS AND PLOTS';
TITLE2 'VIA PROC UNIVARIATE';

These statistics are given on the printout (the circled numbers correspond to numbers on the printout):

①   Sample size   ⑦ q_1
② $\bar{x}$ ⑧   range
③ s ⑨   iqr
④ s^2 ⑩   stem-and-leaf
⑤ $\tilde{x}$ ⑪   box plot
⑥ q_3

```
                        BASIC STATS AND PLOTS
                        VIA PROC UNIVARIATE

                        Univariate Procedure

Variable=DAYS


                              Moments

①  N                      21    Sum Wgts            21
②  Mean             42.61905    Sum                895
③  Std Dev           22.613    Variance       511.3476  ④
   Skewness         1.420384    Kurtosis       3.131485
   USS                 48371    CSS            10226.95
   CV               53.05843    Std Mean        4.93456
   T:Mean=0         8.636848    Pr>|T|           0.0001
   Num ^= 0             21    Num > 0             21
   M(Sign)             10.5    Pr>=|M|          0.0001
   Sgn Rank           115.5    Pr>=|S|          0.0001
```

Quantiles(Def=5)

100%	Max	108	99%	108
⑥ 75%	Q3	47	95%	89
⑤ 50%	Med	40	90%	61
⑦ 25%	Q1	32	10%	20
0%	Min	8	5%	12
			1%	8

⑧	Range	100
⑨	Q3-Q1	15
	Mode	40

Extremes

Lowest	Obs	Highest	Obs
8(	1)	50(	17)
12(	2)	52(	18)
20(	3)	61(	19)
27(	4)	89(	20)
30(	5)	108(	21)

Stem	Leaf	#	Boxplot
10	8	1	*
8	9	1	0
⑩ 6	1	1	│ ⑪
4	0000125702	10	+--+--+
2	070256	6	+-----+
0	82	2	0

```
    ----+----+----+----+
```
Multiply Stem.Leaf by 10**+1

2

Introduction to Probability and Counting

In Chapter 1 we introduced many of the methods used to describe a data set. If the aim of the experimenter is just that, to describe the results of one particular experiment, then the methods of Chapter 1 might be sufficient. However, if the purpose of the experiment is to use the information obtained to draw broad conclusions concerning all objects of the type studied, then the methods of Chapter 1 constitute only the beginning of the analysis. To draw valid conclusions and make accurate predictions concerning a population based on observing only a portion of that population, inferential statistical methods must be employed. These methods entail the intelligent use of probability theory.

Probability theory is an interesting branch of mathematics and is the foundation upon which statistical inference is based. In Sections 2.2 to 2.6 counting techniques and their use in calculating classical probabilities are discussed. Chapter 3 presents the basic definitions, axioms, and theorems that govern the behavior of probabilities. If time permits, these sections should be covered. However, Sections 2.1 and 2.2 provide a sufficient background for understanding the use of probability in data analysis. Hence, after you read these sections it is possible to skip to Chapter 4 without loss of continuity.

2.1
INTERPRETING PROBABILITIES

When asked the question, Do you know anything about probability? most people are quick to answer "no!" But usually that is not the case at all. The ability to correctly interpret probabilities, at least on the intuitive level, is assumed in our culture. One hears the phrases "the probability of rain today is 95%" or "there is a 10% chance of rain today." It is assumed that the general public knows how to interpret these values.

Briefly, the interpretation of probabilities can be summarized as follows:

1. Probabilities are numbers between 0 and 1, inclusive, that reflect the chances of a particular physical event occurring.
2. Probabilities near 1 indicate that the event involved is expected to occur. They do not mean that the event will occur, only that the event is considered to be a common occurrence.
3. Probabilities near 0 indicate that the event is not expected to occur. They do not mean that the event will fail to occur, only that the event is considered to be rare.
4. Probabilities near $\frac{1}{2}$ indicate that the event is just as likely to occur as not.

The interval [0, 1] can be thought of as a scale that is used to assess the likelihood of the occurrence of an event. The closer the probability is to 1, the more confidence we have that the event will occur. An event that is certain to occur is assigned a probability of 1. The closer a probability is to 0, the more sure we are that the event will not occur. An event that is physically impossible is assigned a probability of 0.

What constitutes a large or small probability? Certainly a probability of 1 is large and a probability of 0 is small. How close must a probability lie to these extremes to be considered large or small? There is no clear-cut answer to this question. The interpretation of probabilities is somewhat subjective, and the interpretation given can depend on the consequences of being wrong. A probability that is deemed large in one setting might seem small in another. For example, suppose that I have an opportunity to go on an outdoor field trip and I hear that the probability of rain is .1. I would consider this probability to be small and conclude that it most likely will not rain. If I am wrong, I will be inconvenienced only. However, suppose that I am told that I have been selected to be the first civilian to descend to the ocean floor in a new minisubmarine and that the probability is .1 that the vehicle will fail. I would decline this offer! The consequences of failure are too serious to accept. In the first case a probability of .1 is considered to be small; in the second case, it appears to be large.

The preceding comments offer guidelines for interpreting probabilities once these numbers are available, but they do not indicate how to actually go about assigning probabilities to events. Three methods are commonly used: the *personal* approach, the *relative frequency* approach, and the *classical* approach. Each method has its uses, advantages, and disadvantages.

EXAMPLE 2.1.1. A patient is suffering from kidney stones, and his condition has not been improved by ordinary means. His physician is contemplating an operation and must answer the question, What is the probability that the operation will be a success? Many factors come into play, among them the patient's age, general health, and attitude toward the operation. These factors make this patient unique. The physician has not faced this *exact* problem before and will not face it again. It is a "one-shot" situation, and its solution calls for a value judgment to be made. Any probability assigned to the event "the operation is a success" is a *personal opinion.*

This example illustrates both the advantages and disadvantages of the personal approach. Its main advantage is that it is always applicable. Anyone can have a personal opinion about anything. Its main disadvantage is obvious: its accuracy depends on the accuracy of the information available and the ability of the scientist to correctly assess that information.

EXAMPLE 2.1.2. A researcher is developing a new drug to be used in desensitizing patients to bee stings. Of 200 subjects tested, 180 showed a lessening in the severity of symptoms upon being stung after the treatment was administered. It is natural to assume, then, that the probability of this occurring in another patient receiving treatment is at least *approximately*

$$\frac{180}{200} = .90$$

On the basis of this study, the drug is reported to be 90% effective in lessening the reaction of sensitive patients to stings. This probability is *not* simply a personal opinion. It is a figure based on repeated experimentation and actual observation. It is in fact a *relative frequency*.

Example 2.1.2 illustrates the characteristics of the relative frequency approach to probability. It arises in any situation in which the experiment can be repeated many times and the results observed. Then the approximate probability of the occurrence of event *A*, denoted P[*A*], is given by

$$P[A] \doteq \frac{f}{n} = \frac{\text{number of times event } A \text{ occurred}}{\text{number of times experiment was run}}$$

where the symbol $\doteq$ means "approximately equal to." The disadvantage in this approach is that the experiment cannot be a one-shot situation; it must be repeatable. The advantage in this approach over the personal approach is that usually it is more accurate, because it is based on actual observation rather than personal opinion. Keep in mind the fact that any probability obtained by using the relative frequency approach is an approximation or an estimate. It is a value based on *n* trials. Further testing might result in a different approximate value. However, as the number of trials increases, the changes in the approximate values obtained tend to become slight. Thus for a large number of trials, the approximate probability obtained by using the relative frequency approach is usually quite accurate.

We dealt with relative frequency probabilities in Section 1.3. The relative frequency distribution and the relative cumulative frequency distribution found there can be viewed as giving relative frequency probabilities. For example, Table 1.19 shows that the onset of the reaction to an insect sting occurred between 8.2 and 10.3 minutes in 10 of the 40 patients studied. We can use this information to say that the probability is approximately $\frac{10}{40}$ that a future patient will experience a reaction in this time period. That is, we expect roughly 1 of every 4 patients to experience a reaction in the interval from 8.2 to 10.3 minutes. Notice that the relative cumulative frequency for category 5 is $\frac{38}{40}$. From this we can say that the approximate probability that a reaction will take at most 14.7 minutes to appear is $\frac{38}{40}$. The relative frequency and relative cumulative frequency distributions can be used to approximate the future behavior of a random variable. We cannot say for certain what values will be assumed in some future trial of the experiment, but we can anticipate which values are likely to arise and which are considered to be rare.

EXAMPLE 2.1.3. What is the probability that a child born to a couple, each with genes for both brown and blue eyes, will be brown-eyed? To answer this question, we note that since the child receives one gene from each parent, the possibilities for the child are (brown, blue), (blue, brown), (blue, blue), and (brown, brown), where the first member of each pair represents the gene received from the father. Since each parent is just as likely to contribute a gene for brown eyes as for blue eyes, all four possibilities are equally likely. Since an individual with a gene for brown eyes will have brown eyes, three of the four possibilities lead to a brown-eyed child. Hence, the probability that the child is brown-eyed is $\frac{3}{4} = .75$.

The above probability is not a personal opinion, nor is it based on repeated experimentation. In fact, we found this probability by the *classical method*. This method is appropriate whenever the possible outcomes of the experiment are *equally likely*. In this case, the probability of the occurrence of even A is given by

$$P[A] = \frac{n(A)}{n(S)} = \frac{\text{number of ways } A \text{ can occur}}{\text{number of ways the experiment can proceed}}$$

This method, too, has advantages and disadvantages. Its main drawback is that it is not always applicable; it does require that the possible outcomes be equally likely. Its main advantage is that, when applicable, the probability obtained is exact. Furthermore, it requires neither experimentation nor data gathering and so is easy to use.

All three methods come into play at times and are used frequently in upcoming discussions.

EXERCISES 2.1

In each of Exercises 1 to 10 a probability is sought. What method—personal, relative frequency, or classical—do you think is most appropriate in solving the problem? Be ready to defend your choice. Where possible, find the exact or approximate probability called for.

1. A woman contracts German measles while pregnant. What is the probability that her child will be born with a birth defect?
2. A drug is being tested for use in the treatment of poison ivy. Of 190 people tested, 150 gained some relief from the drug. What is the probability that the drug will be effective on the next patient who uses it?
3. A behavioral zoologist studies a large colony of baboons in the wild. She notes that of the 150 animals in the colony, 5 have unusually light-colored fur. What is the probability that the next baboon infant born will be light-colored?
4. A biochemist plans to isolate and purify a newly discovered enzyme from spinach leaves. He consults the literature for guidance in designing a purification procedure, but since this particular enzyme has never been isolated before, no specific guidelines are available. What is the probability that his newly designed purification procedure will be successful?

5. A husband is left-handed, and his wife is right-handed. Two children are born to the couple. Each child is just as likely to be left-handed as right-handed. What is the probability that both children will be left-handed?

6. A laboratory makes an error in cross-matching blood only about once in every 2000 cross-matches. What is the probability that a reported cross-match will be in error?

7. A chemist knows from experience that about 8 out of every 100 samples she receives to test for phosphate have too little phosphate to detect with routine analysis. What is the probability that she will have to use an alternative, more sensitive procedure on the next sample she is asked to assay?

8. An excess number of asbestos bodies were found in 98 of 140 construction workers studied. What is the probability that a randomly selected construction worker will have an undue number of asbestos bodies in the lungs?

9. A blood bank has available five units of blood labeled A^+. One unit is mislabeled and is, in fact, type O. A unit is selected at random from the five for use in a transfusion. What is the probability that the mislabeled unit will be selected?

10. A blight that attacks pines is such that 50% of all trees affected die within 1 year. Three trees are affected. What is the probability that all three will die? What is the probability that at least one will die?

11. Based on the information found in Table 1.19 approximate each of these probabilities:

    (a) The probability that the onset of reaction will occur within 12.5 minutes.

    (b) The probability that no reaction will occur in the first 5.9 minutes.

    (c) The probability that a reaction will occur in the interval from 12.6 to 14.7 minutes.

12. Use the data of Exercise 7 of Section 1.3 to approximate the probability that the percentage of ash in a future peat moss sample is at most 1.8%.

13. It is known that the HIV virus can be contracted by nurses, emergency technicians, doctors, and others by accidental needle sticks. Suppose that the probability of this occurring for each stick is .05. Do you think that this represents a high or a low probability of occurrence? Explain.

14. One method of fighting a forest fire is to deliberately set a backfire. Suppose that in a particular instance it is estimated that the probability that this method will succeed is .05. Do you think that this represents a high or a low probability of occurrence? Explain.

2.2
TREE DIAGRAMS AND ELEMENTARY GENETICS

The problems in Section 2.1 are simple because the number of possibilities in each case is very small. When experiments become more complex, it is helpful to have a systematic method for listing possible outcomes. One method for doing so is the *tree diagram*. This technique works well when the experiment can be visualized as taking place in a small number of distinct steps or stages. Each step in the experiment is represented as a branching point on the tree. The tree is constructed by first determining how many stages are involved. At each stage the tree branches to represent the possibilities at that particular point. Once the tree is complete, sequences of events can be read by following what are called "paths" through the tree. The method is demonstrated in Example 2.2.1.

EXAMPLE 2.2.1. A woman is a carrier for classic hemophilia. This means that although the woman does not have hemophilia, she can pass the disease on to her son. She gives birth to three sons. What are the possibilities for this experiment?

Since we are primarily concerned with whether each son has the disease, we need to generate a tree that gives that information. In this case, we have three natural stages, one to represent the birth of each son. The first son born either does (yes) or does not (no) have the disease. This is indicated in the tree diagram of Figure 2.1a, where yes = y and no = n. Likewise, the second son either does or does not have the disease. This fact is shown in Figure 2.1b. Finally, the third son either does or does not have the disease. Therefore the tree is completed as illustrated in Figure 2.1c. A path through the tree is found by starting at the far left side of the tree and tracing your way to the far right without backing up or picking up your pencil. Thus, the first path through the tree is *yyy*, which corresponds to the fact that all three sons have classical hemophilia.

The set of possibilities for the experiment can be read from the tree by following each of the eight distinct paths through the tree. This set is

$$\{yyy, yyn, yny, ynn, nyy, nyn, nny, nnn,\}$$

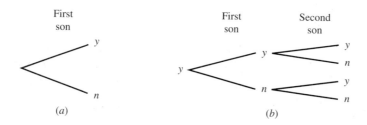

(a)

(b)

(c)

FIGURE 2.1

Constructing a tree diagram.

When the physical context of the problem guarantees that each path through the tree is just as likely to occur as any other, then the tree can be used to calculate probabilities using the classical approach. For instance, in Example 2.2.1 it is known that a carrier of classic hemophilia is just as likely to pass the disease to a son as she is to fail to do so. For this reason, we are just as likely to branch one way as the other at each stage in the diagram of Figure 2.1. This implies that each of the eight paths through the tree is equally likely. This fact can be used to calculate the probability of various events associated with the experiment. Example 2.2.2 demonstrates how this is done.

> **EXAMPLE 2.2.2.** What is the probability that a woman with three sons who is a carrier of classic hemophilia will not pass on her disease to any of her sons? We know that there are eight paths through the tree of Figure 2.1. Hence this experiment has eight equally likely outcomes. From the tree, we can see that one path, *nnn*, represents the event in question. Hence
>
> $$P[\text{none of the three has the disease}] = \tfrac{1}{8}$$

In a similar way, we can say that the probability that exactly two of the three sons have hemophilia is $\tfrac{3}{8}$. The three paths corresponding to the occurrence of this event are *yyn*, *yny*, *nyy*.

In Chapter 4 we will consider how to calculate probabilities using trees in which the paths are not equally likely.

Elementary Genetics (Optional)

The hereditary characteristics of an organism are determined by units called *genes*. Genes occur in pairs in an individual and come in contrasting forms. These forms are called *alleles*. For example, consider the gene that determines the height of a pea plant. This gene has two alleles, *T* for tallness and *t* for dwarfism. Thus there are three possible genetic compositions, or *genotypes*, with respect to this trait. They are *TT*, *Tt*, and *tt*. When the two genes are of the same form, we say that the organism is *homozygous* for the given trait; otherwise, it is *heterozygous*. A trait that will appear when the allele for the trait is present is called a *dominant* trait, and the allele is the dominant allele. Its contrasting trait or allele is said to be *recessive*. In the case of pea plants, the allele for tallness is dominant. Thus the genotypes *TT* and *Tt* will result in a tall plant, while the genotype *tt* will result in a dwarfed plant. Notationally, dominant alleles are denoted by capital letters, and recessive alleles are written as lowercase letters. For each trait the offspring inherits one gene randomly from each parent.

Tree diagrams can be used to solve simple problems in genetics. To illustrate, we reconsider Example 2.1.3.

> **EXAMPLE 2.2.3.** Each member of a couple has alleles for both brown and blue eyes. In genetic terms they are heterozygous for eye color. In the case of eye color, the allele for brown eyes, which we denote by *B*, is dominant over that for blue eyes, *b*. That is, anyone with the *B* allele will have brown eyes. At conception, each parent contributes one allele for eye color. Hence we can view the experiment of determining the eye color of a child as a two-stage process. Stage 1 represents the inheritance of an allele from the mother; stage 2

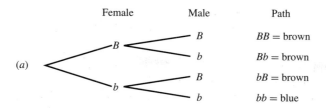

Female   Male   Path

BB = brown
Bb = brown
bB = brown
bb = blue

Female gametes

		B	b
Male gametes	B	BB (brown)	bB (brown)
	b	Bb (brown)	bb (blue)

FIGURE 2.2

(*a*) Tree diagram for the inheritance of eye color from a couple, each of whom is heterozygous for eye color. (*b*) A biologist's representation of the problem as a Punnett square.

represents the inheritance from the father. The tree for the two-stage process is shown in Figure 2.2*a*. Notice that since alleles are inherited at random, at each step we are just as likely to inherit a *B* as we are a *b* allele. Each of the four paths through the tree is equally likely. Since three of the four paths result in a brown-eyed child, we can use classical probability to conclude that

$$P[\text{brown-eyed child}] = \tfrac{3}{4}$$

You might have seen this problem solved in a biology text using what is called a Punnett square or a checkerboard. The checkerboard for the problem is shown in Figure 2.2*b*. Notice that it gives the same information as the tree.

In the previous example one allele, that for brown eyes, is dominant over the other. Hence, the presence of the *B* allele produces a brown-eyed individual. Sometimes two alleles exist but neither is dominant over the other. Our next example illustrates a situation of this sort.

EXAMPLE 2.2.4. The plant known as the four-o'clock can have red, white, or pink flowers. The allele for redness is denoted by *R* and that for white by *r*. A red flower has two *R* alleles and is said to be homozygous for color; a white flower is homozygous with genotype *rr*. When pure white plants are bred to pure red ones, the resulting flower has genotype *Rr*. Since there is no dominant allele, the resulting flower is pink. When two of these heterozygous plants are bred, the outcomes given in the tree of Figure 2.3 result. Each of the four paths through the tree is equally likely. By using classical probability we can conclude that the probability of obtaining a white flower from the cross-match is $\tfrac{1}{4}$.

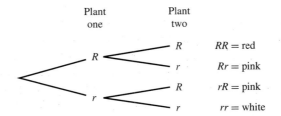

■ **FIGURE 2.3**

Outcomes that result when two heterozygous four-o'clock
flowers are cross-matched.

Trees can be used in a genetic setting to study more than one trait simultaneously.
To do so, we simply extend the idea developed in the previous two examples.

EXAMPLE 2.2.5. In humans, the allele for normal skin pigmentation S is dominant over
that for albinism s. The allele for free earlobes F is dominant over that for attached lobes f.
A woman has genotype $SsFF$, and her husband has genotype $ssFf$. Hence the woman has
normal skin pigmentation and free earlobes; her husband is albino with free earlobes. What
are the possible outcomes for their offspring? We visualize this as a four-stage experiment
with the following stages:

1. Inherit an allele for skin pigmentation from the mother
2. Inherit an allele for skin pigmentation from the father
3. Inherit an allele for ear formation from the mother
4. Inherit an allele for ear formation from the father

The resulting tree is given in Figure 2.4. From the tree, we see that there are four equally
likely outcomes. The tree can be used to see that the probability that the child is albino is $\frac{1}{2}$;
the probability of having free earlobes is 1; and the probability of having normal skin and
free earlobes is $\frac{1}{2}$.

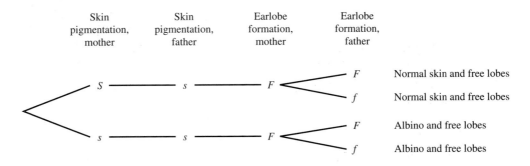

■ **FIGURE 2.4**

A four-stage tree used to study two traits simultaneously.

Notice that classical probability can be used to solve these problems because of the fact that at each step in the game an offspring is just as likely to inherit one gene as the other from each parent. This guarantees that the paths through the tree are equally likely. We consider trees for which this is not true in Chapter 3.

EXERCISES 2.2

1. A family has four children. Identifying each child by sex only, use a tree to find the 16 possible birth orders of the children. Assume that each child is just as likely to be a boy as a girl. Find the probability of each of these events.

   A: The first child is a boy

   B: Exactly two of the four are boys

   C: The oldest and youngest are boys

   D: Two are girls and three are boys

2. A bioactive tetrapeptide (a compound consisting of four amino acids linked into a chain) has the following amino acid composition: alanine (A), glutamic acid (G), lysine (L), and histidine (H). For example, ALGH and LGHA are typical four acid chains.

   (a) Draw a tree to represent the 24 possible ways in which these four amino acids can link to form a four-acid chain.

   (b) If each chain is equally likely, find the probability of event A: glutamic acid is found at one or the other end of the chain.

   (c) Find the probability of event B: lysine is not found at either end of the chain.

3. An experiment is being planned to study the effect of three types of fertilizer on the growth of wheat. A plot of ground is prepared and divided into three strips of equal size. One fertilizer is to be applied to each strip. Denote the fertilizers by A, B, and C.

   (a) Draw a tree to represent the six ways in which fertilizers can be assigned to strips.

   (b) If the assignment is done randomly so that each path of the tree is equally likely, what is the probability that the first strip will receive fertilizer A?

4. Mountain lions living on public grazing lands can pose a threat to cattle and sheep. It is of interest to estimate the number of these lions living in a particular area. Ten are caught, tagged, and released. Later, four mountain lions are captured and each is classified as being either tagged (t) or untagged (u). Thus a typical outcome of the experiment is *tuut* in which the first and last animals are tagged while the second and third are not.

   (a) Draw a tree to represent the 16 possible outcomes of this experiment.

   (b) List the paths that correspond to the occurrence of event A: the first and last animals caught are tagged.

   (c) List the paths that correspond to event B: exactly three animals are tagged.

   (d) List the paths that correspond to the simultaneous occurrence of events A and B.

   (e) If there are, in fact, 100 mountain lions living in the region, are the 16 paths through the tree equally likely? If not, which path is most likely to occur? Which is least likely to occur?

5. In examining a patient a physician notes the presence (p) or absence (a) of four symptoms: headache, fever, body rash, or muscle soreness.
   (a) Construct a tree to represent the sixteen combinations of symptoms that are possible.
   (b) For the diagnosis to be systemic food allergy, a body rash must be present. List the paths for which this diagnosis is feasible.
   (c) For the diagnosis to be flu, the patient must experience fever *and* muscle soreness. List the paths for which this diagnosis is feasible.
   (d) Do any paths allow for either flu or food allergy to be a possible diagnosis? If so, which?
   (e) List paths for which neither flu nor a food allergy is a possible diagnosis.

6. In a particular area of the Smoky Mountains many of the evergreens have been attacked by the pine beetle. Four evergreens are randomly selected for study. Assume that each has a 50% chance of being infected.
   (a) Draw a tree diagram to represent the sixteen ways that this experiment can proceed. (Let y denote the fact that a given evergreen is infected; let n denote that it is not infected.)
   (b) Use the tree to find the probability that no evergreens are infected; that at least one is infected.
   (c) Would it be unusual to find exactly three of the four evergreens to be infected? Explain.

7. One way to measure the progress of the treatment of an AIDS patient is to measure the T4 cell count. An AIDS patient is tested three times. Each time the cell count is denoted as n (normal) or l (low).
   (a) Draw a tree to represent the eight ways in which this series of three tests can occur.
   (b) Under what conditions would the eight paths through the tree be equally likely? From what you know about AIDS, do you think that this condition is likely to be met?

8. Sickle-cell anemia is a fatal condition in which the red blood cells tend to assume a sickle shape in the blood vessels. This results in the clogging of the capillaries, which eventually leads to death. Let us represent the allele responsible for the formation of normal red blood cells by S and that which leads to the formation of sickle cells by s. An individual will have sickle-cell anemia if and only if his or her genotype is ss. In each case below construct a tree to represent the possible outcome(s) for a child born to the parents described. Use the tree to find the probability that the child will have sickle-cell anemia.
   (a) The mother is Ss and the father is Ss.
   (b) The mother is SS and the father is Ss.

9. Consider the experiment of Example 2.2.5. Suppose that the parents are each genotype $SsFf$.
   (a) Draw the tree to represent the possible outcomes for the offspring.
   (b) Use the tree to find the probability that
       i. The child will be albino with attached earlobes
       ii. The child will have normal skin and free earlobes
       iii. The child will be albino
       iv. The child will have free earlobes

10. In guinea pigs, short hair (L) is dominant to long hair (l) and black fur (B) is dominant to albino fur (b). A female which is black with short hair is mated to a male that is albino with long hair.
    (a) What are the possible genotypes for the female? What are the possible genotypes for the male?
    (b) For each possible genotype for the female, construct a tree to represent the possible outcomes for the offspring.
    (c) Find the probability of obtaining an albino with short hair in each case.

11. In the pea plant, tallness (T) is dominant to shortness (t). Yellow seeds (Y) are dominant to green (y), and the round shape (W) is dominant to wrinkled (w). Suppose that two plants are cross-matched. One has genotype $TTYYWw$ and the other $TtYyWw$.
    (a) Describe each of the parent plants relative to the three characteristics mentioned.
    (b) Draw a tree to represent the possible ways in which the cross-match can occur. (*Hint:* Extend the idea of Example 2.2.5 to a six-stage process.)
    (c) Describe the plant associated with each path through the tree.
    (d) Use the tree to find the probability that the cross-match will result in a tall pea plant.
    (e) What is the probability that the cross-match will result in a tall, yellow, wrinkled pea plant?
    (f) What is the probability that the cross-match will produce a green pea plant?

12. Peach trees have fuzzy fruits and nectarines are smooth. The allele for fuzziness is dominant. Each type of fruit can be either yellow or white with yellow dominant. A white peach tree is crossed with a yellow nectarine tree.
    (a) What are the possible genotypes for the peach tree?
    (b) What are the possible genotypes for the nectarine tree?
    (c) There are four possible ways to match the genotypes for the two trees. Draw separate tree diagrams for each.
    (d) Use the trees of part c to find the probability of obtaining a white peach tree in each case.

13. Two body colors, gray (E) and ebony (e), are recognized in fruit flies with gray being dominant. Two wing types are also noted, normal (V) and short, or vestigial (v), with normal being dominant. Homozygous flies ($EEVV$ and $eevv$) are mated to form double-heterozygous offspring ($EeVv$). These are allowed to mate.
    (a) Draw a tree to demonstrate the possible outcomes for the offspring.
    (b) How many of the paths result in an ebony fruit fly?
    (c) How many of the paths result in a normal winged fruit fly?
    (d) If a fly is selected at random from among a large number of flies resulting from the above experiment, what is the probability that it will have normal wings? What is the probability that it will be ebony and have short wings? What is the probability that it will *not* be ebony with short wings?

14. Alleles determining albinism are denoted A and a, with A dominant and leading to a normal individual with respect to this trait. In order to be an albino, one must receive the recessive gene a from each parent. Individuals of the type Aa, although normal themselves, can pass on the trait to their offspring and are called *carriers*.

(*a*) A normal couple gives birth to an albino son. What is the genotype of each parent?

(*b*) What is the probability that the next child born to the couple also will be an albino? What is the probability that the child will be a carrier of albinism?

(*c*) A woman has a normal mother and an albino father. Her maternal grandmother is also albino. What is the probability that the woman is a carrier of albinism?

2.3
PERMUTATIONS AND COMBINATIONS (OPTIONAL)

As indicated in Section 2.1, there are various ways to determine the probability of a physical event. The classical approach, when applicable, has the advantage of being exact. Recall that to apply the classical method, you must be dealing with an experiment in which the possible physical outcomes are equally likely. In this case, the probability of the occurrence of a specific event A is given by

$$P[A] = \frac{n(A)}{n(S)}$$

Thus to compute a probability by using the classical approach, you must be able to count two things: $n(A)$, the number of ways in which event A can occur, and $n(S)$, the number of ways in which the experiment can proceed. When the experiment involved is rather simple, each can be found by listing or by use of a tree diagram. However, as the experiment becomes more complex, these methods are cumbersome and time-consuming. Alternative methods for counting must be developed. In the remainder of this chapter we introduce some counting techniques and demonstrate their use in calculating classical probabilities. These methods are applicable to many problems in the biological sciences and underlie much of the elementary theory of genetics.

Two widely encountered types of problems can be solved by using the classical approach, namely, those involving permutations and those involving combinations. Before we consider how to mathematically handle the two, it is necessary to distinguish one from the other.

DEFINITION 2.3.1. Permutation. A *permutation* is an arrangement of objects in a definite order.

DEFINITION 2.3.2. Combination. A *combination* is a selection of objects without regard to order.

It is evident from Definitions 2.3.1 and 2.3.2 that the characteristic that distinguishes a permutation from a combination is *order.* If the order in which some action is taken is important, then the problem is a permutation problem and can be solved by using the multiplication principle discussed in Section 2.4. If order is irrelevant, then it is a "combination" problem and it involves the use of the combination formula developed in Section 2.6.

EXAMPLE 2.3.1

(*a*) Write your social security number. Is this a permutation of numbers or a combination of numbers? It is obviously a permutation. The number 239-62-5558 is *not* the same as the number 329-62-5558. The order in which the digits are written is important.

(*b*) Twenty different amino acids are commonly found in peptides and proteins. A pentapeptide consisting of the five amino acids

alanine–valine–glycine–cysteine–tryptophan

has different properties and is, in fact, a different compound from the pentapeptide

alanine–glycine–valine–cysteine–tryptophan

which contains the same amino acids. Are peptides permutations or combinations of amino acid units? They are permutations because the sequence, or order, of the amino acids in the chain is important.

(*c*) A biologist has 10 plants with which to experiment. Only eight are needed in the experiment. The eight to be used are selected at random. Does this collection of plants represent a combination or a permutation of plants? It is a combination since interest centers only on which plants are selected and not on the order in which they were chosen.

Example 2.3.1 is intended only to convey an intuitive notion of the difference between permutations and combinations. Their significance in the analysis of scientific data is illustrated shortly.

EXERCISES 2.3

1. Write your name. Does this string of letters constitute a permutation of letters or a combination of letters?

2. Consider all families with exactly 5 children. If the gender of each child is considered, there are 32 possible birth orders. For example, MMMFF represents a situation in which the first three children born are male and the last two are female. Give an example of another birth order in which there are exactly three males and two females. Are the strings of five letters that represent birth orders permutations of letters or combinations of letters?

3. A scientist has six different cages of white rats in the animal room and wants to select three of the six to use in an experiment. Is the set of animals chosen a permutation of animals or a combination of animals?

4. Eight patients, each allergic to insect stings, are to be desensitized. Four are to be selected at random and treated with a compound consisting of insect venom. For comparative purposes, the other four are to be treated with a compound made from insect bodies. Is the set of four patients chosen to receive the insect venom a permutation of patients or a combination of patients?

5. In running a glucose tolerance test, the blood sugar level of a patient is observed and recorded every half hour for $2\frac{1}{2}$ hours. Each reading is recorded as being normal (*n*), high (*h*), or low (*l*). Consider the string *nhhnl*. Explain the way in which the test proceeded for this patient. Give an example of another possible string that consists of two normal, two high, and one low reading. Are these strings of letters permutations or combinations of letters?

6. A chemist has 10 water samples taken from the wastewater of a paper factory. Three are randomly selected and tested for acidity. Does the set of three water samples chosen for testing represent a permutation of samples or a combination of samples?

7. Two of the paths of the tree found in Exercise 4 of Section 2.2 are *tutu* and *tuut*. Each of these is a permutation consisting of *two t*'s and two *u*'s. Explain the difference between the two in the context of the experiment described in Exercise 4.

8. In opening a locker, we dial a "combination" lock. Is the sequence of numbers or letters dialed a combination in the mathematical sense?

9. A forester selects four pink and four white dogwoods from among the trees available at a wholesale supplier. At this point do the trees constitute a combination of pink and white trees or a permutation of trees? The trees are to be planted in a row along the entrance road to a national park campground. Give an example of two ways to plant the trees in such a way that the first and last tree in the row are pink. Keeping color in mind, does the row of trees now form a permutation of colors or a combination of colors?

10. A forester wants to estimate the number of species of trees in a large stand of timber. A map of the area is obtained and 10- by 10-meter squares are marked and numbered. Fifteen of these squares are chosen randomly, and the number of species per square is determined by inspection. Do the 15 squares represent a combination of squares or a permutation of squares?

2.4

MULTIPLICATION PRINCIPLE (OPTIONAL)

Once a problem has been identified as being one in which order is important, the next question to be answered is, How many permutations or arrangements of the given objects are possible? This question usually can be answered by means of the *multiplication principle.*

To apply the principle we first ask, How many stages or steps are there in the experiment as a whole? or How many decisions must I make in the course of the experiment? One slot is drawn to represent each stage or decision. For each stage we ask, In how many ways can this step in the experiment be done? These numbers are placed in the slots. The total number of ways to do the entire experiment is the product of the slot values.

This principle is easy to use, and most people apply it intuitively even if they have had little formal mathematical training. We illustrate its use in Example 2.4.1.

EXAMPLE 2.4.1. Biologists are interested in the order in which the four ribonucleotides adenine (A), uracil (U), guanine (G), and cytosine (C) combine to form small chains. These nucleotides provide the principal subunits of RNA, the intermediate information-carrying molecule involved in translating the DNA genetic code. How many chains, each consisting of two *different* nucleotides, can be formed? This question can be answered easily by means of the tree of Figure 2.5.

The answer is evidently 12. Note that we are considering the chain AC to be different from CA. That is, the order in which the nucleotides are arranged is important. Hence we have shown that there are 12 permutations of four distinct objects when used two at a time.

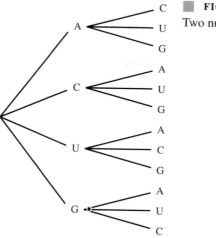

FIGURE 2.5
Two nucleotide chains.

This result could have been predicted without recourse to a tree by asking three simple questions.

1. How many stages or steps are involved in the experiment as a whole? Answer: two. Stage 1 corresponds to the first nucleotide falling into place; stage 2 corresponds to a second, *different* nucleotide linking with the first. Represent the fact that two stages are involved by drawing two slots.

$$\underline{\hspace{3cm}} \qquad \underline{\hspace{3cm}}$$
$$\text{1st} \qquad\qquad \text{2d}$$
$$\text{nucleotide} \qquad \text{nucleotide}$$

2. In how many ways can the first stage of the experiment be performed? Answer: four. There are four nucleotides available, any one of which could fall into the first position. Indicate this by placing a 4 in the first slot.

$$\underline{\quad 4 \quad} \qquad \underline{\hspace{3cm}}$$
$$\text{1st} \qquad\qquad \text{2d}$$
$$\text{nucleotide} \qquad \text{nucleotide}$$

3. After the first stage is complete, in how many ways can stage 2 be performed? Answer: three. Since each chain is to consist of two different nucleotides, repetition is not allowed. The nucleotide appearing first in the chain is no longer in contention. The second member of the chain must be one of the three remaining. Indicate this by placing a 3 in the second slot.

$$\underline{\quad 4 \quad} \qquad \underline{\quad 3 \quad}$$
$$\text{1st} \qquad\qquad \text{2d}$$
$$\text{nucleotide} \qquad \text{nucleotide}$$

The multiplication principle says that to determine the total number of possible permutations, you need only multiply these two numbers, once again obtaining an answer of 12. Note that the 4 in the first slot corresponds directly to the first-stage branching in the tree diagram and the 3 to the second-stage branching.

The multiplication principle can be used to solve problems that arise in everyday life. Example 2.4.2 demonstrates its use.

EXAMPLE 2.4.2

(a) How many computer passwords can be formed that consist of five different letters? This is a five-step process. There are 26 choices for the first letter of the password. Since letters cannot be used more than once, the number of choices drops by 1 in successive stages. Hence the total number of passwords is

$$26 \cdot 25 \cdot 24 \cdot 23 \cdot 22 = 7,893,600$$

(b) How many license tags can be formed that consist of three different letters followed by three different digits? This is a six-stage process. We first choose three different letters in succession from among the 26 letters of the alphabet.

$$\underset{\text{Letters}}{26 \cdot 25 \cdot 24} \quad \underset{\text{Digits}}{\underline{\quad} \ \underline{\quad} \ \underline{\quad}}$$

We next chose three different digits in succession from among the digits 0, 1, 2, 3, 4, 5, 6, 7, 8, 9. Altogether there are

$$\underset{\text{Letters}}{26 \cdot 25 \cdot 24} \quad \underset{\text{Digits}}{10 \cdot 9 \cdot 8} = 11,232,000$$

possible tags that meet the stated conditions.

(c) In how many ways can a five-question true-false test be answered? This is a five-step process. Since each question can be marked either true or false, there are two possibilities at each stage of the game. Thus there are

$$2 \cdot 2 \cdot 2 \cdot 2 \cdot 2 = 32$$

ways to answer the test.

(d) How many 10-digit telephone numbers can be formed if the area code of each is 703 and the local code cannot begin with 0 or 1? This is a 10-step process. Since the area code must be 703, we have only one choice for each of the first three stages. The first must be a 7, the second a 0, and the third a 3.

$$\underset{\text{Area code}}{1 \ 1 \ 1} \quad \underset{\text{Local code}}{\underline{\quad} \ \underline{\quad} \ \underline{\quad}} \quad \underset{\text{Number}}{\underline{\quad} \ \underline{\quad} \ \underline{\quad} \ \underline{\quad}}$$

Since the local code cannot begin with 0 or 1, the fourth steps has eight possibilities.

$$\underset{\text{Area code}}{1 \ 1 \ 1} \quad \underset{\text{Local code}}{8 \ \underline{\quad} \ \underline{\quad}} \quad \underset{\text{Number}}{\underline{\quad} \ \underline{\quad} \ \underline{\quad} \ \underline{\quad}}$$

There are no special restrictions on the other positions, and so there are 10 choices in each case. The total number of possibilities is

$$\underset{\text{Area code}}{1 \ 1 \ 1} \quad \underset{\text{Local code}}{8 \ 10 \ 10} \quad \underset{\text{Number}}{10 \ 10 \ 10 \ 10} = 8,000,000$$

There are several guidelines to consider when you apply the multiplication principle. These are following.

Guidelines for Using the Multiplication Principle

1. Watch out for repetition versus nonrepetition. Sometimes objects can be repeated (such as the digits in a telephone number); at other times they cannot (as specified in Examples 2.4.2a and 2.4.2b). Usually the physical context of the problem either allows or precludes repetition.
2. Watch for subtraction. Consider event A. Occasionally it will be difficult, if not impossible, to find $n(A)$ directly. However, we might be able to find the total $n(S)$ and the number of ways that A can fail to occur rather easily. Let us denote the latter by $n(A')$ [the prime (') is read "not"]. Since event A either will occur or else it will not, the total is the sum of the numbers $n(A)$ and $n(A')$. That is, $n(S) = n(A) + n(A')$. This implies that $n(A) = n(S) - n(A')$.
3. If there is a stage in the experiment with a special restriction, then you should worry about the restriction first (as in Example 2.4.2d).

These points are illustrated in Example 2.4.3.

> **EXAMPLE 2.4.3.** The DNA-RNA code is a molecular code in which the sequence of molecules provides significant genetic information. Each segment of RNA is composed of "words." Each word specifies a particular amino acid and is composed of a chain of three ribonucleotides that are not necessarily all different. For example, the word UUU corresponds to the amino acid phenylalanine, whereas AUG identifies methionine.
>
> (a) Consider the experiment of forming an RNA word. How many words can be formed? That is, what is $n(S)$? Each of the three ribonucleotides in the chain is one of the four mentioned in Example 2.4.1, namely, adenine (A), uracil (U), guanine (G), and cytosine (C). Notice that repetition is allowed. Thus this is a three-stage experiment with four possibilities at each stage. By the multiplication principle, $n(S) = 4 \cdot 4 \cdot 4 = 64$.
>
> (b) How many of the words of part a have at least two identical nucleotides? This question is easily answered by subtraction. Let R denote the event that the word contains repeated nucleotides. The event R' is the event that there is no repetition of nucleotides. Consider the diagram of Figure 2.6. We already know that $n(S) = 64$. By the multiplication principle, $n(R') = 4 \cdot 3 \cdot 2 = 24$. Hence, by subtraction, the number of words involving some repetition is
>
> $$n(R) = n(S) - n(R') = 64 - 24 = 40$$

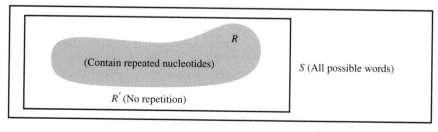

FIGURE 2.6

Since each word does (R) or does not (R') have repetition, $n(S) = n(R) + n(R')$. Hence $n(R) = n(S) - n(R')$.

(c) If a word is formed at random, what is the probability that it will contain some repetition of nucleotides? Using classical probability, we have

$$P[R] = \frac{n(R)}{n(S)} = \frac{40}{64} = .625$$

(d) Consider event B that a randomly formed word ends with U (uracil) and involves no repetition. Find $P[B]$. Since the last position in the word must be filled by uracil, there is only one choice for that position, as indicated:

$$\underline{\hspace{2em}} \quad \underline{\hspace{2em}} \quad \underline{\hspace{1em} 1 \hspace{1em}}$$

Once this restriction has been taken care of, we note that repetition is not allowed. So the first position can be filled with any of the three remaining nucleotides and the second position by either of two.

$$\underline{\hspace{1em} 3 \hspace{1em}} \quad \underline{\hspace{1em} 2 \hspace{1em}} \quad \underline{\hspace{1em} 1 \hspace{1em}}$$

Thus, $n(B) = 6$ and

$$P[B] = \frac{n(B)}{n(S)} = \frac{6}{64}$$

We have not given a formula for solving permutation problems because most problems involving order are complex enough that no single formula is appropriate. Rather, we have suggested that when order is important you should think "multiplication principle." In some cases, however, there is a permutation formula that can be used. This formula is discussed in Exercise 15.

■ EXERCISES 2.4

1. A satellite dish can receive signals from 20 different telecommunications satellites. Each satellite handles 15 stations. How many stations are available to the owner of this dish?
2. A physician has four patients waiting to be seen. One case is an emergency, but the patient does not make this fact known to the physician.
   (a) In how many orders can the patients be seen?
   (b) In how many of these orders will the emergency case be seen first?
   (c) If the order is selected at random, what is the probability that the emergency case will be seen first?
3. How many computer passwords can be formed that consist of five different letters if each word must begin with a vowel (A, E, I, O, U) and end with a consonant?
4. Four persons check in at an airline counter. The ticket agent assigns seats and then places each ticket at random in a ticket folder which has a traveler's name on it. In how many ways can this be done? Draw a tree to illustrate the problem. What is the probability that no one will receive his or her own ticket?
5. (a) How many RNA words can be formed that begin with U (uracil) and end with A (adenine) or G (guanine)? (Remember that four ribonucleotides may be

used—A, U, G, and C—and that a word consists of three of these, not necessarily all different.)

(b) How many of the words of part *a* have no repetition?

(c) What is the probability that a randomly formed word will begin with U, end with A or G, but involve repetition?

(d) Check your answers by constructing the tree diagrams corresponding to parts *a* and *b*.

6. Of the possible 64 RNA words, 61 are known to code for the 20 existing amino acids. The other three code "stops," which cause termination of the peptide. If a word is formed at random, what is the probability that it will code for an amino acid?

7. A word codes for threonine if and only if it begins AC. How many synonyms (words that have identical meanings) are there for threonine?

8. Consider the RNA segment UUUAUUUUA. This segment involves the three nonoverlapping words UUU (phenylalanine), AUU (isoleucine), and UUA (leucine). Note that if a mutation occurs and the string of nucleotides is changed to read UUAAUUUUA, then the segment no longer codes the same sequence of amino acids. There are two synonyms for phenylalanine, three for isoleucine, and six for leucine. In how many different but equivalent ways can the above three-amino-acid sequence be expressed?

9. Consider any segment of three nonoverlapping words. In how many ways could such a segment be expressed? How many of these segments have no repeated words? If a segment is selected at random, what is the probability that it will have some repetition of words? What is the probability that each word will be different and each code an amino acid? (See Exercise 6.)

10. In treating a patient for high blood pressure, a physician has a choice of five different drugs, two of which are experimental. She can also select any one of four exercise programs, of which two involve indoor activities and the other two outdoor activities. Three choices of diet are available, one of which is completely salt-free.

(a) How many treatments consisting of one drug, one exercise program, and one diet are possible?

(b) How many of the treatments in part *a* involve the use of an experimental drug?

(c) All treatments in part *a* are assumed to be equally desirable. If a treatment is selected at random, what is the probability that it will involve an experimental drug and an outdoor exercise program?

(d) If, in fact, a specific one of the experimental drugs is dangerous when used in conjunction with the salt-free diet, what is the probability that such a treatment will nevertheless be prescribed by chance?

11. Seven drugs are being tested for their effectiveness in controlling acne. A researcher is asked to rank the drugs from 1 to 7, with the most effective drug receiving a rank of 1.

(a) In how many ways can the seven ranks be assigned to the seven drugs?

(b) Drugs A and B are manufactured by the company running the test, although this is not known by the researcher. If, in fact, the researcher cannot distinguish among the products and actually randomly assigns ranks, what is the probability that these two drugs will receive the top two ranks?

(*c*) If the experiment is run and drugs A and B are ranked in the top two positions, do you think that the company has evidence that its products are more effective than the competitor's? Explain on the basis of your answer to part *b*.

12. A study is being designed to investigate the effect of polymer type, temperature, radiation dose, radiation dose rate, and pH on the ability to remove trace quantities of benzene from water. There are two polymer types (A and B), three temperatures (high, medium, low), three radiation doses, three radiation dose rates, and three pH levels (acidic, basic, neutral).

(*a*) How many experimental conditions are to be studied?

(*b*) If each experimental condition is to be replicated (repeated) 5 times, how many experimental runs must be made?

(*c*) How many runs are made with polymer A at low temperature?

(*d*) How many runs are made with polymer B at high or medium temperature and low pH?

13. The basic storage unit of a digital computer is a *bit.* A bit is a storage position that can be designated as either on (1) or off (0) at any given time. In converting picture images to a form that can be transmitted electronically, a picture element called a *pixel* is used. Each pixel is quantized into gray levels and coded using a binary code. For example, a pixel with four gray levels can be coded using 2 bits by designating the gray levels 00, 01, 10, 11.

(*a*) How many gray levels can be quantized using a 4-bit code?

(*b*) How many bits are necessary to code a pixel quantized to 32 gray levels?

14. An experiment is designed to investigate the effect of ground temperature on the rate of germination of a new variety of grass seed. Only one environmental room is available for conducting the experiment; hence, only one temperature can be considered at a time. Temperatures are coded as H = high, M = moderate, L = low. In how many orders can temperatures be run? Draw a tree to verify your answer and list the possible experimental conditions.

15. *Permutation of* n *distinct objects arranged* r *at a time:* $_nP_r$. Consider *n* distinct objects and assume that $r \leq n$ of these objects are to be used in an arrangement. No repetition is allowed and there are no restrictions on any position in the arrangement. The number of possible arrangements is denoted by $_nP_r$. To derive a formula for $_nP_r$, the multiplication principle is used. We begin by writing *r* slots as shown below:

$$\underline{\qquad} \quad \underline{\qquad} \quad \underline{\qquad} \quad \cdots \quad \underline{\qquad}$$

Slot 1   Slot 2   Slot 3   Slot *r*

(*a*) In how many ways can slot 1 be filled? Slot 2? Slot 3? Slot *r*?

(*b*) Via the multiplication principle, argue that

$$_nP_r = n(n-1)(n-2)\cdots(n-r+1)$$

(*c*) Let $n = 10$ and $r = 4$. Use these numbers to verify the formulas derived in part *b*.

(*d*) Find a formula for $_nP_n$.

(*e*) A pharmacist has 10 different brands of headache remedy. There is room on the top shelf for only three. In how many ways can the remedies be arranged on the top shelf?

◼ 2.5

PERMUTATIONS OF
INDISTINGUISHABLE OBJECTS (OPTIONAL)

Thus far we have been concerned with fairly simple problems that may or may not involve repetition. Now we consider situations in which repetition is inevitable. The question to be answered is, How many distinct arrangements of n objects are possible if some of the objects are identical and therefore cannot be distinguished one from the other? To answer this question, first we must consider a shorthand notation called *factorial notation*. This notation is used extensively throughout the remainder of this text.

DEFINITION 1.5.3. n factorial. Let n be a positive integer. The product $n(n-1)(n-2) \cdots 3 \cdot 2 \cdot 1$ is called n *factorial* and is denoted by $n!$.

EXAMPLE 2.5.1. $6! = 6 \cdot 5 \cdot 4 \cdot 3 \cdot 2 \cdot 1 = 720$.

DEFINITION 2.5.2. Zero factorial

$$0! = 1$$

Now we return to the problem at hand, that of determining the number of possible permutations when some of the objects being permuted are indistinguishable from others.

EXAMPLE 2.5.2. Consider the two nucleotides adenine (A) and uracil (U). How many words—chains of three ribonucleotides not necessarily all different—can be formed by using only these two symbols? Since a word involves three symbols and only two distinct symbols are to be used, repetition is inevitable. By the multiplication principle, there are $2 \cdot 2 \cdot 2 = 8$ possible words. This is not new. However, if we now ask, How many of the eight involve uracil twice and adenine once? the question is new. We are arranging a total of $n = 3$ objects, but two are identical (namely, two U's) and therefore are indistinguishable from each other. To answer the question, let us list the possibilities.

$$AUU \qquad UAU \qquad UUA$$

The answer is 3. How could this have been predicted without the use of a list? We note that

$$3 = \frac{3 \cdot 2 \cdot 1}{(2 \cdot 1)(1)} = \frac{3!}{2! \, 1!}$$

The 3 factorial in the numerator represents the fact that a total of three objects are being permuted. There are two factorials in the denominator because there are two types of objects involved, namely, two U's and one A.

The above pattern is not coincidental. It can be shown to hold in any situation in which n objects are to be arranged with some objects indistinguishable from others. Theorem 2.5.1 formalizes this idea.

THEOREM 2.5.1. Permutations of indistinguishable objects. Consider n objects where n_1 are of type 1, n_2 of type 2, . . . , n_k of type k. The number of ways in which the n objects can be arranged is given by

$$\frac{n!}{n_1! \, n_2! \, \cdots \, n_k!} \qquad n_1 + n_2 + \cdots + n_k = n$$

EXAMPLE 2.5.3. Fifteen patients are to be used in an experiment to test a standard drug, an experimental drug, and a placebo. Each patient is to be randomly assigned a treatment. In how many different ways can the three treatments be assigned to the 15 patients? What is the probability that a random assignment of treatments would result in 10 patients receiving the placebo, 3 receiving the experimental drug, and 2 receiving the standard?

The first question is now new. There are $3 \cdot 3 \cdot 3 \cdots 3 = 3^{15} = 14{,}348{,}907$ ways to assign treatments to patients. The second question is new. To find the desired probability, we must determine how many of the above arrangements involve the placebo 10 times, the experimental drug three times, and the standard drug twice. This is easily found by Theorem 2.5.1 to be

$$\frac{15!}{10! \, 3! \, 2!} = \frac{15 \cdot 14 \cdot 13 \cdot 12 \cdot 11 \cdot \cancel{10!}}{\cancel{10!}(3 \cdot 2 \cdot 1 \cdot 2 \cdot 1)} = 30{,}030$$

The desired probability is therefore

$$\frac{30{,}030}{14{,}348{,}907} \doteq .0021$$

▨ EXERCISES 2.5

1. In how many ways can the letters of the word BOO be arranged to form distinguishable patterns?

2. A researcher has eight plants with which to experiment. Two different watering regimens are being investigated. They are tap water (T) and water that is slightly acidic (A) so as to approximate acid rain. Four plants are to receive tap water and the rest the acid solution. A typical assignment of treatments to plants is *ATTTAATA*. How many such assignments are possible?

3. A medical laboratory contains a machine that is used to determine the white blood cell count in a patient's blood. Each morning a test slide, one for which the proper count is known, is run. If the machine gives a count that is acceptably close to the true count, then the machine is assumed to be "in control" or working properly; otherwise, it is "out of control" and must be adjusted. A technician reports that on 4 of the last 14 days the machine was out of control. In how many ways could this have occurred?

4. In how many ways can the letters in your last name be rearranged to form distinguishably different patterns?

5. In observing biorhythms in mice, a mouse is isolated in a cage that contains an exercise wheel. The mouse is kept in 24-hour light, and its activity is monitored over a 24-hour period via a computerized monitor attached to the wheel. It is reported that there are 16 recognizable time segments with the following breakdown: R = rest (8), SA = short period of activity (4), MA = moderate period of activity (2), LA = long period of activity (2). Activity periods are always followed by a period of rest. In how many ways could this experiment have proceeded? If the activity of the mouse is random so that each of the possible outcomes is equally likely, what is the probability that the two periods of long activity will occur consecutively?

6. Consider the experiment of Exercise 9 of Section 2.3. If a tree is distinguished by color only, in how many ways can the eight dogwoods be planted? How many of these arrangements have at least two trees of the same color side by side?

7. A 10-word RNA sequence is to be formed. It involves the word ACU (threonine) three times, GGU (glycine) twice, GAA (glutamic acid) four times, and UAA (stop) once. How many 10-word sequences with this composition are possible? What is the probability that a randomly selected sequence from this group will have the stop somewhere other than at the end of the sequence?

8. Fifteen experimental animals are available to use in a study to compare three different diets. Each diet is to be used on five randomly selected animals. In how many ways can the diets be assigned to the experimental subjects?

9. Show that $_nP_r$ can be written as

$$_nP_r = \frac{n!}{(n-r)!}$$

■ 2.6

COMBINATIONS (OPTIONAL)

Thus far we have considered counting problems in which order, either natural or imposed, was important. The words *order* or *arrange* usually appear in the wording of these problems. They signal the use of the multiplication principle or the formula for permutations of indistinguishable objects in their solution. We now turn our attention to situations in which order is irrelevant. That is, we now consider problems involving combinations rather than permutations.

The key words that identify a combination are the words *select, choose,* or *pick.* Combinations will be solved by means of a combination formula. The pattern involved in the formula is easy to spot. Example 2.6.1 illustrates the idea.

EXAMPLE 2.6.1. Five people have volunteered to take part in an experimental program. Only two are needed to complete the study. In how many ways can two people be selected from five?

Order is not important here. Interest centers only on which two are selected, not on the order of selection. Thus we are asking, How many combinations are there of five objects, selected two at a time? The question can be answered by labeling the volunteers $A, B, C, D,$ E and then listing all possible subsets of size two as follows:

{A, B}   {A, E}   {B, E}   {D, E}
{A, C}   {B, C}   {C, D}
{A, D}   {B, D}   {C,E}

There are obviously 10 combinations. We write $_5C_2 = 10$, where the 5 indicates the number of objects available, the 2 shows the number selected, and the C indicates a combination is involved. Alternatively, we may write $\binom{5}{2} = 10$. How could the value 10 have been obtained without the use of the list? We note simply that

$$10 = \frac{5!}{2!\,3!}$$

The numerator of this expression is 5! because there are five objects from which to choose. There are two factorials in the denominator, 2! and 3!. This is due to the fact that the five objects are split into two groups, namely, those selected for the study (2) and those omitted from the study $(5 - 2 = 3)$.

The pattern noted above is not coincidental and is generalized in Theorem 2.6.1.

THEOREM 2.6.1. The number of combinations of n distinct objects, selected r at a time, denoted $_nC_r$, or $\binom{n}{r}$, is given by

$$_nC_r = \binom{n}{r} = \frac{n!}{r!(n-r)!}$$

Example 2.6.2 illustrates the use of the combination formula in the solution of probability problems.

EXAMPLE 2.6.2. A blood bank has available 10 units of A$^+$ blood. In fact, four are contaminated with serum hepatitis. Three units are randomly selected for use with three patients. What is the probability that exactly one patient will be exposed to hepatitis from this source?

This question involves combinations, since we are interested in only the final units selected, not the order in which they are selected. Consider the diagram of Figure 2.7. The total number of ways to select three units from the 10 available is

$$_{10}C_3 = \frac{10!}{3!\,7!} = 120$$

In order for exactly one patient to be exposed to hepatitis from this source, we must select exactly one unit from the four contaminated units and the other two from the six that are not contaminated. The contaminated unit can be selected in

$$_4C_1 = \binom{4}{1} = \frac{4!}{1!\,3!} = 4 \text{ ways}$$

The uncontaminated units can be selected in

$$_6C_2 = \binom{6}{2} = \frac{6!}{2!\,4!} = 15 \text{ ways}$$

Altogether, there are $(4)(15) = 60$ ways to make the selection in such a way that exactly one patient will be exposed to hepatitis from this source. Assuming that each of the 120 possible ways to select three units from 10 is just as likely to occur as any other, we may use classical methods to conclude that

$$P[\text{exactly one patient exposed to risk}] = \tfrac{60}{120} = .5$$

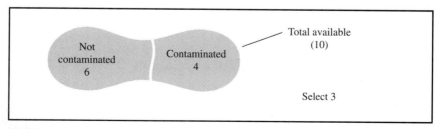

FIGURE 2.7
Partitioning the set of blood units.

■ EXERCISES 2.6

1. Evaluate:
   (a) $_6C_2$ (c) $\binom{4}{0}$ (d) $\binom{3}{3}$
   (b) $_8C_5$
   (e) If $_nC_2 = 21$, what is n?
   (f) If $_nC_3 = 20$, what is n?
   (g) Show that $_5C_3 = _5C_2$.

2. A group of 12 patients is available for use in a study. Five are to be selected to receive an experimental treatment; the other seven are to receive the standard treatment and are to serve as a control. In how many ways can the control group be selected? What is the probability that a specific individual A will be selected into the control group? *Hint:* Think of the group as being split as shown in Figure 2.8.

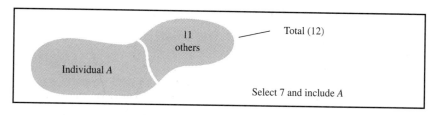

■ **FIGURE 2.8**
Partitioning the set of patients.

3. A new compound has been developed to help reduce skin dryness. Fifteen women, all about the same age with the same skin type, are asked to take part in a test. Seven are randomly selected and asked to use the product on their hands for 2 weeks. The others serve as a control. At the end of the experiment, an impartial judge is asked to select the seven whose hands appear to be in the best condition. If, in fact, the treatment has had no effect at all, what is the probability that by chance alone the judge will select all seven who used the experimental compound? What is the probability that she will select exactly five of those who used the experimental compound?

4. A scientist has six different cages of white rats in the animal room. Of the six cages, two contain some rats which are diseased. What is the probability in a random selection of three cages that none of the cages containing diseased animals will be selected? What is the probability that exactly one cage with diseased animals will be selected?

5. A chemist has 10 water samples taken from the wastewater of a paper factory. Unknown to the chemist, four samples are excessively acidic. In a random selection of three samples, what is the probability that exactly two will have excess acid?

6. Ten bears have been captured, tagged, and released into the wild. Later, a sample of eight bears is to be caught and the number tagged is to be counted. It is assumed that no bear is more likely than another to be caught, so every set of size eight

occurs with equal probability. Assume that the bear population in the region numbers 100.

   (*a*) How many subsets of size eight can be selected?

   (*b*) Would you be surprised if no tagged bears were caught? Explain based on the probability of this occurring.

   (*c*) What is the probability that all eight bears will be tagged?

7. A pharmacist has a supply of 100 penicillin tablets. Unknown to her, five have lost their potency. A prescription is filled by randomly selecting 15 tablets from the stock on hand. What is the probability that none of the tablets chosen will have lost their potency? What is the probability that exactly one will have lost its potency? What is the probability that at most one will have lost its potency?

8. The Delta project is a project to determine if large-scale agricultural production can succeed in Alaska. In this project 22 persons are to be selected from a pool of 103 qualified applicants and awarded the right to purchase land parcels to be developed for agricultural purposes. (Based on information from "Expanding Subarctic Agriculture," *Interdisciplinary Science Reviews,* vol. 7, no. 3, 1982, pp. 178–187.)

   (*a*) In how many ways can the 22 persons be selected? (Provide problem setup only.)

   (*b*) Assume that you are one of the persons in the applicant pool. In how many of the subgroups of part *a* will you be included? (Provide problem setup only.)

   (*c*) If the selection process is done randomly, each of the subgroups of part *a* is equally likely. If your name is in the applicant pool, what is the probability that you will be given the right to purchase land?

9. Consider Exercise 10 of Section 2.3. In how many ways can the 15 squares to be sampled be selected if the map contains a total of 50 squares?

10. A study is conducted to compare the effectiveness of 10 different over-the-counter headache compounds. If the compounds are tested in pairs, how many different comparisons are possible?

TECHNOLOGY TOOLS

VI. $n!, \, _nC_r, \, _nP_r$

The TI83 calculator has the formula for $n!$, $_nC_r$, and $_nP_r$ in memory. We illustrate the use of the calculator by finding $10!$, $_{10}C_3$, and $_{10}P_3$.

TI83 Keystroke	Purpose
1. 10	1. Enter the number 10
2. MATH	2. Calculate 10! and clear the screen
◁	
4	
ENTER	
CLEAR	

3. 10
   MATH
   ◁
   3
   3
   ENTER
   CLEAR

3. Calculate $_{10}C_3$ and clear the screen

4. 10
   MATH
   ◁
   2
   3
   ENTER
   CLEAR

4. Calculate $_{10}P_3$ and clear the screen

3

Probability and
Problem Solving (Optional)

In Chapter 2 we considered the interpretation of probabilities and some elementary methods for determining them. In this chapter we continue our study by discussing some of the theorems that are useful in problem solving in settings that are more complex than those seen in Chapter 2.

3.1
VENN DIAGRAMS AND THE AXIOMS OF PROBABILITY

Venn Diagrams

Before we begin to develop the basic rules that govern the behavior of probabilities, let us introduce a diagram that is useful in organizing probabilities. The diagram, called a *Venn diagram,* is named after John Venn (1834–1923). In such a diagram, we represent the set of possibilities for an experiment by a rectangle. We refer to this set as the *sample space* and denote it by the capital letter S (Figure 3.1a). An event of interest is represented by a closed curve within the rectangle and is denoted by a capital letter other than S. In Figure 3.1b the event A is pictured. The event that A does not occur is denoted by A' and is represented by the region of the rectangle that lies outside of A (Figure 3.1c). The event A' is called the *complement* of event A. When two events A_1 and A_2 are associated with the same experiment, they divide the rectangle into four separate regions. Each region represents a unique way of combining the two events. These are shown in Figure 3.1d to g. An example will illustrate the idea.

> **EXAMPLE 3.1.1.** A study is designed to investigate weight and smoking habits of patients with hypertension. Here S represents all patients with hypertension. Let A_1 denote those patients who are overweight and A_2 those that smoke. Figure 3.1d represents patients who are overweight but who do not smoke; Figure 3.1e pictures those who smoke but are not overweight. Figure 3.1f shows those patients who are overweight and smoke, while those who neither smoke nor are overweight are represented in Figure 3.1g.

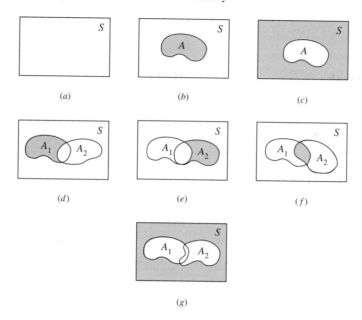

FIGURE 3.1

(a) The sample space is denoted by a rectangle; (b) the event A is represented by a closed curve within the rectangle; (c) event A' is the event that A does not occur; (d) A_1 occurs, but A_2 does not occur; (e) A_2 occurs, but A_1 does not occur; (f) both A_1 and A_2 occur; (g) neither A_1 nor A_2 occurs.

The English word *or* has two different meanings. When used inclusively, it means one or the other or perhaps both; in the exclusive sense it means one or the other but not both. In this text the word *or* is used inclusively unless specified otherwise. For example, if we say that a hypertensive patient is overweight or smokes, we mean that the patient exhibits at least one of these characteristics. He or she is (1) overweight but does not smoke, or (2) smokes but is not overweight, or (3) smokes and is overweight. The Venn diagram for the event A_1 *or* A_2 is shown in Figure 3.2.

Axioms of Probability

We begin by considering three axioms of probability. These axioms, which are statements that are assumed to be true and require no proof, are intuitive in nature. Most people apply them quite naturally without even being aware that they are doing so.

Before stating the axioms, let us develop one definition. Consider the two events, A_1: patient A recovers from open heart surgery, and A_2: patient A dies on the operating table. It is evident that these events cannot occur simultaneously. The occurrence of one precludes the occurrence of the other. When this occurs, we say that events A_1 and A_2 are *mutually exclusive*. The Venn diagram representation of two mutually exclusive

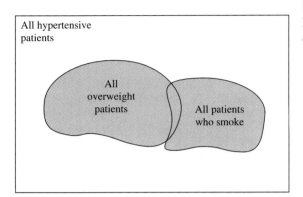

FIGURE 3.2

Patients who smoke *or* are overweight.

events is shown in Figure 3.3*a*. Notice that in this special case the curves representing the two events do not overlap. The idea is extended to a collection of mutually exclusive events in Figure 3.3*b*.

Three axioms are used to lay the foundation for the basic problem-solving theorems of this chapter. They are as follows:

Axioms of probability

1. Let *S* denote a sample space for an experiment. Then $P[S] = 1$.

2. $P[A] \geq 0$ for every event *A*.

3. Let $A_1, A_2, A_3, \ldots$ be a finite or infinite collection of mutually exclusive events. Then $P[A_1 \text{ or } A_2 \text{ or } A_3 \text{ or } \cdots] = P[A_1] + P[A_2] + P[A_3] + \cdots$.

Axiom 1 states a fact that was regarded as obvious in Chapter 2, namely, that the probability assigned to a sure, or certain, event is 1. Axiom 2 ensures that probabilities

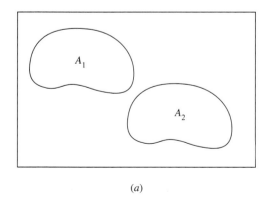
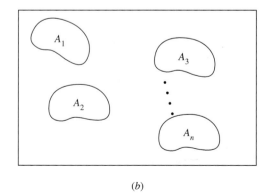

(*a*)   (*b*)

FIGURE 3.3

(*a*) The events A_1 and A_2 are mutually exclusive. If one occurs, the other cannot.

(*b*) A collection of *n* mutually exclusive events.

can never be negative. Axiom 3 guarantees that when one deals with mutually exclusive events, the probability of one *or* the other of the events occurring can be found by adding the individual probabilities. These axioms lead quite easily to Theorem 3.1.1.

THEOREM 3.1.1. $P[\varnothing] = 0$.

This theorem states that the probability associated with the "impossible" event, $\varnothing$, is 0. Since the impossible event corresponds to a physical event that cannot occur, we would want our axioms to assign a probability of 0 to such an event. For example, consider the experiment that consists of rolling a single ordinary six-sided die. The faces on the die show the numbers 1 through 6 inclusive. If we ask, What is the probability that on a single toss the number 8 will be obtained? the answer is 0. The event described is physically impossible. The proof of the theorem is outlined in Exercise 13 of this section.

Axiom 3 is especially important because it gives us the ability to find the probability of an event when the sample points in the sample space for the experiment are not equally likely. To understand this idea, consider Example 3.1.2.

EXAMPLE 3.1.2. The distribution of blood types among whites in the United States is roughly as follows:

A: 40%   AB: 4%
B: 11%   O: 45%

A white man is brought into the emergency room after an automobile accident. He is to be blood-typed. What is the probability that he will be of type A, B, or AB? Axiom 3 can be used to find the desired probability. Let A_1, A_2, and A_3 denote the events that the patient has type A, B, and AB blood, respectively. We are looking for $P[A_1 \text{ or } A_2 \text{ or } A_3]$. Since it is impossible for one individual to have two different blood types, these events are mutually exclusive. By Axiom 3,

$$P[A_1 \text{ or } A_2 \text{ or } A_3] = P[A_1] + P[A_2] + P[A_3]$$

$$= .40 + .11 + .04$$

$$= .55$$

There is a 55% chance that the patient will have one of the three blood types mentioned. (Based on information from *Technical Manual,* American Association of Blood Banks, 1985.)

Suppose that the probability that event A will occur is known, and we want to find the probability that A will not occur. This can be done easily by subtraction from 1. For example, based on recently conducted research, it is estimated that the probability of "curing" childhood leukemia is $\frac{1}{3}$. ("Cure" means that the child is free from disease for at least 4 years after treatment ended.) Thus the probability that the disease will not be cured is $1 - \frac{1}{3} = \frac{2}{3}$.

This idea, which seems evident, is justified by Theorem 3.1.2, whose proof is outlined in Exercise 14 of this section. Remember that A' denotes the event that A does *not* occur.

THEOREM 3.1.2. $P[A'] = 1 - P[A]$.

Note that this theorem gives a way to determine the probability of the complement of event *A*.

▧ EXERCISES 3.1

1. Let *L* denote the event that a patient has leukemia and *W* denote the event that his or her white blood cell count is high. Consider the Venn diagrams given in Figure 3.4. In each case describe the patients represented by the shaded region.
2. Let *H* denote the event that a tree is found at a high elevation and let *G* denote the event that the tree's growth is stunted. Consider the Venn diagrams given in Figure 3.5. In each case describe the trees represented by the shaded region.
3. In a study of immunization in preschool children, interest centers on the mumps and measles vaccines. Let *P* represent the event that a child has received the mumps vaccine and *M* represent the event that a child has received the measles vaccine.
    (*a*) Describe the children in the event *P* and *M*.
    (*b*) Draw a Venn diagram to represent the collection of children who have received the measles vaccine but not the mumps vaccine.
    (*c*) Draw a Venn diagram to represent the collection of children who have received neither vaccine.
    (*d*) Draw a Venn diagram to represent the collection of children who have received the mumps or the measles vaccine.
    (*e*) Draw a Venn diagram to represent the collection of children who have received the mumps or the measles vaccine but have not received both.

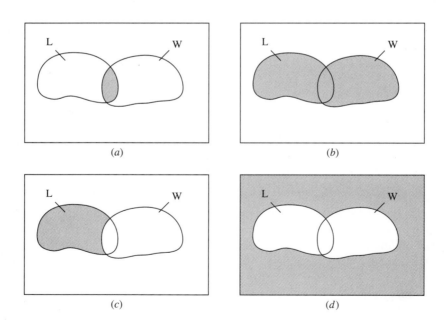

(*a*)   (*b*)

(*c*)   (*d*)

▧ **FIGURE 3.4**

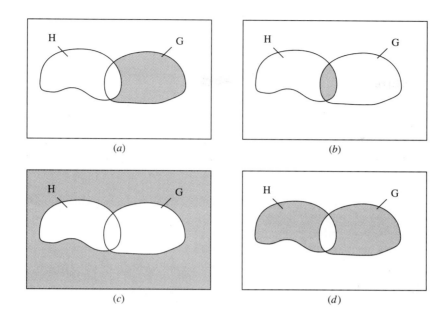

FIGURE 3.5

4. In a study of the effects of sulfur dioxide on trees along major roadways in the Smokies, two events are identified. They are L, the tree has leaf damage, and T, the tree is stunted.
   (*a*) Draw a Venn diagram to represent the collection of trees that are not stunted.
   (*b*) Draw a Venn diagram to represent the collection of trees that are stunted but show no leaf damage.
   (*c*) Draw a Venn diagram to represent the collection of trees that exhibit neither characteristic.
   (*d*) Draw a Venn diagram to represent the collection of trees that are stunted or show leaf damage.
   (*e*) Draw a Venn diagram to represent the collection of trees that are stunted or show leaf damage but do not have both problems.
5. Which of the following are sets of mutually exclusive events?
   (*a*) *A*: Jane Doe's son has hemophilia.
        B: Jane Doe's daughter is a carrier of hemophilia.
   (*b*) *A*: 65% of pea seeds planted germinate.
        B: 50% of pea seeds fail to germinate after planting.
   (*c*) *A*: José is suffering from hypothermia.
        B: José's temperature is 102°F.
   (*d*) *A*: The pH of a topsoil sample is equal to 7.0.
        B: The sample of topsoil is alkaline.
   (*e*) *A*: A patient has AIDS.
        B: A patient has had a blood transfusion.

(*f*) *A*: The animal is a mammal.

   B: The animal is a dolphin.

   C: The animal is fur bearing.

(*g*) *A*: The tree is an evergreen.

   B: The tree is an oak.

   C: The tree is a dogwood.

(*h*) *A*: The forest is a virgin stand.

   B: The forest was clear-cut 10 years ago.

6. In the treatment of premature babies, the amount of oxygen babies received can affect their vision. Each child treated can be classified as having normal vision, having a mild lesion, having a moderate lesion, having a severe lesion, or being blind. A study shows that the probabilities of each of these events occurring are .80, .10, .06, .02, and .02, respectively.

   (*a*) Find the probability that a child is born with a vision defect.

   (*b*) Find the probability that a child is born with normal vision.

7. A particular chemical analysis has a rather limited range. Typically, 15% of the samples are too concentrated to be assayed without dilution, and 20% are contaminated with an interfering material that must be removed before analysis. The rest may be analyzed without pretreatment. Assume that samples both too concentrated and contaminated never occur. What is the probability that a randomly selected sample can be assayed without pretreatment?

8. Diabetes in pregnancy constitutes a major problem in maternal and child welfare. Among pregnant diabetics, toxemia occurs in 25% of the cases, hydramnios in 21% of the cases, and fetal wastage in 15%. Other complications occur in 6% of the cases. Assume that no two of these complications can occur in a single pregnancy. What is the probability that a randomly selected pregnant diabetic will have a normal pregnancy? What is the probability that a randomly selected pregnant diabetic will have some sort of complication?

9. The weather bureau's air pollution index classifies each day as being extremely good, good, fair, poor, or extremely poor. Past experience indicates that 50% of the days are classified as extremely good, 22% as good, 18% as fair, 8% as poor, and 2% as extremely poor. A warning is issued on days that are classified as poor or extremely poor. What is the probability that a warning is issued on a randomly selected day?

10. Studies on depression indicate that a particular course of treatment improves the condition of 72% of those on whom it is used, does not affect 10%, and worsens the condition of the rest. A patient suffering from depression is treated by using this method. What is the probability that his condition will worsen? What is the probability that the treatment is not detrimental to his condition?

11. Trees on Mount Mitchell and other areas in the southern Appalachian mountains have been affected by pollution. Suppose that in a particular area 40% of the evergreens show mild damage, 15% show moderate damage, 10% are severely damaged, 8% are dead, and the rest are unaffected. If a tree is selected at random for study, what is the probability that it is

   (*a*) Unaffected?

   (*b*) At most mildly damaged?

(c) Severely damaged or dead?

(d) Neither severely damaged nor dead?

12. The blood type distribution among blacks in the United States is

O: 49%   B: 20%

A: 27%   AB: 4%

If a black woman is brought into an emergency room, what is the probability that she will be of type A, B, or AB? (Based on information from *Technical Manual, American Association of Blood Banks, 1985.*)

13. Prove Theorem 3.1.1. *Hint:* Notice that $S = S$ or $\varnothing$ and that S and $\varnothing$ are mutually exclusive. Apply Axioms 3 and 1.

14. Prove Theorem 3.1.2. *Hint:* Notice that $S = A$ or A' and that A and A' are mutually exclusive. Apply Axioms 1 and 3.

15. Let A and B be events such that A is contained in B (see Figure 3.6). Note that

$$B = A \text{ or } (B \text{ but NOT } A)$$

and that the events on the right of the above equation are mutually exclusive.

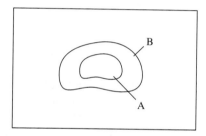

FIGURE 3.6

Venn diagram showing event A contained in event B.

(a) Use this information and the theorems and axioms developed in this section to prove that

$$P[A] \le P[B]$$

(b) Let C denote any event. Use part a and the theorems and axioms developed in this section to prove that $P[C] \le 1$. You have thus proved the claim made in Chapter 2 that probabilities cannot exceed 1.

3.2

GENERAL ADDITION RULE

In Section 3.1 we saw how to handle questions concerning the probability of one or another event's occurring if those events were mutually exclusive. In this section we discuss the general addition rule. Its purpose is to allow us to handle the more general case of finding the probability that at least one of two events will occur when the events themselves are not necessarily mutually exclusive.

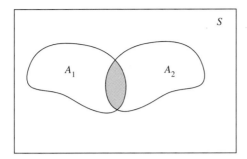

■ **FIGURE 3.7**

A_1 and A_2 are not mutually exclusive. The shaded region is not empty.

We begin by considering the Venn diagram of Figure 3.7. Note that A_1 and A_2 are *not* mutually exclusive. Therefore, the shaded region shown is not empty. If we computed $P[A_1 \text{ or } A_2]$ as in Section 3.1, we would conclude that

$$P[A_1 \text{ or } A_2] = P[A_1] + P[A_2]$$

However, since the shaded region is contained in both A_1 and A_2, we included $P[A_1 \text{ and } A_2]$ twice in the above calculation. In order to correct for this, $P[A_1 \text{ and } A_2]$ must be subtracted from the right-hand side of the equation. The resulting expression is the general addition rule.

THEOREM 3.2.1. General addition rule. Let A_1 and A_2 be events. Then

$$P[A_1 \text{ or } A_2] = P[A_1] + P[A_2] - P[A_1 \text{ and } A_2]$$

The key word to watch for in identifying a problem as one in which the general addition rule applies is the word *or*. Due to the third axiom of probability and the general addition rule, it is safe to say that when you see the word *or* in a probability question, addition is almost always involved. In Sections 3.5 and 3.6 you will see that the word *and* typically signals that numbers will be multiplied to solve the problem at hand. The use of the rule is illustrated in Example 3.2.1.

EXAMPLE 3.2.1. It is thought that 30% of all people in the United States are obese (A_1) and that 3% suffer from diabetes (A_2). Two percent are obese and suffer from diabetes. What is the probability that a randomly selected person is obese *or* suffers from diabetes?

We have been given $P[A_1] = .3$, $P[A_2] = .03$, and $P[A_1 \text{ and } A_2] = .02$. We are asked to find $P[A_1 \text{ or } A_2]$. Applying the general addition rule, we obtain

$$P[A_1 \text{ or } A_2] = P[A_1] + P[A_2] - P[A_1 \text{ and } A_2]$$
$$= .30 + .03 - .02$$
$$= .31$$

The general addition rule not only is useful in computing $P[A_1 \text{ or } A_2]$, but given the proper information, it can be used to find $P[A_1 \text{ and } A_2]$. Example 3.2.2 illustrates how this is done.

EXAMPLE 3.2.2. It was recently reported that 18% of all college students at some point in their college careers suffer from depression (A_1), that 2% consider suicide (A_2), and that 19% suffer from depression or consider suicide. What is the probability that a randomly

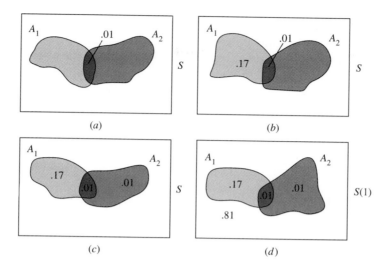

FIGURE 3.8

Computing probabilities by using Venn diagrams. (*a*) $P[A_1 \text{ and } A_2] = .01$; (*b*) $P[A_1] = .18$; (*c*) $P[A_2] = .02$; (*d*) $P[A_1 \text{ or } A_2] = .19$, implying that $P[(A_1 \text{ or } A_2)'] = .81$.

selected college student suffers from depression *and* has considered suicide? What is the probability that a randomly selected student has suffered from depression *but* has not considered suicide?

We know that $P[A_1] = .18$, $P[A_2] = .02$, and $P[A_1 \text{ or } A_2] = .19$. We are asked, first, to find $P[A_1 \text{ and } A_2]$. Applying the general addition rule, we get

$$P[A_1 \text{ or } A_2] = P[A_1] + P[A_2] - P[A_1 \text{ and } A_2]$$

or
$$P[A_1 \text{ and } A_2] = P[A_1] + P[A_2] - P[A_1 \text{ or } A_2]$$

$$= .18 + .02 - .19$$

$$= .01$$

To answer the second question posed, we display the information given in a Venn diagram. Since $P[A_1 \text{ and } A_2] = .01$, we know that 1% of the total area in the diagram lies in the region representing A_1 and A_2, as shown in Figure 3.8*a*. Since $P[A_1] = .18$, of the total area 18% lies in the region labeled A_1; since A_1 and A_2 is contained in A_1, 17% of the area lies in the region shown in Figure 3.8*b*. Similarly, since $P[A_2] = .02$ and A_1 and A_2 is contained in A_2, 1% of the area lies in the region shown in Figure 3.8*c*. Since $P[S] = 1$ and we have accounted for $17 + 1 + 1 = 19\%$ of the area, the remaining 81% lies in the region shown in Figure 3.8*d*. Now we can answer the second question by looking for the appropriate region in the Venn diagram, namely, A_1 and A_2'. It can be seen that the probability associated with the region is .17. Thus, the probability that a randomly selected college student has suffered from depression but has not considered suicide is .17.

Notice that if the percentages reported in problems such as these are based on population data, then the probabilities calculated by use of the general addition rule are exact. However, if the percentages reported are based on samples drawn from a larger population, then the probabilities computed are relative frequency probabilities. They are *approximations* to the true probability of the occurrence of the event in question. Since most percentages reported in the literature are based on samples, most are properly viewed as being relative frequency probabilities. We use the word *probability* with the understanding that the probabilities given and computed by using the theorems in this chapter are, in most cases, only approximations.

▓ EXERCISES 3.2

1. Suppose that $P[A_1 \text{ and } A_2] = .04$, $P[A_1] = .06$, $P[A_2] = .10$. Find
   (a) $P[A_1 \text{ or } A_2]$
   (b) $P[A_1 \text{ and } A_2']$
   (c) $P[A_1' \text{ and } A_2]$
   (d) $P[A_1' \text{ and } A_2']$
   (e) Construct a Venn diagram to show the breakdown of probabilities within the sample space as demonstrated in Figure 3.8.
2. Suppose that $P[A_1 \text{ or } A_2] = .30$, $P[A_1] = .15$, $P[A_2] = .20$. Find
   (a) $P[A_1 \text{ and } A_2]$
   (b) $P[A_1 \text{ and } A_2']$
   (c) $P[A_1' \text{ and } A_2]$
   (d) $P[A_1' \text{ or } A_2']$
   (e) $P[(A_1 \text{ or } A_2)']$
   (f) Construct a Venn diagram to show the breakdown of probabilities within the sample space as demonstrated in Figure 3.8.
3. To meet the demand by farmers for white pine saplings to use as windbreaks, forestry service employees sampled farmers in the state. They found that 30% had acquired trees from the service in prior years, 40% anticipated ordering trees in the coming year, and 10% had acquired trees in the past and anticipated ordering additional ones in the coming year. What is the probability that a randomly selected farmer has acquired trees in the past or anticipates ordering them during the coming year? What is the probability that a randomly selected farmer acquired trees in the past but does not anticipate ordering others during the coming year? If each farmer that requests trees is allowed at most 100 and there are 5000 farmers in the state, approximate the maximum number of saplings needed to fill all requests for the coming year.
4. Data gathered at a particular blood center show that .1% of all donors test positive for human immunodeficiency virus (HIV) and 1% test positive for herpes. If 1.05% test positive for one or the other of these problems, what is the probability that a randomly selected donor will have neither problem? Would you be surprised to find a donor with both problems? Explain based on the estimated probability of this occurring.
5. It has been reported that 62% of all health services are financed through private (nongovernment) funds, that 70% are financed by a combination of employer and employee working together, and that 50% are financed both privately and by the

employer and employee. What is the probability that a randomly selected patient will have health services that are funded privately or by the employer and employee? What is the probability that a randomly selected patient will have health services that are funded by the employer and employee but are not funded privately?

6. Studies show that 12% of all persons treated by physicians are admitted to the hospital. Of the persons treated, 1% have an adverse drug reaction of some sort, and 12.4% are admitted to the hospital or have an adverse drug reaction. What is the probability that a randomly selected patient will be admitted to the hospital and have a drug reaction? What is the probability that a randomly selected patient will be admitted to the hospital but have no adverse drug reaction? What is the probability that a randomly selected patient will have an adverse reaction to a drug but will not be admitted to the hospital?

7. A chemist analyzes seawater samples for two heavy metals: lead and mercury. She finds that 38% of the samples taken from near the mouth of a river on which numerous industrial plants are located contain toxic levels of lead or mercury, and 32% contain toxic levels of lead. Of these samples, 10% contain high levels of both metals. What is the probability that a given sample will contain a high level of mercury? What is the probability that a given sample will contain only lead?

8. If Swiss mice are given a dose of 1 mg of compound A per kilogram of body weight, then 50% of the animals die (a dose that kills 50% of the test animals is known as the LD_{50} for a drug or poison) and 40% of the treated animals, whether surviving or not, are cyanotic (that is, their skin has a bluish appearance, indicating inadequate oxygenation of the blood). One-fourth of the animals die and exhibit obvious cyanosis at death. What is the probability that an animal to whom compound A was administered (the LD_{50} dose) dies *or* is observed to be cyanotic? What is the probability than an animal to whom compound A was administered lives *and* is observed to be cyanotic?

3.3
CONDITIONAL PROBABILITY

In this section we introduce the notion of conditional probability. The name itself is indicative of what is to be done. We wish to determine the probability that some event A_2 will occur, "conditioned on" the assumption that some other event A_1 has occurred already. The key words to look for in identifying a conditional question are *if* and *given that*. We use the notation $P[A_2 \mid A_1]$ to denote the conditional probability of event A_2 occurring given that event A_1 has occurred. Note that although this expression involves two events, it represents only one probability. The first event listed is the event whose occurrence is in doubt; the slash is read "given that"; the second event listed is assumed to have occurred already.

> **EXAMPLE 3.3.1.** A woman has three children. What is the probability that the first two are boys (A_1)? What is the probability that exactly two of the three are boys (A_2)? What is the probability that both conditions are satisfied?

First   Second   Third   ■ **FIGURE 3.9**
child   child   child   Birth orders in a three-child family.

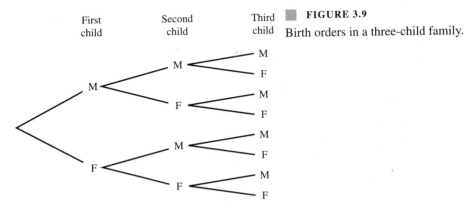

These questions are not conditional and can be easily answered by using a tree diagram (see Figure 3.9. If we assume that each child is just as likely to be a boy as a girl, then the eight sample points represented in the tree are equally likely. Therefore, the classical approach can be used to compute the desired probabilities. In particular,

$$P[A_1] = \tfrac{2}{8}$$

$$P[A_2] = \tfrac{3}{8}$$

$$P[A_1 \text{ and } A_2] = \tfrac{1}{8}$$

Suppose we are told that the first two children are boys. Now, what is the probability that there are exactly two boys in the family? That is, what is $P[A_2 \mid A_1]$? Since we know that the first two children are boys, the sample space for the experiment no longer logically consists of eight points but, in fact, now contains only the two points MMM and MMF. The remaining six points are inconsistent with the known information. The conditional question posed is answered via this new two-point sample space. Since these points are equally likely and only one of them corresponds to having exactly two boys in the family,

$$P[A_2 \mid A_1] = P[\text{exactly two boys} \mid \text{first two are boys}] = \tfrac{1}{2}$$

In this case note that $\tfrac{1}{2} = P[A_2 \mid A_1] \neq P[A_2] = \tfrac{3}{8}$. Receipt of the new information did affect the probability assigned to the event that exactly two of the children are boys.

Example 3.3.1 is an oversimplification of the general problem. Most conditional questions are asked relative to situations for which it is not convenient to work directly with an explicitly restricted sample space. Thus, it is necessary to develop a formula for conditional probability that, in essence, automatically reduces the sample space to be consistent with the given information and computes the desired probability relative to this reduced sample space. To discover the formula, we need only look for some pattern in Example 3.3.1. Numerically, the pattern is easy enough to spot. Just note that

$$P[A_2 \mid A_1] = \frac{1}{2} = \frac{\tfrac{1}{8}}{\tfrac{2}{8}} = \frac{P[A_1 \text{ and } A_2]}{P[A_1]}$$

This relationship is not unique to this problem. In fact, it is the general definition for the conditional probability of event A_2 and A_1.

DEFINITION 3.3.1. Conditional probability. Let A_1 and A_2 be events such that $P[A_1]$ $\neq 0$. The conditional probability of A_2 given A_1, denoted $P[A_2 \mid A_1]$, is defined by

$$P[A_2 \mid A_1] = \frac{P[A_1 \text{ and } A_2]}{P[A_1]}$$

Practically speaking, note that the condition that $P[A_1] \neq 0$ is not restrictive. If A_1 has occurred, it must have had nonzero probability originally. Definition 3.3.1 is remembered easily as

$$\boxed{\text{Conditional probability} = \frac{P[\text{both events}]}{P[\text{given event}]}}$$

EXAMPLE 3.3.2. It is estimated that 15% of the adult population has hypertension, but that 75% of all adults feel that personally they do not have this problem. It is also estimated that 6% of the population has hypertension but does not think that the disease is present. If an adult patient reports thinking that he or she does not have hypertension, what is the probability that the disease is, in fact, present?

Letting A_1 denote the event that the patient does not feel that the disease is present and A_2 the event that the disease is present, we are given that $P[A_1] = .75$, $P[A_2] = .15$, and $P[A_1 \text{ and } A_2] = .06$. We are asked to find $P[A_2 \mid A_1]$.

By Definition 3.3.1,

$$P[A_2 \mid A_1] = \frac{P[\text{both}]}{P[\text{given}]} = \frac{P[A_1 \text{ and } A_2]}{P[A_1]}$$

$$= \frac{.06}{.75} = .08$$

There is an 8% chance that a patient who expresses the opinion that she or he has no problem with hypertension does, in fact, have the disease. Similarly, we might ask, If the disease is present, what is the probability that the patient will suspect its presence? That is, what is $P[A_1' \mid A_2]$? Before applying Definition 3.3.1, we organize these data into a Venn diagram, as shown in Figure 3.10. By Definition 3.3.1,

$$P[A_1' \mid A_2] = \frac{P[\text{both}]}{P[\text{given}]} = \frac{P[A_1' \text{ and } A_2]}{P[A_2]}$$

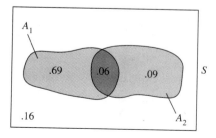

FIGURE 3.10

$A_1 =$ Does not think the disease is present and $A_2 =$ Disease is present.

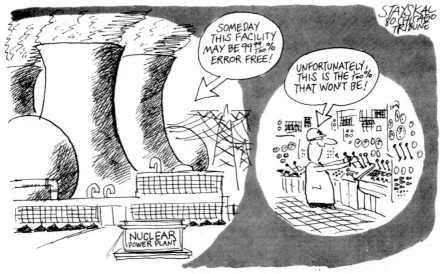

Reading from the Venn diagram, we have

$$\frac{P[A_1' \text{ and } A_2]}{P[A_2]} = \frac{.09}{.15} = .60$$

That is, if the patient expresses the opinion that he or she has hypertension, there is a 60% chance of the patient's being right.

◼ EXERCISES 3.3

1. Suppose a family has four children.
   (a) Find the probability that exactly two are male.
   (b) What is the probability that exactly two are male if the first child born is male?
   (c) Find the probability that the last child born is male.
   (d) What is the probability that the last child born is male if the first three are female?
2. Assume that 50% of all dogwood trees in a given area are blighted. Three trees are sampled and each is classified as being affected by blight (y) or unaffected (n). Since $P[\text{affected}] = P[\text{unaffected}]$, each of the eight possible outcomes of the experiment is equally likely.
   (a) Draw a tree to represent the eight sample points.
   (b) Find $P[\text{at least two are affected}]$.
   (c) Find $P[\text{at least two are affected} \mid \text{first is affected}]$.
   (d) Find $P[\text{exactly two are affected} \mid \text{first is affected}]$.
3. A study indicates that 10% of the population in the United States is 65 years old or older and that 1% of the total population is afflicted with mild heart failure. Fur-

thermore, 10.4% of the population is age 65 or older or suffers from mild heart failure. An individual is selected at random.

(a) Find the probability that the individual is 65 or older and suffering from mild heart failure.

(b) Use the answer to part a to organize the data into a Venn diagram.

(c) If an individual is 65 or older, what is the probability that the person will suffer mild heart failure?

(d) If an individual is under age 65, what is the probability that he or she will suffer mild heart failure?

4. In a study of alcoholics, it was found that 40% had alcoholic fathers and 6% had alcoholic mothers. Forty-two percent had at least one alcoholic parent. What is the probability that a randomly selected alcoholic will

(a) Have both parents alcoholic?

(b) Have an alcoholic mother if the father is alcoholic?

(c) Have an alcoholic mother but not an alcoholic father?

(d) Have an alcoholic mother if the father is not alcoholic?

5. In a study of senility, patients thought to be suffering from either senile dementia or arteriosclerotic cerebral degeneration were identified. Upon death, autopsies were performed on their brains. It was found that 35% had changes principally associated with senile dementia, 45% had changes associated with arteriosclerotic cerebral degeneration, and 20% showed evidence of both. Based on this information, what is the probability that a patient with brain damage resulting from arteriosclerotic cerebral degeneration also will have brain changes characteristic of senile dementia? What is the probability that a patient who does not have changes owing to senile dementia will have arteriosclerotic cerebral degeneration?

6. In a study of waters located near power plants and other industrial plants that release wastewater into the water system, it was found that 5% showed signs of chemical and thermal pollution, 40% showed signs of chemical pollution, and 35% showed evidence of thermal pollution. Assume that the results of the study accurately reflect the general situation. What is the probability that a stream that shows some thermal pollution also will show signs of chemical pollution? What is the probability that a stream showing chemical pollution will now show signs of thermal pollution?

7. Studies have shown that snowshoe hares die off periodically, even in the absence of predators and known diseases. Two identifiable causes of death are low blood sugar and convulsions. It is estimated that 7% of the animals dying exhibit both symptoms, 40% have low blood sugar, and 25% suffer from convulsions. What percentage die from causes other than the two mentioned? What is the probability that a randomly selected animal that has low blood sugar also will have suffered from convulsions?

8. Use the data of Exercise 3 of Section 3.2 to find the probability that a farmer will order trees in the coming year given that he or she had acquired trees in the past. Find the probability that a farmer will not order trees in the coming year given that he or she had acquired trees in the past. What is the mathematical relationship between your two answers? Explain why this occurred.

9. Use the data of Exercise 4 of Section 3.2 to find the probability that a randomly selected donor will test negative for HIV. Find the probability that a randomly selected donor will test negative for HIV given that he or she tests negative for herpes.

▨ 3.4

DIAGNOSTIC TESTS AND RELATIVE RISK

One of the most useful applications of probability in a medical or biological setting is in the area of diagnostic testing. A diagnostic test is a test given to detect the presence of some specific condition in an experimental unit. In a medical setting we are usually trying to detect the presence of a disease, genetic factor, or some other specified condition in a human being. It would be nice if such tests were foolproof in the sense that they would always detect the condition when it is in fact present and would never indicate its presence in an individual who does not have the condition. Unfortunately, this is not the case. We can only hope that the tests in use do not often give erroneous results.

In a diagnostic test, either each subject is a true positive, meaning that the condition that the test is designed to detect is present, or the subject is a true negative. The test itself can be positive, meaning that the presence of the condition has been detected, or not. This guarantees that each subject will fall into exactly one of four categories. These are

1. The condition is present and the test detects its presence. That is, a true positive subject tests positive. In this case no error has been made.
2. The condition is present but the test does not detect its presence. When a true positive subject tests negative, we say that we have obtained a *false-negative* result. An error has been made in this case.
3. The condition is not present but the test detects its presence. When a true negative subject tests positive, we say that a *false-positive* result has been obtained. An error has been made.
4. The condition is not present and the test does not indicate its presence. A true negative tests negative. No error has been made.

Notice that two errors are possible. We hope that neither error will be made, but each is possible. An ideal test is one for which the probability of committing each error is small. These probabilities, called error rates, are defined below.

> **DEFINITION 3.4.1. False-positive rate.** The *false-positive rate* of a test is denoted by α (alpha) and is given by
>
> $$\alpha = P[\text{test results are positive} \mid \text{subject is a true negative}]$$

> **DEFINITION 3.4.2. False-negative rate.** The *false-negative rate* of a test is denoted by β (beta) and is given by
>
> $$\beta = P[\text{test results are negative} \mid \text{subject is a true positive}]$$

TABLE 3.1

Terminology associated with diagnostic tests

		True state	
		Condition absent (−)	**Condition present (+)**
Test results	Condition found (+)	True − but tests + False-positive result P [false positive] $= \alpha$	True + and tests + No error
	Condition not found (−)	True − and tests − No error	True + but tests − False = negative result P[false negative] $= \beta$

Table 3.1 summarizes the terminology introduced thus far.

In screening for a disease, an error that results from a high false-positive rate can result in inconvenience and expense to the individual involved. He or she is found to have a condition that is not present and as a result will probably seek treatment for the nonexistent problem. An error that results from a high false-negative rate is potentially dangerous. In this case, the subject is unaware of an existing condition and hence will not seek needed treatment. Given a frequency table, these rates can be approximated by the technique demonstrated in Example 3.4.1.

EXAMPLE 3.4.1. The serum of a pregnant woman can be analyzed by using a procedure known as starch gel electrophoresis. This test may reveal the presence of a protein zone called the pregnancy zone which is thought to be an indicator that the child is female. To investigate the properties of this test 300 women were selected for study. The results of the test and the subsequent sexes of the children born are given in Table 3.2. Notice that in this case the only value in the table that is predetermined or fixed by the experimenter is the overall sample size. Row totals, column totals, and cell frequencies are all random. By definition the false-positive rate is

$$\alpha = P[\text{test} + \mid \text{true} -]$$

To estimate this conditional probability we must estimate $P[\text{true} -]$ and $P[\text{test} +$ and are true $-]$. Using the relative frequency approach to probability, $P[\text{true} -] \doteq 147/300$ and $P[\text{test} +$ and true $-] \doteq 51/300$. The definition of conditional probability yields

$$\alpha \doteq \frac{51/300}{147/300} = \frac{51}{147} = .3469$$

TABLE 3.2

	Sex		
Pregnancy Zone	**Male (true −)**	**Female (true +)**	
Present (test +)	51	78	129 (Random)
Absent (test −)	96	75	171 (Random)
	147 (Random)	153 (Random)	300 (Fixed)

This result could have been obtained from Table 3.2 at a glance by realizing that once we know that the subject is a true negative, attention is immediately restricted to the 147 cases in column 1. Of these, 51 tested positive. Hence common sense points to 51/147 as the estimated false-positive rate. To estimate β, note that of the 153 true-positive subjects, 75 tested negative. Hence

$$\beta \doteq \frac{75}{153} = .4902$$

Since these are estimated error rates, the test does not appear to be effective in determining the sex of a child. (Based on data reported in *Human Heredity,* vol. 20, 1970, p. 530.)

Two other rates, the *specificity* and the *sensitivity,* can also be approximated. These rates give the probability of making correct decisions in a diagnostic setting. They are defined in Exercises 5 and 6 of this section.

The technique demonstrated in Example 3.4.1 can be used to estimate conditional probabilities in settings other than diagnostic tests. However, a word of caution is in order. If all row and column totals are random, then *any* conditional probability can be approximated. If not, then the only probabilities that can be approximated are those for which the sample sizes for the *given events are fixed* by the researcher. The reason for this is explained in Example 3.4.2.

> **EXAMPLE 3.4.2.** Suppose that a new home-pregnancy test has been developed. An experiment is conducted to approximate the false-positive and false-negative rates of the test. Five women who are known to be pregnant and 10 women who are not pregnant are selected to participate in the study. The new test is used on each and the results are given in Table 3.3 (data are fictitious).
>
> Some conditional probabilities can be reliably approximated from these data whereas others cannot. For instance,

$$P[\text{are pregnant} \mid \text{test pregnant}]$$

cannot be approximated, but

$$P[\text{test pregnant} \mid \text{are pregnant}]$$

can be. What is the difference between the two? Simply this: In finding the former, one must approximate from the data the probability of a randomly selected individual's being pregnant and testing pregnant. Since the experimenter fixed the number of pregnant women in the experiment at 5, the approximated probability of this event was forced to be at most $\frac{5}{15}$. Because of this artificial constraint, the probability that an individual who tests pregnant is pregnant cannot be approximated from this experiment. However, in finding

TABLE 3.3

	True state		
	Not pregnant (true −)	**Pregnant (true +)**	
Pregnant (+)	5	1	6 (Random)
Not pregnant (−)	5	4	9 (Random)
	10 (Fixed)	5 (Fixed)	15 (Fixed)

the latter, the five pregnant women randomly selected by the experimenter can be viewed as being a random sample from the population of all pregnant women. Thus we can use the relative frequency approach to approximate the probability that a pregnant woman will test pregnant to be $\frac{1}{5}$.

We have seen that the false-positive and false-negative rates for a diagnostic test can be approximated from a table with all row and column totals free to vary. Example 3.4.2 shows that these can also be approximated whenever the row (or column) totals are fixed as long as the totals that are fixed relate to the number of true-positive and true-negative subjects in the study.

Relative Risk

Some studies are designed to investigate a factor that the researcher believes might be associated with the development of a specific disease or condition. Such a factor is called a *risk* factor. To conduct the study two samples are selected. One sample, denoted by E, consists of subjects who have been exposed to the risk factor; the others, denoted by E', have not been exposed to the risk factor.

At an appropriate time each subject is classified as either having the disease, D, or not having it, D'. Two conditional probabilities are of interest. They are the probability that the disease is present given that the subject was at risk, $P[D \mid E]$, and the probability that the disease is present given that the subject was not at risk, $P[D \mid E']$. Since the sample sizes for events E and E' are fixed, each of these probabilities can be approximated using the idea demonstrated in Example 3.4.2. A measure of the impact of the risk factor can be approximated from these conditional probabilities. This measure, called *relative risk* (RR), is estimated by

$$\text{RR} \doteq \frac{P[D \mid E]}{P[D \mid E']}$$

Remember that since the probabilities used in the calculation are approximate, the ratio obtained is only an estimate of the true relative risk. If $\text{RR} = 1$, then there appears to be no association between the risk factor and the development of the disease. If $\text{RR} > 1$, then an individual exposed to risk is assumed to be more likely to develop the disease than one not at risk. A value of $\text{RR} < 1$ means that an individual at risk appears to be less likely to develop the disease than one not at risk. Example 3.4.3 demonstrates the idea.

EXAMPLE 3.4.3. A study of age of the mother at the birth of the child as a risk factor in the development of sudden infant death syndrome (SIDS) is conducted. A total of 7330 women who were under the age of 25 when the child was born were selected for study. Of these, 29 had children afflicted with SIDS. Of the 11,256 women selected for study who were 25 or older when their children were born, 15 had children with SIDS. These data are shown in Table 3.4. From this table we see that

$$P[D \mid E] = \frac{29}{7330} \quad \text{and} \quad P[D \mid E'] = \frac{15}{11,256}$$

▓ **TABLE 3.4**

Age as a risk factor in the development of SIDS

		SIDS		
		Yes	No	
Age	Under 25 years	29	7,301	7,330 (Fixed)
	25 years or over	15	11,241	11,256 (Fixed)

The estimated relative risk is

$$\text{RR} \doteq \frac{P[D\,|\,E]}{P[D\,|\,E']} = \frac{29/7330}{15/11,256} = 2.96$$

We can conclude that the child of a younger mother (under 25) is approximately 2.96 times more likely to develop SIDS than one born to an older mother. (Based on data reported in Norman Lewak, Bea van der Berg, and Bruce Beckwith, "Sudden Infant Death Syndrome Risk Factors: Prospective Data Review," *Clinical Pediatrics,* vol. 18, 1979, pp. 404–411.)

Since $P[D\,|\,E]$ and $P[D\,|\,E']$ can be approximated from tables in which all row and column totals are random, relative risk can be approximated from such tables. Exercise 14 of this section is an example of this setting.

▓ **EXERCISES 3.4**

1. In a study of 300 pairs of twins, the twins were questioned as to whether they were identical. Then other factors such as ABO blood group, MN blood type, and Rh blood type were considered. On the basis of these traits, the twins were classified as identical (+) or nonidentical (−). The latter classification procedure is considered to be the true classification. The purpose of the study is to test the ability of twins to self-classify. The results are shown in Table 3.5. All row and column totals are random. Approximate the false-positive and false-negative rates of the self-classification procedure.

▓ **TABLE 3.5**

Self-classification	True classification		
	Nonidentical (−)	Identical (+)	
+	12	54	
−	130	4	
			200

2. A study is run to investigate the association between flower color and fragrance in wild azaleas found in the Great Smoky Mountains. A 5-acre tract of mountain terrain was selected and found to contain 200 blooming plants. Each was classified both by color and by the presence or absence of fragrance. The results are shown in Table 3.6. Using these data, approximate, if possible, each of the following

TABLE 3.6

		Color	
		No	Yes
Fragrance	Yes	12	118
	No	50	20
			200

probabilities. If it is not possible to approximate a particular probability from the given data, explain why.

(a) P[a randomly selected azalea has a fragrance]
(b) P[a randomly selected azalea is colored]
(c) P[a randomly selected azalea is colored and has a fragrance]
(d) P[a randomly selected azalea is colored given that it has a fragrance]
(e) P[a randomly selected azalea has a fragrance given that it is colored]

3. The results shown in Table 3.7 were obtained in a study designed to test the ability of a surgical pathologist to correctly score surgical biopsy samples as malignant or benign. From the data approximate α and β.

TABLE 3.7

Pathologist report	True state	
	Benign (−)	Malignant (+)
+	7	79
−	395	19
		500

4. A study was conducted to investigate a procedure for detecting renal disease in patients with hypertension. Using the new procedure, experimenters screened 137 hypertensive patients. Then the presence or absence of renal disease was determined by another method. The data obtained are shown in Table 3.8. Use the data to approximate the false-positive and false-negative rates for the test.

5. *Definition:* The *specificity* of a test is the probability that the test results will be negative given that the subject is a true negative. Approximate the specificity of the test of Exercise 1. In general, would you want the specificity of a test to be high or low? Explain.

TABLE 3.8

Disease detected	True state	
	Disease absent (−)	Disease present (+)
Yes (+)	23	44
No (−)	60	10
		137

6. *Definition:* The *sensitivity* of a test is the probability that the test results will be positive given that the subject is a true positive. Approximate the sensitivity of the test of Exercise 1. In general, would you want the sensitivity of a test to be high or low? Explain.

7. One hundred patients and 75 normal subjects were given a diagnostic urine test. Sixty percent were reported positive. There were eight false negatives. What was the approximate false-positive rate?

8. Approximate the specificity and sensitivity of the test of Example 3.4.1. In general, what is the relationship between the specificity and the false-positive rate? What is the relationship between the sensitivity and the false-negative rate?

9. A study of an enzyme-linking immunoassay (EIA) technique for screening blood donors for HIV antibodies is conducted. Subjects are tested for HIV using the EIA technique, and the presence or absence of the antibodies is then confirmed at a later date. Data are given in Table 3.9.

▨ **TABLE 3.9**

	True state	
EIA test	**Antibodies absent (−)**	**Antibodies present (+)**
+	1,000	30
−	98,969	1
		100,000

(*a*) Estimate the false-positive rate of the test. Use this to find the specificity of the test.

(*b*) Estimate the false-negative rate of the test. Use this to find the sensitivity of the test.

(Based on information found in Richard Eisenstaedt and Thomas Getzen, "Screening Blood Donors for HIV Antibody: Cost Benefit Analysis," *American Journal of Public Health,* vol. 78, no. 4, April 1988, pp. 450–454.)

10. The *positive predictive value* of a test is defined to be the probability that an individual is a true positive given that the test result is positive. This can be approximated from a table in which all row and column totals are free to vary. Approximate the positive predictive value of the self-classification test of Exercise 1.

11. The *negative predictive value* of a test is defined to be the probability that an individual is a true negative given that the test result is negative. This can be approximated from a table in which all row and column totals are free to vary. Approximate the negative predictive value of the self-classification test of Exercise 1.

12. Approximate the positive and negative predictive values of the test for renal disease of Exercise 4.

13. A study is conducted to determine clinical symptoms that aid in the identification of whooping cough. One symptom investigated is acute cough of any duration. Data obtained on 233 children studied are shown in Table 3.10. Approximate the false-positive rate and the positive predictive value of the test. Does it appear that the presence of acute cough alone is a good indicator of the presence of whooping

TABLE 3.10

	True state	
Cough present	No whooping cough (−)	Whooping cough present (+)
Yes (+)	83	116
No (−)	32	2
		233

cough? Explain. (Based on information found in Peter Patriaca et al., "Sensitivity and Specificity of Clinical Case Definition of Pertussis," *American Journal of Public Health,* vol. 78, no. 7, July 1988, pp. 833–835.)

14. In 1985, many Asian children were adopted by American families. Some of these children had been exposed to the hepatitis B virus and were capable of transmitting the virus to others. In a study of the risk involved, the data of Table 3.11 were obtained. Cell entries represent the number of close family members found with the virus, and all row and column totals are random. Approximate the relative risk. (Based on information found in Andrew Friede et al., "Transmission of Hepatitis B Virus from Adopted Asian Children to Their American Families," *American Journal of Public Health,* vol. 78, no. 1, January 1988, pp. 26–29.)

TABLE 3.11

		Virus present	
		Yes	No
Exposed to risk	Yes	7	70
	No	4	228

15. It is known that AIDS patients often develop tuberculosis. A study of the risk factors associated with the development of tuberculosis in these patients is conducted. One factor considered is the abuse of intravenous drugs. Of the 1992 patients in the study, 307 had abused intravenous drugs. Forty-six of the patients had tuberculosis, and of these 11 had abused intravenous drugs. (Based on data reported in Timothy Cote et al., "The Present and the Future of AIDS and Tuberculosis in Illinois," *American Journal of Public Health,* vol. 80, no. 8, August 1990, pp. 950–953.)

    (*a*) Construct a 2 × 2 table to display these data.

    (*b*) Find and interpret the relative risk.

16. In a study of the relationship between the regular use of hair dye and the development of leukemia, 577 leukemia patients and 1245 persons free from the disease (controls) were selected and questioned concerning their use of hair dye. Forty-three patients and 55 controls claimed to have had significant exposure to hair dye. (Based on information found in Kenneth Cantor et al., "Hair Dye Use and Risk of

▓ **TABLE 3.12**

		Leukemia present	
		Yes	**No**
Use hair dye	Yes	43	55
	No		
		577 (Fixed)	1245 (Fixed)

Leukemia and Lymphoma," *American Journal of Public Health,* vol. 78, no. 5, May 1988, pp. 570–571.)

(*a*) Complete Table 3.12.

(*b*) In this case, is it possible to approximate relative risk using the definition given in this section? Explain.

(*c*) Some idea of the impact of hair dye use can be obtained by considering the ratio

$$\frac{P[E \mid D]}{P[E \mid D']}$$

where E is the event that the individual was exposed to risk and D the event that leukemia is present. Can each of the conditional probabilities involved in this ratio be estimated? If so, evaluate and interpret the ratio.

▓ 3.5
INDEPENDENCE

Two important relationships may exist between events. The first, being mutually exclusive, is discussed in Section 3.1; the second, being *independent,* is described here. The mathematical term has virtually the same meaning as its English counterpart. Webster defines *independent* objects as objects acting "irrespective of each other." Thus two events are independent if one may occur irrespective of the other. That is, the occurrence or nonoccurrence of one has no effect on the occurrence or nonoccurrence of the other. In many cases, we can determine on a purely intuitive basis whether two events are independent. For example, events A_1, the patient has tennis elbow, and A_2, the patient has appendicitis, are intuitively independent. The fact that the patient has appendicitis should have no bearing on whether she or he has tennis elbow, and vice versa!

In some instances, however, the issue is not clear-cut. Then we need a precise mathematical definition of the term to be able to determine without a doubt whether two events are, in fact, independent. The definition is easy to develop. For example, suppose that, based on the symptoms described, you feel that the probability that the patient has appendicitis is .9 (A_2). Now, suppose you are suddenly given the additional information that the patient has tennis elbow (A_1). What do you think is the probability of the patient's having appendicitis? Obviously, the answer is still .9! Since A_1 and A_2 are independent, the new information is irrelevant and has no effect at all on the original probability. Thus independence between two events A_1 and A_2 results in the conditional probability $P[A_2 \mid A_1]$ being equal to the probability originally assigned to event A_2. This characterization is taken as the definition of the term *independent events*.

DEFINITION 3.5.1. Independent events. Let A_1 and A_2 be events such that $P[A_1] \neq 0$. These events are *independent* if and only if

$$P[A_2 \mid A_1] = P[A_2]$$

EXAMPLE 3.5.1. Assume that among the U.S. population as a whole, 55% are overweight (A_1), 20% have high blood pressure (A_2), and 60% are overweight or have high blood pressure. Is the fact that a person is overweight independent of the state of his or her blood pressure? The answer to this question is not obvious. Using the general addition principle yields

$$P[A_1 \text{ and } A_2] = P[A_1] + P[A_2] - P[A_1 \text{ or } A_2]$$

or, in this case,

$$P[A_1 \text{ and } A_2] = .55 + .20 - .60 = .15$$

Thus
$$P[A_2 \mid A_1] = \frac{P[A_1 \text{ and } A_2]}{P[A_1]}$$

$$= \frac{.15}{.55} = \frac{15}{55} = .27$$

Since $P[A_2 \mid A_1] = .27 \neq .20 = P[A_2]$, we may conclude that the events are not independent. Practically speaking, the fact that a person is overweight increases the probability of his or her having high blood pressure.

Notice that we are assuming that the probabilities given in Example 3.5.1 are based on population data and are therefore exact. In this setting Definition 3.5.1 can be used to test two events for independence. In practice, this situation seldom arises. Rather, we are usually dealing with relative frequency probabilities obtained from samples drawn from the population. In this case, Definition 3.5.1 cannot be used to test for independence. However, a test that is appropriate for samples is developed in Chapter 12.

Definition 3.5.1 is logical and easy to understand. However, it is not the definition commonly given for the term *independent events*. The usual definition can be derived by noting the following:

$$P[A_2 \mid A_1] = \frac{P[A_1 \text{ and } A_2]}{P[A_1]} \qquad \text{is always true as long as } P[A_1] \neq 0$$

$$P[A_2 \mid A_1] = P[A_2] \qquad\qquad \text{if } P[A_1] \neq 0 \text{ and the events are independent}$$

Thus if A_1 and A_2 are independent, both equations hold simultaneously. So we have two expressions for $P[A_2 | A_1]$, which can be equated to yield

$$\frac{P[A_1 \text{ and } A_2]}{P[A_1]} = P[A_2]$$

Multiplying both sides of this equation by $P[A_1]$, we obtain $P[A_1 \text{ and } A_2] = P[A_1]P[A_2]$, the usual definition of the term *independent events*.

> **DEFINITION 3.5.2. Independent events.** Let A_1 and A_2 be events. Then A_1 and A_2 are *independent* if and only if $P[A_1 \text{ and } A_2] = P[A_1]P[A_2]$.

Notice that when events are independent, to find the probability that both A_1 *and* A_2 occur, we multiply. Thus, as mentioned in Section 3.2, the word *and* is typically a signal that probabilities will be multiplied.

> **EXAMPLE 3.5.2.** Studies in population genetics indicate that 39% of the available genes for determining the Rh blood factor are negative. Based on this information, what is the probability that a randomly selected individual will have Rh-negative blood? Rh-negative blood occurs if and only if the individual involved has two negative genes. Since one gene is inherited from each parent, it may be assumed that the gene type of the first gene is independent of that of the second. Hence the probability that an individual has two negative genes is $(.39)(.39) \doteq .15$. (Based on information from William Keeton and Carol McFadden, *Elements of Biological Science,* W. W. Norton, New York, 1983.)

The idea of independence can be extended to more than two events. A collection of events is said to be independent whenever any subcollection of events satisfies the property that the probability of their simultaneous occurrence is equal to the product of the individual event probabilities. Example 3.5.3 demonstrates this idea in the context of a problem involving a tree diagram. Notice that we are now in a position to calculate path probabilities in a setting in which the paths are not equally likely.

> **EXAMPLE 3.5.3.** During the course of a day, a particular diagnostic test is run on three unrelated patients. The test is 90% accurate on both those who do and those who do not have the condition that the test is designed to detect. What is the probability that exactly two of the three test results are in error?
>
> A tree diagram will help answer this question. Within the tree, C represents a correct decision and E an error. Appropriate probabilities are listed in Figure 3.11. Starred paths represent cases of interest. A typical path represents the simultaneous occurrence of three

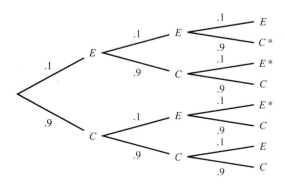

FIGURE 3.11

Results of a diagnostic test (three patients).

distinct events. For example, the path EEC represents the occurrence of an error with the first patient (E_1) and an error with the second (E_2) and a correct decision with the third (C_3). Since the tests are run independently on different patients, we can assume that the results are independent. By Definition 3.5.2, the probability along each path can be found by *multiplying* the probabilities that appear along the path. Thus, for instance, $P[E_1$ and E_2 and $C_3] = P[E_1]P[E_2]P[C_3] = (.1)(.1)(.9) = .009$. Since there are three paths which involve exactly two errors, the probability of obtaining exactly two errors in some order is $3(.009) = .027$.

Definition 3.5.2 must be used with care. One must be certain that it is reasonable to assume that events are independent before applying the definition to compute the probability that a series of events will occur. The danger of erroneously assumed independence is illustrated in Example 3.5.4.

EXAMPLE 3.5.4. An Atomic Energy Commission Study, WASH 1400, reported the probability of a nuclear accident such as that which occurred at Three Mile Island in March 1978 to be 1 in 10 million. Yet, the accident did occur. According to Mark Stephens, "The methodology of WASH 1400 made use of event trees—sequences of actions that would be necessary for accidents to take place. These event trees did not assume any interrelation between events—that they might be caused by the same error in judgment or as part of the same mistaken action. The statisticians who assigned probabilities in the writing of WASH 1400 said, for example, that there was a one-in-a-thousand risk of one of the auxiliary feed-water control valves—the twelves—being closed. And if there is a one-in-a-thousand chance of one valve being closed, the chances of both valves being closed is one-thousandth of that, or a million to one. But both of the twelves were closed by the same man on March 26—and one had never been closed with the other." The events A_1: the first valve is closed and A_2: the second valve is closed were not independent. However, they were treated as such when calculating the probability of an accident. This, among other things, led to an underestimate of the accident potential (from *Three Mile Island* by Mark Stephens, Random House, 1980).

EXERCISES 3.5

1. Which of the following pairs of events do you think are independent? Which are mutually exclusive?

   A_1: A mother has rubella during the first 3 months of pregnancy.
   B_1: A mother's child is born dead or deformed.
   A_2: A man is sterile.
   B_2: A man contracts mumps as an adult.
   A_3: A male and female rat are caged together.
   B_3: The female rat is sterile.
   A_4: A child is nearsighted.
   B_4: A child is farsighted.
   A_5: An area has been strip-mined.
   B_5: The area experiences frequent floods.
   A_6: A rabbit is inoculated with polio virus.
   B_6: The rabbit's blood contains antibodies to polio.

A_7: A rabbit is inoculated with polio virus.

B_7: The rabbit's blood contains antibodies to measles.

2. Argue on an intuitive level that if two events that are not impossible are mutually exclusive, then they cannot be independent. Prove this result mathematically. *Hint:* Show that, under the stated conditions, Definition 3.5.2 cannot be satisfied.

3. The most common water pollutants are organic. Since most organic materials are broken down by bacteria that require oxygen, an excess of organic matter may result in a depletion of available oxygen. In turn, this can be harmful to other organisms living in the water. The demand for oxygen by the bacteria is called the *biological oxygen demand* (BOD). Assume that among streams located near industrial complexes 35% have a high BOD, 10% show high acidity, and 4% have both characteristics. Are the events a stream has a high BOD and a stream has high acidity independent? Find the probability that a stream has high acidity given that it has a high BOD.

4. Approximately 50% of the population is male, 68% drinks to some extent, and 38.5% drinks and is male. Given that a randomly selected individual is male, find the probability that he drinks. Is a person's drinking status independent of gender?

5. The probability of contracting serum hepatitis from a unit of blood is .01. A patient receives two units of blood during a hospital stay. What is the probability that he will not contract serum hepatitis from this source?

6. Even though tetanus is rare in the United States, it is fatal 70% of the time. If three persons contract tetanus during one year, what is the probability that at least two of the three will die? (*Hint:* Use a tree.)

7. Consider the tree diagram of Exercise 5 of Section 2.2. Assume that the probabilities of a patient's exhibiting headache, fever, body, rash or muscle soreness are .7, .8, .1, and .2, respectively. Assume also that the appearances of these symptoms are independent of one another.

   (*a*) Find the path probability for each of the 16 paths of the tree.

   (*b*) Find the probability that the diagnosis could be systemic food allergy

   (*c*) Find the probability that the diagnosis could be flu.

   (*d*) Find the probability that the diagnosis could be neither a food allergy nor flu.

8. *Hardy–Weinberg Principle.* The Hardy–Weinberg principle from population genetics is named after G.H. Hardy, an English mathematician, and G. Weinberg, a German physician. Basically, the principle states that a population is genetically stable in succeeding generations. The mathematical basis for this principle relies on the notion of independence in two ways: independent mating and independent inheritance of one gene from each parent in offspring. Consider the distribution of a single pair of genes A and a. Each member of the population will have two of these genes. Thus we have three genotypes: AA, Aa, and aa. Suppose that these genotypes are present in the population in the ratio $\frac{1}{4}AA$, $\frac{1}{2}Aa$, $\frac{1}{4}aa$. If we assume that members of the population mate at random, the nine possible mating types are as listed in Table 3.13. Each mating type leads to one or more possible genotypes among offspring. Given independence, the first few rows are as shown. Complete the table. Once it is complete, verify that one-fourth of the offspring are of genotype AA, half are of Aa, and one-fourth are of aa, which verifies the Hardy–Weinberg principle.

◼ **TABLE 3.13**

Mating type		Probability of match	Possible offspring genotype	Probable offspring genotype	Path probability
Male	**Female**				
AA	AA	$\frac{1}{4} \cdot \frac{1}{4}$	AA	1	$\frac{1}{16}$
AA	Aa	$\frac{1}{4} \cdot \frac{1}{2}$	AA	$\frac{1}{2}$	$\frac{1}{16}$
			Aa	$\frac{1}{2}$	$\frac{1}{16}$
AA	aa	$\frac{1}{4} \cdot \frac{1}{4}$	Aa	1	$\frac{1}{16}$
Aa	AA				
Aa	Aa				
Aa	aa				
aa	AA				
aa	Aa				
aa	aa				

9. Some characteristics in animals are said to be sex-influenced. For example, the production of horns in sheep is governed by a pair of alleles, H and h. The allele H for the production of horns is dominant in males but recessive in females. The allele h for hornlessness is dominant in females and recessive in males. Thus, given a heterozygous male (Hh) and a heterozygous female, the male will have horns and the female will be hornless. Assume that two such animals mate.

(a) Draw a tree to represent the possible genotypes relative to the gene determining horn production.

(b) Assume that each offspring of this mating is just as likely to be male as female. Find the probability that a given offspring will be male and have horns. Find the probability that a given offspring will be female and have horns.

(c) Find the probability that a given offspring will have horns. Show that events A, the offspring is male, and B, the offspring has horns, are not independent.

10. Verify that the probability that a randomly selected individual is Rh-positive homozygous ($+\ +$) is approximately .37 and that the probability that he or she is Rh-positive heterozygous ($+\ -$ or $-\ +$) is approximately .48.

11. An individual's blood group (A, B, AB, O) is independent of the Rh factor classification.

(a) Find the probability that a randomly selected individual will have AB negative blood given that the individual is a white American (see Examples 3.5.2 and 3.1.2).

(b) Find the probability that a randomly selected individual has AB negative blood given that the individual is a black American (see Example 3.5.2 and Exercise 12 of Section 3.1).

(c) Is having AB negative blood independent of the racial group, black or white, to which the individual belongs? Explain.

(d) Is having A negative blood independent of the racial group, black or white, to which the individual belongs? Explain.

12. Consider the relative risk defined in Section 3.4. Prove that if RR = 1, then events D, the disease is present, and E, the patient is exposed to risk, are independent. *Hint:* Set $P[D \mid E]$ equal to $P[D \mid E']$ and apply the definition of conditional probability to each side of the equation. Remember that $P[E'] = 1 - P[E]$. Show that $P[D \text{ and } E] = P[D]P[E]$.

13. A physician orders 10 independent diagnostic tests to be run on the same patient. The false-positive rate for each test is .05. What is the probability of obtaining at least one erroneous positive result?

14. If the false-positive rate of each test in a battery of tests is .05, how many independent tests can be included in the battery if we want the probability of obtaining at least one false-positive result to be at most .20?

▪ 3.6
THE MULTIPLICATION RULE

We can find $P[A_1 \text{ and } A_2]$ if the events are independent. Furthermore, if the proper information is given, the general addition rule can be used to find this quantity. Is there any other way to find the probability of the simultaneous occurrence of two events if the events are not independent? The answer is yes, and the method used is easy to derive. We know that

$$P[A_2 \mid A_1] = \frac{P[A_1 \text{ and } A_2]}{P[A_1]}$$

regardless of whether the events are independent. Multiplying each side of this equation by $P[A_1]$, we obtain the following formula, called the *multiplication rule:*

$$\boxed{P[A_1 \text{ and } A_2] = P[A_2 \mid A_1]P[A_1] \quad \text{multiplication rule}}$$

The use of this rule is illustrated in Example 3.6.1.

EXAMPLE 3.6.1. The use of plant appearance in prospecting for ore deposits is called geobotanical prospecting. One indicator of copper is a small mint with a mauve-colored flower. Suppose that, for a given region, there is a 30% chance that the soil has a high copper content and a 23% chance that the mint will be present there. If the copper content is high, there is a 70% chance that the mint will be present. What is the probability that the copper content will be high and the mint will be present? If we let A_1 denote the event that the copper content is high and A_2 the event that the mint is present, we are asked to find $P[A_1 \text{ and } A_2]$. We are given that $P[A_1] = .30$, $P[A_2] = .23$, and $P[A_2 \mid A_1] = .70$. By the multiplication rule

$$P[A_1 \text{ and } A_2] = P[A_2 \mid A_1]P[A_1]$$

$$= .70(.30)$$

$$= .21$$

The use of the multiplication rule in a genetics setting is illustrated in Example 3.6.2.

EXAMPLE 3.6.2. When a mother is Rh negative and her child is Rh positive, a blood incompatibility exists that may lead to erythroblastosis fetalis, a condition in which the mother forms an antibody against fetal Rh which leads to the destruction of fetal red blood cells. What is the probability that a randomly selected child will have this condition?

One way for the child to have this problem is for the father to be Rh-positive heterozygous ($+-$ or $-+$) and pass a positive gene to the child while the mother is Rh negative. To find the probability of this combination of events we must find $P[(A_1$ and $A_2)$ and $A_3]$ where A_1 denotes the event that the father is Rh-positive heterozygous, A_2 that the father passes a positive gene to the child, and A_3 that the mother is Rh negative. Notice that events A_1 and A_2 are not independent; the fact that the father is positive heterozygous does have a bearing on the child's ability to obtain a positive gene from this source. Via the multiplication rule,

$$P[A_1 \text{ and } A_2] = P[A_2 \mid A_1]P[A_1]$$

From Exercise 10 of Section 3.5, we know that $P[A_1] \doteq .48$. Since one gene is inherited at random from the father, $P[A_2 \mid A_1] = .5$. Hence

$$P[A_1 \text{ and } A_2] \doteq .5(.48) = .24$$

Since the mother's gene type has no effect on the father or on his ability to convey a positive gene to the child, A_3 is independent of A_1 and A_2. From Example 3.5.2, we know that $P[A_3] \doteq .15$. Hence by definition of independence,

$$P[(A_1 \text{ and } A_2) \text{ and } A_3] \doteq .24(.15) = .0360$$

There are other ways for the condition to be present. Exercise 1 outlines these and allows you to compute the probability that a child will contract the problem from any source.

EXERCISES 3.6

1. A child will have erythroblastosis fetalis if the mother is Rh negative and the father is Rh-positive homozygous ($++$). Use the information given in Exercise 10 of Section 3.5 to find the probability of this occurring. Find the probability that a randomly selected child will have the condition by combining this result with that obtained in Example 3.6.2.
2. Studies indicate that 82% of all professional men drink. If they drink, 18% are heavy drinkers. What is the probability that a randomly selected professional man drinks and drinks heavily?
3. Of all cancer patients, 52% are male. Overall 40% of all patients survive for at least 5 years after the original diagnosis. However, for males the 5-year survival rate is only 35%. What is the probability that a randomly selected cancer patient will be male and survive for at least 5 years?
4. The probability that a unit of blood was donated by a paid donor is .67. If the donor was paid, the probability of contracting serum hepatitis from the unit is .0144. If the donor was not paid, this probability is .0012. A patient receives a unit of blood. What is the probability of the patient's contracting serum hepatitis from this source?

5. Two percent of the general population has diabetes. Of these, only half are aware of their condition. If an individual is selected at random, what is the probability that he or she has diabetes but is unaware of the condition?

6. It is known that the false-positive rate for a test for a specific disease is 4% and that the false-negative rate is 6%. The test shows 15% of the people to be positive. What is the probability that a randomly selected individual actually has the disease? *Hint:* Let $x = P$[true positive] and $1 - x = P$[true negative]. Note that

$$P[\text{test positive}] = P[\text{test positive and are true positive}]$$
$$+ P[\text{test positive and are true negative}]$$

7. In DNA replication, occasionally errors occur that can lead to observable mutations in the organism. Sometimes these errors are chemically induced. Growing bacteria are exposed to a chemical that has a probability of .4 of inducing an error. However, 65% of the errors are "silent" in that they do not lead to an observable mutation. What is the probability of observing a mutated colony? *Hint:* Find P[error and observable].

8. The ability to observe and recall details is important in science. Unfortunately, the power of suggestion can distort memory. A study of recall is conducted as follows: Subjects are shown a film in which a car is moving along a country road. There is no barn in the film. The subjects are then asked a series of questions concerning the film. Half of the subjects are asked: "How fast was the car moving when it passed the barn?" The other half of the subjects are not asked the question. Later, each subject is asked: "Is there a barn in the film?" Of those asked the first question concerning the barn, 17% answer "yes"; only 3% of the others answer "yes." What is the probability that a randomly selected participant in this study claims to have seen the nonexistent barn? Is claiming to see the barn independent of being asked the first question about the barn? *Hint:*

$$P[\text{yes}] = P[\text{yes and asked about barn}] + P[\text{yes and not asked about barn}]$$

(Based on a study reported in *McGraw-Hill Yearbook of Science and Technology,* 1981, pp. 249–251.)

9. *Randomized response method of getting honest answers to sensitive questions.* This is a method used to guarantee an individual that answers to sensitive questions will be anonymous, thus encouraging a truthful response. It operates as follows. Two questions A and B are posed, one of which is sensitive and the other not. The probability of receiving a yes to the nonsensitive question must be known. For example, one could ask

  A: Does your Social Security number end in an odd digit? (Nonsensitive)

  B: Have you ever intentionally filed a fraudulent insurance claim? (Sensitive)
  We know that $P[\text{answer yes} \mid \text{answered } A] = \frac{1}{2}$. We wish to approximate P[answer yes | answered B]. The subject is asked to flip a coin and answer A if the coin comes up heads and answer B if it is tails. In this way, the interviewer does not know which question the subject is answering. Thus a yes answer is not incriminating. There is no way for the interviewer to know whether the subject is saying, "Yes, my Social Security number ends in a odd digit," or "Yes, I have intention-

ally filed a fraudulent claim." The percentage of subjects in the group answering yes is used to approximate P[answer yes].

(a) Use the fact that the event "answer yes" is the event "answer yes and answered A" or "answer yes and answered B" to show that P[answer yes | answered B] equals

$$\frac{P[\text{answer yes}] - P[\text{answer yes} \mid \text{answered } A]P[\text{answered } A]}{P[\text{answered } B]}$$

(b) If this technique is tried on 100 subjects and 60 answered yes, find the approximate probability that a person randomly selected from the group has intentionally filed a fraudulent claim.

10. In a study of high school students, each subject was asked to roll a die and then flip a coin. If the coin came up heads, the subject was to answer question A below and if tails, question B.

A: Did the die land on an even number?

B: Have you ever smoked marijuana?

In a group of 50 subjects, 35 answered yes. Use this information to approximate the probability that a student randomly selected from this group has smoked marijuana.

3.7
BAYES' THEOREM

The topic of this section is the theorem formulated by the Reverend Thomas Bayes (1761). It deals with conditional probability. Bayes' theorem is used to find P[A | B] when the available information is not directly compatible with that required in Definition 3.3.1. That is, it is used to find P[A | B] when P[A and B] and P[B] are not immediately available.

Bayes' problems can be solved with the aid of a tree diagram. We illustrate the idea before stating the theorem formally.

EXAMPLE 3.7.1. A test has been developed to detect a particular type of arthritis in individuals over 50 years old. From a national survey, it is known that approximately 10% of the individuals in this age group suffer from this form of arthritis. The proposed test was given to individuals with confirmed arthritic disease, and a correct test result was obtained in 85% of the cases. When the test was administered to individuals of the same age group who were known to be free of the disease, a 4% false-positive rate was obtained.

For the test to be useful as a screening test for arthritis, it is necessary that a positive test result be a strong indicator that the disease is present. Let D denote the event that the disease is present and T+ the event that the test result is positive. We want to find P[D | T+], the positive predictive value, and we want it to be high. Since this probability is conditional, the first impulse is to try to use Definition 3.3.1 to find it. However, P[D and T+], the probability that the disease is present and the test result is positive, and P[T+], the probability of obtaining a positive result, are not given. Hence Definition 3.3.1 cannot be used directly; another method is needed to compute the desired probability.

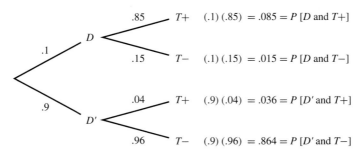

Path probability

FIGURE 3.12

Paths and path probabilities.

To solve the problem, note that these probabilities are given ($T-$ denotes the event that the test result is negative):

$$P[D] = .10 \qquad P[T+ \mid D] = .85 \qquad P[T+ \mid D'] = .04$$
$$P[D'] = .90 \qquad P[T- \mid D] = .15 \qquad P[T- \mid D'] = .96$$

Since we know $P[D]$ and $P[D']$, we begin the tree by listing these events along with their corresponding probabilities. If the disease is present, then we can assign probabilities of .85 and .15 to the events $T+$, the test result is positive, and $T-$, the test result is negative, respectively. If the disease is not present, these conditional probabilities are, respectively, .04 and .96. All these probabilities are shown in Figure 3.12. Notice that the first path probability is $P[D]P[T+ \mid D]$ which, by the multiplication rule, yields $P[D$ and $T+]$.

To find $P[D \mid T+]$, the positive predictive rate, we apply Definition 3.3.1 to obtain

$$P[D \mid T+] = \frac{P[D \text{ and } T+]}{P[T+]}$$

From the tree, we see that $P[D$ and $T+] = .085$. The event $T+$ is represented by paths 1 and 3 and hence $P[T+] = .085 + .036 = .121$. Upon substitution we see that

$$P[D \mid T+] = \frac{.085}{.121} = .70$$

That is, if the test results are positive, there is about a 70% chance that the disease is actually present.

In solving Example 3.7.1 with a tree, we are actually using Bayes' theorem quite naturally. The theorem itself is a formal statement of the technique employed when using a tree. We assume that there is a collection of mutually exclusive events, A_1, $A_2, \ldots, A_n$, such that $P[A_1], P[A_2], \ldots, P[A_n]$ are known and $\sum_{i=1}^{n} P[A_i] = 1$. Such a collection is called a *partition of the sample space*. These events produce the first branching of the tree diagram. We assume that another event B occurs and that $P[B \mid A_i]$ is known for each i. This event produces the second-stage branching of the tree. We want to find the probability that a specific partitioning event A_j occurs given that B has occurred. By Definition 3.3.1,

$$P[A_j \mid B] = \frac{P[A_j \text{ and } B]}{P[B]}$$

In the statement of Bayes' theorem the numerator and denominator are expressed in alternative form by applying the multiplication rule to each. The numerator corresponds to the jth path probability; the denominator is the sum of the path probabilities that correspond to the occurrence of event B. The formal statement of the theorem is given in Theorem 3.7.1. Its proof is outlined in Exercise 6.

THEOREM 3.7.1. Bayes' theorem. Let $A_1, A_2, A_3, \ldots, A_n$ be a collection of events which partition S. Let B be an event such that $P[B] \neq 0$. Then for any of the events, $A_j, j = 1, 2, 3, \ldots, n$,

$$P[A_j \mid B] = \frac{P[B \mid A_j]P[A_j]}{\displaystyle\sum_{i=1}^{n} P[B \mid A_i]P[A_i]}$$

Bayes' theorem is much easier to use in a practical problem than to state formally. To see this, let us reconsider Example 3.7.1 and solve it without use of the tree.

EXAMPLE 3.7.2. In Example 3.7.1 we are asked to find $P[D \mid T+]$, where D is the event that an individual has arthritis and $T+$ is the event that the test result is positive. The two events D and D' partition S. (An individual either does or does not have arthritis.) The event $T+$ occurs with nonzero probability. We are given

$$P[D] = .10 \qquad P[T+ \mid D] = .85 \qquad P[T+ \mid D'] = .04$$
$$P[D'] = .90 \qquad P[T- \mid D] = .15 \qquad P[T- \mid D'] = .96$$

Applying Bayes' theorem, we get

$$P[D \mid T+] = \frac{P[T+ \mid D]P[D]}{P[T+ \mid D]P[D] + P[T+ \mid D']P[D']}$$

$$= \frac{(.85)(.10)}{(.85)(.10) + (.04)(.90)} \doteq .70$$

Note that this is the same result as that obtained by using the tree.

Example 3.7.3 illustrates the use of Bayes' theorem when S is partitioned by more than two events.

EXAMPLE 3.7.3. The blood type distribution in the United States at the time of World War II was thought to be type A, 41%; type B, 9%; type AB, 4%; and type O, 46%. It is estimated that during World War II, 4% of inductees with type O blood were typed as having type A; 88% of those with type A blood were correctly typed; 4% with type B blood were typed as A; and 10% with type AB were typed as A. A soldier was wounded and brought to surgery. He was typed as having type A blood. What is the probability that this was his true blood type?

Let

A_1: He has type A blood.
A_2: He has type B blood.
A_3: He has type AB blood.
A_4: He has type O blood.
 B: He is typed as type A.

We want to find $P[A_1 \mid B]$. We are given that

$P[A_1] = .41 \qquad P[B \mid A_1] = .88$
$P[A_2] = .09 \qquad P[B \mid A_2] = .04$
$P[A_3] = .04 \qquad P[B \mid A_3] = .10$
$P[A_4] = .46 \qquad P[B \mid A_4] = .04$

The tree diagram used to answer this question is shown in Figure 3.13. Notice that by Definition 3.3.1, $P[A_1 \mid B] = P[A_1 \text{ and } B]/P[B]$. The numerator of this probability is the path probability for path 1, namely, .3608. The denominator is the sum of the path probabilities for paths 1, 3, 5, and 7 or .3868. Hence $P[A_1 \mid B] = .3608/.3868 \doteq .93$. By the formal statement of Bayes' theorem we obtain

$$P[A_1 \mid B] = \frac{P[B \mid A_1]P[A_1]}{\sum_{i=1}^{4} P[B \mid A_i]P[A_i]}$$

$$= \frac{(.88)(.41)}{(.88)(.41) + (.04)(.09) + (.10)(.04) + (.04)(.46)}$$

$$\doteq .93$$

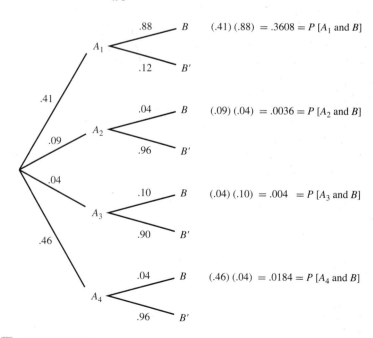

FIGURE 3.13

$P[A_1 \text{ and } B] = .3608; P[B] = .3608 + .0036 + .004 + .0184 = .3868;$
$P[A_1 \mid B] = .3608/.3868 \doteq .93.$

Practically speaking, this means that there is a 93% chance that the blood type is A if it has been typed as A. There is a 7% chance that it has been mistyped as A when it is actually some other type.

■ EXERCISES 3.7

1. Statistics indicate that the probability that a mother will die during childbirth in the United States is .00022. If the mother is not black, the probability of death is .00017, whereas the figure is .00064 if she is black. Assume that 10% of the births recorded are to blacks.
   (a) Draw a tree indicating these probabilities, and find the path probabilities for each of the four paths. (Let D denote the event that the mother dies and B the event that the mother is black.)
   (b) Use the tree of part a to find the probability that a mother who dies in childbirth is black.
   (c) Using Bayes' theorem, find the probability that a mother who dies in childbirth is black, and compare your answer to that obtained in part b.

2. A screening test for cancer of the cervix has a false-negative rate and a false-positive rate, each of .05. Of a certain population of women, 4% have this form of cancer. What is the probability that a randomly selected woman from the population has cancer of the cervix given that she reacts positively to the test?

3. A cancer patient is being treated with a combination of three drugs. It has been observed that when they are used in combination, often two of the three drugs will be inhibited so that, in fact, only one will be actively fighting the tumor. Assume that when this occurs the probability that drug A is acting alone is the same as that for drug B and drug C, namely $\frac{1}{3}$. The effectiveness of each drug alone in producing remission is different. Drug A has been observed to be effective 50% of the time; drug B, 75% of the time; and drug C, 60% of the time. Suppose that the three drugs are used in combination and only one is actively fighting the tumor. The patient has gone into remission. What is the probability that drug B alone was actually responsible for the remission?

4. Duchenne muscular dystrophy is a disease of the muscle that affects young boys. The nature of the disorder is such that it prevents transmission by affected males, but it is spread by carrier females who themselves rarely exhibit any symptoms of the disease. Consider a woman who is the daughter of a known carrier of the disease. She has exactly three sons, all normal. Use Bayes' theorem to find the probability that the woman is a carrier. That is, find P[carrier | three normal sons].

5. It is claimed that the positive predictive value of a test is influenced more by the specificity than the sensitivity. (See Exercises 5, 6, and 10 of Section 3.4.) To demonstrate this, calculate the positive predictive value in each of the settings given in parts a, b, d, and e.
   (a) Sensitivity = .95
       Prevalence (P[true +]) = .10
       Specificity = 1.00
   (b) Sensitivity = .95
       Prevalence = .10
       Specificity = .50

(c) What is the difference in the positive predictive rates as specificity decreases from 1.0 to .5?

(d) Specificity = .95
    Prevalence = .10
    Sensitivity = 1.00

(e) Specificity = .95
    Prevalence = .10
    Sensitivity = .50

(f) What is the difference in the positive predictive rates as sensitivity decreases from 1.00 to .5?

(Based on information found in Victoria Wells, William Halperin, and Michael Thun, "Estimated Predictive Value of Screening for Illicit Drugs in the Workplace," *American Journal of Public Health,* vol. 78, no. 7, July 1988, pp. 817–823.)

6. To derive Bayes' theorem consider Figure 3.14.

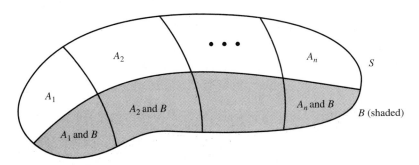

FIGURE 3.14

Events $A_1, A_2, \ldots, A_n$ partition S.

(a) Find an expression for $P[B]$.

(b) Use the multiplication rule to find expressions for $P[A_1 \text{ and } B]$, $P[A_2 \text{ and } B]$, ..., $P[A_n \text{ and } B]$ in which $A_1, A_2, \ldots, A_n$ are the given events.

(c) Use part b to find an alternative expression for $P[B]$.

(d) Apply Definition 3.3.1 to find an expression for $P[A_j \mid B]$.

(e) Substitute into the expression of part d to obtain Bayes' theorem.

Discrete Random Variables

In Chapter 1, we considered some of the methods currently used to describe data sets. Some of these data sets represented the entire population under study; others represented only a sample drawn from a larger population. In the latter case, we did not attempt to draw more than rough conclusions about the parent population from the sample. In Chapters 2 and 3, we discussed probability theory. We saw how the axioms and theorems of probability can be used to answer many questions of a fairly complex nature. We have not yet considered the implications of probability theory to data analysis. That is, we have not yet begun to show how probability theory can be utilized to draw precise conclusions about a population based on a sample drawn from that population. To do this, first we must turn our attention to a topic that provides the link between probability theory and applied statistics. In particular, we reconsider the notion of a *random variable*. This idea was introduced in Chapter 1, and we saw that the random variables of interest to us fall into one of two broad categories. They are either discrete or continuous. We begin by reviewing these definitions.

4.1

DISCRETE AND CONTINUOUS VARIABLES

The concept of a random variable is not difficult. In fact, many of the problems already presented involve random variables even though the term itself was not used at the time. Intuitively, a random variable is a variable whose actual numerical value is determined by chance. Random variables are denoted by uppercase letters and their observed numerical values by lowercase letters.

> **EXAMPLE 4.1.1.** Consider variable Y, the number of oil spills per year affecting U.S. coastal waters. This is a random variable. It does not assume exactly the same value every year. It many vary widely from year to year, and the variability is due to chance. If in a particular year there are five spills, we write $y = 5$.

EXAMPLE 4.1.2. Let Z denote the number of cc's of a drug that should be prescribed for a patient to control epileptic seizures. This variable changes in value from patient to patient as a result of metabolic and other differences among patients. In fact, its value can change in the same patient from time to time; hence it must be considered a random variable.

EXAMPLE 4.1.3. The cephalopods (the "head-foots") are the most highly developed mollusks. One, the octopus, contrary to popular belief, is not large. Variable D, the body diameter of an adult octopus, is a random variable. Not all octopuses are the same size. The variability in size is due to both genetic and environmental factors.

EXAMPLE 4.1.4. Consider variable B, the number of babies born in a given maternity ward before the birth of the first set of Siamese twins. A priori (before the fact), no upper bound can be firmly placed on the set of possible values for B. Conceivably, B can assume any of the values $\{0, 1, 2, 3, 4, \ldots\}$. It is a random variable since chance plays a major role in the birth of Siamese twins.

There are two easily identifiable types of random variables: discrete and continuous. In the material that follows, you must be able to distinguish the two, for computationally they are handled somewhat differently.

DEFINITION 4.1.1. A random variable X is *discrete* if it can assume at most a finite or a countably infinite number of possible values.

In Examples 4.1.1 through 4.1.4, Y, the number of oil spills per year affecting U.S. coastal waters, and B, the number of babies born in a given maternity ward before the birth of the first set of Siamese twins, are both discrete. Variable Y is discrete since the number of possible values for Y is finite. The possible values may reasonably range from 0 to perhaps 50, a finite set of numbers. Variable B is discrete since the set of possible values, $\{0, 1, 2, 3, 4, \ldots\}$, is countably infinite. Usually, discrete variables arise in connection with count data.

DEFINITION 4.1.2. A random variable X is *continuous* if it can assume any value in some interval (or intervals) of real numbers and the probability that it assumes any specific value is 0.

Variables Z, the number of cc's of a drug that should be prescribed for a patient to control seizures, and D, the body diameter of an adult octopus, are both continuous. The amount of drug to be prescribed is not restricted to any finite collection of preset possible values. It may lie anywhere between none at all and, say, .3 cc. That is, Z lies in the interval $[0, .3]$. Similarly, the body diameter of an adult octopus could lie anywhere within reasonable bounds, say, 10 to 30 centimeters. That is, D lies in the interval $[10, 30]$. The statement that the probability that a continuous variable assumes any specific value is 0 is *essential* to the definition. Discrete variables have no such restriction. This restriction is intuitively appealing since if we ask *before* the selection is made, What is the probability that a particular octopus will have a body diameter of *exactly* 12.981 321 069 217 031 2 centimeters? the answer is 0. It is virtually impossible to find an octopus with precisely this diameter—not the slightest bit larger or smaller. We discuss this point further from a mathematical standpoint in Section 4.2. Continuous variables usually arise in connection with measurement data.

▨ EXERCISES 4.1

In each of the following, identify the variable as discrete or continuous.

1. *A*: The number of arms on a chambered nautilus.
2. *V*: The volume of urine output per hour.
3. *B*: The amount of blood lost by a patient during the course of an operation.
4. *H*: The number of hours of light needed per day for a plant to flower.
5. *C*: The number of worker bees in a honeybee society.
6. *R*: The amount of rainfall received per day in a specified region.
7. *S*: The serum bilirubin level in an infant in milligrams per deciliter.
8. *W*: The weight gain of a woman during pregnancy.
9. *T*: The time required for the killer bee infestation to advance 1000 miles.
10. *X*: The number of trials needed to obtain the first successful grafts of a pink dogwood slip onto a white dogwood stem.
11. *C*: Where $C = 1$ if a sampled tree is of suitable size to be cut for lumber and $C = 0$ otherwise.
12. *P*: The systolic blood pressure of a patient with hypertension.
13. *L*: The length of time that a leukemia patient's disease has been in remission.
14. *E*: The elevation at which the tree line ends on a mountain.

▨ 4.2
DISCRETE DENSITY FUNCTIONS AND EXPECTATION

When we are dealing with a variable, it is not enough just to admit that the variable is random. We need to be able to predict in some sense the value that the variable will assume at any time. Since the behavior of a random variable is governed by chance, these predictions must be made in the face of a great deal of uncertainty. The best that can be done is to describe the behavior of the variable in terms of probabilities. Two functions are used to accomplish this, the density function and the cumulative distribution function.

The density function for a discrete random variable gives the probability that the random variable X assumes a specific numerical value x; the cumulative distribution gives the probability of assuming a value up to and including x. The discrete density is defined in Definition 4.2.1.

DEFINITION 4.2.1. Discrete density. Let X be *discrete*. The *density f* for X is

$$f(x) = P[X = x]$$

for x real.

There are several things to note concerning the density in the discrete case. First, f is defined on the entire real line, and for any given real number x, $f(x)$ is the probability that the random variable X assumes the value x. For example, $f(2)$ is the probability that the random variable X assumes the numerical value of 2. Second, since $f(x)$ is a probability, $f(x) \geq 0$ regardless of the value of x. That is, f is never negative. Third, if we sum f over all physically possible values of X, the sum must be 1. That is,

$$\sum_{\text{all } x} f(x) = 1$$

For real values x that are physically impossible, $f(x) = 0$. This fact should be understood in the work to come even if it is not always explicitly stated. Any function that is nonnegative and has the value 1 when summed over its set of possible values can be thought of as being the density for a discrete random variable.

Example 4.2.1 illustrates the use of a tree diagram in generating a density. As you will soon see, the random variable discussed in this example is an example of a random variable that follows a binomial distribution. This distribution arises in practice in diverse settings and for this reason it will be studied in detail in Section 4.4.

EXAMPLE 4.2.1. Batesian mimicry was first described by the British naturalist H. W. Bates in 1862. In Batesian mimicry, an innocuous mimic fools its predator by resembling a stinging or bad-tasting model that the predator has learned to avoid. In an experiment on mimicry, an artificial model is made by dipping mealworms into a solution of quinine to give them a bitter taste. Then they are marked with a green band of cellulose paint, to give them an unusual appearance, and fed to three caged starlings. The starlings learn to associate the special markings with the bitter taste. Next each starling is presented with a mealworm that has not been dipped in quinine but that has been painted to resemble the model. The probability that the mimic will not be eaten by the starling, which normally eats mealworms voraciously, is .8. Let X denote the number of mimics that escape detection. Since it assumes only the values 0, 1, 2, or 3, X is discrete.

To answer probability questions concerning X, we must find its density, $f(x)$. This is done by means of a tree diagram. To construct the tree we let e denote an escape by the mimic and c that the mimic is caught. The tree of Figure 4.1 branches three times to represent the course of action of each of the three starlings used in the experiment. Since the behavior of one starling has no effect on that of any of the others, the probabilities of escape and capture remain .8 and .2, respectively, throughout the experiment. These probabilities

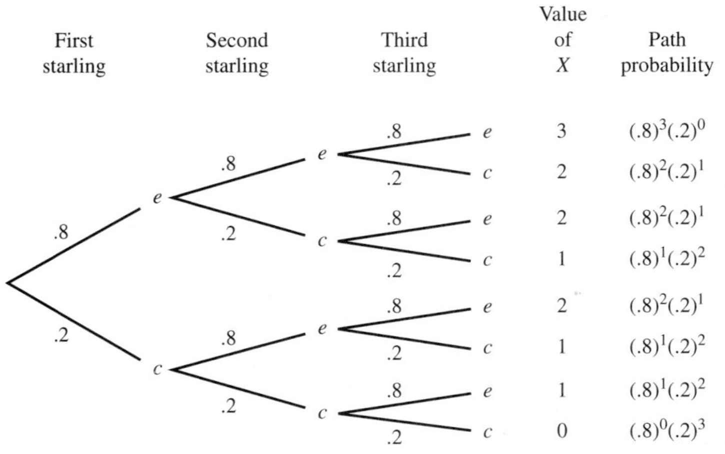

FIGURE 4.1

are listed on the tree. To find the probability of a sequence of events such as *eee*, all three worms escape, we multiply the probabilities along path 1 to obtain $(.8)^3$. To emphasize the fact that this sequence of events guarantees that no worms were caught, we rewrite the path probability in the form $(.8)^3(.2)^0$. Other path probabilities are found in a similar fashion. To find the probability that X assumes a specific value we add the path probability corresponding to that value. The density can be read directly from the tree and is as follows:

x	0	1	2	3
$f(x) = P[X = x]$	$(.2)^3$	$3(.8)^1(.2)^2$	$3(.8)^2(.2)$	$(.8)^3$

or

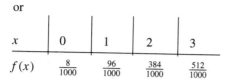

x	0	1	2	3
$f(x)$	$\frac{8}{1000}$	$\frac{96}{1000}$	$\frac{384}{1000}$	$\frac{512}{1000}$

It is understood that $f(x) = 0$ for values of X other than 0, 1, 2, or 3.

Note that, as expected, each entry in row 2 of the table is nonnegative and the entries sum to 1. The table can be used to answer any relevant question posed. For example, the probability that exactly two escape detection is given by $P[X = 2] = f(2) = .384$. The probability that at most two escape is given by

$$P[X \leq 2] = P[X = 0] + P[X = 1] + P[X = 2]$$
$$= f(0) + f(1) + f(2)$$
$$= .008 + .096 + .384 = .488$$

Note also that $P[X < 2] = .104 \neq P[X \leq 2]$. Including or excluding an endpoint in the discrete case can affect the numerical value of the answer.

The above example is intended to illustrate the concept of a discrete density. In practice the theoretical density must often be approximated from sample data. The approximation is given by the relative frequency distribution of the random variable which was discussed in Section 1.3.

Expectation

The density function of a random variable completely describes the behavior of the variable in the ideal, or population, sense. Associated with any random variable when viewed over a population are constants, or "parameters," that are descriptive. Knowledge of the numerical values of these parameters gives the researcher quick insight into the nature of the variables. We mentioned three such parameters: the mean μ, the variance σ^2, and the standard deviation σ in Chapter 1. If the exact density of the variable of interest is known, then the numerical value of each parameter can be found from mathematical considerations. That is the topic of this section. If the only thing available to the researcher is a set of observations on the random variable (a data set), then the values of these parameters cannot be found exactly. They must be approximated by using statistical techniques. That was the topic of Chapter 1 and is the topic of much of the remainder of this text.

To understand the reasoning behind most statistical methods, it is necessary to become familiar with one general concept, namely, the idea of mathematical expectation or expected value. This concept is used in defining most statistical parameters and provides the logical basis for most of the methods of statistical inference presented later in this text. We begin with an intuitive definition of the term.

DEFINITION 4.2.2. Expected value, intuitive. Let X be a random variable. The *expected value* of X, denoted $E[X]$, is the long-run theoretical average value of X.

Recall from Chapter 1 that the theoretical average value of a random variable X is denoted by the Greek letter μ. It is referred to as the population mean. This average value is also called the expected value of X and is denoted $E[X]$. Thus $E[X]$ and μ are interchangeable symbols for the same concept. To get a better understanding of the notion of expected value, consider an experiment in which a single fair die is rolled over and over and each time X, the number obtained, is recorded. A typical sequence of observations might be

$$2, 1, 6, 4, 2, 5, 1, 6, 3, \ldots$$

This sequence generates a corresponding sequence of arithmetic averages:

$$2, \frac{2+1}{2}, \frac{2+1+6}{3}, \frac{2+1+6+4}{4}, \frac{2+1+6+4+2}{5}, \frac{2+1+6+4+2+5}{6}, \ldots$$

or

$$2, 1.5, 3, 3.25, 3, 3.33, \ldots$$

These averages are obviously not constant. They vary as the experiment proceeds, but usually the difference in successive averages decreases as more and more observations are made. That is, as the number of rolls of the die becomes very large, the sequence of averages tends to settle down around some numerical value. This value is the expected value, or the "long-run theoretical average value," for X. Our job is to find a way to determine these expectations from knowledge of the density for X without having to resort to experimentation. Sometimes this can be done by inspection as demonstrated in Example 4.2.2.

EXAMPLE 4.2.2. Consider the experiment of rolling a fair die with the variable X being the number obtained per roll. Variable X is uniformly distributed with density as given:

x	1	2	3	4	5	6
$f(x)$	$\frac{1}{6}$	$\frac{1}{6}$	$\frac{1}{6}$	$\frac{1}{6}$	$\frac{1}{6}$	$\frac{1}{6}$

Notice the symmetry of the density. In the long run, we would expect to roll as many 6s as 1s, as many 2s as 5s, and as many 3s as 4s. Each of these pairs averages to 3.5. Common sense points to 3.5 as the expected value of X. Note also that 3.5 is not a possible value for X. The expected value of a random variable need not be among the physically feasible values of X.

If a density is not symmetric, then its mean cannot be found by inspection. In this case, Definition 4.2.3 is used to compute $E[X]$.

DEFINITION 4.2.3. Expected value, discrete. Let X be a *discrete* random variable with density $f(x)$. The *expected* or *mean value* of X is given by

$$\mu = E[X] = \sum_{\text{all } x} x f(x)$$

Let us compute $E[X]$ for the die problem of Example 4.2.2. Using Definition 4.2.3, we have

$$\mu = E[X] = \sum_{\text{all } x} xf(x)$$

$$= 1 \cdot \tfrac{1}{6} + 2 \cdot \tfrac{1}{6} + 3 \cdot \tfrac{1}{6} + 4 \cdot \tfrac{1}{6} + 5 \cdot \tfrac{1}{6} + 6 \cdot \tfrac{1}{6}$$

$$= 3.5$$

As expected, this result agrees with that found by inspection in Example 4.2.2.

Since the density found in Example 4.2.1 is not symmetric, the expected number of mimics that escape detection cannot be found by inspection. However, $E[X]$ can be computed via Definition 4.2.3.

EXAMPLE 4.2.3. Consider the random variable X, the number of mimics escaping detection in the Batesian mimicry experiment of Example 4.2.1. The density for X is given by

x	0	1	2	3
$f(x)$	$\frac{8}{1000}$	$\frac{96}{1000}$	$\frac{384}{1000}$	$\frac{512}{1000}$

This density is not symmetric, so it is impossible to predict $E[X]$ by inspection. Using Definition 4.2.3, we have

$$\mu = E[X] = 0 \cdot \tfrac{8}{1000} + 1 \cdot \tfrac{96}{1000} + 2 \cdot \tfrac{384}{1000} + 3 \cdot \tfrac{512}{1000}$$

$$= \tfrac{2400}{1000} = \tfrac{12}{5} = 2.4$$

That is, in repeated trials of the same experiment, we would expect the average number of mimics escaping detection to be 2.4.

Given the density for X, it is possible to find the expected value of functions of X such as X^2 or $(X - \mu)^2$. These are particularly important since they allow us to compute σ^2, the variance of X, from knowledge of the density. Exercises 7 to 10 discuss this idea.

EXERCISES 4.2

1. The following table shows the density for the random variable X, the number of persons seeking emergency room treatment unnecessarily per day in a small hospital.

x	0	1	2	3	4	5
$f(x)$	.01	.1	.3	.4	.1	?

(a) Find $f(5)$. What probability does this represent in the context of this problem? 0.09
(b) Find $P[X \leq 2]$. Interpret this probability in the context of this problem. 0.41
(c) Find $P[X < 2]$. 0.11
(d) Find $P[X > 3]$. 0.19

2. The following table shows the density for the random variable X, the number of wing beats per second of a species of large moth while in flight.

x	6	7	8	9	10
$f(x)$	.05	.1	.6	.15	?

(a) Find $f(10)$.
(b) Find $P[X \leq 8]$. Interpret this probability in the context of this problem.
(c) Find $P[X < 8]$.
(d) Find $P[X \geq 7]$.
(e) Find $P[X > 7]$.

3. A compound is developed to give relief from migraine headache. The manufacturer claims that it is 90% effective. It is tried on four patients. Let X denote the number of patients obtaining relief. Use a tree diagram to solve these problems.
(a) Find the density for X, assuming that the claim is correct.
(b) Find $P[X \leq 1]$. Interpret this probability in the context of this problem.
(c) If no one receives relief from the compound, do you think that there is reason to suspect the company's claim of a 90% cure rate? Explain on the basis of the probability involved.

4. An outbreak of mumps among primary school children is in progress. Ten percent of all primary school age children are affected. A pediatrician sees three children of this age during the first hour of her working day. Let X denote the number with mumps. Assume independence and use a tree diagram to find the density for X. Use this to find the probability that among these three children none will have the mumps and then to find the probability that at most one will have the mumps.

5. Consider the following density:

x	-2	-1	0	1	2
$f(x)$	.1	.2	.3	.2	.2

Find $E[X]$ and μ.

6. The following table shows the density for random variable X, the number of adult females in a band of howler monkeys:

x	1	2	3	4	5
$f(x)$	.1	.15	.5	.15	.1

Find the average number of adult females per band.

7. *Expected value of functions of X.* If X is a random variable, then X^2, $X - 1$, $\sqrt{X}$, and any other variable that can be expressed in terms of X are also random variables. Each will have an expected or long-run theoretical average value. If we let $H(X)$ denote some function of X, then its expected value is given by

$$E[H(X)] = \sum_{\text{all } x} H(x)f(x)$$

We illustrate the idea by finding $E[X]^2$ for the single die problem of Example 4.2.2. For this problem,

$$E[X^2] = \sum_{\text{all } x} x^2 f(x)$$

$$= 1^2 \cdot \tfrac{1}{6} + 2^2 \cdot \tfrac{1}{6} + 3^2 \cdot \tfrac{1}{6} + 4^2 \cdot \tfrac{1}{6} + 5^2 \cdot \tfrac{1}{6} + 6^2 \cdot \tfrac{1}{6}$$

$$= \tfrac{91}{6}$$

(a) Find $E[X^2]$ for the random variable of Exercise 1.
(b) Find $E[X^2]$ for the random variable of Exercise 2.
(c) Find $E[X^2]$ for the random variable of Exercise 3.
(d) Find $E[X^2]$ for the random variable of Exercise 4.
(e) Find $E[(X - \mu)^2]$ for the random variable of Exercise 5.
(f) Find $E[(X - \mu)^2]$ for the random variable of Exercise 6.

8. *Variance.* Recall from Section 1.5 that the most common measure of variability in the population is the population variance. We denoted this parameter by the Greek letter σ^2. Its value, like μ, cannot be determined from a sample although it can be estimated via s^2. However, if we have the true density for X available, we can compute σ^2 where σ^2 is defined by $\sigma^2 = \text{Var } X = E[(X - \mu)^2]$. Consider the density

x	1	2	3
$f(x)$	.4	.2	.4

Here $\mu = 2$ by inspection. Hence

$$\sigma^2 = E[(X - 2)^2]$$

$$= (1 - 2)^2(.4) + (2 - 2)^2(.2) + (3 - 2)^2(.4)$$

$$= .8$$

(a) What is the variance of the random variable X of Exercise 5?
(b) What is the variance of the random variable X of Exercise 6?
(c) Find the variance of the random variable X of Example 4.2.2.
(d) Find the variance of the random variable X of Example 4.2.3.

9. *Computational shortcut for computing σ^2.* Exercise 8 defines the variance of a random variable X. It is easy to calculate σ^2 via the definition if the mean value of X is an integer and there are not many values for X. In this exercise, we present an alternative way to find σ^2 that is arithmetically easier to use than the definition. This shortcut formula is given by

$$\sigma^2 = E[(X - \mu)^2] = E[X^2] - (E[X])^2$$

To illustrate, consider the density of Exercise 8. In this case

$$E[X^2] = (1)^2(.4) + (2^2)(.2) + 3^2(.4)$$

$$= 4.8$$

and
$$\sigma^2 = 4.8 - (2)^2 = .8$$

(a) Use the shortcut to verify your answers to parts a to d of Exercise 8.

(b) Consider the density of Exercise 1. Find Var X.

(c) Consider the density of Exercise 2. Find σ^2.

10. *Standard deviation.* Recall from section 1.5 that the sample standard deviation is the nonnegative square root of the sample variance. In the theoretical setting, the standard deviation σ is defined to be the nonnegative square root of σ^2. That is, $\sigma = \sqrt{\sigma^2}$.

(a) Consider the density of Exercise 1. Find σ.

(b) Consider the density of Exercise 2. Find σ.

(c) What physical measurement unit is associated with σ in part a? in part b?

11. Three patients receive injections to desensitize them to insert stings. The serum used is said to be 95% effective. Let X denote the number of patients who actually become desensitized.

(a) Use a tree to derive the table for $f(x)$.

(b) Find and interpret $E[X]$.

(c) Find μ.

(d) Find $E[X^2]$.

(e) Find Var X and σ.

12. Certain genes produce such a tremendous deviation from normal that the organism is unable to survive. Such genes are called lethal genes. An example is the gene that produces a yellow coat in mice, Y. This gene is dominant over that for gray, y. Normal genetic theory predicts that when two yellow mice that are heterozygous for this trait (Yy) mate, $\frac{1}{4}$ of the offspring will be gray and $\frac{3}{4}$ will be yellow. Biologists have observed that these predicted proportions do not, in fact, occur, but that the actual percentages produced are $\frac{1}{3}$ gray and $\frac{2}{3}$ yellow. It has been established that this shift is caused by the fact that $\frac{1}{4}$ of the embryos, those homozygous for yellow (YY), do not develop. This leaves only two genotypes, Yy and yy, occurring in a ratio of 2 to 1, with the former producing a mouse with a yellow coat. For this reason, the gene Y is said to be lethal.

(a) Use a tree diagram to verify that normal genetic theory predicts a 3 to 1 ratio of yellow mice to gray when two heterozygous yellow mice mate.

(b) A mating experiment is conducted in which a pair of heterozygous yellow mice are to be mated. Consider three offspring of this mating. Let X denote the number of yellow mice among the offspring. The density for X is

x	0	1	2	3
$f(x)$	$\frac{1}{27}$	$\frac{6}{27}$	$\frac{12}{27}$	$\frac{8}{27}$

Verify the values in this table.

(c) Find the expected number of yellow mice in a litter of size 3. Find the variance and standard deviation for X.

13. *Chebyshev's inequality.* This inequality points out another useful property of the standard deviation. In particular, it states that "The probability that any random variable X falls within k standard deviations of its mean is at least $1 - 1/k^2$." For example, if we know that X has mean 3 and standard deviation 1, then we can conclude that the probability that X lies between 1 and 5 ($k = 2$ standard deviations from the mean) is at least $1 - 1/2^2 = .75$.

(*a*) Let X denote the amount of rainfall received per week in a region. Assume that $\mu = 1.00$ inch and $\sigma = .25$ inch. Would it be unusual for this region to receive more than 2 inches of rain in a given week? Explain on the basis of Chebyshev's inequality.

(*b*) Let X denote the number of cases of rabies reported in a given state per week. Assume that $\mu = \frac{1}{2}$ and $\sigma^2 = \frac{1}{25}$. Would it be unusual to observe two cases in a given week? Explain on the basis of Chebyshev's inequality.

14. Two drugs are being compared for use in maintaining a steady heart rate in patients who have suffered a mild heart attack. Let X denote the number of heartbeats per minute obtained by using drug A and Y the number per minute with drug B. Consider the following hypothetical and simplified densities:

x	40	60	68	70	72	80	100
$f(x)$	.01	.04	.05	.80	.05	.04	.01

y	40	60	68	70	72	80	100
$f(y)$	.40	.05	.04	.02	.04	.05	.40

(*a*) By inspection, find the mean heart rate for each drug. Is there a difference in the average heart rate produced by the two drugs?

(*b*) By inspection, which drug produces a higher variability in heart rate? Verify your answer by computing Var X and Var Y and comparing the values of these parameters.

(*c*) Find σ_X and σ_Y. What physical measurement unit is associated with these standard deviations?

(*d*) By Chebyshev's inequality, 75% of the patients using drug A will experience a heart rate between what two values? What are these values for drug B? (See Exercise 13.)

4.3
CUMULATIVE DISTRIBUTION FUNCTION

A second function used to calculate probabilities is the cumulative distribution function F. This is the theoretical counterpart of the relative cumulative frequency distribution discussed in Section 1.3. In the discrete case, it is found by summing values found in the density table. It is important to understand this function since the statistical tables that are used throughout the text are cumulative tables. The definition of F is given below.

DEFINITION 4.3.1. **Cumulative distribution function.** Let X be a random variable with density f. The *cumulative distribution function* for X, denoted F, is defined by

$$F(x) = P[X \leq x] \quad \text{for } x \text{ real}$$

Consider a specific real value x_0. In the discrete case, $P[X \leq x_0] = F(x_0)$ is found by summing the density f over all possible values of X that are less than or equal in value to x_0. That is,

$$F(x_0) = \sum_{x \le x_0} f(x)$$

EXAMPLE 4.3.1. Consider the random variable X, the number of mimics escaping detection, of Example 4.2.1. The density f for X is given by

x	0	1	2	3
$P[X = x] = f(x)$	$\frac{8}{1000}$	$\frac{96}{1000}$	$\frac{384}{1000}$	$\frac{512}{1000}$

The cumulative distribution function (or just the distribution function) for X is given by

x	0	1	2	3
$P[X \le x] = F(x)$	$\frac{8}{1000}$	$\frac{104}{1000}$	$\frac{488}{1000}$	$\frac{1000}{1000}$

Suppose we wish to use the cumulative distribution function to find the probability that between 1 and 3 mimics escape detection. That is, we want to find $P[1 \le X \le 3]$. First, we rewrite the expression as shown:

$$P[1 \le X \le 3] = P[X \le 3] - P[X \le 0]$$

In this form, it is evident that

$$P[1 \le X \le 3] = F(3) - F(0)$$

$$= \frac{1000}{1000} - \frac{8}{1000} = \frac{992}{1000} = .992$$

To find $P[X \ge 2]$, next we rewrite the expression as

$$P[X \ge 2] = 1 - P[X \le 1]$$

$$= 1 - F(1)$$

$$= 1 - \frac{104}{1000} = \frac{896}{1000}$$

Note that F does what its name, cumulative distribution function, implies. It sums or accumulates probabilities up to and including the point of interest.

EXERCISES 4.3

1. The following table shows the density for the random variable X, the number of wing beats per second of a species of large moth while in flight:

x	6	7	8	9	10
$f(x)$	.05	.1	.6	.15	.1

(a) Find the table for the cumulative distribution function F.

(b) Use F to find $P[X \le 8]$.

(c) Use F to find $P[X > 7]$. $= 1 - P[X \leqslant 7] = 1 - 0.15 = 0.85$

(d) Use F to find $P[7 \leq X \leq 9]$. $P[X \leqslant 9] - P[X \leqslant 6] = 0.9 - 0.05 = 0.85$

2. The density for the random variable X, the number of persons seeking emergency room treatment unnecessarily per day in a small hospital, is given by

x	0	1	2	3	4	5
$f(x)$	.01	.1	.3	.4	.1	.09

(a) Find the table for the cumulative distribution function.

(b) Find $P[X \leq -2]$.

(c) Using, F, find $P[2 \leq X \leq 4]$.

(d) Find $P[X \leq 6]$.

(e) Find $P[X = 3]$.

(f) Using F, find the probability that more than two will seek emergency room help unnecessarily.

3. Cells in sections of damaged tissue being examined under the microscope are graded for extent of damage by following scale: 0, undamaged; 1, slightly damaged; 2, moderately damaged; 3, extensively damaged. Cells of tissue exposed to 20 minutes of anoxia, an abnormally low oxygen supply, before preparation for microscopic study exhibit the following density, where X is the classification value for damage:

x	0	1	2	3
$f(x)$	0.15	0.25	0.50	0.10

(a) Find the table for the cumulative distribution function F.

(b) Use F to find the probability that a randomly selected cell will be only slightly damaged or undamaged.

(c) Use F to obtain the probability that at least moderate damage is observed in a randomly selected cell.

4. Grafting, the uniting of the stem of one plant with the stem or root of another, is widely used commercially to grow the stem of one variety that produces fine fruit on the root system of another variety with a hardy root system. Most Florida sweet oranges grow on trees grafted to the root of a sour orange variety. An experiment is done with five grafts of this type. The density for X, the number of grafts that fail, is given by

x	0	1	2	3	4	5
$f(x)$	.7	.2	.05	.03	.01	.01

(a) Find the table for F.

(b) Use F to find the probability that at most three grafts fail.

(c) Use F to find the probability that at least two grafts fail.

(d) Use F to verify that the probability of three failures is .03.

5. Let X denote the number of new AIDS cases diagnosed per day at a large metropolitan hospital. Assume that the cumulative distribution for X is

x	0	1	2	3	4	5	6
$F(x)$	.1	.2	.3	.6	.8	.9	1.00

(a) Find the probability that on a randomly selected day,
    i. At most three new cases will be diagnosed.
    ii. At least one new case will be diagnosed.
    iii. No new cases will be diagnosed.
    iv. Between two and four new cases inclusive will be diagnosed.
(b) Find the density for X.
(c) Find the average number of cases diagnosed per day.
(d) Find σ^2.
(e) Find the standard deviation of X. What physical measurement unit is associated with σ?

6. Let F be the cumulative distribution function for a discrete random variable X and let x_0 be the largest possible value that X can assume. What is the numerical value of $F(x_0)$? Explain your reasoning.

4.4
BINOMIAL DISTRIBUTION

We considered the general properties of discrete random variables in some detail in Section 4.1 to 4.3. Here we discuss a specific type of discrete variable, the binomial random variable. Binomial variables arise in connection with experiments that may, on the surface, appear to be quite different in nature. However, upon careful examination, certain common underlying traits become evident. Consider the following experiments.

EXAMPLE 4.4.1

(a) A man and woman, each with one recessive (blue) and one dominant (brown) gene for eye color, parent three children. What is the probability distribution for the number of blue-eyed children?
(b) A carrier of tuberculosis has a 10% chance of passing the disease on to anyone with whom he comes into close contact who has had no prior exposure. During the course of a day, a carrier comes into contact with 10 such individuals. How many would you expect to contract the disease from this source?
(c) A new variety of corn is being developed at an agricultural experimental station. It is hoped that it has 90% germination rate. To verify this figure, 20 seeds are planted in soil of identical composition and given the same care. If the 90% figure is correct, how many seeds are expected to germinate? If 15 or fewer seeds do germinate, is there reason to suspect the 90% figure?
(d) A survey is being conducted to determine public opinion concerning the construction of a dam to control flooding in the New River Valley. Fifteen residents of the area are to be randomly selected and surveyed. If, in fact, 80% of the people living in the area oppose the dam, what is the probability that a majority of those surveyed will be in opposition? What is the probability that between 10 and 14, inclusive, will oppose the construction?

What do these seemingly unrelated experiments have in common? There are essentially four points to be noted:

1. *Each can be viewed as consisting of a fixed number of identical trials* n. In Example 4.4.1a, a trial consists of the birth of a child; $n = 3$. In Example 4.4.1b, a trial is

observing an individual who has come into contact with a carrier of tuberculosis to see whether the individual contracts the disease; $n = 10$. A trial in Example 4.4.1c consists of observing a corn seed to see whether it will germinate; $n = 20$. In Example 4.4.1d, a trial consists of determining a resident's opinion concerning the construction of the dam; $n = 15$.

2. *The outcome of each trial can be classified as a "success" or a "failure."* Here, *success* is defined as observing that characteristic which is being counted. Thus in Example 4.4.1, success consists of obtaining a blue-eyed child, observing an individual who does contract tuberculosis, observing a corn seed that does germinate, and finding a resident of the New River Valley who opposes construction of the dam.

3. *The trials are independent in the sense that the outcome of one trial has no effect on the outcome of any other trial and the probability of success* p *remains the same from trial to trial.* In Example 4.4.1a, these conditions are obviously satisfied with $p = \frac{1}{4}$. Since the fact that one person is susceptible to tuberculosis should have no influence on another's susceptibility, independence may be assumed in Example 4.4.1b with $p = .1$. If we assume that the seeds in Example 4.4.1c are planted so that the growth of one does not impede the growth of any other, then the trials are independent, with $p = .9$. There is some room for debate in Example 4.4.1d. Opinion polling involves sampling without replacement. Once an individual has been polled, he or she is removed from the population. Thus the composition of the population changes, and the probability of success changes slightly from trial to trial. However, if the group being sampled is large, as is usually the case, then the change is so slight as to be negligible. We conclude that for all practical purposes, we have independence with $p = .8$.

4. *The random variable of interest is the number of successes in* n *trials.*

The four trials listed are the general assumptions underlying the *binomial model.* Any random variable X that represents the number of successes in n independent, identical trials, with probability of success p remaining constant from trial to trial, is called a *binomial random variable* with parameters n and p. Notice that to completely identify a binomial random variable, the number of trials and the probability of success must be identified. This is the information that must be known to use binomial tables or to find binomial probabilities via computer packages or statistical calculators. Notice also that p, the probability of success, also represents the proportion of trials that are expected to result in success.

Before considering the density for a binomial random variable let us review two ideas presented in Section 2.5. In particular, we need to recall the meaning of the term *n factorial* (Definition 2.5.1) and the formula for counting the number of arrangements of objects when some of the objects are indistinguishable from one another (Theorem 2.5.1).

DEFINITION 4.4.1. Let n be a positive integer. By *n factorial,* which we denote by $n!$, we mean $n(n - 1)(n - 2) \cdots 3 \cdot 2 \cdot 1$. *Zero factorial,* denoted by $0!$, is defined to be 1.

For example, $5! = 5 \cdot 4 \cdot 3 \cdot 2 \cdot 1 = 120$ and $7! = 7 \cdot 6 \cdot 5 \cdot 4 \cdot 3 \cdot 2 \cdot 1 = 5040$.

Now consider a sequence of n objects of which x are of one type and the rest, $n - x$, are of another. The number of ways to arrange these n objects to form recognizably different patterns is given by

$$\frac{n!}{x! \, (n-x)!}$$

As an example, consider an experiment in which 10 patients are screened for high cholesterol. If we let h denote a high reading and n a normal reading, then the sequence $hnnhhhnhhh$ represents one way in which a 7-high and 3-normal split can occur. Another way to obtain this split is to observe the sequence $nnhhhhnhhhh$. The above formula implies that there are

$$\frac{10!}{7! \, 3!} = \frac{10 \cdot 9 \cdot 8 \cdot 7!}{7! \, 3 \cdot 2 \cdot 1} = 120$$

such sequences. This idea will come into play in the derivation of the binomial density.

To answer the questions posed in Example 4.4.1 or any other probabilistic questions concerning these variables, we must have available the appropriate densities. To see what these densities are, we consider in detail Example 4.1.4a in which the number of trials is small. If a pattern can be found, then this pattern can be generalized to obtain the densities for the variables of the remaining experiments.

EXAMPLE 4.4.2. A man and woman, each with one recessive and one dominant gene for eye color, parent three children. What is the probability distribution for X, the number of blue-eyed children?

This can be viewed as a three-stage process. The sample space and the density for X can be found by considering the tree of Figure 4.2. In the tree, b denotes the birth of a blue-eyed child and B denotes the birth of a brown-eyed child. Since the eye color of one child has no effect on the eye color of any other, the trials are independent and the path probability can be found by multiplying the probabilities that appear along the path. The density

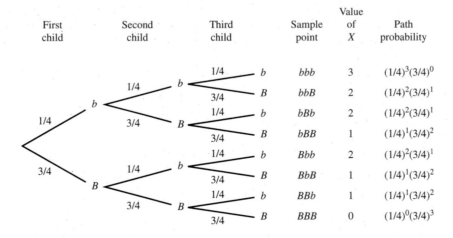

FIGURE 4.2
Eye color in a three-child family.

for X is given by

x	0	1	2	3
$f(x)$	$1\left(\frac{1}{4}\right)^0\left(\frac{3}{4}\right)^3$	$3\left(\frac{1}{4}\right)^1\left(\frac{3}{4}\right)^2$	$3\left(\frac{1}{4}\right)^2\left(\frac{3}{4}\right)^1$	$1\left(\frac{1}{4}\right)^3\left(\frac{3}{4}\right)^0$

To express this density as an equation, we need only look for patterns. It is evident that the success rate of $\frac{1}{4}$ and the failure rate of $\frac{3}{4}$ appear in each probability listed, with the exponent of the success rate being x. Also the sum of the two exponents in each case is 3, the number of trials. Thus, in general, the exponent associated with the failure rate is $3 - x$. The general form of the density is therefore

$$f(x) = k(x)\left(\tfrac{1}{4}\right)^x\left(\tfrac{3}{4}\right)^{3-x} \qquad x = 0, 1, 2, 3$$

where $k(x)$ is a coefficient whose value depends on the value of X in question. That is, the coefficients are not necessarily the same for each value of x. In the example above, when $x = 0$ or $x = 3$, $k(x) = 1$; when $x = 1$ or $x = 2$, $k(x) = 3$. The question to be answered is, What is $k(x)$? Is there a formula for this coefficient? Notice that the coefficient is "path counter." It gives the number of paths through the tree that involve a specified value of X. A path is just a permutation of three letters, x of them being b's and $3 - x$ being B's. By using the formula for finding the number of recognizable arrangements of indistinguishable objects, it is easy to see that

$$k(x) = \frac{3!}{x!\,(3 - x)!}$$

Thus the expression for the density for X is

$$f(x) = \frac{3!}{x!\,(3 - x)!}\left(\frac{1}{4}\right)^x\left(\frac{3}{4}\right)^{3-x} \qquad x = 0, 1, 2, 3$$

The method used to derive the density for X in Example 4.4.2 is independent of both the number of trials involved and the actual numerical value of the success rate. Given any number of trials n and any success rate p, similar reasoning can be employed to find the density. The density found will have the same general form as that of Example 4.4.2, with the number of trials, 3, being replaced by n and the success rate of $\frac{1}{4}$ being replaced by p. This fact is summarized in Theorem 4.4.1.

THEOREM 4.4.1. Let X be a binomial random variable with parameters n and p. The density for X is given by

$$f(x) = \frac{n!}{x!\,(n - x)!}p^x(1 - p)^{n-x} \qquad x = 0, 1, 2, 3, \ldots, n$$

Expected Value and Variance: Binomial

Consider the second type of question posed in Example 4.4.1. Namely, given a binomial random variable X with parameters n and p, what is the expected value of X? Once again, we turn to a numerical example to guide our thinking.

EXAMPLE 4.4.3. Ten individuals, each susceptible to tuberculosis, come into contact with a carrier of the disease. The probability that the disease will be passed from the carrier to any given subject is .10. How many are expected to contract the disease?

Since each individual has a 10% chance of contracting the disease, common sense leads us to expect that 10% of those so exposed will become infected. That is, common sense points to $10(.1) = 1$ for the expected number contracting tuberculosis. Note that this value is obtained by multiplying the number of trials, 10, by the success rate, .1.

Once again, the reasoning used to answer the question is independent of the actual number of trials involved or of the numerical value of the success rate. This suggests at least a portion of Theorem 4.4.2. The fact that the variance is as stated cannot be seen from an intuitive argument. Since the derivation of the variance formula is not particularly instructive, we will use the result without proof. Exercise 11 asks you to verify the formula in a numerical setting.

THEOREM 4.4.2. Let X be binomial with parameters n and p. Then $E[X] = np$ and Var $X = np(1 - p)$.

Calculating Binomial Probabilities: Cumulative Distribution

The density for a discrete random variable gives the probability that the random variable assumes a specific value. In the case of a binomial random variable X, we have a formula for the density. In practice, we usually want to know the probability that X will be at most a given value or at least a given value. That is, questions of interest often entail calculating $P[X \leq x]$ or $P[X \geq x]$. These probabilities can be found by evaluating the density for each x and adding the individual probabilities as was done in Section 4.2. However, an easier way to find such probabilities is to use the cumulative distribution function. Recall that this function, denoted by F, parallels the notion of the relative cumulative frequency given in Section 1.3. It is a function that gives the probability that X will assume a value less than or equal to a specified value x. Its value is found by summing the density for X over all values less than or equal to the value of interest.

Since the binomial random variable has universal appeal, extensive tables and computer and calculator software exist for evaluating F for binomial random variables. Thus, the primary task of researchers is to recognize the fact that they are dealing with a binomial random variable so they can frame their questions in terms of appropriate probabilities and then use available resources to evaluate these probabilities correctly. Table I of Appendix B is an abbreviated binomial table. It shows values of the cumulative distribution function for binomial variables with $n = 5$ to 20 and $p = .1, .2, .25,$ .3, .4, .5, .6, .7, .75, .8, .9. Other more extensive tables are available. They are all similar to the one presented, and mastery of the use of Table I in Appendix B should enable you to adjust to the use of more complete tables with little difficulty. We illustrate the use of Table I in Example 4.4.4.

EXAMPLE 4.4.4. A new variety of corn is being developed at an agricultural experimental station. It is hoped that 90% of all seed from this corn will germinate. To verify this figure, 20 seeds are planted in soil of identical composition and given the same care. If the 90% figure is correct, how many seeds are expected to germinate?

This question is not new. We are being asked to find $E[X]$, where X is the number of seeds that germinate. From Theorem 4.4.2, $E[X] = np = 20(.9) = 18$. If the 90% figure is correct, we would expect to see about 18 seeds germinate. If at most 15 seeds germinate, is there reason to suspect the 90% figure? On the surface, there appears to be some reason for doubt, because 15 is somewhat below the expected figure of 18. The question is, If the 90% success rate is correct, what is the probability of seeing 15 or fewer seeds germinate? If this probability is fairly large, then there is no reason to suspect the 90% figure. However, if this probability is small, there are two possible explanations. Either a rare event has occurred, or the actual rate of germination is smaller than the rate claimed. Thus our decision is clearly based on determining and interpreting $P[X \leq 15]$. Using the cumulative distribution function, we have

$$P[X \leq 15] = F(15) = \sum_{x=0}^{15} f(x) = \sum_{x=0}^{15} \frac{20!}{x!\,(20-x)!}(.9)^x(.1)^{20-x}$$

Evaluating this probability directly entails a prohibitive amount of arithmetic. So we turn to Table I in Appendix B. Since Table I lists directly the cumulative distribution function, we can find the answer to our question by looking at the group of values labeled $n = 20$. The desired probability of .0432 is found in the column labeled .9 and the row labeled 15. That is,

$$P[X \leq 15] = F(15) = .0432$$

Is this value large or small? The answer is not clear-cut. Most researchers would tend to consider this small and would conclude that the stated germination rate of .9 was too high.

Questions not of the form $P[X \leq x]$ cannot be answered directly from Table I. They must be first rewritten in terms of the cumulative distribution function and then answered by means of the table. This point is illustrated in Example 4.4.5.

EXAMPLE 4.4.5. A survey is being conducted to determine public opinion concerning the construction of a dam to control flooding in the New River Valley. Fifteen residents of the area are to be randomly selected and surveyed. If, in fact, 80% of the people living in the area oppose the dam, what is the probability that a majority of those surveyed will be in opposition? Since a majority consists of eight or more individuals, we are being asked to find $P[X \geq x]$.

The desired probability is pictured in Figure 4.3. Notice that we want to find the probability associated with the points that are starred. To do so, we recognize that the total probability associated with the points $0, 1, 2, 3, \ldots, 15$ is 1. We can obtain the desired probability by subtracting the probability associated with the unwanted points, 0 to 7 inclusive, from 1.

In terms of the cumulative distribution function,

$$P[X \geq 8] = 1 - P[X \leq 7] = 1 - F(7)$$

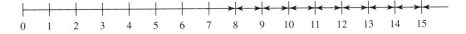

■ **FIGURE 4.3**

Total probability is 1. $P[X \geq 8]$ is the probability associated with points that are marked. $P[X \geq 8] = 1 - P[X \leq 7]$.

From Table I with $n = 15$ and $p = .8$, it can be seen that $F(7) = .0042$. Thus the probability that a majority of those sampled will be in opposition to the dam is $1 - .0042 = .9958$. What is the probability that between 10 and 14, inclusive, will oppose the construction? Expressing this question in terms of the cumulative distribution function, we see that

$$P[10 \leq X \leq 14] = P[X \leq 14] - P[X \leq 9]$$
$$= F(14) - F(9)$$
$$= .9648 - .0611$$
$$= .9037$$

EXERCISES 4.4

1. In each of the following, a random variable is described. For each decide whether the variable is binomial, approximately binomial or not binomial. If the variable is binomial or approximately so, determine the numerical values of n and p. If the variable is not binomial, what binomial assumption is violated? (By *approximately binomial* we mean that even though p may vary slightly from trial to trial, the change is so small as to be negligible. Thus probabilities computed by using the binomial density, though not exact, are good approximations to the actual probabilities involved.)

(a) An accident has occurred, and some units of AB negative blood are needed. There is none in the laboratory. Five unrelated employees are contacted as possible donors, and their blood types are determined. The probability that a randomly selected individual has AB negative blood is .006. The number of employees with AB negative blood is X.

(b) In the RNA code, UGG codes tryptophan and UGA codes a stop. In a particular segment, the word UGA appears 5 times. Assume that nucleotides U and G will not mutate but that nucleotide A (adenine) will mutate to G (guanine) .1% of the time. The number of mutations in the sequence in which the word *stop* (UGA) is mutated to tryptophan (UGG) is X.

(c) A chemical reaction is run in which the usual yield is 70%. A new process has been devised that should improve the yield. Proponents of the new process claim that it produces better yields than the old process 90% of the time. The new process is tried 10 times, and the yields are recorded. Variable X is the number of times that the yield has improved over the 70% figure.

(d) A biologist has eight plants available for experimentation. The experiment calls for the use of only four plants. Unknown to the biologist, three of the plants are diseased. She randomly selects four plants to use in the experiment. Variable X is the number of diseased plants selected.

(e) In a study of the migratory habits of Canadian geese, approximately 5% of the entire population has been tagged. During a given day eight geese are captured. The number that are tagged is X.

(f) A couple is determined to have a daughter. They decide to continue having children until a daughter is born, at which time they will produce no more children. The number of children born before the birth of the first daughter is X.

2. Consider the random variable described in Example 4.2.1.
   (a) Argue that, as claimed, X is binomial.
   (b) What are the numerical values of n and p?
   (c) What is the formula for the density for X?
   (d) Use the formula for the density found in part c to verify the probabilities given in Example 4.2.1.
   (e) Find $E[X]$ and compare your answer to that found in Example 4.2.3.

3. An oil company has 10 offshore rigs scattered throughout a wide area in the Gulf of Mexico. Officials feel that under normal operating conditions, each rig has only a 1% chance of having an oil spill during the year. Let X denote the number of rigs experiencing a spill during the year.
   (a) Argue that X is binomial.
   (b) Find the expression for the density.
   (c) Find $E[X]$, Var X, and σ.
   (d) If the rigs were located close together and some unusual situation occurred (such as a hurricane or an earthquake), is it safe to assume that X was binomial? Explain.

4. For each of the binomial or approximate binomial variables X of Exercise 1 find
   (a) The expression for the density
   (b) The mean of X
   (c) The variance of X
   (d) The standard deviation of X

5. Let X be binomial with $n = 4$ and $p = .2$.
   (a) Find the expression for the density.
   (b) Use the density to find $P[X = 0]$.
   (c) Use the density to find $P[X \leq 1]$. Why can this probability not be found from Table I of Appendix B?

6. A forester is interested in the spread of pine blight in the Great Smoky Mountains. After surveying five key areas, the forester records 0 if no blight is found in the area and 1 if the disease is present. These data are fed into a computer that has probability .001 of reversing a digit upon transmission (reading a 0 as a 1, or vice versa). The number of transmission errors is X.
   (a) Find the expression for the density for X.
   (b) Find $E[X]$, σ^2, and σ.
   (c) Use the density for X to find the probability that no transmission errors were made.
   (d) Use the density for X to find $P[X \leq 1]$.

7. Let X be binomial with $n = 10$ and $p = .4$. In each case sketch a diagram similar to that shown in Figure 4.3 and evaluate the given probability using Table I of Appendix B.
   (a) $P[X \leq 4]$
   (b) $P[X < 4]$
   (c) $P[X = 4]$
   (d) $P[X \geq 5]$
   (e) $P[X > 6]$
   (f) $P[3 \leq X \leq 6]$

(g) $P[4 \leq X \leq 7]$
(h) $P[3 \leq X < 6]$
(i) $P[4 < X \leq 7]$

8. In humans, geneticists have identified two sex chromosomes, R and Y. Every individual has an R chromosome, and the presence of a Y chromosome distinguishes the individual as male. Thus the two sexes are characterized as RR (female) and RY (male). Color blindness is caused by a recessive allele on the R chromosome, which we denote by r. The Y chromosome has no bearing on color blindness. Thus relative to color blindness, there are three genotypes for females and two for males:

Female	Male
RR (normal)	RY (normal)
Rr (carrier)	rY (color-blind)
rr (color-blind)	

A child inherits one sex chromosome randomly from each parent.
(a) A carrier of color blindness parents a child with a normal male. Construct a tree to represent the possible genotypes for the child.
(b) What is the probability that a given child born to this couple will be a color-blind male?
(c) If the couple has three children, what is the probability that exactly two are color-blind males?
(d) If the couple has five children, what is the expected number of color-blind males? What is the probability that at most two will be color-blind males? What is the probability that three or more will be color-blind males?

9. A nuclear power plant is to be built. Local public opinion is sought. A random sample of 20 individuals is selected and polled. It is thought that 60% of the local inhabitants favor the project. If this is true, how many would you expect to express a favorable opinion? If nine or fewer express such an opinion, do you think that there is strong reason to suspect the 60% figure? Explain on the basis of the probability involved.

10. Albino rats used to study the hormonal regulation of a metabolic pathway are injected with a drug that inhibits body synthesis of protein. Usually, 4 out of 20 rats die from the drug before the experiment is over. If 10 animals are treated with the drug, what is the probability that at least 8 will be alive at the end of the experiment?

11. Use Exercises 7 and 9 of Section 4.2 to verify that the variance of the random variable X of Example 4.4.2 is $3 \cdot \frac{1}{4} \cdot \frac{3}{4} = \frac{9}{16}$ as indicated in Theorem 4.4.2.

■ 4.5

POISSON DISTRIBUTION (OPTIONAL)

The second discrete family considered is the Poisson family, named for the French mathematician Siméon Denis Poisson (1781–1840). Poisson random variables arise in connection with what are termed *Poisson processes*. Poisson processes involve observing discrete events in a continuous "interval" of time, length or space. We use the word *interval* in describing the general Poisson process with the understanding that we may not be dealing with an interval in the usual mathematical sense. For example, we might observe the number of white blood cells in a drop of blood. The discrete event of interest is the observation of a white cell, whereas the continuous "interval" involved is a drop of blood. We might observe the number of times radioactive gases are emitted from a nuclear power plant during a 3-month period. The discrete event of concern is the emission of radioactive gases. The continuous interval consists of a period of 3 months. We could observe the number of emergency calls received by a rescue squad per hour. Here the discrete event of interest is the arrival of a call. The observation period is an hour.

The random variable of interest in a Poisson process is X, the number of occurrences of the event in an interval of size s units. To determine the density for X we ask three questions.

1. What is the basic physical unit of measurement in the problem?
2. What is the average number of occurrences of the event per unit? This average is denoted by λ.
3. What is the size of the observation period? This value is denoted by s.

Calculate techniques can be used to show that the density for X is given by

$$f(x) = \frac{e^{-\lambda s}(\lambda s)^x}{x!} \qquad x = 0, 1, 2, 3, \ldots$$

where $e \doteq 2.7183$, and that its expected value is λs. As you can see, once the numerical values of λ and s have been determined from the physical context of the problem, desired probabilities can be found by means of the above density. A random variable whose density assumes this form is called a *Poisson random variable*. Example 4.5.1 illustrates this idea.

> **EXAMPLE 4.5.1.** The white blood cell count of a healthy individual can average as low as 6000 per cubic millimeter of blood. To detect a white cell deficiency, a .001-cubic-millimeter drop of blood is taken and the number of white cells X is found. How many white cells are expected in a healthy individual? If at most two are found, is there evidence of a white cell deficiency?
>
> This experiment can be viewed as a Poisson process. The discrete event of interest is the occurrence of a white cell; the continuous interval is a drop of blood. Let the measurement unit be a cubic millimeter; then $s = .001$, and λ, the average number of occurrences of the event per unit, is 6000. Thus X is a Poisson random variable with $E[X] = \lambda s = 6000(.001) = 6$. In a healthy individual, we would expect, on the average, to see six white cells. How rare is it to see at most two? That is, what is $P[X \leq 2 \mid \lambda s = 6]$?
>
> To answer this question we use the density which is given by
>
> $$f(x) = \frac{e^{-6}6^x}{x!} \qquad x = 0, 1, 2, 3, \ldots$$

By substitution,

$$P[X \leq 2] = \sum_{x=0}^{2} f(x) = \sum_{x=0}^{2} \frac{e^{-6}6^x}{x!}$$

$$= \frac{e^{-6}6^0}{0!} + \frac{e^{-6}6^1}{1!} + \frac{e^{-6}6^2}{2!}$$

Evaluating this type of expression directly does entail some arithmetic.

Once again, because of the wide appeal of the Poisson model, the values of the cumulative distribution function for selected values of the parameter λs have been tabled. Table II in Appendix B is one such table. The desired probability of .062 is found by looking under the column labeled $\lambda s = 6$ in the row labeled 2. Is there evidence of a white cell deficiency? Since .062 seems moderate in size, there appears to be no clear-cut answer to this question.

One other important application of the Poisson density should be mentioned. Consider a binomial variable with large n and small p. In this case, it can be shown that the Poisson density with parameter $\lambda s = np$ gives a good approximation to the desired binomial density. A rule of thumb is that the Poisson approximation is good if $n \geq 20$ and $p \leq .05$ and very good if $n \geq 100$ and $np \leq 10$. Since the approximation is used whenever the probability of success p is small, often the Poisson density is referred to as the distribution of "rare" events.

EXAMPLE 4.5.2. In *Escherichia coli*, a bacterium often found in the human digestive tract, 1 cell in every 10^9 will mutate from streptomycin sensitivity to streptomycin resistance. This mutation can cause the individual involved to become resistant to the antibiotic streptomycin. In observing 2 billion (2×10^9) such cells, what is the probability that none will mutate? What is the probability that at least one will mutate?

This problem is actually binomial, with $n = 2 \times 10^9$ and $p = 1/10^9$. Since $1/10^9$ is extremely small, the mutation of a cell is a very rare event. Thus X, the number of cells mutating, can be thought of as being approximately Poisson with $\lambda s = np = (2 \times 10^9)(1/10^9) = 2$. From Table II in Appendix B, $P[X = 0] = .135$. The probability of at least one mutation is $P[X \geq 1]$. This probability is found by subtraction. That is, $P[X \leq 1] = 1 - P[X = 0] = 1 - .135 = .865$.

◼ EXERCISES 4.5

1. A Poisson random variable X has parameter $\lambda s = 10$.
    (a) Find $E[X]$
    (b) Find the expression for the density for X.
    (c) Find $P[X \leq 4]$.
    (d) Find $P[X \geq 6]$.
    (e) Find $P[4 \leq X \leq 12]$.
    (f) Find $P[X = 9]$.
2. In studying sleep patterns in humans, five stages of sleep (drowsiness, light, intermediate, deep, REM) are recognized by using the electroencephalogram. Intermediate sleep is characterized by the presence of high-amplitude waves averaging about 2 waves per second. What is the probability that during intermediate sleep none of these waves will occur during a 5-second period? What is the probability that at most 15 such waves will appear in a 5-second period? If 20 or more such waves appeared during a 5-second period, would you suspect that the subject was not in the intermediate sleep stage? Explain on the basis of the probability involved.
3. A particular nuclear plant releases a detectable amount of radioactive gases twice a month on the average. Find the probability that there will be no such emissions during a 3-month period. Find the probability that there will be at most four such

emissions during the period. What is the expected number of emissions during a 3-month period? If, in fact, 12 or more emissions are detected, do you feel that there is reason to suspect the reported average figure of twice a month? Explain on the basis of the probability involved.

4. The average number of deaths from lung cancer in a certain population per year has been observed to be 12. If the number of deaths from the disease follows the Poisson distribution, what is the probability that during the current year
   (a) There will be exactly 10 deaths from lung cancer?
   (b) Fifteen or more people will die from the disease?
   (c) Ten or fewer people will die from the disease?

5. In a certain culture, the average number of *Rickettsia typhi* cells (cells which cause typhus) is 5 per 20 square micrometers (1/10,000 of a centimeter). How many such cells would you expect to find in a culture of size 16 square micrometers? What is the probability that none will be found in a 16-square-micrometer culture? What is the probability that at least nine such cells will be found in a culture of this size?

6. Many samples of water, all the same size, are taken from the Hillbank River, suspected of having been polluted by irresponsible operators at a sewage treatment plant. The number of coliform organisms in each sample was counted. The average number of organisms per sample was 15. Assuming the number of organisms to be Poisson-distributed, find the probability that
   (a) That next sample will contain at least 17 organisms
   (b) That next sample will contain 18 or fewer organisms
   (c) That next sample will contain exactly two organisms

7. Some strains of paramecia produce and secrete "killer" particles that will cause the death of a sensitive individual if contact is made. All paramecia unable to produce killer particles are sensitive. The mean number of killer particles emitted by a killer paramecium is 1 every 5 hours. What is the probability that a killer paramecium would emit no such particles in a $2\frac{1}{2}$-hour period? What is the probability that it would emit at least one killer particle?

8. A rescue squad spokesperson claims that the squad receives an average of 3 calls per hour. If at most 6 calls were received over a 5-hour period, would you suspect that the spokesperson was overestimating the average number of calls received per hour? Explain based on the probability of this occurring.

9. Let X be binomial with $n = 20$ and $p = .1$. Use the binomial table to complete the second row of the table shown in Figure 4.4. Notice that the guidelines for

x	0	1	2	3	4	5	6	7	8	9	10	$\cdots$
Binomial cumulative distribution	.1216	.3917	.6769	?	?	?	?	?	?	?	?	?
Poisson approximation	.135	.406	.677	?	?	?	?	?	?	?	?	?

FIGURE 4.4
A comparison of the binomial distribution with $n = 20$ and $p = .1$ to the Poisson distribution with $\lambda s = np = 2$.

approximating a binomial distribution via the Poisson distribution are not met in this case. However, try the approximation by using the Poisson table with $\lambda s = 2$ to complete row 3 of Figure 4.4. Is the approximation fairly good?

10. In fruit flies, 4 sperm cells in every 10^5 carry a mutation for red eye to white eye, or vice versa. How many mutations would you expect to occur in 200,000 sperm cells? What is the probability that at most 10 would occur? What is the probability that between 6 and 10, inclusive, would occur?

11. In human beings, mutations for Huntington's disease occur in about 5 of every 10^6 gametes. What is the probability that in 2 million gametes there will be at least one mutation?

12. It is estimated that only 1 in every 50 parrots captured in the Amazon Basin for use as household pets will survive the transition. During the course of a day, 700 birds are captured. What is the expected number of survivors? What is the probability that at most 10 birds will survive? During a given 3-day period, 700 birds are captured each day. What is the probability that on each of the 3 days at most 10 birds will survive?

13. By damaging the chromosomes in the egg or sperm, mutations can be caused which lead to abortions, birth defects, or other genetic defects. The probability that such a mutation is produced by radiation is .10. Of the next 150 mutations caused by damage to the chromosomes, how many would you expect to have been produced by radiation? What is the probability that exactly 10 were produced by radiation?

14. The probability that a randomly selected baby will be albino is $1/20,000$. Of the next 40,000 babies born, what is the probability that none will be albino? What is the probability that at least one will be albino?

TECHNOLOGY TOOLS

TI83

The TI83 calculator has the capability of evaluating the density and the cumulative distribution for both the binomial and Poisson distribution. In each case, the user must supply the numerical values of the parameters that identify the distribution and the value of x of interest.

VII.   Binomial density

We illustrate the use of the TI83 in finding binomial probability by reconsidering Example 4.4.5. In this example, $n = 15$ and $p = .8$. We begin by finding the probability that $x = 12$. Recall that to do this by hand, the binomial density is evaluated at $x = 12$. Thus

$$P[X = 12] = \frac{15!}{12!\, 3!}(.8)^{12}(.2)^3 = f(12)$$

The following keystrokes will evaluate this expression:

TI83 Keystroke		Purpose	
1.	2ND DISTR $\emptyset$	1.	Displays the binomial density screen, binomial pdf (
2.	15 ,	2.	Enters the numerical value of n
3.	.8 ,	3.	Enters the numerical value of p
4.	12) ENTER	4.	Enters the numerical value of x; calculates $f(12) = .2501388953$

VIII. Cumulative distribution binomial

Here we find $P[10 \leq X \leq 14]$. As noted in Example 4.4.5, this is done by subtracting $F(9)$ from $F(14)$. These cumulative probabilities are found easily via the calculator.

TI83 Keystroke		Purpose	
1.	2ND DISTR ALPHA A	1.	Displays the cumulative binomial distribution screen; binomial cdf (
2.	15 ,	2.	Enters the numerical value of n
3.	.8 ,	3.	Enters the numerical value of p
4.	14) ENTER	4.	Enters the first value of x desired; calculates and displays $F(14) = .9648156279$
5.	CLEAR	5.	Clears screen
6.	2ND DISTR ALPHA A	6.	Displays the cumulative distribution screen again
7.	15 ,	7.	Enters the numerical value of n
8.	.8 ,	8.	Enters the numerical value of p
9.	9) ENTER	9.	Enters the second value of x desired; calculates and displays $F(9) = .0610514296$

To complete the calculation use the calculator to find $F(14) - F(9)$.

IX.   Poisson density

The Poisson density can be evaluated by identifying the numerical value of λs and the numerical value of x involved in the calculation. To illustrate, we reconsider Example 4.5.1. In this example, $\lambda s = 6$. Let us use the TI83 to evaluate $P[X = 0]$.

TI83 Keystroke	Purpose
1. 2ND DISTR ALPHA B	1. Displays the Poisson density screen; Poisson pdf (
2. 6 ,	2. Enters the numerical value of λs
3. 0) ENTER	3. Enters the numerical value of x; calculates and displays the value of $f(0) = .0024787522$

X.   Cumulative poisson distribution

Here we find $P[X \leq 2]$. When computing by hand this is given by

$$F(2) = P[X \leq 2] = f(0) + f(1) + f(2)$$

The answer, as obtained in Example 4.5.1, is about .062.

TI83 Keystroke	Purpose
1. 2ND DISTR ALPHA C	1. Displays the Poisson cumulative distribution screen; Poisson cdf (
2. 6 ,	2. Enters the numerical value of λs
3. 2) ENTER	3. Enters the numerical value of x; calculates and displays the value of $F(2) = .0619688044$

SAS Package

VI.   Cumulative binomial distribution

SAS can be used to generate the cumulative tables given in the appendix portion of this text. We demonstrate by generating the cumulative probabilities shown in Table I, Appendix B, for $n = 10$ and $p = .5$. This program can be adjusted to generate other probabilities.

SAS Code	**Purpose**
OPTIONS LS = 80 PS = 60 NODATE;	Sets printing specifications
DATA BINOMIAL;	Names data set
DO X = 0 to 10;	Generates the cumulative binomial distribution for a binomial random variable with $p = .5$, $n = 10$ via the SAS function named PROBBNML
P = PROBBNML (.5, 10, X);	
CUMPROB = ROUND (P, .0001);	Rounds the probabilities generated to four decimal places to match the table in the textbook
OUTPUT;	Outputs both P and CUMPROB to a SAS data set
END;	Ends the "DO" loop
PROC PRINT;	Prints the results

The results of this program are given below. The variable OBS is a SAS-produced variable that gives the observation number. The variable X is the value of the random variable X whose cumulative probability is being found. P is the cumulative probability as calculated by the SAS function PROBBNML; CUMPROB is this probability rounded to four-decimal-place accuracy.

The SAS System

OBS	X	P	CUMPROB
1	0	0.00098	0.0010
2	1	0.01074	0.0107
3	2	0.05469	0.0547
4	3	0.17188	0.1719
5	4	0.37695	0.3770
6	5	0.62305	0.6230
7	6	0.82812	0.8281
8	7	0.94531	0.9453
9	8	0.98926	0.9893
10	9	0.99902	0.9990
11	10	1.00000	1.0000

5

Continuous Random Variables

$\mathbf{R}$ecall that a continuous random variable is a random variable that can conceivably assume *any* value in some interval or continuous span of real numbers. It does *not* assume its values only at isolated points. We saw some examples of continuous random variables in Section 4.1 and noted there that, before the fact, the probability that a continuous random variable assumes any specific value is 0. Since this is not true in the discrete case, this property most clearly distinguishes a continuous random variable from one that is discrete. We also noted that continuous random variables arise in practice in connection with measurement-type data.

In this chapter we parallel the concepts presented in Chapter 4. In particular, we will define the notion of a continuous density and will explain how the density is used to compute probabilities. We will interpret the expected value of X geometrically and will also consider the cumulative distribution function from a geometric viewpoint. We will then introduce the family of normal random variables, one of the most commonly encountered continuous distributions.

5.1
CONTINUOUS DENSITY FUNCTIONS AND EXPECTATION

Density functions in the discrete case often are presented in table form. The table lists the possible values of X along with $f(x)$, the probability that X assumes the value x. The continuous case is more complex. Since a continuous random variable has an infinite number of possible values, we cannot possibly list them all. Furthermore, there is no point in trying to find an equation which, when evaluated at a specific value x, will yield the probability that X assumes the value x since we know that this probability is 0. However, we do need to find a function that will allow us to compute probabilities. In the continuous case we are interested in finding the probability that X will lie in some specific interval of values.

For example, consider the random variable T, the time in hours between the observation of harmonic tremors and the next eruption of the Kilauea volcano. We would like to find the probability that T is less than 24 hours ($P[T < 24]$). Computation of probabilities in the continuous case is done geometrically by equating probabilities with areas. Definition 5.1.1 shows how this is done.

DEFINITION 5.1.1. Continuous density. Let X be a *continuous* random variable. The *density* for X is a function f defined on the entire real line such that

1. $f(x) \geq 0$ (nonnegative).
2. The area bounded by the graph of f and the x axis is equal to 1.
3. For any real numbers a and b, $P[a \leq X \leq b]$ is given by the area bounded by the graph of f, the lines $x = a$, $x = b$, and the x axis.

This definition looks formidable, but it is not, as we show shortly. Notice that there are similarities between Definitions 5.1.1 and 4.2.1. In both instances, the functions involved are nonnegative, both "sum" to 1 in some sense, and both are used to calculate probabilities. Graphs of some typical continuous densities are shown in Figure 5.1.

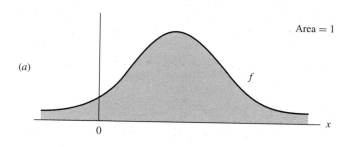

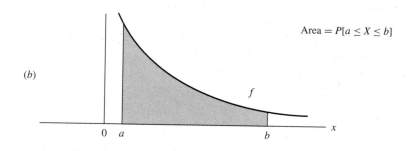

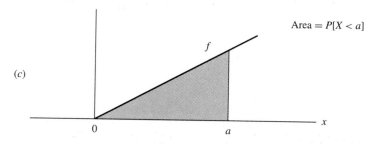

FIGURE 5.1

Some continuous densities. (*a*) The total area under the graph of f is 1. (*b*) The probability that X lies between a and b is the area under the graph of f between points a and b. (*c*) The area under the graph of f to the left of a gives the probability that X is at most a.

The first task of the experimental scientist is to determine the proper density for the random variable under consideration. If the variable has been studied extensively in the past, then an acceptable density might have been developed earlier by others. This density can be used to answer the questions posed. If the variable is being studied for the first time, then the proper density must be discovered from experimental data. In Chapter 1, two methods for doing so were presented. They are stem-and-leaf diagrams and histograms. For example, the data on the circumference at birth of a male child's head in centimeters (Example 1.2.2) form a rough bell. This implies that a density such as that shown in Figure 5.1*a* could be used in the future to compute probabilities concerning this variable; data such as the earthquake data of Example 1.2.1 suggest a density of the form pictured in Figure 5.1*b*. In this chapter we are concerned with how to use a density to compute probabilities once its shape has been determined.

> EXAMPLE 5.1.1. Assume that past experience with volcanic eruptions indicates that T, the time in hours between the observation of harmonic tremors and the eruption of the volcano, has a bell-shaped density centered at 36 hours. The density is pictured in Figure 5.2*a*. It is assumed that the shaded area has value 1. To find the probability that T is less than 24 hours, $P[T < 24]$, we must find the area of the shaded region pictured in Figure 5.2*b*. Notice that by definition $P[T = 24] = 0$. This can be seen geometrically by realizing that the area in question is the area of the dotted line at $T = 24$ shown in Figure 5.2*c*. Since lines have length but no width, their area is 0. Since probability corresponds to area, $P[T = 24]$ is also 0. One implication of this fact is that $P[T \leq 24]$ is the same as $P[T < 24]$. In the *continuous* case adding or deleting an endpoint of an interval makes no difference to the final probability because the endpoint itself occurs with zero probability. This is certainly not true in the discrete case where endpoints occur with positive probability.
>
> Areas such as that pictured in Figure 5.2*b* are not easy to find. To do so, the exact equation for the curve must be known and calculus techniques applied. Thus, at this point, even though we can picture $P[T < 24]$, we cannot compute its exact numerical value.

Expectation

Recall that the expected value of X is its theoretical average value. This average value is denoted by $E[X]$ or μ. In the discrete case, we found that μ can be calculated from the density by means of Definition 4.2.3.

Without calculus we cannot compute the expected value of a continuous random variable in any but the simplest cases. However, it is possible to view $E[X]$ geometrically. Consider the graph of the density f for X. Imagine cutting the region bounded by the graph of f and the x axis out of a piece of thin, rigid metal and attempting to balance this region on a knife-edge held parallel to the vertical axis of the graph. The point at which the region would balance is $E[X]$. Typical examples of these "balance points" are shown in Figure 5.3. Notice that in Figure 5.2 the symmetric bell-shaped curve pictured is centered at 36 hours. Because of the symmetry of the curve, 36 is the balance point, and we can conclude that the average time that elapses between the observation of harmonic tremors and the eruption of a volcano is 36 hours.

■ EXERCISES 5.1

1. Assume that the density for the random variable Z, the number of cc's of a drug to be prescribed for the control of epileptic seizures, is as shown in Figure 5.4a.
   (a) Verify that for the area under the graph of f to be 1, h, the height of the triangle, must be $\frac{20}{3}$. *Hint:* The formula for the area of a triangle is $A = \frac{1}{2}$(base)(height).
   (b) In Figure 5.4a shade the area corresponding to the probability that at least .1 cc should be prescribed.
   (c) What probability is represented by the shaded area of Figure 5.4b?

(a)

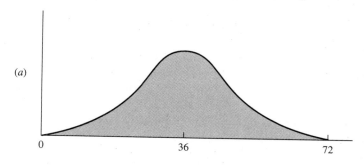

(b)

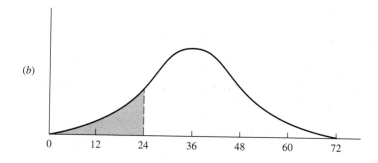

(c)

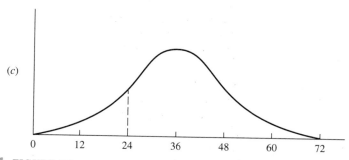

■ FIGURE 5.2

(a) T has a bell-shaped distribution centered at 36. (b) $P[T < 24]$ is given by the area of the shaded region. (c) $P[T = 24] = 0$ since the line at $T = 24$ has no area.

(d) What probability is represented by the shaded area of Figure 5.4c?

(e) What probability is represented by the shaded area of Figure 5.4d?

(f) If you knew the areas in parts c and d, how would you find the area in part e?

(g) Approximate the average dosage required by estimating the balance point by inspection.

(h) It can be shown that the equation of the density for Z is

$$f(z) = 200z/9 \qquad 0 \le z \le .3$$

Use this information to find the value of $f(z)$ when $z = .2$. Now find the area of the shaded region in Figure 5.4b, thus finding the probability that at most .2 cc of drug should be prescribed to control seizures.

(i) Use the method of part h to find the probability that at most .1 cc of the drug should be prescribed.

(j) Use the information from parts h and i to find the probability that between .1 cc and .2 cc of the drug should be prescribed.

2. Let X denote the percentage of body fluid lost during the first 24 hours by a person suffering from a severe burn. Assume that X has the density shown in Figure 5.5.

(a) What probability is represented by the shaded area in Figure 5.5?

(b) What is the probability that $X = 15\%$?

(c) Shade the area corresponding to $P[X \ge 20\%]$.

(d) What is the average percentage lost in this situation?

3. Let X denote the survival time in years after the diagnosis of acute leukemia. The density for X is shown in Figure 5.6.

(a) Shade the area corresponding to the probability that the patient will survive less than 6 months.

(b) If the area in part a has value $\frac{7}{16}$, what is the probability that a patient will survive for at least 6 months?

(c) What is the probability that the patient will survive exactly 6 months?

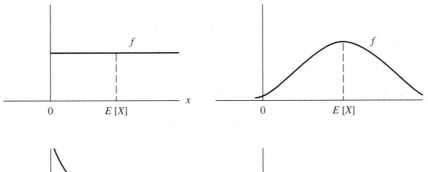

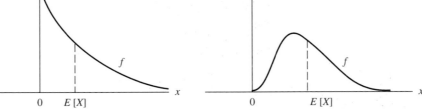

FIGURE 5.3

$\mu = E[X] =$ balance point.

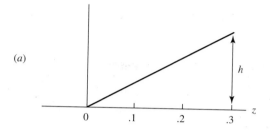

(a)

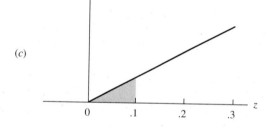

(b)

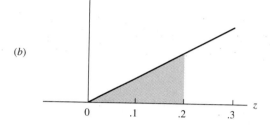

(c)

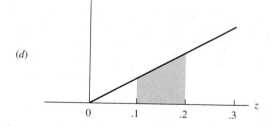

(d)

FIGURE 5.4

Density for Z, the number of cc's of a drug
needed to control epileptic seizures.

4. Chemical communication among animals is widespread. The major chemical communication in insects is by means of externally released hormones called pheromones. Such a hormone is used as a trail marker by ants. As an ant goes from the nest to a source of food and back, it leaves a chemical trail by touching its abdomen to the ground. Once no more food is available, the ants using the trail

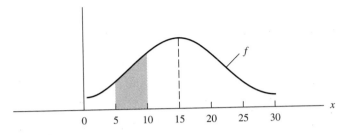

FIGURE 5.5
Density for X, the percentage of body fluid lost during the first
24 hours by a person suffering from a severe burn. The density
is symmetric.

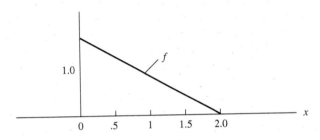

FIGURE 5.6
Density for X, the survival time of patients diagnosed
with acute leukemia.

FIGURE 5.7
Density for X, the time in
minutes that a pheromone
trail persists. The density is
symmetric.

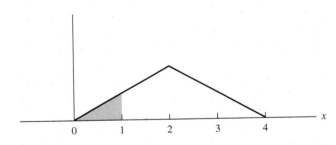

secrete no more markers and the trail dissipates. Assume that the density for X, the
time in minutes that a pheromone trail persists after the last secretion of hormone,
is as shown in Figure 5.7.

(a) What probability is represented by the shaded area?
(b) If the probability of part a is $\frac{1}{8}$, what is the probability that the trail will persist
between 1 and 2 minutes?
(c) What is the probability that the trail will persist for more than 3 minutes?
(d) What is the probability that the trail will persist for exactly 2 minutes?
(e) What is the average length of time that a trail persists?

5. *Uniform distribution.* A random variable whose density is flat is said to be *uniformly* distributed. The equation for the curve is $f(x) = c$ where c is a constant. Such densities are easy to handle because the areas involved are always rectangular. The equation for the area of a rectangle is *area = base · height.* Assume that the random variable X, the time is minutes that it takes a nurse to respond to a patient's call, is uniformly distributed over the interval 0 to 5 minutes. The density is shown in Figure 5.8.

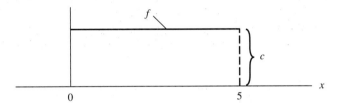

FIGURE 5.8

The random variable X, the time required for a nurse to respond to a patient's call, is uniformly distributed over a 5-minute interval.

(*a*) Verify that in this case $c = \frac{1}{5}$.
(*b*) Shade the area corresponding to the probability that the response time exceeds 3 minutes.
(*c*) Find the probability pictured in part *b*.
(*d*) What is the average response time?

5.2
CUMULATIVE DISTRIBUTION FUNCTION

The cumulative distribution function, denoted by F, was defined in Section 4.3. Recall that this function gives the probability that the random variable will assume a value less than or equal to the value specified. That is, $F(x) = P[X \le x]$. In the discrete case this function is evaluated for a specific point x_0 by summing the density over all possible values of X that are less than or equal to x_0; in the continuous case, we evaluate $F(x_0)$ by finding the area under the graph of the density to the *left of and including the point* x_0. Since this is difficult to do without calculus in all but the simplest cases, tables and computer and calculator software have been developed to provide cumulative probabilities for the random variables most often used in applied settings. Your job in the future will be to learn how to read these tables or use the software to evaluate the cumulative distribution. To solve problems, you must be able to picture the probabilities desired and be able to express them in terms of F. An example will illustrate the idea.

> **EXAMPLE 5.2.1.** The random variable X, the tree line or upper limit of tree growth in mountainous regions in meters, is influenced by temperature, soil conditions, and rainfall. Assume that X has the bell-shaped distribution shown in Figure 5.9a. Suppose that we want to find the probability that the tree line on a randomly selected mountain lies between 3000

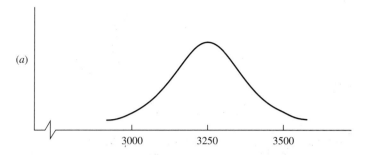

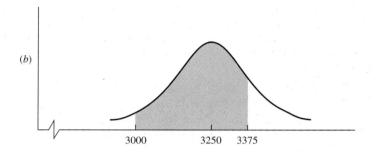

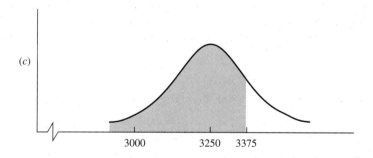

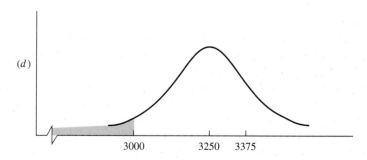

FIGURE 5.9

(a) Assumed density for X, tree line in meters; (b) area =
P[3000 ≤ X ≤ 3375]; (c) area = P[X ≤ 3375] = F(3375);
(d) area = P[X < 3000] = P[X ≤ 3000] = F(3000).

and 3375 meters inclusive. The area corresponding to this probability is shown in Figure 5.9*b*. This area can be found by subtraction. We first find the area to the left of and including 3375 (Figure 5.9*c*). We then find the area to the left of 3000 (Figure 5.9*d*). The desired area is found by subtracting the second area from the first one found. These steps can be expressed in terms of F as follows:

$$P[3000 \leq X \leq 3375] = P[X \leq 3375] - P[X < 3000]$$

$$= F(3375) - P[X < 3000]$$

Remember that in the continuous case $P[X = 3000] = 0$. Hence $P[X \leq 3000] = P[X < 3000]$. Substitution yields

$$P[3000 \leq X \leq 3375] = F(3375) - P[X \leq 3000]$$

$$= F(3375) - F(3000)$$

If a table of cumulative probabilities were available, we could find the desired probability by locating 3375 and 3000 in the table and subtracting the tabled probabilities. (Based on information found in William Keeton and Carol Hardy McFadden, *Elements of Biological Science,* 3d ed., W. W. Norton, New York, 1984.)

The major point of this section is that when dealing with a continuous random variable, F is given by the area to the left of the point in question. All the cumulative tables in this text are constructed so that these areas can be read directly from the tables. Other areas must be found by subtraction.

EXERCISES 5.2

1. Let X denote the time in years to failure of an artificial pacemaker. The density for X is shown in Figure 5.10.

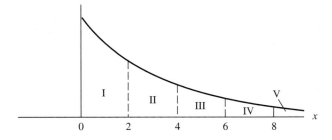

FIGURE 5.10
Hypothetical density for X, the time in years to failure of an artificial pacemaker.

(*a*) Which region(s) represents $F(4)$?
(*b*) What probability is represented by regions II and III together? Express this probability in terms of F.
(*c*) What probability is represented by region V? Express this probability in terms of F.
(*d*) Express $P[X \leq 4]$ and $P[X < 4]$, each in terms of F.

2. Figure 5.11 shows the graph of the density for random variable X, the time in minutes required for a sedative to take effect.

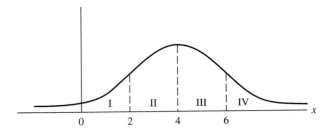

FIGURE 5.11
Hypothetical density for X, the time in minutes required for a sedative to take effect.

(a) Which region(s) in the diagram corresponds to $F(2)$?
(b) Which region(s) in the diagram corresponds to $F(6)$?
(c) Express region III in terms of F.
(d) Express region IV in terms of F.

3. Consider random variable X, the effective lifetime in months of a pH electrode. Its density is pictured in Figure 5.12.

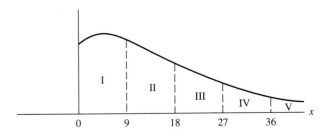

FIGURE 5.12
Hypothetical density for X, the lifetime in months of a pH electrode.

(a) Which regions in the graph correspond to $F(27)$?
(b) Express, in terms of F, the probability that a randomly selected pH electrode will work effectively for at least 18 months. What regions correspond to this probability?
(c) Express, in terms of F, the probability that a randomly selected pH electrode will have an effective lifetime of 27 to 36 months. What regions correspond to this probability?

4. When heated coolant from a power plant is released suddenly into a stream, thermal shock, a sudden shift in stream temperature, can occur. Often this results in the death of organisms living in the stream. Let X denote the river temperature in degrees Celsius at a point $\frac{1}{4}$ mile downstream from a power plant just before coolant is released into the stream. Let Y denote the river temperature at the same point 5 minutes after the coolant is released. Let $D = Y - X$, the change in river temper-

ature attributed to the release of heated coolant into the system. Figure 5.13 gives the graph of the density f for D.

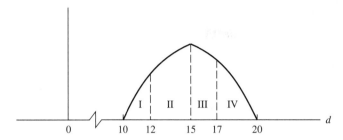

FIGURE 5.13

Hypothetical density for D, the change in river temperature due to the release of heated coolant from a power plant.

(*a*) Which region(s) represents $F(12)$?

(*b*) What probability is represented by the combined areas of regions I and II? Assuming that f is symmetric about 15, what is the numerical value of the probability represented by the area of regions I and II?

(*c*) What probability is represented by region III?

(*d*) What regions represent $F(17) - F(12)$? What probability corresponds to $F(17) - F(12)$?

(*e*) What is $F(5)$?

(*f*) What is the probability that the temperature change will be at most 25°C?

5.3

NORMAL DISTRIBUTION

The normal family is a family of continuous random variables. The normal distribution was first described in 1733 by Abraham De Moivre as being the limiting form of the binomial density as the number of trials becomes infinite. This discovery did not get much attention, and the distribution was "discovered" again by both Pierre-Simon Laplace and Carl Friedrich Gauss a half-century later. Both men dealt with problems of astronomy, and each derived the normal distribution as a distribution that seemingly described the behavior of errors in astronomical measurements.

The normal distribution is of tremendous importance in the analysis and evaluation of every aspect of experimental data in science and medicine. In fact, the majority of the basic statistical methods that we study in the next chapters is based on the normal distribution.

Recall that in the discrete case there are many different binomial distributions. Each has a density of the form

$$f(x) = \frac{n!}{x!\,(n-x)!}\,p^x(1-p)^{n-x} \quad \text{where} \quad x = 0, 1, 2, \ldots, n$$

Thus to identify a particular binomial distribution it is only necessary to determine the numerical values of n and p. The same situation holds here. There are many different normal distributions. Each has a density of the form

$$f(x) = \frac{1}{\sigma\sqrt{2\pi}}\, e^{-1/2[(x-\mu)/\sigma]^2} \quad (x \text{ is real})$$

where σ is the standard deviation of the random variable and μ is its mean. To identify a particular normally distributed random variable we need only determine the numerical values of μ and σ. The above equation is not simple. Since we will be working with tabled probabilities rather than with the equation itself, its complexity is of no importance.

Techniques of elementary calculus can be used to verify the following properties.

Properties of Normal Curves

1. The graph of the density of any normal random variable is a symmetric, bell-shaped curve centered at its mean, μ. See Figure 5.14. Note that, as mentioned in Chapter 1, μ is a location parameter in the sense that it indicates where the curve is centered or located along the horizontal axis.
2. The points of inflection, or "dips" in the curve, occur for values of X one standard deviation to either side of the mean ($x = \mu \pm \sigma$). The location of these points determines the shape of the curve. the larger the value of σ, the farther the inflection points will lie from the mean and thus the flatter the curve will be. Hence, as indicated in Chapter 1, σ is a shape parameter. See Figure 5.15.

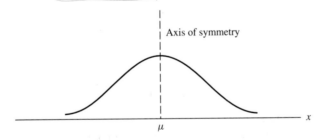

FIGURE 5.14

The bell is centered at μ, the average value of the random variable.

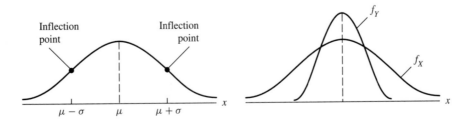

FIGURE 5.15

σ determines the points of inflection (left); $\mu_X = \mu_Y$ and $\sigma_X > \sigma_Y$ (right).

3. Every normal random variable is continuous. All the general properties of continuous variables discussed in Section 5.1 apply here. In particular, for any normal density, f, $f(x) \geq 0$ and the area bounded by the graph of f and the horizontal axis is 1. Probabilities can be found by finding appropriate areas.

EXAMPLE 5.3.1. One of the major contributors to air pollution is hydrocarbons emitted from the exhaust systems of automobiles. Let X denote the number of grams of hydrocarbons emitted by an automobile per mile. Assume that X is normally distributed with a mean of 1 gram and a standard deviation of .25 gram. The density for X is given by

$$f(x) = \frac{1}{.25\sqrt{2\pi}} \cdot e^{-1/2[(x-1)/.25]^2}$$

The graph of this density is a symmetric, bell-shaped curve centered at $\mu = 1$ with inflection points at $\mu \pm \sigma$, or $1 \pm .25$. A rough sketch of the density is given in Figure 5.16.

One point must be made. Theoretically speaking, a normal random variable must be able to assume any value whatsoever. This is clearly unrealistic here. It is impossible for an automobile to emit a negative amount of hydrocarbons. When we say that X is normally distributed, we mean that over the range of physically reasonable values of X, the given normal curve yields acceptable probabilities. With this understanding we can at least approximate the probability that a randomly selected automobile will emit between .9 and 1.5 grams of hydrocarbons by finding the area under the graph of f bounded by the horizontal axis and the lines $x = .9$ and $x = 1.5$, as shown in Figure 5.17.

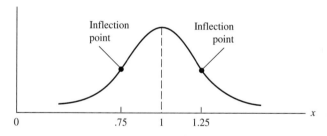

FIGURE 5.16

Graph of the density of X, the number of grams of hydrocarbons emitted by an automobile per mile. Points of inflection occur at $\mu \pm \sigma$, or $1 \pm .25$.

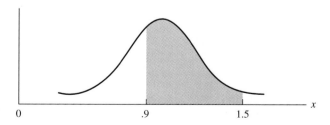

FIGURE 5.17

Shaded area $= P[.9 \leq X \leq 1.5]$.

Standard Normal Distribution

There are infinitely many normal random variables, each uniquely characterized by the two parameters μ and σ^2. To calculate probabilities associated with a specific normal curve directly requires the use of calculus. A simple algebraic transformation is employed to overcome this problem. By means of this transformation, called the *standardization procedure,* any question about any normal random variable can be transformed to an equivalent question concerning a normal random variable with mean 0 and variance 1. This particular normal variable is denoted by Z and is called the *standard normal* random variable. The cumulative distribution function for Z is given in Table III of Appendix B. That is, Table III gives $P[Z \leq z]$ for selected values of z. The use of Table III is illustrated in Example 5.3.2.

EXAMPLE 5.3.2

(a) Find $P[Z \leq 1.56] = F(1.56)$. Graphically, we are looking for the area shown in Figure 5.18a. Table III of Appendix B gives the values of F directly. So $F(1.56)$ is found by locating the first two digits (1.5) in the column headed z; since the third digit is 6, the desired probability of .9406 is found in the row labeled 1.5 and the column labeled .06.

(b) Find $P[Z \geq -1.29]$. the desired area is shown in Figure 5.18b. This probability is found by subtraction. Note that

$$P[Z \geq -1.29] = 1 - P[Z < -1.29]$$
$$= 1 - P[Z \leq -1.29] \quad (Z \text{ is continuous})$$
$$= 1 - F(-1.29)$$

From Table III, $F(-1.29) = .0985$ is found in the row labeled -1.2 and the column labeled .09. The desired probability is therefore $1 - .0985 = .9015$.

(c) Find $P[-1.72 \leq Z \leq 1.80]$. This probability is shown in Figure 5.18c. In terms of the cumulative distribution function,

$$P[-1.72 \leq Z \leq 1.80] = P[Z \leq 1.80] - P[Z < -1.72]$$
$$= P[Z \leq 1.80] - P[Z \leq -1.72] \quad (Z \text{ is continuous})$$
$$= F(1.80) - F(-1.72)$$
$$= .9641 - .0427 = .9214$$

(d) Find the point z such that $P[Z \leq z] = .025$. The question is of a different type from those asked previously. The former involved finding the probability associated with a given point; the latter involves finding a point associated with a given probability. We are asked to find the point z shown in Figure 5.18d. To do so, Table III is read in reverse. That is, we go into the body of the table and locate the probability .025. This probability is found in the row labeled -1.9 and the column labeled .06. Thus the desired point is $z = -1.96$.

(e) Find the point z such that $P[-z \leq Z \leq z] = .90$. This point is shown in Figure 5.18e. Note that the point z has the property that the area to the left of z is $.90 + .05 = .95$. Thus z is the point such that $P[Z \leq z] = .95$. To find z, we try to locate the probability .95 in the body of Table III. This value is not listed exactly. However, there are two values, namely, .9495 corresponding to $z = 1.64$ and .9505 corresponding to $z = 1.65$, which are equidistant from the desired value of .9500. Thus we are in the following situation:

Area to the left	Point
.9495	1.64
.9500	?
.9505	1.65

Since the desired probability is halfway between the two probabilities that can be read from the table, we shall estimate the point z to be the point halfway between 1.64 and 1.65. We take z to be 1.645.

(*f*) Find the point z such that $P[Z \leq z] = .10$. This point is shown in Figure 5.18*f*. When we look for .1000 in the body of Table III it is not there. It is also not halfway between two listed areas as was the case in part *e*. In this situation, we shall estimate z by finding the area closest to .1000. No interpolation will be done. In this instance, the area closest to .1000 is .1003; the z value associated with this area is $z = -1.28$.

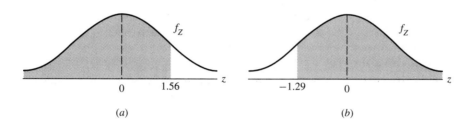

(a)   (b)

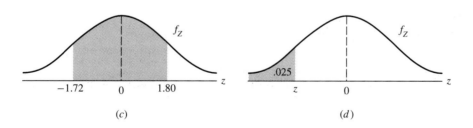

(c)   (d)

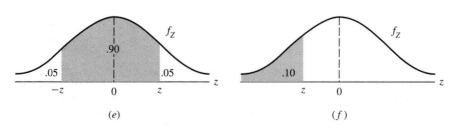

(e)   (f)

FIGURE 5.18

(a) $P[Z \leq 1.56]$; (b) $P[Z \geq -1.29]$; (c) $P[-1.72 \leq Z \leq 1.80]$;
(d) $P[Z \leq z] = .025$; (e) $P[-z \leq Z \leq z] = .90$; (f) $P[Z \leq z] = .10$.

Standardization

To use the standard normal table to answer questions about any normal random variable X, we must first rewrite the question in terms of Z. This process is called *standardization,* and it is accomplished by subtracting the mean of X and dividing by its standard deviation. The idea is stated formally in Theorem 5.3.1, and its use is illustrated in Example 5.3.3.

THEOREM 5.3.1. Standardization theorem. Let X be normal with mean μ and variance σ^2. The variable $(X - \mu)/\sigma$ is standard normal.

EXAMPLE 5.3.3. Lead, like most other elements, is present in the natural environment. The industrial revolution and the advent of the automobile have increased the background of lead in the environment to the extent that in some individuals, the lead concentration may reach dangerous levels. Let X denote the lead concentration in parts per million in the bloodstream of an individual. Assume that X is normal with mean .25 and standard deviation .11. A concentration of .6 or more is considered to be extremely high. What is the probability that a randomly selected individual will fall in the extremely high range?

To answer this question, we must find $P[X \geq .6]$. This can be done by standardizing X, that is, by subtracting the mean of .25 and dividing by the standard deviation of .11 on both sides of the inequality. Thus,

$$P[X \geq .6] = P\left[\frac{X - .25}{.11} \geq \frac{.6 - .25}{.11}\right]$$

$$= P[Z \geq 3.18]$$

$$= 1 - P[Z \leq 3.18]$$

$$= 1 - .9993 = .0007$$

Concentration between .4 and .6 represent occupational exposure to lead. The probability that a randomly selected individual will fall into this range is

$$P[.4 \leq X \leq .6] = P\left[\frac{.4 - .25}{.11} \leq Z \leq \frac{.6 - .25}{.11}\right]$$

$$= P[1.36 \leq Z \leq 3.18]$$

$$= .9993 - .9131 = .0862$$

In Example 5.3.3 we are given a value, namely .6, and are asked to find a probability. In the next example, we work in reverse. We are given a probability and are asked to find the number associated with the probability.

EXAMPLE 5.3.4. Let X denote the amount of radiation that can be absorbed by an individual before death ensues. Assume that X is normal with a mean of 500 roentgens and a standard deviation of 150 roentgens. Above what dosage level will only 5% of those exposed survive?

Here we are asked to find the point x_0 shown in Figure 5.19. In terms of probabilities, we want to find the point x_0 such that

$$P[X \geq x_0] = .05$$

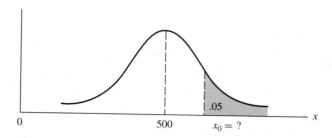

FIGURE 5.19

$P[X \geq x_0] = .05.$

Standardizing gives

$$P[X \geq x_0] = P\left[\frac{X - 500}{150} \geq \frac{x_0 - 500}{150}\right]$$

$$= P\left[Z \geq \frac{x_0 - 500}{150}\right] = .05$$

Thus $(x_0 - 500)/150$ is the point on the standard normal curve with 5% of the area under the curve to the right and 95% to the left. From Table III in Appendix B, the numerical value of this point is 1.645. Equating these, we get

$$\frac{x_0 - 500}{150} = 1.645$$

Solving this equation for x_0 gives the desired dosage level:

$$x_0 = 150(1.645) + 500 = 746.75 \text{ roentgens}$$

■ EXERCISES 5.3

1. A random variable X is normal with mean 5 and variance 4.
   (a) Find the equation for the density f for X.
   (b) At what values of X are the inflection points of the graph of f located?
   (c) Give a rough sketch of the graph of f.
   (d) Shade in the region in the sketch corresponding to $P[3 \leq X \leq 7]$.
2. Blood clams are an important product harvested off the coast of Virginia. Studies are being conducted to estimate the population size and to determine the physical and reproductive properties of these clams. In a recent study it was shown that the random variable clam height, H, is approximately normally distributed with mean 20.3 millimeters and standard deviation 1.4 millimeters (see Figure 5.20). (Based on information found in "Population Structure of the Arkshell Clams," by Katherine McGraw and Sally Dennis, Department of Biology, Radford University, and Michael Castagna, Virginia Institute of Marine Science, College of William and Mary, 1996, a technical report prepared for National Oceanic and Atmospheric Administration: National Marine Fisheries Service.)

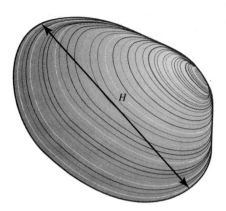

FIGURE 5.20
The distance shown is defined to be the height of the clam.

(a) Sketch the graph of the density of H. Label the mean and the points of inflection.
(b) Shade the area corresponding to the probability that the next clam found will have a height that exceeds 23 millimeters.
(c) What is the probability that the next clam found will have a height of exactly 20 millimeters?

3. Use Table III of Appendix B to find each of the following:
   (a) $P[Z \leq -1.52]$
   (b) $P[Z \leq 1.37]$
   (c) $F(1.37)$
   (d) $P[Z \geq -1.42]$
   (e) $P[Z \geq 1.98]$
   (f) $P[-1.21 \leq Z \leq 1.73]$
   (g) $P[Z = 1.50]$
   (h) The point z such that $P[Z \leq z] \doteq .05$
   (i) The point z such that $P[Z \leq z] \doteq .75$
   (j) The point z such that $P[Z \geq z] \doteq .10$
   (k) The point z such that $P[Z \geq z] \doteq .80$
   (l) The point z such that $P[-z < Z \leq z] \doteq .95$
   (m) The point z such that $P[-z \leq Z \leq z] \doteq .99$

4. Let X be normal with mean 4 and variance 9. What is the distribution of the variable $(X - 4)/3$?

5. The number of Btu's of petroleum and petroleum products used per person in the United States in 1975, X, was normally distributed with mean 153 million Btu and standard deviation 25 million Btu.
   (a) Find $P[X \leq 100$ million$]$.
   (b) Find $P[X \geq 180$ million$]$.
   (c) Find $P[100$ million $\leq X \leq 175$ million$]$.
   (d) Find $P[128$ million $\leq X \leq 178$ million$]$.
   (e) Find the point x_0 such that $P[X \leq x_0] \doteq .10$.
   (f) Find the point x_0 such that $P[X \geq x_0] \doteq .06$.

6. In 1969, pheasants in Montana were found to have an appreciable mercury conta-
   mination that was thought to have been caused by their eating seed from plants
   grown from seed treated with methyl mercury. Let X denote the mercury level of
   a bird in parts per million. Assume that X is normally distributed with mean .25
   and standard deviation .08. A pheasant is killed, and the mercury level is determined. Find $P[X \leq .3]$, $P[X \geq .17]$, $P[.2 \leq X \leq .4]$, and $P[.01 \leq X \leq .49]$.

7. Among diabetics, the fasting blood glucose level X may be assumed to be approximately normally distributed with mean 106 mg/100 ml and standard deviation
   8 mg/100 ml.
   (a) Find $P[X \leq 120$ mg/100 ml$]$.
   (b) What percentage of diabetics have levels between 90 and 120 mg/100 ml?
   (c) Find $P[106 \leq X \leq 110]$.
   (d) Find $P[X \geq 121$ mg/100 ml$]$.
   (e) Find the point x_0 that has the property that 25% of all diabetics have a fasting
       glucose level X lower than x_0.

8. Among a certain population of primates, the volume of the cranial cavity X is approximately normally distributed with mean 1200 cc and standard deviation 140 cc.
   (a) Find the probability that a randomly chosen member of the population will
       have a cranial cavity larger than 1400 cc.
   (b) Find $P[1000 \leq X \leq 1050]$.
   (c) Find $P[X \leq 1060]$.
   (d) Find $P[X \leq 920]$.
   (e) Find the point x_0 such that 20% of these primates have a cranial cavity smaller
       than x_0.
   (f) Find the point x_0 such that 10% of these primates have a cranial cavity larger
       than x_0.

9. The bulk density of soil is defined as the mass of dry solids per unit bulk volume.
   A high bulk density implies a compact soil with a few pores. Bulk density is an important factor in influencing root development, seedling emergence, and aeration.
   Let X denote the bulk density of Pima clay loam. Studies show that X is normally
   distributed with $\mu = 1.5$ and $\sigma = .2$ g/cm^3. (*McGraw-Hill Yearbook of Science
   and Technology,* 1981, p. 361.)
   (a) What is the density for X? Sketch a graph of the density function. Indicate on
       this graph the probability that X lies between 1.1 and 1.9. Find this probability.
   (b) Find the probability that a randomly selected sample of Pima clay loam will
       have bulk density less than .9 g/cm^3.
   (c) Would you be surprised if a randomly selected sample of this type of soil has
       a bulk density in excess of 2.0 g/cm^3? Explain, based on the probability of this
       occurring.

10. Most galaxies take the form of a flattened disk with the major part of the light
    coming from this very thin fundamental plane. The degree of flattening differs
    from galaxy to galaxy. In the Milky Way galaxy, most gases are concentrated near
    the center of the fundamental plane. Let X denote the perpendicular distance from
    this center to a gaseous mass. X is normally distributed with mean 0 and standard
    deviation 100 parsecs. (A parsec is equal to approximately 19.2 trillion miles.)
    (*McGraw-Hill Encyclopedia of Science and Technology,* vol. 6, 1971, p. 10.)

(a) Sketch a graph of the density for X. Indicate on this graph the probability that a gaseous mass is located within 200 parsecs of the center of the fundamental plane. Find this probability.

(b) Approximately what percentage of the gaseous masses is located more than 250 parsecs from the center of the plane?

(c) What distance has the property that 20% of the gaseous masses are at least this far from the fundamental plane?

5.4

NORMAL PROBABILITY RULE AND MEDICAL TABLES (OPTIONAL)

In Chapter 4 Chebyshev's inequality was introduced. This inequality states that "the probability that a random variable will assume a value within k standard deviations of its means is at least $1 - 1/k^2$." Notice that there are no restrictions on the random variables to which the rule applies. If we let $k = 2$, the inequality guarantees that the probability that the random variable lies within two standard deviations of its mean is at least $1 - 1/2^2 = .75$. In other words, we can conclude that for any random variable X

$$P[\mu - 2\sigma < X < \mu + 2\sigma] \doteq .75$$

If X is normally distributed, a stronger statement can be made based on a rule known as the normal probability rule. The rule is as follows:

NORMAL PROBABILITY RULE. Let X be normally distributed with mean μ and variance σ^2. Then

(a) The probability that X lies within one standard deviation of its mean is approximately .68 ($P[\mu - \sigma < X < \mu + \sigma] \doteq .68$).

(b) The probability that X lies within two standard deviations of its mean is approximately .95 ($P[\mu - 2\sigma < X < \mu + 2\sigma] \doteq .95$).

(c) The probability that X lies within three standard deviations of its mean is approximately .99 ($P[\mu - 3\sigma < X < \mu + 3\sigma] \doteq .99$).

Notice that if X is normally distributed

$$P[\mu - 2\sigma < X < \mu + 2\sigma] \doteq .95$$

rather than .75, the figure guaranteed by Chebyshev's inequality. The rule is easy to derive

EXAMPLE 5.4.1. To verify part a of the normal probability rule, we first subtract μ to obtain

$$P[\mu - \sigma < X < \mu + \sigma] = P[\mu - \sigma - \mu < X - \mu < \mu + \sigma - \mu]$$
$$= P[-\sigma < X - \mu < \sigma]$$

To complete the standardization, each piece of the inequality is divided by σ and $(X - \mu)/\sigma$ is replaced by Z. We conclude that

$$P[\mu - \sigma < X < \mu + \sigma] = P[-\sigma < X - \mu < \sigma]$$
$$= P\left[\frac{-\sigma}{\sigma} < \frac{X - \mu}{\sigma} < \frac{\sigma}{\sigma}\right]$$
$$= P[-1 < Z < 1]$$

From the standard normal table,

$$P[-1 < Z < 1] = P[Z < 1] - P[Z \leq -1]$$
$$= .8413 - .1587$$
$$= .6826$$

The normal probability rule is pictured in Figure 5.21. This rule is just a quick rule of thumb. It allows one to see whether or not an observed value of a normal random variable is unusually large or small or is a commonly occurring value based on knowledge of the mean and standard deviation of the variable alone. For example, suppose that the average amount of rainfall for the month of June in a particular region is 9 inches with a standard deviation of 2 inches. Suppose also that past data indicate that this random variable is approximately normally distributed. Would a June in which more than

(a)
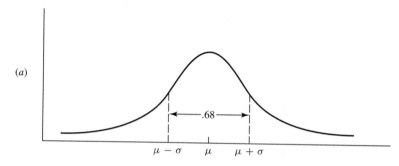

(b)
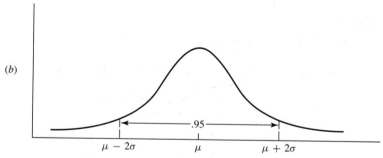

(c)
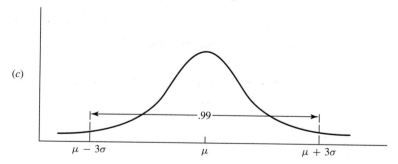

■ **FIGURE 5.21**
The normal probability rule. (a) $P[\mu - \sigma < X < \mu + \sigma] \doteq .68$;
(b) $P[\mu - 2\sigma < X < \mu + 2\sigma] \doteq .95$; (c) $P[\mu - 3\sigma < X < \mu + 3\sigma] \doteq .99$.

13 inches of rain falls be considered to be "unusually" wet? The answer is yes. By the normal probability rule, we know that the rainfall total for June will fall within two standard deviations of its mean with probability .95. In this case there is a 95% chance that the rainfall total will lie in the interval $\mu \pm 2\sigma$ or 9 inches ± 2 (2 inches). That is, there is a high probability that the total will be between 5 and 13 inches. There is only about a 2.5% chance of seeing a value above 13 inches. Since this probability is rather small, a June in which this occurs would be considered to be unusually wet.

One of the most useful applications of the normal probability rule arises in a medical setting. As you know, when a blood sample is drawn, several tests are run on the sample. For example, such things as potassium, sodium, total protein, calcium, and cholesterol levels are measured routinely. Over the years, readings have been taken on a very large number of individuals. This information has been used to establish the average reading and amount of variability to be expected in a healthy individual with a high degree of accuracy. These values can be used to establish what are called "2-sigma limits," $\mu \pm 2\sigma$, on each variable measured. By the normal probability rule, approximately 95% of all healthy individuals fall within these limits; by chance, 5% fall outside the limits, with 2.5% having unusually high readings and 2.5% unusually low ones.

Notice that there are two reasons for observing a value beyond the 2-sigma limits of an established medical table. The person might be perfectly healthy but simply be one whose "normal" level is usually high or unusually low compared to the general population; or the person might, in fact, have a problem. The presence of an unusual reading sends up a red flag that further investigation is in order.

> **EXAMPLE 5.4.2.** The potassium level in a healthy individual has mean 4.4 and standard deviation .45 meq/l. By the normal probability rule approximately 95% of all healthy individuals have readings that lie between $\mu - 2\sigma = 3.5$ and $\mu + 2\sigma = 5.3$. If the reading for a particular individual falls within these bounds, then the physician assumes that there is no problem with respect to this variable. If the reading falls below 3.5 or above 5.3, then an unusual value has been observed. This does not necessarily mean that there is a problem since 5% of all healthy individuals will exhibit these unusual values. However, it does send a signal to the physician that there might be a problem. A follow-up of some sort is probably in order. (Taken from laboratory chemistry reports currently in use at Baptist Medical Center, Columbia, S.C.)

Laboratory reports that are sent to the physician come in a variety of forms. Such reports typically list the 2-sigma limits for each variable and flag readings that are considered to be unusual. In Figure 5.22a, the 2-sigma bounds are shaded so that a reading in the shaded region is acceptable; one outside the shaded region is considered to be unusual. For example, the reading of 4.0 for potassium is acceptable and is graphed as shown. In Figure 5.22b, the 2-sigma limits are listed to the right of the report. An out-of-range value is flagged by printing the value in the shaded center column of the chart. The unusually high potassium reading is flagged by printing 5.7 H in the shaded region as shown.

Out-of-range values are not necessarily bad. For example, a lower-than-normal cholesterol reading might be of no concern, whereas a higher-than-normal reading is not desirable. This type of judgment is one that must be made by the physician.

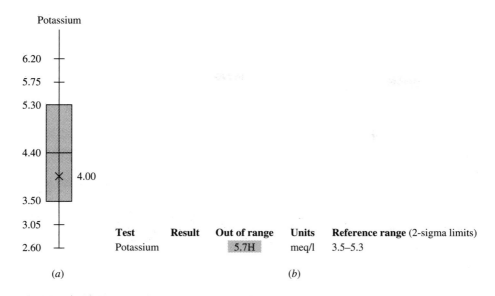

Test	Result	Out of range	Units	Reference range (2-sigma limits)
Potassium		5.7H	meq/l	3.5–5.3

    (a)   (b)

FIGURE 5.22
(a) Values lying within the shaded region are considered to be normal. The value 4.0 is acceptable. (b) Values lying in the shaded region are unusual and might call for further investigation. The value 5.7 is unusually high.

EXERCISES 5.4

1. Consider the data of Exercise 2 of Section 5.3. Based on the normal probability rule, do you think that it would be unusual to sample a blood clam whose height is between 18.9 and 21.7 millimeters? Explain.
2. Consider the random variable X of Example 5.3.4. Use the normal probability rule to find $P[350 \leq X \leq 650]$.
3. Consider the random variable X of Example 5.3.3. Without using the normal table, what is the approximate probability that the lead concentration in a randomly selected individual will lie between .03 and .47?
4. The sodium level in healthy individuals has mean 141.5 and standard deviation 3.25 meq/l.
   (a) What are the 2-sigma limits for this variable?
   (b) Construct a table similar to that of Figure 5.22a and graph the reading 149 on the table. Is this reading considered to be unusual?
   (Taken from laboratory chemistry reports currently in use at Baptist Medical Center, Columbia, S.C.)
5. The cholesterol level in healthy individuals is age and sex dependent. For males under 21, the average reading is 160 mg/dl with a standard deviation of 10 mg/dl; for males 21 to 29, the mean is 200 with a standard deviation of 30; males 30 or over have a mean reading of 220 with a standard deviation of 30.

(a) What are the 2-sigma limits for each of these three age groups?
(b) Construct a table similar to that of Figure 5.22b and graph the readings for these males:

Age	Cholesterol level
20	125
20	200
18	165
25	200
28	160
35	200
38	210
60	270

(c) Flag and discuss any readings that are unusual.
(Taken from laboratory chemistry reports currently in use at Baptist Medical Center, Columbia, S.C.)

6. For females, the 2-sigma limits for cholesterol for various age groups are

Age	2-sigma limits
Less than 21	140–180
21 to 49	140–280
50 or over	180–280

(a) Find the average reading and standard deviation being used in each case.
(b) Construct a 2-sigma table similar to that of Figure 5.22a and graph the readings for each of these females:

Age	Cholesterol level
20	125
20	200
18	165
25	200
28	160
35	200
38	210
60	270

(c) Flag and discuss any readings that are unusual.
(d) Compare your results to those of Exercise 5.
(Taken from laboratory chemistry reports currently in use at Baptist Medical Center, Columbia, S.C.)

TECHNOLOGY TOOLS

TI83

The TI83 calculator is programmed to find areas and points associated with any normal curve. The values found will agree closely with those found in the textbook examples. Where slight differences exist, the calculator values are the more accurate values.

XI. Calculating Z probabilities

To use the TI83 to calculate Z probabilities, a lower and an upper boundary for Z must be specified. To find the area to the left of a point, use -5 as the lower boundary and the point itself as the upper boundary; to find the area to the right of a point, use the point itself as the lower boundary and 5 as the upper boundary; to find the area between two given Z values, use these values as the boundaries. As an illustration we will find $P[Z \leq 1.56]$, $P[Z \geq -1.29]$, and $P[-1.72 \leq Z \leq 1.80]$. Apart from rounding differences the answers obtained will agree with those found in Example 5.3.2.

TI83 Keystroke	**Purpose**
1. 2ND DISTR 2	1. Displays the normal cumulative distribution screen; normalcdf(
2. $(-)5$,	2. Enters -5 as the lower boundary
3. 1.56) ENTER	3. Enters 1.56 as the upper boundary; calculates and displays $P[Z \leq 1.56] = .9406197625$
4. CLEAR	4. Clears screen
5. 2ND DISTR 2	5. Displays normal cumulative distribution screen
6. $(-)1.29$,	6. Enters -1.29 as the lower boundary
7. 5) ENTER	7. Enters 5 as the upper boundary; calculates and displays $P[Z \geq -1.29] = .9014743186$
8. CLEAR	8. Clears screen
9. 2ND DISTR 2	9. Displays normal cumulative distribution screen
10. $(-)1.72$,	10. Enters -1.72 as the lower boundary

11.	1.80	11.	Enters 1.80 as the upper boundary; calculates and displays $P[-1.72 \leq Z \leq 1.80] = .9213535499$
	)		
	ENTER		

XII.   Finding *Z* points

The TI83 calculator can find the z value corresponding to a given area to its left. To illustrate, we find the points z such that $P[Z \leq z] = .025$, $P[Z \leq z] = .95$, and $P[Z \leq z] = .10$. These are the points whose values were estimated from the Z table in Example 5.3.2. As you will see, the estimates given in the example are quite good.

TI83 Keystroke		**Purpose**	
1.	2ND	1.	Displays the inverse normal screen; invNorm(
	DISTR		
	3		
2.	.025	2.	Enters .025; finds and displays the z point with .025 area to its left; $z = -1.959963986$
	)		
	ENTER		
3.	CLEAR	3.	Clears screen
4.	2ND	4.	Displays the inverse normal screen
	DISTR		
	3		
5.	.95	5.	Enters .95; finds and displays the z point with .95 area to its left; $z = 1.644853626$
	)		
	ENTER		
6.	2ND	6.	Displays the inverse normal screen
	DISTR		
	3		
7.	.10	7.	Enters .10; finds and displays the z point with .10 area to its left; $z = -1.281551567$
	)		
	ENTER		

XIII.   Calculating normal probabilities directly

The TI83 calculator will enable you to find probabilities without standardizing the normal random variable X first. To do so, we must specify a lower and an upper boundary for X; we must then identify the mean and standard deviation of X. We illustrate by reconsidering Example 5.3.3. In this example, $\mu = .25$ and $\sigma = .11$. Let us find $P[X \geq .6]$ and $P[.4 \leq X \leq .6]$.

TI83 Keystroke		**Purpose**	
1.	2ND	1.	Displays the normal cumulative distribution screen; normalcdf(
	DISTR		
	2		
2.	.6	2.	Enters .6 as the lower boundary
	,		

3.	.80	3.	Enters .8 as the upper boundary; we are using 5 standard deviations above the mean as a reasonable upper boundary; $.25 + 5(.11) = .80$
	,		
4.	.25	4.	Enters .25 as μ
	,		
5.	.11	5.	Enters .11 as σ; calculates and displays $P[X \geq .6] = .0007315462284$
	)		
	ENTER		
6.	CLEAR	8.	Clears screen
7.	2ND	7.	Displays the normal cumulative distribution screen
	DISTR		
	2		
8.	.4	8.	Enters .4 as the lower boundary
	,		
9.	.6	9.	Enters .6 as the upper boundary
	,		
10.	.25	10.	Enters .25 as μ
	,		
11.	.11	11.	Enters .11 as σ; calculates and displays $P[.4 \leq X \leq .6] = .0856092456$
	)		
	ENTER		

XIV.   Finding normal points

The value of X corresponding to a given area to its left can be found via the TI83 calculator. To do so, we must identify the area desired as well as the numerical value of μ and σ. Consider Example 5.3.4. We know that $\mu = 500$ and $\sigma = 150$. We want the point x_0 such that $P[X \geq x_0] = .05$ or $P[X \leq x_0] = .95$. This point is found as follows:

TI83 Keystroke		**Purpose**	
1.	2ND	1.	Displays the inverse normal screen; invNorm(
	DISTR		
	3		
2.	.95	2.	Enters .95 as the desired area to the left
	,		
3.	500	3.	Enters 500 as μ
4.	150	4.	Enter 150 as σ; finds and displays the points x_0 with 95% of the area to its left; $x_0 = 746.7280439$
	)		
	ENTER		

6

Inferences on the Mean

Recall that the purpose of a statistical study is twofold. We want to describe the sample at hand, and we want to draw conclusions or inferences about the population from which the sample is drawn. The techniques introduced in Chapter 1 are sufficient to accomplish the first goal. The techniques introduced in the remainder of the text will allow us to accomplish the second. Decisions made concerning the population based on sample information are based on probability. The ideas concerning discrete and continuous random variables introduced in Chapters 4 and 5 will be used extensively in the work to come.

6.1

RANDOM SAMPLING AND RANDOMIZATION

As indicated in Chapter 1, inferences concerning a population are made based on information obtained from a sample of objects drawn from the population. The sample is viewed as a miniature population. We hope that the behavior of the random variable over the sample is an accurate description of its behavior over the population. For this reason, we view the observed values of the statistics evaluated for the sample as approximations for the corresponding population parameters. This idea is illustrated in Figure 6.1.

How does one obtain a random sample? This is not an easy question to answer. There are many different sampling schemes available to the researcher. The scheme chosen in a particular study depends on many things. Factors such as population size, type of population, questions to be answered, available time and resources, and accuracy desired all contribute to the choice of a sampling technique. It is not reasonable to assume that a procedure designed to sample records from a hospital's files will work equally well when sampling trees in a national forest or when sampling a species of endangered whales in the Pacific Ocean. At the *design stage* of a study the researcher must consult a statistician for help in choosing an appropriate sampling scheme. Advice will be given on how to draw the sample, what information to obtain from each object sampled, and how large the sample must be to accomplish the goals of the study.

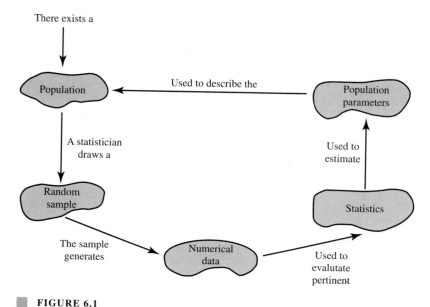

There exists a

Population

Used to describe the

Population parameters

A statistician draws a

Used to estimate

Random sample

Statistics

The sample generates

Numerical data

Used to evalutate pertinent

FIGURE 6.1

A summary of the manner in which a statistical study is conducted.

Simple Random Sampling

Here we consider *simple random sampling*. This type of sampling works well in many cases and is easy to use and to understand. It is the type of sampling that most laypersons assume when they hear the term *sample*. In simple random sampling, objects are selected "at random" in the sense that the choice of objects sampled is controlled by some random mechanism. The researcher does not deliberately include a particular object in the sample or purposely exclude one from the sample. Each object in the population has the same chance of being chosen for study as every other one. The random mechanism used to accomplish this could be as simple as drawing names from a hat or as complex as using an electronic random number generator.

One of the easiest ways to select a simple random sample from a finite population is by means of a table of random digits. This table is generated in such a way that each of the digits 0 to 9 has the same probability of appearing in a given position in the table as every other digit. One such table is Table IV of Appendix B. Its use is illustrated in Example 6.1.1. The sample size chosen in the example is small so that the use of the table can be demonstrated quickly. Do not interpret this example as implying that inferences about large populations are routinely made using small samples. This is certainly not the case.

EXAMPLE 6.1.1. There has been some concern recently that doctors are ordering an excessive number of laboratory tests for their hospitalized patients. A hospital administrator is interested in studying the situation at her institution. One question to be answered is, What was the mean number of tests ordered per patient visit in this hospital last year?

▓ **TABLE 6.1**

77921	06907	11008
99562	72905	⑤642
96301	91977	05463
89579	14342	63661
85475	36857	43342
28918	69578	88231
63553	40961	48235
09429	93969	52636
10365	61129	87529
07119	97336	71048

Suppose that a total of 8000 patient visits are on file. How can we randomly select five files to be studied? To do so, first note that the records of patient visits are listed in the files and can be numbered from 1 to 8000. We use Table IV of Appendix B to obtain five random four-digit numbers (0001 to 8000). Patient records corresponding to the numbers selected are chosen for study and therefore constitute our simple random sample of size 5. In this way, control of the visits sampled has been taken out of our hands, and there can be no charge that we manipulated the results of the study in any way.

To begin, a random starting point is selected. One way to do this is to place the row numbers (01 to 50) on slips of paper in a box and then draw a slip at random. The number drawn determines the row of Table IV containing the random starting point. A random column number from 01 to 14 is selected in a similar way. Suppose that when this is done we obtain row 7 and column 3. The number found in this position in Table IV is 56420. The portion of the table containing this value is shown in Table 6.1. We begin reading the table at this point. The table may be read in a variety of ways: across the row, down the column, every other digit down the column, or by any other arbitrary scheme desired. The easiest way is to read the first four digits across the row to obtain the random number 5642. Thus patient visit 5642 has been selected as the first member of our simple random sample. Reading down the column, we find the next random four-digit number is 0546, corresponding to visit number 546. The third and fourth visits selected are numbers 6366 and 4334, respectively. As we continue down the column, the next random number is 8823. Since we have only 8000 patient visits, this number is too large and is discarded. Thus the final member of the random sample corresponds to the next number in the table, 4823. If the same random number had been obtained more than once, it would have been discarded after the first selection. At this point we have a simple random sample that consists of the *files on five patient visits*. These files can be examined to obtain a sample of five observations on the random variable X, the number of laboratory tests ordered per patient visit. These observations can then be averaged to find $\bar{x}$, the mean of the sample and the approximation for the mean of the population from which the sample was drawn.

As demonstrated, simple random samples can be drawn using a random digit table. These samples can also be selected via random number generators written for computers or random number generators programmed into handheld calculators. The use of the TI83 calculator to generate a random sample is illustrated in the Technology Tools section of this chapter; a SAS program for this purpose is also given.

The term *random sample* is used in three different ways. For example, suppose that I want to conduct a study of the random variable X, the birth weight of babies born to mothers addicted to cocaine. Suppose that I intend to draw a random sample of size

10. Before any babies are actually chosen for study, I know that I am dealing with 10 random variables $X_1, X_2, \ldots, X_{10}$ where X_i denotes the birth weight of the ith baby selected for study. Each of these random variables can conceivably assume any value between perhaps $\frac{1}{2}$ and 20 pounds. These 10 random variables are referred to as being a random sample from the distribution of X. Capital letters, our notation for random variables, are used to emphasize the fact that at this point each member of the sample is a random variable. I then select 10 babies for study. These babies are referred to as being a random sample of babies drawn from the population of babies born to mothers addicted to cocaine. Here each member of the sample is a baby. Once the babies have been identified and their birth weights recorded, 10 numbers, $x_1, x_2, \ldots, x_{10}$, are available. These numbers, which represent observations on the random variables $X_1, X_2, \ldots, X_{10}$, are also referred to as being a random sample. In this setting each member of the sample is a number. Figure 6.2 illustrates these three uses of the term *random sample*. In practice, it is clear from the context which usage is intended.

A statistician has a population about which to draw inferences.

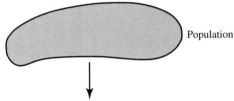

Population

Prior to the selection of the objects for study, interest centers on the n random variables $X_1, X_2, X_3, \ldots, X_n$.

A set of n *objects* is selected from the population for study.

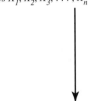
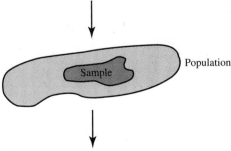

Sample

Population

The objects selected generate n *numbers* $x_1, x_2, x_3, \ldots, x_n$, which are the observed values of the random variables $X_1, X_2, X_3, \ldots, X_n$.

FIGURE 6.2

Three ways to view the term *random sample*.

Randomization

The random digit table can be used to "randomize" sequences of events or to randomly assign treatments to experimental units. For example, suppose that a study is to be conducted to compare the effects of four different sulfate concentrations on the growth of pines. Typically, the researcher obtains a collection of seedlings and divides them into four groups with each group receiving a different sulfate treatment. It is assumed that the seedlings are identical at the beginning of the experiment. During the course of the experiment they are treated alike in all respects other than the level of sulfate received. Any differences that are observed at the end of the experiment are attributed to the fact that different sulfate levels were used. Notice that even though we assume that the seedlings are identical at the beginning of the experiment, we know that this is not true. Some slight differences in height, or weight, or general health of the plant are present. To spread these differences across treatments and to protect against charges that a systematic bias is present in the experiment, we randomly assign treatments to seedlings. The random digit table can be used to do this. For example, suppose that we have 20 seedlings and we want to assign 5 seedlings to each of the four treatments at random. To accomplish this, we number the seedlings from 01 to 20. We then choose random two-digit numbers from the random number table. The first five numbers between 01 and 20 selected receive treatment A, the second five receive treatment B, the third five are assigned to treatment C, and the remainder receive treatment D. Example 6.1.2 illustrates this idea.

> **EXAMPLE 6.1.2.** Figure 6.3a shows 20 pine seedlings numbered from 01 to 20. Suppose that the technique explained in Example 6.1.1 is used to obtain the random starting point 27958 shown in Table 6.2 (row 36, column 3 of Table IV of Appendix B). We read the first two digits down the column from that point. We then move to the bottom of column 4 and read up. The first five numbers found are 18, 06, 20, 07, and 12. The seedlings with these numbers will receive treatment A. See Figure 6.3b. The next five numbers chosen are 14, 09, 08, 03, and 10. These seedlings receive treatment B. Seedlings 16, 02, 17, 13, and 19 receive treatment C, and the rest treatment D. The complete assignment of treatments is shown in Figure 6.3c.

This technique can be used in other settings. For example, it can be used to randomly assign experimental protocols to patients in a medical setting, to randomly assign experimental drug treatments to laboratory mice, or to randomly form groups so that they can be assigned specific tasks as members of a research team.

▧ EXERCISES 6.1

1. Use the technique explained in Example 6.1.1 to find a random starting point in Table IV of Appendix B. Use this starting point to randomly assign treatments to the 20 pine seedlings of Example 6.1.2. How many of the seedlings were assigned the same treatment as that assigned by the randomization of Example 6.1.2?
2. *Species diversity.* The species diversity index is a comparative index used to measure the effect of a disturbance, such as water pollution, on living organisms. The diversity of the population prior to and after the disturbance can be determined and

a comparison made. In general, a lower index after the disturbance is an indication that the disturbance has had a negative effect. The following example illustrates the technique used to determine the index for a given sample.

EXAMPLE. Suppose that a water sample is examined under the microscope and is found to contain three members of species A, four of species B, and seven of species C for a total of 14 organisms. We mark off positions as shown below:

— — — — — — — — — — — — — —

Now select 14 random two-digit numbers, 01 to 14, from the random number table. The first three chosen determine the positions assigned to species A, the next four are assigned to species B, and the last seven to species C. Suppose that our random starting point is row 11, column 5. Reading down from this point in Table 6.2, we see that the first three numbers chosen are 09, 13, 04. These positions are assigned to species A as shown below.

— — — A — — — — A — — — A —

The next four numbers chosen are 02, 01, 14, 10, and these positions are assigned to species B.

B B — A — — — — A B — A B
— — — — — — — — — — — — —

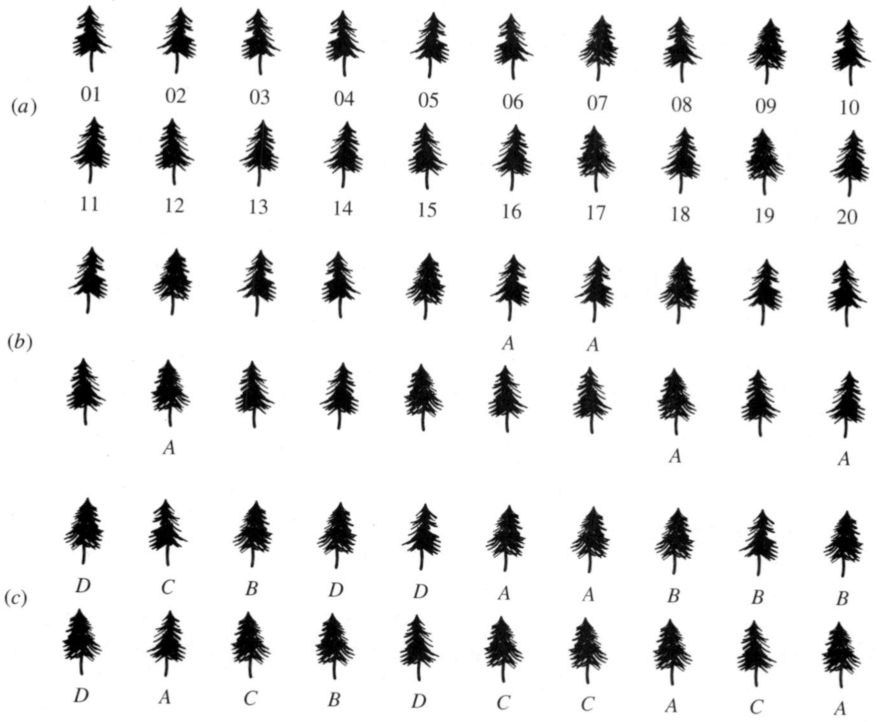

FIGURE 6.3

(*a*) Seedlings are numbered 01 to 20. (*b*) The seedlings numbered 18, 06, 20, 07, and 12 are selected first and receive treatment A. (*c*) Complete assignment of treatments.

■ TABLE 6.2

The number 27958 found in row 36 and column 3 provides the random starting point for selecting random two-digit numbers from 01 to 20

Row/Col.	(1)	(2)	(3)	(4)	(5)	(6)	(7)	(8)	(9)	(10)	(11)	(12)	(13)	(14)
1	10480	15011	01536	02011	81647	91646	69179	14194	62590	36207	20969	99570	91291	90700
2	22368	46573	25595	85393	30995	89198	27982	53402	93965	34095	52666	19174	39615	99505
3	24130	48360	22527	97265	76393	64809	15179	24830	49340	32081	30680	19655	63348	58629
4	42167	93093	06243	61680	07856	16376	39440	53537	71341	57004	00849	74917	97758	16379
5	37570	39975	81837	16656	06121	91782	60468	81305	49684	60672	14110	06927	01263	54613
6	77921	06907	11008	42751	27756	53498	18602	70659	90655	15053	21916	81825	44394	42880
7	99562	72905	56420	69994	98872	31016	71194	18738	44013	48840	63213	21069	10634	12952
8	96301	91977	05463	07972	18876	20922	94595	56869	69014	60045	18425	84903	42508	32307
9	89579	14342	63661	10281	17453	18103	57740	84378	25331	12566	58678	44947	05585	56941
10	85475	36857	43342	53988	53060	59533	38867	62300	08158	17983	16439	11458	18593	64952
11	28918	69578	88231	33276	70997	79936	56865	05859	90106	31595	01547	85590	91610	78188
12	63553	40961	48235	03427	49626	69445	18663	72695	52180	20847	12234	90511	33703	90322
13	09429	93969	52636	92737	88974	33488	36320	17617	30015	08272	84115	27156	30613	74952
14	10365	61129	87529	85689	48237	52267	67689	93394	01511	26358	85104	20285	29975	89868
15	07119	97336	71048	08178	77233	13916	47564	81056	97735	85977	29372	74461	28551	90707
16	51085	12765	51821	51259	77452	16308	60756	92144	49442	53900	70960	63990	75601	40719
17	02368	21382	52404	60268	89368	19885	55322	44819	01188	65255	64835	44919	05944	55157
18	01011	54092	33362	94904	31273	04146	18594	29852	71585	85030	51132	01915	92747	64951
19	52162	53916	46369	58586	23216	14513	83149	98736	23495	64350	94738	17752	35156	35749
20	07056	97628	33787	09998	42698	06691	76988	13602	51851	46104	88916	19509	25625	58104
21	48663	91245	85828	14346	09172	30168	90229	04734	59193	22178	30421	61666	99904	32812
22	54164	58492	22421	74103	47070	25306	76468	26384	58151	06646	21524	15227	96909	44592
23	32639	32363	05597	24200	13363	38005	94342	28728	35806	06912	17012	64161	18296	22851
24	29334	27001	87637	87308	58731	00256	45834	15398	46557	41135	10367	07684	36188	18510
25	02488	33062	28834	07351	19731	92420	60952	61280	50001	67658	32586	86679	50720	94953

26	81525	72295	04839	96423	24878	82651	66566	14778	76797	14780	13300	87074	79666	95725
27	29676	20591	68086	26432	46901	20849	89768	81536	86645	12659	92259	57102	80428	25280
28	00742	57392	39064	66432	84673	40027	32832	61362	98947	96067	64760	64584	96096	98253
29	05366	04213	25669	26422	44407	44048	37937	63904	45766	66134	75470	66520	34693	90449
30	91921	26418	64117	94305	26766	25940	39972	22209	71500	64568	91402	42416	07844	69618
31	00582	04711	87917	77341	42206	35126	74087	99547	81817	42607	43808	76655	62028	76630
32	00725	69884	62797	56170	86324	88072	76222	36086	84637	93161	76038	65855	77919	88006
33	69011	65797	95876	55293	18988	27354	26575	08625	40801	59920	29841	80150	12777	48501
34	25976	57948	29888	88604	67917	48708	18912	82271	65424	69774	33611	54262	85963	03547
35	09763	83473	73577	12908	30883	18317	28290	35797	05998	41688	34952	37888	38917	88050
36	91567	42595	27958	30134	04024	86385	29880	99730	55536	84855	29080	09250	79656	73211
37	17955	56349	90999	49127	20044	59931	06115	20542	18059	02008	73708	83517	36103	42791
38	46503	18584	18845	49618	02304	51038	20655	58727	28168	15475	56942	53389	20562	87338
39	92157	89634	94824	78171	84610	82834	09922	25417	44137	48413	25555	21246	35509	20468
40	14577	62765	35605	81263	39667	47358	56873	56307	61607	49518	89656	20103	77490	18062
41	98427	07523	33362	64270	01638	92477	66969	98420	04880	45585	46565	04102	46880	45709
42	34914	63976	88720	82765	34476	17032	87589	40836	32427	70002	70663	88863	77775	69348
43	70060	28277	39475	46473	23219	53416	94970	25832	69975	94884	19661	72828	00102	66794
44	53976	54914	06990	67245	68350	82948	11398	42878	80287	88267	47363	46634	06541	97809
45	76072	29515	40980	07391	58745	25774	22987	80059	39911	96189	41151	14222	60697	59583
46	90725	52210	83974	29992	65831	38857	50490	83765	55657	14361	31720	57375	56228	41546
47	64364	67412	33339	31926	14883	24413	59744	92351	97473	89286	35931	04110	23726	51900
48	08962	00358	31662	25388	61642	34072	81249	35648	56891	69352	48373	45578	78547	81788
49	95012	68379	93526	70765	10593	04542	76463	54328	02349	17247	28865	14777	62730	92277
50	15664	10493	20492	38391	91132	21999	59516	81652	27195	48223	46751	22923	32261	85653

The remaining positions are allocated to species C to obtain the random sequence

$$B \quad B \quad C \quad A \quad C \quad C \quad C \quad C \quad A \quad B \quad C \quad C \quad A \quad B$$

We now count the number of runs in the sequence where a run is a sequence of like organisms. The runs in the above sequence are shown below.

$$B \quad B \quad C \quad A \quad C \quad C \quad C \quad C \quad A \quad B \quad C \quad C \quad A \quad B$$

The sequence contains nine runs. The *sequential comparison index* (SCI) is defined by

$$\text{SCI} = \frac{\text{number of runs}}{\text{number of specimens}}$$

In this case,

$$\text{SCI} = \frac{9}{14} = .64$$

This measure of diversity can be refined to produce a second diversity measure, *the diversity index* (DI), by multiplying the SCI by the number of different species found in the sample. Thus

$$\text{DI} = (\text{SCI})(\text{number of species})$$

In our example,

$$\text{DI} = .64(3) = 1.92$$

The randomization procedure is repeated to obtain a second SCI and a second DI. The diversity index for the sample is taken as the average of the two DI scores. Experience has shown that when this procedure is applied to streams, a diversity index greater than 12 is an indication of a healthy stream; values of 8 or less indicate serious pollution; and other values are of a marginal nature. (Information from James Brower, Jerrold Zar, and Carl Von Ende, *Field and Laboratory Methods for General Ecology*, Wm. C. Brown, Publishers, Dubuque, Iowa, 1990, pp. 51–52.)

(a) Obtain a second randomization for the above example and compute its SCI and DI. Average the two available DI's to obtain the diversity index for the sample.
(b) In a study of the effect of a sewage treatment plant on the microorganisms living in a river, water samples were taken above and below the plant. These data were obtained:

Microorganism	Above	Below
Diatoms	12	5
Spirochetes	2	1
Protists	4	1

For each sample obtain two SCI and DI readings. Find the diversity index for each sample by averaging the two DI readings. Is there an indication that the sewage treatment plant might be affecting the diversity of organisms in the river? (Based on a study conducted by Joseph Hutton, Department of Biology and the Statistical Consulting Service, Radford University, Radford, Virginia, 1990.)

3. A forester wants to sample loblolly pines in a large wooded tract so that the mean diameter at breast height (MDBH) of the trees can be estimated. To do so, a topographical map of the area is obtained. Grid lines are marked on the map in such a way that 200 squares each of size 10 by 10 meters are defined. A random sample of 20 squares is to be selected, and the diameter of each loblolly pine within each square is obtained.

    (*a*) Use the random number generator to obtain 20 random three-digit numbers lying between 001 and 200.

    (*b*) Table V of Appendix B gives information on the pines in the 200 squares. For your sample, compute $\bar{x}$, the average diameter at breast height of the trees in your sample. Is this value the MDBH for the entire stand? Explain. Compare your average with those obtained by some of your colleagues.

    (*c*) For your sample, compute $\bar{n}$, the average number of trees per square. Multiply $\bar{n}$ by 200 to estimate the total number of trees in the stand. Is your estimate close to 600, the actual number of trees listed in Table V?

    (Data based on Harold Burkhart et al., *Yields of Old-Field Loblolly Pine Plantations,* Division of Forestry and Wildlife Resources, Pub. FWS-3-72, VPI and SU, Blacksburg, Va.)

4. Table XIII of Appendix B gives the sex and systolic and diastolic blood pressure of the 120 patients seen at a particular clinic. Use the random digit table to draw a simple random sample of size 20 from this population. Record the sex and each of the blood pressures of the individuals selected.

5. A biologist is investigating the effect of pH on the growth of pea plants. Thirty pots each containing two plants are to be used. Three pH levels will be used with 10 pots receiving treatment *A*, 10 treatment *B*, and the rest treatment *C*. The 30 pots are arranged in six rows on a table in the greenhouse as shown below:

    (*a*) Why would it be rather risky from a practical point of view to treat all pots in the first two rows with level 1 pH, all pots in rows 3 and 4 with level 2 pH, and the rest with level 3 pH?

    (*b*) Use the random number table or a random number generator to determine the assignment of pH levels to the 30 pots of plants.

6. Two drugs, A and B, are to be compared to a placebo P. Thirty persons are to be used in the drug trial with the three drugs being randomly assigned to 10 persons each. Use the technique explained in Example 6.1.1 to randomize the drugs to subjects. Compare your randomization to that of a classmate. Suppose that you are subject number 12. What treatment will you receive via your randomization? via your classmate's randomization? In how many cases did the two randomizations assign the same treatment to subjects?

▓ 6.2

POINT ESTIMATION OF THE MEAN AND INTRODUCTION TO INTERVAL ESTIMATION: CENTRAL LIMIT THEOREM

Recall from the discussion in Section 1.4 that the sample mean serves two purposes. It gives the average value of the sample at hand and it approximates or estimates the mean of the population from which the sample was drawn. Recall also that the sample mean is a random variable; its value varies from sample to sample even when sampling from the same population. To emphasize this point we will use a capital letter $\bar{X}$ to denote the sample mean in a general setting. Once a sample has been drawn and a numerical value obtained for the sample mean, we will switch to a lowercase letter as in the past. Example 6.2.1 illustrates the notation.

> **EXAMPLE 6.2.1.** Researchers at the Environmental Protection Agency (EPA) are interested in air quality. One indicator of air quality is the mean number of micrograms of particulates per cubic meter of air. That is, interest centers on μ, the mean of the random variable X where X is the number of micrograms of particulates per cubic meter of air. To monitor the situation, a reading is taken every 6 days by drawing a cubic meter of air through a filter and determining the number of micrograms of particulates trapped. Over a 30-day period, a random sample X_1, X_2, X_3, X_4, X_5 of size 5 is generated. Assume that the observed values of these variables for a given 30-day period are
>
> $x_1 = 58 \qquad x_3 = 57 \qquad x_5 = 59$
>
> $x_2 = 70 \qquad x_4 = 61$
>
> The observed value of the statistic $\bar{X}$ is found by averaging these five values. In this case
>
> $$\bar{x} = \frac{58 + 70 + 57 + 61 + 59}{5} = 61$$
>
> Notice that once we have evaluated the statistic $\bar{X}$ for this particular sample, we switch to a lowercase letter.

Some new terminology must be introduced at this time. A statistic used to approximate a population parameter is called an *estimator* for the parameter. The number obtained when the estimator is evaluated for a particular sample is called an *estimate* for the parameter. In Example 6.2.1, $\bar{X}$ is an estimator for μ; the number 61 is the estimate for μ based on the given sample. The statistic $\bar{X}$ is called a *point estimator* for μ because when evaluated for a particular sample, it yields a single number or point.

Common sense points to $\bar{X}$ as the most logical estimator for μ. It can be shown that this estimator has some nice mathematical properties also. In particular, it can be shown that in repeated sampling from a population with mean μ the values of $\bar{X}$ will fluctuate about μ as an average value. It can also be shown that for large sample sizes, the values of $\bar{X}$ are fairly consistent. That is, the observed values of $\bar{X}$ are centered at μ, the value that this statistic is trying to estimate, and for large samples, most of the observed values are expected to fall close to μ. This means that if we have a moderately sized sample and estimate μ via $\bar{x}$, this estimate is likely to be fairly accurate. These facts are proved in Appendix A. They are illustrated in Example 6.2.3.

Interval Estimation

We have seen that the statistic $\bar{X}$ provides a good, commonsense point estimate for a population mean μ. Its major drawback is that any single observed value of $\bar{X}$ is usually not exactly equal to μ; there will be some difference between $\bar{x}$ and μ. It would be comforting to be able to get an idea of how close our estimate is to the true population mean. It would also be good to be able to report how sure or confident we are of the accuracy of our estimate.

To get an idea of not only the value of the mean but also the accuracy of the estimate, researchers turn to the method of interval estimation, or *confidence intervals*. An interval estimator is what the name implies. It is a random interval, an interval whose endpoints L_1 and L_2 are each statistics. It is used to determine a numerical interval based on a sample. It is hoped that the numerical interval obtained will contain the population parameter being estimated. By expanding from a point to an interval, we create a little room for error and in so doing gain the ability, based on probability theory, to report the confidence that we have in the estimator.

A confidence interval on μ is an interval $[L_1, L_2]$ which traps the mean with some stated degree of certainty. For example, a 95% confidence interval is an interval such that $P[L_1 \leq \mu \leq L_2] \doteq .95$; a 99% confidence interval satisfies the condition that $P[L_1 \leq \mu \leq L_2] \doteq .99$. To say that an interval is a 95% confidence interval on μ means that when it is used in repeated sampling from the population, 95% of the intervals that result should contain μ; by chance, 5% will fail to trap the true population mean. The degree of confidence desired is controlled by the researcher. Figure 6.4 illustrates the idea.

To create a confidence interval on μ we must first find a random variable whose expression involves μ and whose distribution is known at least approximately. To do

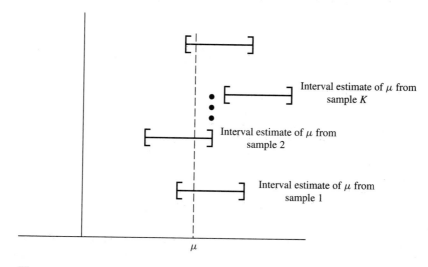

FIGURE 6.4

Of the intervals constructed by using $[L_1, L_2]$, 95% are expected to contain μ, the true but unknown population mean.

this we must consider further the distribution of $\bar{X}$. Recall that since $\bar{X}$ is a random variable, it has a distribution. What we are asking is, What is the shape of the distribution of $\bar{X}$? What is its mean? What is its variance? Theorem 6.2.1 answers these questions in the case in which sampling is from a normal distribution. This theorem is partially proved in Appendix A. Theorem 6.2.2 answers the questions for cases in which sampling is from nonnormal distributions.

THEOREM 6.2.1. Let $X_1, X_2, \ldots, X_n$ be a random sample of size n, from a distribution that is normal with mean μ and variance σ^2. Then $\bar{X}$ is normal with mean μ and variance σ^2/n. Furthermore, the random variable

$$\frac{\bar{X} - \mu}{\sigma/\sqrt{n}}$$

is *standard normal*.

Note that the random variable $(\bar{X} - \mu)/(\sigma/\sqrt{n})$ involves the parameter μ, and its distribution is known to be standard normal. This variable can be used to determine the general formula for a confidence interval on μ. We illustrate the method by considering first the construction of a 95% confidence interval. The technique used can be generalized easily to obtain any desired degree of confidence.

EXAMPLE 6.2.2. Let us find a 95% confidence interval on μ, the mean number of micrograms of particulate per cubic meter of air, based on the random sample of size 5 given in Example 6.2.1. From Example 6.2.1 it is known that a point estimate for μ is $\bar{x} = 61$. Assume that from past experience X, the number of micrograms of particulate per cubic meter of air, is *known* to be normally distributed with variance $\sigma^2 = 9$. We want to extend the point estimate to an interval of real numbers in such a way that we can be 95% confident that the interval obtained contains the true value of μ. That is, we want to determine L_1 and L_2 so that $P[L_1 \leq \mu \leq L_2] = .95$. (See Figure 6.5.)

To do so, consider the partition of the standard normal curve shown in Figure 6.6. It can be seen that

$$P[-1.96 \leq Z \leq 1.96] = .95$$

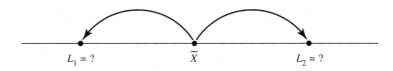

FIGURE 6.5

L_1 and L_2 are statistics such that $P[L_1 \leq \mu \leq L_2] \doteq .95$.

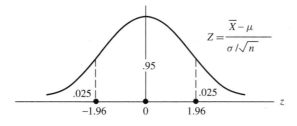

$$Z = \frac{\bar{X} - \mu}{\sigma/\sqrt{n}}$$

FIGURE 6.6

Partition of Z needed to obtain a 95% confidence interval on μ.

$P[-1.96 \leq Z \leq 1.96] = .95$.

In this case, $Z = (\bar{X} - \mu)/(\sigma/\sqrt{n})$, and hence we may conclude that

$$P\left[-1.96 \le \frac{\bar{X} - \mu}{\sigma/\sqrt{n}} \le 1.96\right] = .95$$

To find the endpoints for a 95% confidence interval on μ, we algebraically isolate μ in the center of the preceding inequality:

$$P\left[-1.96 \le \frac{\bar{X} - \mu}{\sigma/\sqrt{n}} \le 1.96\right] = .95$$

$$P\left[\frac{-1.96\sigma}{\sqrt{n}} \le \bar{X} - \mu \le \frac{1.96\sigma}{\sqrt{n}}\right] = .95$$

$$P\left[-\bar{X} - \frac{1.96\sigma}{\sqrt{n}} \le -\mu \le -\bar{X} + \frac{1.96\sigma}{\sqrt{n}}\right] = .95$$

$$P\left[\bar{X} + \frac{1.96\sigma}{\sqrt{n}} \ge \mu \ge \bar{X} - \frac{1.96\sigma}{\sqrt{n}}\right] = .95$$

$$P\left[\bar{X} - \frac{1.96\sigma}{\sqrt{n}} \le \mu \le \bar{X} + \frac{1.96\sigma}{\sqrt{n}}\right] = .95$$

From this we see that the lower and upper bounds for the 95% confidence interval are

$$L_1 = \bar{X} - \frac{1.96\sigma}{\sqrt{n}} \qquad L_2 = \bar{X} + \frac{1.96\sigma}{\sqrt{n}}$$

Since it is assumed that σ^2 is known to be 9, L_1 and L_2 are statistics. Their observed values for the sample at hand are

$$\bar{x} - 1.96\left(\frac{3}{\sqrt{5}}\right) = 61 - 2.63 = 58.37$$

$$\bar{x} + 1.96\left(\frac{3}{\sqrt{5}}\right) = 61 + 2.63 = 63.63$$

(See Figure 6.7.) Since this interval was generated by using a procedure that, in repeated sampling, will trap the mean 95% of the time, we can be 95% confident that μ actually lies between 58.37 and 63.63.

To generalize this procedure to any desired degree of confidence we need only substitute an appropriate point from the Z table for the value 1.96. For example, to find a 99% confidence interval on μ, we begin with the partition of the Z curve shown in

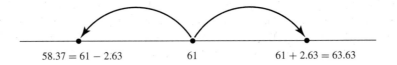

$$58.37 = 61 - 2.63 \qquad\qquad 61 \qquad\qquad 61 + 2.63 = 63.63$$

FIGURE 6.7
The 95% confidence interval on μ.

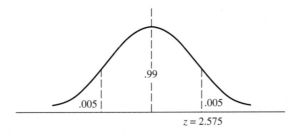

$z = 2.575$

■ **FIGURE 6.8**
Partition of Z needed to obtain a 99% confidence
interval on μ. The point needed is $z = 2.575$.

Figure 6.8. The bounds for the interval are

$$\bar{x} - 2.575 \left(\frac{3}{\sqrt{5}} \right) = 61 - 3.45 = 57.55$$

$$\bar{x} + 2.575 \left(\frac{3}{\sqrt{5}} \right) = 61 + 3.45 = 64.45$$

We can be 99% confident that μ actually lies between 57.55 and 64.45. In general, any confidence interval on μ with σ^2 known takes the form

$$\bar{X} \pm z \frac{\sigma}{\sqrt{n}}$$

Several things are evident from this formula. First, each confidence interval on μ will be centered at $\bar{x}$, the sample mean. Second, the length of the interval depends on three things: (1) the confidence desired, (2) the standard deviation, (3) the sample size. You are asked to investigate the effect of these factors on interval length in Exercises 2 through 4.

Central Limit Theorem

There is one further point to be made. The bounds $\bar{X} \pm z(\sigma/\sqrt{n})$ are derived assuming that the variable X is normal. If this condition is not satisfied, then the confidence bounds given can be used as long as the sample is not too small. Empirical studies have shown that for samples as small as 25, the above bounds are usually satisfactory even though approximate. This is because of a remarkable theorem, first formulated in the early nineteenth century by Laplace and Gauss. This theorem, known as the Central Limit Theorem, is stated now.

THEOREM 6.2.2. Central Limit Theorem. Let $X_1, X_2, \ldots, X_n$ be a random sample of size n from a distribution with mean μ and variance σ^2. Then for large n, $\bar{X}$ is approxi-

TABLE 6.3

Density for X, the number obtained in the toss of a single die

x	1	2	3	4	5	6
$f(x)$	$\frac{1}{6}$	$\frac{1}{6}$	$\frac{1}{6}$	$\frac{1}{6}$	$\frac{1}{6}$	$\frac{1}{6}$

mately normal with mean μ and variance σ^2/n. Furthermore, for large n, the random variable $(\bar{X} - \mu)/(\sigma/\sqrt{n})$ is approximately standard normal.

The proof of this theorem is beyond the scope of this text. Basically it states that even if sampling is from a nonnormal distribution, $\bar{X}$ will be approximately normal as long as the sample size is not too small. Example 6.2.3 illustrates the Central Limit Theorem.

EXAMPLE 6.2.3. Consider the random variable X, the number obtained on the toss of a single die. The density for X is shown in Table 6.3. Notice that X is discrete and uniformly distributed. This distribution is vastly different from normal, which is continuous and bell-shaped. Therefore, if we want to construct confidence intervals on μ based on the bounds

$$\bar{X} \pm z \left(\frac{\sigma}{\sqrt{n}} \right)$$

we must rely on the Central Limit Theorem. This means that the sample size used must not be too small. Consider an experiment in which the die is tossed $n = 25$ times and the average $\bar{x}$ is obtained.

According to the Central Limit Theorem, the random variable $\bar{X}$ is approximately normally distributed. This means that if we repeat this experiment a large number of times and graph the $\bar{x}$ values observed, the histogram obtained should form a rough bell. Since $E[\bar{X}] = \mu$, the average value of the $\bar{x}$ values observed should be close to the true average value of X. In Section 4.2, this true mean was shown to be 3.5. That is, the observed $\bar{x}$ values are expected to fluctuate about the value 3.5. The Central Limit Theorem implies that Var $\bar{X} = \sigma^2/n$ where σ^2 is the true variance of X. Methods of Section 4.2 can be used to show that Var $X = \sigma^2 = 2.916$. This, in turn, implies that $\sigma = \sqrt{2.916} \doteq 1.708$. Thus, in this case, Var $\bar{X} = 2.916/25 = .116$.

SAS was used to simulate the die toss experiment 50 times. The results of this simulation are shown in Figure 6.9. In this simulation, SAS was allowed to choose its own classes. Notice that the histogram does not form a perfect bell, but the bell shape is suggested strongly by the plot. The average value of the 50 $\bar{x}$ values is 3.51; this average is very close to the theoretical value of 3.5. The variance of the 50 $\bar{x}$ values is .143; this variance is somewhat larger than the theoretical value of .116.

Figure 6.10 shows some additional simulations. In Figure 6.10a the 50 $\bar{x}$ values are each based on samples of size $n = 5$; in Figure 6.10b, on samples of size $n = 10$; and in Figure 6.10c, on samples of size $n = 40$. Notice that as n increases, the class boundaries and the number of classes change as these characteristics are a function of the data itself; the bell shape becomes somewhat more pronounced; the average value of the $\bar{x}$ values gets closer to the true value of 3.5; and the variance in the $\bar{x}$ values decreases. All of these things are anticipated by the Central Limit Theorem.

Computer simulation can also be used to gain a better understanding of the notion of a confidence interval. The 50 $\bar{x}$ values obtained in the simulation of Example 6.2.3

```
   XBAR                                            Cum.               Cum.
 Midpoint                            Freq  Freq  Percent  Percent

    2.7    |****                        2     2     4.00     4.00

    3.0    |*********                    5     7    10.00    14.00

    3.3    |*****************************  15    22    30.00    44.00

    3.6    |*****************************  15    37    30.00    74.00

    3.9    |*****************             9    46    18.00    92.00

    4.2    |********                      4    50     8.00   100.00

           |---+---+---+---+---+---+---+--
             2   4   6   8  10  12  14
                    Frequency
```

DISTRIBUTION OF XBAR

Analysis Variable : XBAR

	Mean	Variance	Std Dev	Std Error	N
	3.510	0.143	0.378	0.053	50

FIGURE 6.9
Simulation based on 50 samples each of size 25.

```
   XBAR                                            Cum.               Cum.
 Midpoint                            Freq  Freq  Percent  Percent

    1.8    |**********                    5     5    10.00    10.00

    2.4    |************                  6    11    12.00    22.00

    3.0    |*********************        11    22    22.00    44.00

    3.6    |*********************        11    33    22.00    66.00

    4.2    |***********************      12    45    24.00    90.00

    4.8    |**********                    5    50    10.00   100.00

           |---+---+---+---+---+---+
             2   4   6   8  10  12
                    Frequency
```

DISTRIBUTION OF XBAR

Analysis Variable : XBAR

	Mean	Variance	Std Dev	Std Error	N
	3.412	0.693	0.832	0.118	50

FIGURE 6.10a
Simulation based on 50 samples each of size (a) $n = 5$, (b) $n = 10$, and (c) $n = 40$.

```
    XBAR                                        Cum.                Cum.
  Midpoint                             Freq     Freq   Percent    Percent

    1.5     |**                          1       1     2.00       2.00

    2.0     |**                          1       2     2.00       4.00

    2.5     |******                      3       5     6.00      10.00

    3.0     |******************************   15   20    30.00      40.00

    3.5     |***************************   14   34    28.00      68.00

    4.0     |************************    12      46    24.00      92.00

    4.5     |********                     4      50     8.00     100.00

            ----+---+---+---+---+---+---+--
                2   4   6   8  10  12  14
                         Frequency
```

DISTRIBUTION OF XBAR

Analysis Variable : XBAR

Mean	Variance	Std Dev	Std Error	N
3.428	0.374	0.612	0.087	50

FIGURE 6.10*b*

```
    XBAR                                        Cum.                Cum.
  Midpoint                             Freq     Freq   Percent    Percent

   2.875   |**                          1       1     2.00       2.00

   3.125   |********                     4       5     8.00      10.00

   3.375   |****************************************   20   25    40.00      50.00

   3.625   |*************************************   19   44    38.00      88.00

   3.875   |********                     4      48     8.00      96.00

   4.125   |****                         2      50     4.00     100.00

           ----+---+---+---+---+---+---+---+---+
               2   4   6   8  10  12  14  16  18  20
                         Frequency
```

DISTRIBUTION OF XBAR

Analysis Variable : XBAR

Mean	Variance	Std Dev	Std Error	N
3.482	0.064	0.253	0.036	50

FIGURE 6.10*c*

■ **TABLE 6.4**

95% Confidence intervals on the mean of X, the number obtained on the toss of a single die

OBS	XBAR	L1	L2	STATUS	OBS	XBAR	L1	L2	STATUS
1	3.64	2.97046	4.30954	trapped	26	3.48	2.81046	4.14954	trapped
2	3.24	2.57046	3.90954	trapped	27	3.32	2.65046	3.98954	trapped
3	3.52	2.85046	4.18954	trapped	28	3.40	2.73046	4.06954	trapped
4	3.88	3.21046	4.54954	trapped	29	3.40	2.73046	4.06954	trapped
5	3.60	2.93046	4.26954	trapped	30	4.00	3.33046	4.66954	trapped
6	2.88	2.21046	3.54954	trapped	31	3.16	2.49046	3.82954	trapped
7	2.96	2.29046	3.62954	trapped	32	3.72	3.05046	4.38954	trapped
8	4.16	3.49046	4.82954	trapped	33	4.12	3.45046	4.78954	trapped
9	3.32	2.65046	3.98954	trapped	34	3.60	2.93046	4.26954	trapped
10	3.48	2.81046	4.14954	trapped	35	3.84	3.17046	4.50954	trapped
11	2.88	2.21046	3.54954	trapped	36	3.64	2.97046	4.30954	trapped
12	3.20	2.53046	3.86954	trapped	37	2.60	1.93046	3.26954	missed
13	2.68	2.01046	3.34954	missed	38	4.12	3.45046	4.78954	trapped
14	3.96	3.29046	4.62954	trapped	39	3.36	2.69046	4.02954	trapped
15	4.12	3.45046	4.78954	trapped	40	3.72	3.05046	4.38954	trapped
16	3.44	2.77046	4.10954	trapped	41	3.92	3.25046	4.58954	trapped
17	3.72	3.05046	4.38954	trapped	42	3.80	3.13046	4.46954	trapped
18	3.44	2.77046	4.10954	trapped	43	3.80	3.13046	4.46954	trapped
19	3.44	2.77046	4.10954	trapped	44	3.52	2.85046	4.18954	trapped
20	3.68	3.01046	4.34954	trapped	45	3.52	2.85046	4.18954	trapped
21	3.64	2.97046	4.30954	trapped	46	3.40	2.73046	4.06954	trapped
22	2.92	2.25046	3.58954	trapped	47	3.44	2.77046	4.10954	trapped
23	3.24	2.57046	3.90954	trapped	48	3.24	2.57046	3.90954	trapped
24	3.80	3.13046	4.46954	trapped	49	3.68	3.01046	4.34954	trapped
25	3.96	3.29046	4.62954	trapped	50	2.92	2.25046	3.58954	trapped

where $n = 25$ are shown in Table 6.4. Each of the $\bar{x}$ values was plugged into the formula

$$\bar{x} \pm z \left(\frac{\sigma}{\sqrt{n}} \right) \quad \text{or} \quad \bar{x} \pm 1.96 \left(\frac{1.708}{\sqrt{25}} \right)$$

to form a 95% confidence interval on μ. The numerical bounds for these intervals are given by L_1 and L_2 in the table. Theory indicates that about 95% of the intervals produced will trap the true mean value of 3.5; by chance about 5% will fail to do so. In this case, we expect 5% of 50 (about 2.5) intervals to miss the mean. Notice that, in fact, 2 of the 50 missed. This agrees quite well with what theory predicts.

Keep in mind the fact that in an actual study, only *one* confidence interval is found. It either does or does not succeed in trapping μ. We always hope that the interval found in our study is one of the intervals that does successfully catch μ between the lower and upper bounds rather than one of the few unusual intervals that, due to the chance nature of sampling, leads to a miss. Also keep in mind that to use the formula given in this section, σ, the true standard deviation of X, *must be known*. If it is not known and must be estimated from the data then the formula in this section is not appropriate.

■ **EXERCISES 6.2**

1. A random sample of size 9 yielded the following observations on the random variable X, the coal consumption in millions of tons by electric utilities for a given year:

406	395	400	450	390
410	415	401	408	

   Find a point estimate for μ, the mean coal consumption of electric utilities. Is the value that you got necessarily exactly equal to the average coal consumption of all electric utilities for the year in question? Explain.

2. Find a 90% confidence interval on the mean number of micrograms of particulate per cubic meter of air based on the data of Example 6.2.1. It this interval longer or shorter than the interval found earlier?

3. In general, would you expect a 90% confidence interval on μ to be longer or shorter than a 95% confidence interval based on the same sample?

4. Sample size plays a role in determining the length of a confidence interval. Consider two 95% confidence intervals on μ based on samples of size n_1 and n_2 drawn from the same population. If $n_1 > n_2$, which confidence interval will be longer?

5. Conduct the experiment described in Example 6.2.3 10 times. Do your $\bar{x}$ values vary around the value 3.5 as expected? Average your 10 $\bar{x}$ values. Does this average lie fairly close to the number 3.5? Calculate the variance of your 10 $\bar{x}$ values. Is the answer obtained close in value to the number .116 as expected? Use each of your 10 $\bar{x}$ values to form a 95% confidence interval on μ. Do any of your intervals fail to trap the true mean of 3.5?

6. *Standard error of the mean*. Since $\bar{X}$ is a random variable, it has a mean and a variance. We know that $\text{Var } \bar{X} = \sigma^2/n$. The standard deviation of $\bar{X}$ is called the "standard error of the mean."

   (a) What is the formula for the standard error of the mean?

   (b) What role does the standard error of the mean play in forming a confidence interval on μ?

7. (a) Draw five simple random samples from the MDBH data of Table V of Appendix B each of size 10. Find $\bar{x}$ for each sample. The true mean for the population of Table V is 6.254 with a variance of .4829. Do your $\bar{x}$ values vary around the value of 6.254 as expected? Is the average of your five $\bar{x}$ values fairly close to 6.254?

   (b) What is the theoretical Var X? Find the variance of your five $\bar{x}$ values. Is your variance close to the value expected?

   (c) Compute the theoretical standard error of the mean.

   (d) Use your smallest $\bar{x}$ value to construct a 99% confidence interval on μ. Does your numerical interval trap μ as hoped? If not, would a 90% confidence interval trap the mean?

   (e) Repeat part *d* using your largest $\bar{x}$ value.

8. Most species of conifers have both pollen cones and seed cones. Pollen released by the male cone is carried by the wind to the female cone where the ovules are fertilized. Consider variable X, the elapsed time between pollination and fertilization.

Assume that for pines X is normally distributed with a mean of 6 months and a standard deviation of 2 months. Consider the statistic $\bar{X}$ based on a random sample of 25 female cones. What is $E[\bar{X}]$? Var $\bar{X}$? Standard error of the mean?

9. Acute myeloblastic leukemia is among the most deadly of cancers. Consider variable X, the time in months that a patient survives after the initial diagnosis of the disease. Assume that X is normally distributed with a standard deviation of 3 months. Studies indicate that $\mu = 13$ months. Consider the sample mean $\bar{X}$ based on a random sample of size 16. If the above information is correct, what are the numerical values of $E[\bar{X}]$, Var $\bar{X}$, and the standard error of the mean?

10. Consider 200 samples each of size 25 drawn from a population with unknown mean μ. Assume that the 200 sample means obtained are used to create two hundred 90% confidence intervals on μ. Approximately how many of these intervals would you expect to fail to trap μ?

11. An experiment is conducted by flipping a fair coin 30 times. Let X_i, $i = 1, 2, 3, \ldots,$ 30, be defined by

$$X_i = \begin{cases} 1 & \text{if the coin lands heads} \\ 0 & \text{otherwise} \end{cases}$$

(a) Use the methods of Section 4.2 to verify that the mean of $X_i = \frac{1}{2}$ and that its variance is $\frac{1}{4}$. Thus $X_1, X_2, \ldots, X_{30}$ is a random sample from a distribution with $\mu = \frac{1}{2}$ and variance $= \frac{1}{4}$.

(b) Consider the random variable $\bar{X} = \sum X_i/30$. Argue that $\bar{X}$ gives the proportion of tosses which results in heads.

(c) By the Central Limit Theorem, what is the distribution of $\bar{X}$?

(d) What is the distribution of the following random variable?

$$\frac{\bar{X} - .5}{\sqrt{.5(.5)/30}}$$

6.3
CONFIDENCE INTERVAL ON THE POPULATION MEAN AND THE T DISTRIBUTION

Note that to obtain a point estimate for a population mean μ, it is not necessary to know the population variance; the sample mean $\bar{X}$ provides a reasonable estimate for μ regardless of the value of σ^2. However, the bounds for a confidence interval on μ given in Section 6.2 are $\bar{X} \pm z\sigma/\sqrt{n}$. It is assumed that, even though the population mean is unknown, the population variance is known. Practically speaking, this assumption is unrealistic. In most instances, when a statistical study is being conducted, it is being done for the first time; there is no way to know prior to the study either the mean or the variance of the population of interest. We consider in this section the more realistic problem of making inferences on a population mean when the population variance is assumed to be *unknown* and must be estimated from the available data.

To derive a general formula for a confidence interval on μ under these circumstances, it is natural to begin by considering the random variable used earlier, namely,

$$\frac{\bar{X} - \mu}{\sigma/\sqrt{n}}$$

Now there are two problems to overcome:

1. The value of σ is not known and must be estimated.
2. The distribution of the variable obtained by replacing σ by an estimator is not known.

The first problem was solved in Section 1.5. Recall that we first posed the statistic

$$\frac{\sum (X_i - \bar{X})^2}{n}$$

as an estimator for σ^2. This estimator was rejected because, on the average, it tends to underestimate σ^2. To obtain an estimator whose observed values are centered at σ^2, we divide by $n - 1$. Thus the sample variance is defined by

$$S^2 = \frac{\sum (X_i - \bar{X})^2}{n - 1}$$

The sample standard deviation is given by $S = \sqrt{S^2}$. To solve the second problem, consider again the random variable $(\bar{X} - \mu)/(\sigma/\sqrt{n})$, which is at least approximately standard normal. Replace the population standard deviation σ, now assumed to be unknown, by its estimator S to obtain the random variable $(\bar{X} - \mu)/(S/\sqrt{n})$. To use this random variable to derive a general formula for a confidence interval on μ when σ^2 is unknown, one question must be answered: What is the distribution of this variable? It can be shown that the distribution is no longer standard normal. In fact, if the variable X is normal, then the random variable $(\bar{X} - \mu)/(S/\sqrt{n})$ follows what is called a T distribution with $n - 1$ degrees of freedom. We pause briefly to consider the general characteristics of T random variables.

Properties of T Random Variables

1. There are infinitely many T random variables, each identified by one parameter γ, called *degrees of freedom*. The parameter γ is always a positive integer. The notation T_γ denotes a T random variable with γ degrees of freedom.
2. Each T random variable is continuous.
3. The graph of the density of each T random variable is a symmetric bell-shaped curve centered at zero.
4. The parameter γ is a shape parameter in the sense that as γ increases, the variance of the T_γ random variable decreases. Thus, the larger the number of degrees of freedom, the more compact the bell curve associated with the variable becomes.
5. As the number of degrees of freedom increases, the T curve approaches the standard normal curve. (See Figure 6.11.)

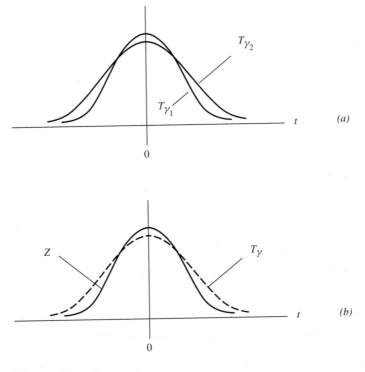

FIGURE 6.11
(a) Typical relationship between two T curves with $\gamma_1 > \gamma_2$, (b) typical relationship between a T curve and the standard normal curve.

A partial summary of the cumulative distribution function F for selected T variables is given in Table VI of Appendix B. Table VI is constructed so that the degrees of freedom are listed as row headings, selected probabilities are listed as column headings, and the points associated with those probabilities are listed in the body of the table.

As the degrees of freedom increase, the changes in the listed values become slight. The last row, labeled ∞, is used when γ exceeds 100. Example 6.3.1 illustrates the use of this table.

EXAMPLE 6.3.1. Consider the random variable T_{10}.

(a) From Table VI of Appendix B, $P[T_{10} \leq 1.372] = F(1.372) = .90$. (See Figure 6.12.)
(b) Because of the symmetry of the T distribution, the area to the left of -1.372 is the same as the area to the right of 1.372. From Figure 6.12, $P[T_{10} \leq -1.372] = .10$.
(c) Find the point t such that $P[-t \leq T_{10} \leq t] = .95$. Since we want 95% of the area to lie between $-t$ and t, 5% of the area lies below $-t$ or above t. This 5% is split into two equal areas of 2.5% each. To find t, we note from Figure 6.13 that the area to the left of t is $.95 + 0.25 = .975$. The value in row 10 and column .975 of the T table is 2.228. The point t such that $P[-t \leq T_{10} \leq t] = .95$ is $t = 2.228$. (See Figure 6.13.)

The last row in Table VI of Appendix B is labeled ∞. The points listed in that row are actually points associated with the standard normal curve. Note that as γ increases, the values in each column of Table VI approach the value listed in the last row.

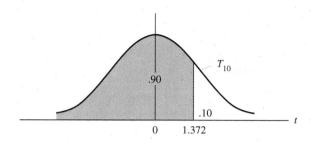

The area to the left of 1.372 is .90; therefore, $F(1.372) =$ $P[T_{10} \leq 1.372] = .90$.

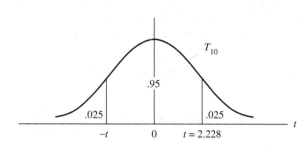

The area to the left of 2.228 is .975; therefore, $P[-2.228 \leq T_{10} \leq 2.228] = .95$.

It is now easy to determine the general form for a confidence interval on μ when σ^2 is unknown and must be estimed from the data. We need only note that the two random variables

$$Z = \frac{\bar{X} - \mu}{\sigma/\sqrt{n}} \quad \text{and} \quad T_\gamma = \frac{\bar{X} - \mu}{S/\sqrt{n}}$$

have the same algebraic structure. Thus the algebraic argument given in Example 6.2.2 will go through exactly as shown, with σ being replaced by S and z being replaced by t. These substitutions result in Theorem 6.3.1.

THEOREM 6.3.1. Confidence interval on μ when σ^2 is estimated. Let $X_1, X_2, X_3, \ldots, X_n$ be a random sample of size n from a normal distribution with mean μ and variance σ^2. Then a confidence interval on μ is given by

$$\bar{X} \pm t \frac{S}{\sqrt{n}}$$

where the t point is based on the T_{n-1} distribution.

EXAMPLE 6.3.2. Wolf packs are territorial with territories of 130 square kilometers or more. Howling in wolves, which communicates information about the location and the composition of the pack, is thought to be related to territoriality. The following observations were obtained on X, the length in minutes of a howling session of a particular pack under study. Assume that X is normally distributed.

1.0	1.8	1.6	1.5	2.0	1.8
1.2	1.9	1.7	1.6	1.6	
1.7	1.5	1.4	1.4	1.4	

A point estimate for the mean length of a howling session for this pack is $\bar{x} = 1.57$ minutes. The sample variance for these data is $s^2 = .066$. An estimate for σ is

$$s = \sqrt{.066} = .26 \text{ minute}$$

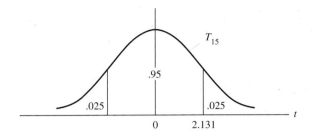

FIGURE 6.14

Partition of T_{15} to obtain a 95% confidence interval on μ.

A 95% confidence interval on μ is found by considering the partition shown in Figure 6.14 of the T_{15} curve obtained from Table VI of Appendix B. The bounds for a 95% confidence interval on μ are

$$\bar{x} \pm t \frac{s}{\sqrt{n}} = 1.57 \pm 2.131 \frac{.26}{\sqrt{16}}$$

$$= 1.57 \pm .14$$

We can be 95% confident that the mean length of a howling session for this particular pack lies between 1.43 and 1.71 minutes inclusive.

Several things should be pointed out. First, the number of degrees of freedom involved in finding a confidence interval on μ when σ^2 is unknown is $n - 1$, the sample size minus 1. For large samples, this value may not be listed in Table VI of Appendix B. In this case, the last line in the table (∞) is used to find points of interest. Second, a normality assumption has been made. The random variable $(\bar{X} - \mu)/(s/\sqrt{n})$ follows a T distribution if the random variable X is itself normally distributed. The validity of this assumption can be checked visually by constructing a histogram or a stem-and-leaf diagram. An analytical method for testing for normality is given in Chapter 13. If X appears to exhibit an approximate bell shape, then methods based on the T distribution usually work quite well. This is true even if X is, in fact, discrete. However, if there is reason to suspect that the variable under study has a distribution that is far from normal, then statistical procedures based on the T distribution should not be used. Rather, some distribution-free technique should be employed. Such techniques are discussed in Chapter 13.

EXERCISES 6.3

1. These data are obtained on the height, in meters, of the eastern white pine, *Pinus strobus*.

17.16	22.00	10.08	15.00
07.02	10.67	11.16	10.92
11.10	04.05	15.93	07.22
08.19	16.45	07.38	10.00
14.10	10.26	11.96	10.00

(a) Sketch a double stem-and-leaf plot for these data. Use stems of 0, 0, 1, 1, and 2, 2. Use the second digit of each number as the leaf. Does the plot form at least a rough bell?

(b) Estimate μ, σ, and σ^2.

(Based on data collected by Sabrina Norton, Department of Biology, Radford University, 1994.)

2. The following is a random sample of 16 observations on random variable X, the number of pounds of beef consumed last year per person in the United States:

118	110	117	120	119	126
115	112	112	113	122	
125	130	115	118	123	

Use these data to estimate μ, σ, and σ^2.

3. Let T_{15} denote a T random variable with 15 degrees of freedom. Use Table VI of Appendix B to find the following:

(a) Point t such that $P[T \le t] = .95$

(b) Point t such that $P[T \ge t] = .025$

(c) Point t such that $P[T \le t] = .05$

(d) Point t such that $P[T \ge t] = .975$

(e) $P[T_{15} \ge 2.602]$

(f) $P[T_{15} \le -1.341]$

(g) $P[-1.753 \le T_{15} \le 1.753]$

(h) Point t such that $P[-t \le T_{15} \le t] = .95$

(i) Point t such that $P[-t \le T_{15} \le t] = .99$

4. Researchers studying photoperiodism used the cocklebur as an experimental plant. The variable observed was X, the number of hours of uninterrupted darkness per day required to produce flowering. The following data were obtained:

15.0	13.0	15.1	16.0	13.5
15.5	13.2	14.9	14.7	

Estimate μ, σ, and σ^2.

5. To set a standard for what is to be considered a "normal" calcium reading, a random sample of 1000 apparently healthy adults is obtained. A blood sample is drawn from each adult. The variable studied is X, the number of milligrams of calcium per deciliter of blood. A sample mean of 9.5 and a sample standard deviation of .5 are found. Assume that X is approximately normally distributed. Find a 95% confidence interval on μ.

6. A study is conducted of the effect of heat on the rate of movement of large land snails. These data are obtained on X, the distance in centimeters traveled by a sample of 20 snails subjected to a temperature 10°F above room temperature (room temperature = 65°F).

$$\bar{x} = 4.855 \qquad s = .7178$$

Construct a 95% confidence interval on the average distance traveled by snails when the temperature is 75°F. What assumption is being made concerning the distribution of X? If the average distance traveled at room temperature is 2.885 centimeters, is there evidence that heat tends to increase the average distance traveled by these snails? Explain. (Based on an experiment conducted by Joseph Christian, Department of Biology, Radford University, 1996.)

7. The following data were obtained on a random sample of size 30 from the distribution of X, the percentage increase in blood-alcohol content after a person drinks four beers.

$$\bar{x} = 41.2 \qquad s = 2.1$$

Find a 90% confidence interval on the average percentage increase in blood-alcohol content after drinking four beers. Would a 95% confidence interval on μ be longer or shorter than the 90% interval just found? If you hear a claim that the average increase is less than 35% would you believe the claim? Explain.

8. In a study of water usage in a small town, a random sample of 25 homes is obtained. The variable of interest is X, the number of gallons of water utilized per day. The following observations are obtained on a randomly selected weekday.

175	185	186	168	158
150	190	178	137	175
180	200	189	200	180
172	145	192	191	181
183	169	172	178	210

(a) Construct a stem-and-leaf plot for these data. Do the data exhibit at least a rough bell shape?

(b) Estimate μ, σ, and σ^2.

(c) Find a 90% confidence interval on μ. The town reservoir is large enough to handle an average usage of 160 gallons per day. Does there appear to be a water shortage problem in the town? Explain your answer on the basis of the confidence interval obtained.

9. Duck farms lining the shores of Great South Bay have seriously polluted the water. One pollutant is nitrogen in the form of uric acid. The following is a random sample of nine observations on X, the number of pounds of nitrogen produced per farm per day:

| 4.9 | 5.8 | 5.9 | 6.5 | 5.5 |
| 5.0 | 5.6 | 6.0 | 5.7 | |

Assume X is normal, and construct a 99% confidence interval on μ.

10. A process called abscission in photobiology is being tested in hopes of increasing the fruit set (the percentage of fruit held on the trees) in orange trees in Florida. The process involves exposing the trees to colored light for 15 minutes each night. The fruit set for 10 experimental trees was obtained first under normal conditions and then after the new treatment. The following observations were obtained on X, the percentage increase in the fruit set from one year to the next:

| 29 | 37 | 32 | 34 | 39 |
| 30 | 36 | 35 | 27 | 40 |

Assume that X is normal, and construct a 95% confidence interval on the mean percentage increase in the fruit set. The developer of the new process claims that it will increase the fruit set by an average of 40%. Do you believe this statement? Explain your answer on the basis of the confidence interval found.

11. Use the data of Exercise 1 to find a 90% confidence interval on the average height of the eastern white pine in the region in which sampling was conducted.

12. The caliper of a tree is the diameter measured 6 inches above ground. A sample of 16 trees between 12 and 14 feet tall grown at a particular nursery is obtained and the caliper of each determined. These data are obtained (data in inches):

2.3	1.9	1.7	2.1	1.5	1.8	1.8	1.1
2.1	1.5	2.0	1.6	1.3	1.6	1.5	1.3

Find a 95% confidence interval on the mean caliper of trees grown at the nursery. To ensure that the size of the tree is proportional to the strength of the trunk, the average caliper for trees of this size should be 2 inches. Do the trees grown here appear to meet this standard? (Based on data found in Gary Moll, "The Best Way to Plant Trees," *American Forests,* April 1990, pp. 61–64.)

■ 6.4

INTRODUCTION TO HYPOTHESIS TESTING

In a hypothesis testing problem, there is a preconceived theory concerning the population characteristic under study. This implies that there are, in fact, two theories, or hypotheses, involved in any statistical study: the hypothesis being proposed by the experimenter and the negation of this hypothesis. The former, denoted H_1, is called the *alternative,* or *research hypothesis,* whereas the latter is denoted by H_0 and is called the *null hypothesis.* The purpose of the experiment is to decide whether the evidence tends to support or refute the null hypothesis. You should keep in mind three general statements when stating H_0 and H_1:

1. The null hypothesis is the hypothesis of "no difference." Practically speaking, this will result in the statement of equality being a part of H_0.
2. Make whatever is to be detected or supported the alternative hypothesis. That is, label your preconceived research theory as H_1.
3. Statistical hypotheses are always set up in hopes of being able to reject H_0 and thereby accept H_1.

   EXAMPLE 6.4.1. A new drug is being developed for use in the treatment of skin cancer. It is hoped that it will be effective on a majority of those patients on whom it is used. The company developing the drug wants to get statistical evidence to support such a claim. Let p denote the proportion of patients for whom the drug will be effective. Since we make whatever is to be supported or detected the alternative hypothesis, the alternative here is that $p > .5$. This automatically implies that the null hypothesis is the negation of H_1, namely, that $p \leq .5$. Thus the two hypotheses involved are

$$H_0: p \leq .5$$

$$H_1: p > .5$$

Note that the statement of equality appears as part of the null hypothesis. Note also that from the manufacturer's point of view, it is hoped that H_0 will be rejected, thus allowing the acceptance of H_1, the manufacturer's claim.

Once a sample has been selected and the data have been collected, a decision must be made. The decision will be either to reject H_0 or to fail to do so. The decision is made by observing the value of some statistic whose probability distribution is known under the assumption that H_0 is true. Such a statistic is called a *test statistic*. If the observed value of the test statistic is unusual when H_0 is true, we reject the null hypothesis in favor of the alternative; if the value observed is a commonly occurring one under the assumption that H_0 is true, then we do not reject the null hypothesis. This means that at the end of any hypothesis testing study, we will be forced into exactly one of the following situations:

1. We will have rejected H_0 when it was true; therefore, we will have committed what is known as a *Type I error*. (effective on less than .5)
2. We will have made the correct decision of rejecting H_0 when the alternative H_1 was true. (more then 0.5)
3. We will have failed to reject H_0 when the alternative H_1 was true; therefore, we will have committed what is known as a *Type II error*. (more than 0.5)
4. We will have made the correct decision of failing to reject H_0 when H_0 was true.

These possibilities are summarized in Table 6.5.

EXAMPLE 6.4.2. Consider the drug testing problem of Example 6.4.1. The hypothesis being tested is

$$H_0: p \leq .5$$

$$H_1: p > .5 \quad \text{(drug is effective for majority of patients)}$$

If a Type I error is made, we will have rejected H_0 when H_0 is true. Practically speaking, we will have concluded that the drug is effective for a majority of users when it is not. This error could lead to the marketing of a drug which is worthless for most patients. A Type II error occurs if we fail to reject H_0 when H_1 is true. Here this amounts to concluding that the effectiveness rate of the drug is 50% or less when, in fact, it would be useful for a majority of the patients on whom it is tried. This error could lead to failure to market a useful drug. Both errors are serious. The Type I error generally would be considered more serious, since it could result in a delay in the proper treatment of the disease.

Note that regardless of what is done, an error is possible. Anytime H_0 is rejected, a Type I error might occur; anytime H_0 is not rejected, a Type II error might occur. There is no way to avoid this dilemma. The job of the statistician is to design methods

TABLE 6.5

Possible ways in which a hypothesis test can proceed

	True state	
Action taken	**H_0 true**	**H_1 true**
Reject H_0	Type I error	Correct decision
Fail to reject H_0	Correct decision	Type II error

for testing hypotheses that will keep the probabilities of making either error reasonably small. There are two ways to distinguish between H_0 and H_1. Each of these will be demonstrated later.

▓ EXERCISES 6.4

1. In 1969 in the United States on the average 8% of household waste was metal. Because of the increase in recycling efforts, it is hoped that this figure has been reduced. An experiment is run to verify this contention.
   (a) Set up the appropriate null and alternative hypotheses for the experiment. Note that the parameter of interest is μ, the average amount of household waste.
   (b) Explain in a practical sense what has occurred if a Type I error has been committed.
   (c) Explain in a practical sense what has occurred if a Type II error has been committed.

2. In 1974, 38% of the females in the United States ages 17 to 24 years old had smoked or were smokers at the time. It is feared that this figure has increased. An experiment is conducted to gain evidence to support this contention.
   (a) Set up the appropriate null and alternative hypotheses for the experiment.
   (b) Explain in a practical sense what has occurred if a Type I error has been committed.
   (c) Explain in a practical sense what has occurred if a Type II error has been committed.

3. Past studies show that the biocide DDT can accumulate in the body. In 1965 the mean concentration of DDT in the body fat of individuals in the United States was 9 ppm. It is hoped that as a result of stricter controls, this concentration has decreased.
   (a) Set up the appropriate null and alternative hypotheses for documenting this claim.
   (b) Explain in a practical sense the consequences of making a Type I error and a Type II error.

4. The mean level of background radiation in the United States is .3 rem per year. It is feared that as a result of the increased use of radioactive materials, this figure has increased.
   (a) Set up the appropriate null and alternative hypotheses to document this claim.
   (b) Explain in a practical sense the consequences of making a Type I error and a Type II error.

5. In running a test to detect the presence of the AIDS virus, the following test is conducted:

$$H_0: \text{virus is not present}$$

$$H_1: \text{virus is present}$$

Explain what has taken place if a Type I error results. What has occurred if a Type II error is made? Which error do you believe is the more serious of the two?

6. It is thought that a majority of smokers begin smoking by age 18. A study is designed to gain support for this theory so that funds can be obtained for an anti-smoking campaign. Let p denote the proportion of smokers who began to smoke by age 18. We are testing

H_0: $p \leq .5$

H_1: $p > .5$ (a majority of smokers begin to smoke by age 18)

Explain the financial consequences of making a Type I error. Explain the health consequences of making a Type II error. Which error do you believe is the more serious of the two?

7. Many studies have been conducted on the effect of "acid rain" on the growth of plants. In a particular area under normal conditions a dogwood sapling will grow an average of about 8 inches during its first year. It is thought that acid rain will stunt this growth. In statistical notation, what is H_1? H_0? If a Type I error is made, what has occurred in this setting?

6.5

TESTING HYPOTHESES ON THE POPULATION MEAN: T TEST

We consider now the problem of testing a hypothesis on the mean of a population. This means that we have an idea concerning the value of μ prior to running the experiment. We want to gain evidence to support our theory. Notice that in each of the next three examples, our theory, the situation that we want to detect or support, is labeled H_1.

EXAMPLE 6.5.1. The U.S. Department of Health has set an average bacteria count of 70 bacteria per cubic centimeter of water as its maximum acceptable level for clam-digging waters. An average value larger than 70 is felt to be dangerous, for eating clams taken from such waters may cause hepatitis. In monitoring the waters for the government, one would be interested in testing

$$H_0: \mu \leq 70$$

$$H_1: \mu > 70$$

EXAMPLE 6.5.2. A recent study of the ecosystem in a deciduous forest indicated that in the natural forest, the average net change in nitrate nitrogen is an increase of 2 kilograms per hectare per year. Foresters feel that defoliation of forest undergrowth would lead to a decrease in this value. The hypothesis of interest is

$$H_0: \mu \geq 2$$

$$H_1: \mu < 2$$

EXAMPLE 6.5.3. The average total blood protein in a healthy adult is 7.25 grams per deciliter. In running a blood test, the technician is testing

$$H_0: \mu = 7.25$$

$$H_1: \mu \neq 7.25$$

As can be seen from these examples, a hypothesis on μ can take one of three different forms. Let μ_0, called the *null value,* denote the hypothesized value of the population mean. The three general forms are

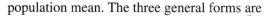

I H_0: $\mu \leq \mu_0$	II H_0: $\mu \geq \mu_0$	III H_0: $\mu = \mu_0$
H_1: $\mu > \mu_0$	H_1: $\mu < \mu_0$	H_1: $\mu \neq \mu_0$

The test statistic used to test each hypothesis is

one sided   *two sided*

$$T_{n-1} = \frac{\bar{X} - \mu_0}{S/\sqrt{n}}$$

Notice that $\bar{X}$ estimates the true population mean. If H_0 is true, $\bar{X}$ is estimating μ_0, and hence the difference between $\bar{X}$ and μ_0 should be small. In each case, a small observed value of the test statistic is an indication that H_0 should *not* be rejected. In case I, the research hypothesis is that $\mu > \mu_0$. If this is true, then $\bar{X}$ is actually estimating a mean value that is larger than the null value. We would expect $\bar{X}$ to exceed μ_0, forcing the difference $\bar{X} - \mu_0$ to be positive. Thus, in case I, we reject H_0 in favor of H_1 for large positive values of the test statistic. Since these values lie on the right-hand side of the number line, the test described in case I is called a *right-tailed test*. A similar argument leads to the conclusion that in case II, H_0 is rejected in favor of H_1 for large negative values of the test statistic. The test is called a *left-tailed test*. In case III, the test is referred to as a *two-tailed test*. The null hypothesis is rejected for unusually large values of the test statistic in either the positive or negative sense. What do we mean by "unusually" large values? These are values of the test statistic that are considered to be rare. It would be surprising to observe these values if H_0 were true. We know that if the null value is correct, then this statistic follows a T distribution with $n - 1$ degrees of freedom. This fact can be used to ascertain whether or not our experiment has produced an unusual result. This is done by calculating the P or probability value of the test where by P value we mean the following:

DEFINITION 6.5.1. The *P value* of a test is the probability that the test statistic will assume a value as extreme as or more extreme than that seen under the assumption that the null value is correct.

Hodges and Lehmann (*Basic Concepts of Probability and Statistics*, Holden-Day, San Francisco, 1970) describe the P value "as giving, in a single convenient number, a measure of the degree of surprise which the experiment should cause a believer of the null hypothesis." For a right-tailed test the P value is the area under the T_{n-1} curve to the right of the observed value of the test statistic; for a left-tailed test it is the area to the left. Two-tailed P values are discussed later. We reject H_0 if the P value is deemed to be too small to have reasonably occurred by chance. The next three examples illustrate the computation of P values.

EXAMPLE 6.5.4. Consider Example 6.5.1. The statistician for the U.S. Department of Health is to monitor the fishing waters. The job is to detect a situation in which the mean bacteria count has risen above the maximum safe level of 70. Since what is to be detected is taken as the alternative hypothesis, we are testing

$$H_0: \mu \le 70 \quad \text{(waters are safe)}$$

$$H_1: \mu > 70 \quad \text{(waters are unsafe)}$$

A random sample of size 9 is drawn, and the bacteria count X for each case is determined. The test statistic is

$$T_{n-1} = \frac{\bar{X} - \mu_0}{S/\sqrt{n}}$$

or

$$T_8 = \frac{\bar{X} - 70}{S/3}$$

Since $\bar{X}$ is a reasonable estimator for the mean, we expect the observed value of X to be close to 70 if H_0 is true. This forces the numerator of the test statistic, $\bar{X} - 70$, to be small, causing the observed value of the test statistic to be small. However, if H_1 is true, we expect $\bar{X}$ to be larger than 70, forcing $\bar{X} - 70$ to be large and *positive*. This, in turn, results in a large positive value for the test statistic. Hence logically we should reject H_0 in favor of H_1 whenever the observed value of the statistic is positive and too large to have reasonably occurred by chance.

The following observations were obtained when the experiment was conducted:

69   74   75   70   72
73   71   73   68

For this data set,

$$\bar{x} = 71.7 \qquad s = 2.3$$

The observed value of the test statistic is

$$\frac{\bar{x} - 70}{s/3} = \frac{71.7 - 70}{2.3/3} = 2.22$$

Is this value unusually large? To answer this question, we calculate the P value of the test. By definition the P value is the probability of observing a value as extreme as or more extreme than that actually obtained. For a right-tailed test "more extreme" means to the right of the value obtained. Hence in this case

$$P = P[T_8 > 2.22]$$

This probability is pictured in Figure 6.15a. To approximate the P value we look for the number 2.22 in row 8 of Table VI of Appendix B.

This value falls between the numbers 1.860 and 2.306. Since $P[T_8 \ge 1.860] = .05$ (Figure 6.15b) and $P[T_8 \ge 2.306] = .025$ (Figure 6.15c), the P value of our test lies between .025 and .05. This is reported by writing $.025 < P < .05$. We now make a value judgment. Is this probability small? Since most people would consider a probability of this magnitude to be so, we reject H_0 and conclude that the waters are unsafe for fishing.

There are no rigid rules concerning how small a P value must be to cause us to reject H_0. Recall that whenever we reject H_0, we are at risk of committing a Type I error. The P value is a measure of the degree of risk that we take when we make our research claim. If the consequences of making such an error are very serious, then P must be very small before we are willing to reject H_0. If making a Type I error causes an

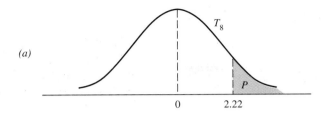

(a)

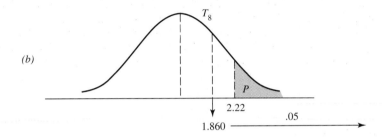

(b)

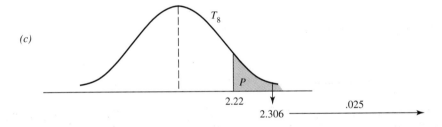

(c)

FIGURE 6.15

(a) $P = P[T_8 \geq 2.22]$, (b) $P[T_8 \geq 1.86] = .05$, (c) $P[T_8 \geq 2.306] = .025$.

inconvenience only, then H_0 can be rejected for larger P values. A rough rule of thumb is that H_0 should not be rejected for P values that exceed .10.

The next example illustrates the computation of the P value for a left-tailed test.

EXAMPLE 6.5.5. The hypothesis

$$H_0: \mu \geq 2 \qquad H_1: \mu < 2$$

of Example 6.5.2 was tested by removing the undergrowth in a 15-hectare area of an experimental forest. The area was sprayed to prevent regrowth. At the end of a year, the change in nitrate nitrogen per hectare was determined by analyzing runoff water at 15 locations within the forest. The following data resulted:

$$\bar{x} = -3 \quad \text{(average } loss \text{ of 3 kilograms per hectare)}$$

$$s = 7.5 \text{ kilograms per hectare}$$

Is this evidence that removal of forest undergrowth results in a decrease in the mean net change in nitrate nitrogen per hectare per year?

The value of the test statistic based on these data is

$$\frac{\bar{x} - \mu_0}{s/\sqrt{n}} = \frac{-3 - 2}{7.5/\sqrt{15}} = -2.58$$

For a left-tailed test a value "more extreme" than that obtained is a value to the left of -2.58. Thus, the P value is given by $P = P[T_{14} \leq -2.58]$. The P value for the test is shown in Figure 6.16a. From Table VI, row 14 we see that the number 2.58 lies between 2.145 and 2.624. Since the T distribution is symmetric, $P[T_{14} \geq 2.145] = P[T_{14} \leq -2.145] = .025$. From Figure 6.16b, it is evident that the P value, the area to the left of -2.58, is smaller than .025. Since $P[T_{14} \leq - 2.624] = .01$ and the area to the left of -2.624 is smaller than that represented by the P value (see Figure 6.16c), we know that $P > .01$. By combining these two results, we see that $.01 < P < .025$. These probabilities are small. We reject H_0 and conclude that the removal of forest undergrowth does result in a decrease in the average nitrate nitrogen concentration.

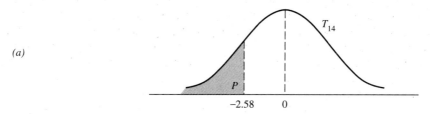

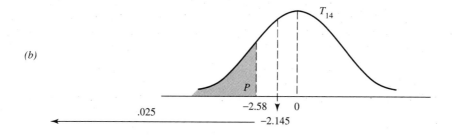

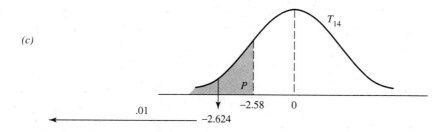

▨ **FIGURE 6.16**

(a) $P = [T_{14} \leq -2.58]$, (b) $P < P[T_{14} \leq -2.145] = .025$,
(c) $P > P[T_{14} \leq -2.624] = .01$.

There has been some controversy as to the correct way to calculate a two-tailed *P* value. If the distribution of the test statistic, under the assumption that H_0 is true, is symmetric, then it is reasonable to double the apparent one-tailed *P* value. Since the *T* distribution is symmetric, this is the natural procedure to use in conducting a *T* test. If the distribution of the test statistic under H_0 is not symmetric, the issue is more complex. Various suggestions have been offered by statisticians, but no consensus has been reached yet. However, the most common procedure is to report a two-tailed *P* value that is twice the one-tailed value.

EXAMPLE 6.5.6. A series of eight blood tests was run on a particular patient over several days. The variable monitored is the total protein level. Since the blood protein level should be neither too large nor too small, it is desirable to detect either situation. Thus we are testing

$$H_0: \mu = 7.25 \quad \text{(normal for healthy adult)}$$

$$H_1: \mu \neq 7.25$$

based on a sample of size 8. The test is two-tailed.

Based on the following observations, what conclusion can be drawn?

7.23	7.25	7.28	7.29
7.32	7.26	7.27	7.24

For these data,

$$\bar{x} = 7.268 \qquad s = .029$$

The observed value of the test statistic is

$$\frac{\bar{x} - 7.25}{s/\sqrt{n}} = \frac{7.268 - 7.25}{.029/\sqrt{8}} = 1.756$$

Since the number 1.756 lies between the values 1.415 and 1.895 in row 7 of Table VI of Appendix B, the *P* value for a right-tailed test would lie between .05 and .10. Since we are conducting a two-tailed test, these values are doubled to obtain $.10 < P < 20$. Based on this fact, we are unable to reject H_0. We do not have sufficient evidence to claim that $\mu \neq 7.25$.

Preset Alpha Values

$\alpha = 0.05$
$\alpha = 0.01$

Some statisticians prefer to take a slightly different approach to hypothesis testing. In particular they carefully consider the consequences of making a Type I error. They then determine the risk that they are willing to take. This determination is made *before* the data are gathered and analyzed. In this way the probability of committing a Type I error is set prior to experimentation. This preset probability of error is called the *level of significance* or the *size of the test*. It is usually denoted by the Greek letter alpha (α). To conduct such a test, we proceed as explained in the previous examples. If the *P* value found is less than or equal to the preset α level, we reject H_0; otherwise, we do not reject H_0.

EXAMPLE 6.5.7. Each species of firefly has a unique flashing pattern. One species has a pattern that consists of one short pulse of light followed by a resting period thought to have an average length of less than 4 seconds. We want to test

$$H_0: \mu \geq 4$$

$$H_1: \mu < 4$$

If we make a Type I error, we will misjudge the average resting period and will probably write a research paper that is misleading. The error will eventually be discovered by other researchers and some embarrassment might ensue. However, the consequences of our error are not life threatening. We can tolerate a fairly high probability of making a Type I error. For this reason let us preset α at the .10 level. The following data were obtained on the resting time between flashes of a sample of 16 fireflies of this species:

3.9   4.1   3.6   3.7   4.0   4.3
3.8   3.2   3.7   4.2   4.0
3.5   3.5   3.8   3.4   3.6

Does the evidence support the proposed mean resting time of less than 4 seconds?
    For this data set,

$$\bar{x} = 3.77 \qquad \frac{\bar{x} - 4}{s/\sqrt{n}} = \frac{3.77 - 4}{.30/4} = -3.06$$

$$s = .30$$

From Table VI of Appendix B, the P value for the text, $P[T_{15} \leq -3.06]$, is less than .005. Since this P value is below the preset α level of .10, we reject H_0 and conclude that the mean resting time is less than 4 seconds.

EXERCISES 6.5

1. In testing

$$H_0: \mu \leq 10$$

$$H_1: \mu > 10$$

based on a random sample of size 20, the observed value of the T statistic is 3. What is the P value of the test? Do you think that H_0 should be rejected?

2. In testing

$$H_0: \mu \geq 5$$

$$H_1: \mu < 5$$

based on a random sample of size 24, the observed value of the T statistic is -2.00. What is the P value of the test? Do you think that H_0 should be rejected?

3. In testing

$$H_0: \mu = 2$$

$$H_1: \mu \neq 2$$

based on a random sample of size 16, the observed value of the T statistic is 1.5. What is the P value of the test? Do you think that H_0 should be rejected?

4. One of the effects of DDT on birds is to inhibit the production of the enzyme carbonic anhydrase. This enzyme controls calcium metabolism. The end result is thought to be the formation of egg shells that are much thinner and weaker than normal. To test this theory, a study was run in which sparrow hawks were fed a mixture of 3 parts per million (ppm) dieldrin and 15 ppm DDT. The thickness of the shells of these birds was compared to the known mean thickness for birds not affected by DDT. The percentage decrease in shell thickness was noted. A random sample of size 16 yielded a sample mean percentage decrease of 8% with a sample standard deviation of 5%. Use this information to test

$$H_0: \mu \leq 0$$
$$H_1: \mu > 0 \quad \text{(shell thickness decreases)}$$

What is the approximate P value for the test? Do you think that the theory has been supported statistically? Explain your answer on the basis of the P value.

5. The mean carbon dioxide concentration in the air is .035%. It is thought that the concentration immediately above the soil surface is higher than this.
   (a) Set up the null and alternative hypotheses required to gain statistical support for this contention.
   (b) One hundred forty-four randomly selected air samples taken from within 1 foot of the soil were analyzed. A sample mean of .09% and sample standard deviation of .25% resulted. What is the P value for this test? Do you think that the stated contention has been supported statistically?

6. It is often difficult to grow plants near black walnut trees because the roots of the tree leach a toxin called juglone into the surrounding soil. It is thought that the average pH of the soil near the roots is .7 points higher than the soil beyond the roots. To support this theory, a sample of 25 black walnut trees is selected and the soil pH at the roots and beyond is determined. The random variable X is the difference in pH with subtraction in this order: roots pH minus beyond-roots pH. The sample mean $\bar{x}$ is found to be .8 with a sample standard deviation of .3. Do these data support the research theory that $\mu > .7$? Explain. If you make this research claim, what is your probability of error? (Based on information from Diane Relf, *Plants at War,* Virginia Cooperative Extension Service, NA: 1-NA, 1983.)

7. An experiment is conducted to study the effect of exercise on the reduction of the cholesterol level in slightly obese patients considered to be at risk for heart attack. Eighty patients are put on a specified exercise regimen while maintaining a normal diet. At the end of 4 weeks the change in cholesterol level will be noted. It is thought that the program will reduce the average cholesterol reading by more than 25 points. At the end of the study these data are reported:

$$\bar{x} = 27 \qquad s = 18$$

Do these data support the research theory? If you make the research claim, what is your probability of error?

8. Bats in flight locate a solid object by emitting shrill squeaks and listening for the echo. It is thought that the mean maximum effective range for this echolocation

system is more than 6 meters. To support this hypothesis, a random sample of 16 bats were selected. Each bat was released in a large, enclosed area that contained only one obstruction. The distance from the object at which the bat was observed to veer away from the obstruction was noted. The experiment was repeated several times for each bat, and the mean veer distance for each was determined. The following observations were obtained:

6.2	6.8	6.1	5.7	6.1	6.3	5.8	6.3
5.9	6.3	6.4	6.0	6.3	6.2	5.9	6.1

Find the P value for this data set. What practical conclusion can you draw from these data? What type of error might you be committing?

9. Consider each of the hypotheses given in Exercises 1 through 3. In each case, could H_0 be rejected at the $\alpha = .05$ level? Explain.

10. The maximum acceptable level for exposure to microwave radiation in the United States is an average of 10 microwatts per square centimeter. It is feared that a large television transmitter may be polluting the air nearby by pushing the level of microwave radiation above the safe limit.

   (a) Set up the null and alternative hypotheses needed to gain evidence to support this contention.

   (b) The following is a random sample of nine observations on X, the number of microwatts per square centimeter, taken at locations near the transmitter:

9	11	14	10	10
12	13	8	12	

   Find the P value of the test.

   Can H_0 be rejected at the $\alpha = .1$ level? What practical conclusion can be drawn? What type of error might be committed?

11. Normally the leaves of the *Mimosa pudica* are horizontal. However, if one of them is touched lightly, the leaflets will fold. It is reported that the mean time from touch to complete closure is 2.5 seconds. An experiment is run to test this value.

   (a) Set up the appropriate two-tailed hypothesis.

   (b) The following observations were obtained on variable X, the elapsed time between touch and closure:

3.0	2.9	2.8	2.7	2.6
2.4	2.5	2.4	2.6	2.7

   Find the P value of the test.

   Can H_0 be rejected at the $\alpha = .10$ level? To what type of error are you now subject?

12. In the past the average number of nursing home days required by elderly patients before they could be released to home care was 17. It is hoped that a new program will reduce this figure. Do these data support the research hypothesis at the $\alpha = .05$ level? Explain based on the P value of the test.

3	5	12	7	22	6	2
18	9	8	20	15	3	36
38	43					

(Based on information found in Julianne Oktay and Patricia Volland, "Post-Hospital Support Program for the Frail Elderly and Their Caregivers," *American Journal of Public Health*, January 1990, pp. 29–45.)

13. In the past, the average number of angina attacks per week among patients was 1.3. A new drug is being tested, and it is hoped that it will reduce this figure. These data are obtained by observing a sample of 20 patients who are using the new drug.

| 1 | 3 | 0 | 1 | 1 | 1 | 0 | 2 | 2 | 0 |
| 0 | 1 | 0 | 0 | 0 | 1 | 1 | 1 | 1 | 0 |

Can the research hypothesis be rejected at the .01 level? Explain based on the *P* value of the test. (Based on information found in an advertisement in the *American Journal of Nursing,* September 1990, p. 13.)

6.6

SAMPLE SIZE: CONFIDENCE INTERVALS AND POWER (OPTIONAL)

In designing an experiment to study the mean, one of the first questions that must be answered is, How large must the sample be to accomplish the goals of the study? This question is fairly easy to answer if the goal is estimation. However, if the intent of the study is hypothesis testing, the situation is more complex. In this section we consider the problem of determining an appropriate sample size in each of these settings.

Sample Size: Estimation

For a confidence interval to be useful it must be short enough to pinpoint the value of μ reasonably well with a high degree of confidence. If an experiment is unplanned or poorly planned, there is a distinct possibility that the resulting confidence interval will be too long to be of any use to the researcher. For example, an experiment that allows us to conclude that "we are 95% confident that the true average weight of a baby at birth lies between 2 and 20 pounds" is clearly not of much value. What factors affect the length of a confidence interval? Consider the confidence interval on the mean pictured in Figure 6.17. The length of the interval is

$$2t\frac{s}{\sqrt{n}}$$

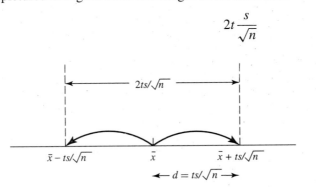

FIGURE 6.17

A confidence interval on μ is given by $\bar{x} \pm ts/\sqrt{n}$. The length of the interval is $2ts/\sqrt{n}$. The value of d is half the length, or $ts/\sqrt{n}$.

If we use $\bar{x}$ as an estimate of μ, this estimate is expected to differ from μ by at most half of this length. That is, the maximum distance between $\bar{x}$ and μ should be at most d, where

$$d = ts/\sqrt{n}$$

The length of the interval and also d is affected by three things. They are

1. The confidence desired, which controls the value of t
2. The variability of the sample, which is measured by s
3. The sample size

To guarantee that the interval is short enough to be informative, we must specify the length and confidence desired. We then choose the sample size in such a way that these specifications will be met. An example will illustrate how this is done.

> **EXAMPLE 6.6.1.** Suppose that a study is to be run to estimate the average birth weight of babies born to mothers addicted to cocaine. How large a sample is needed to estimate this average to within $\frac{1}{2}$ pound with 95% confidence? The phrase "to within $\frac{1}{2}$ pound" means that the difference between the estimated mean $\bar{x}$ and the true mean μ is at most $\frac{1}{2}$ pound. This situation is pictured in Figure 6.18. Since μ should lie in the confidence interval, it will be within $\frac{1}{2}$ pound of $\bar{x}$ if the interval is of length 1 pound. Consider the equation
>
> $$d = t\frac{s}{\sqrt{n}}$$
>
> When this equation is solved for n, we obtain
>
> $$n = \frac{t^2 s^2}{d^2}$$
>
> In this case, where $d = 1/2$,
>
> $$n = \frac{t^2 s^2}{\left(\frac{1}{2}\right)^2}$$
>
> What t point should be used? Remember that the point used in the construction of a confidence interval depends on the confidence and the sample size. Here we know the confidence desired, namely 95%, but we are trying to find the sample size. To get around this problem, recall that, for large samples, t points can be approximated by z points. Since the proper t value cannot be determined until the sample size is known, let us approximate its value by using the z point associated with a 95% confidence interval. This point, 1.96, is

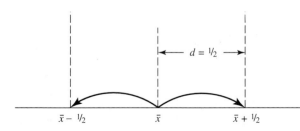

FIGURE 6.18

Since μ should lie within the interval, it will be within $\frac{1}{2}$ pound of $\bar{x}$ if the interval is of length 1.

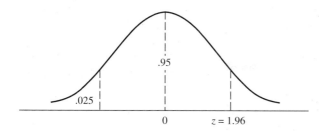

FIGURE 6.19

Partition of the Z distribution
needed to create a 95%
confidence interval.

shown in Figure 6.19. At this point we know that

$$n = \frac{(1.96)^2 s^2}{\left(\frac{1}{2}\right)^2}$$

We have one problem left to solve. What is s^2? What value should be used to estimate the
population variance? There are several ways to answer this question.

1. Use an estimate from a previous study.
2. Run a small preliminary or pilot study and use the value of s^2 found to help plan the
    larger experiment.
3. Recall that the normal probability rule guarantees that X will be within 2 standard
    deviations of its mean 95% of the time. Hence, the range of X is roughly 4 standard
    deviations. We can use the range divided by 4 to approximate s.

Here it is safe to assume that the birth weight of these babies probably lies between 2 and
12 pounds. Hence, the range is 10, and s is approximately $\frac{10}{4} = 2.5$.

The sample size required is

$$n = \frac{(1.96)^2 (2.5)^2}{\left(\frac{1}{2}\right)^2} = 96.04$$

Since we can't sample .04 of a baby, we will take a sample of size 97.

In general, the sample size required to estimate μ to within a stated degree of
accuracy with a stated confidence is

$$n = \frac{z^2 s^2}{d^2}$$

where z is a point from the Z distribution whose value is dependent upon the confidence desired; s^2 is an estimate for the population variance; and d is $\frac{1}{2}$ of the overall
length of the final interval desired.

EXAMPLE 6.6.2. How large a sample is needed to estimate the average diameter at
breast height of a mature stand of loblolly pines to within 6 inches with 90% confidence?
Here, the length of the interval desired is 1 foot and $d = \frac{1}{2}$. From Figure 6.20, we see that
the z point associated with a 90% confidence interval is 1.645. Foresters know from
experience that the diameter at breast height lies between 3 and 8 feet. Hence, the range
of X is 5, and an estimate for the population standard deviation is $\frac{5}{4} = 1.25$. The sample

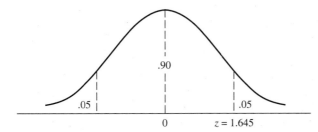

■ **FIGURE 6.20**
Partition of the Z distribution
needed to obtain a 90%
confidence interval.

size required is

$$n = \frac{(1.645)^2(1.25)^2}{\left(\frac{1}{2}\right)^2}$$

$$= 16.9$$

We will sample 17 trees.

Sample Size: Hypothesis Testing

The problem of determining an appropriate sample size to test a hypothesis on the value of the population mean requires careful thought. Example 6.6.3 presents a typical setting in which this problem arises.

> **EXAMPLE 6.6.3.** A researcher is studying a drug which is to be used to reduce the cholesterol level in adult males aged 30 or over. The random variable considered is the change in cholesterol level before and after using the drug with subtraction done in this order: reading before minus reading after. If the drug is effective, the average difference in readings should be positive. The hypothesis to be tested is
>
> $$H_0: \mu \leq 0 \quad \text{(drug is ineffective)}$$
>
> $$H_1: \mu > 0 \quad \text{(drug is effective in reducing the cholesterol level)}$$
>
> How large a sample should be used to conduct the test?

Recall that in testing a hypothesis two errors are possible. We might reject H_0 when in fact H_0 is true, thus committing a Type I error. In our example, we would market an ineffective drug. The probability of making this mistake can be controlled by agreeing to preset α at some acceptably low value as explained in Section 6.5. A Type II error occurs when we fail to reject H_0 even though the research hypothesis is true. In our example, a Type II error leads to the inability to recognize the effectiveness of the drug being studied. The probability of committing a Type II error is called a beta (β). It is evident that ideally in any hypothesis testing setting β should be small. If our research theory is correct, we want to know it. The probability that we will be able to detect a true research theory is called *power*. Computationally, power $= 1 - \beta$. These probabilities are displayed in Table 6.6. Since power is the probability that we will be able to support our research claim when we are right, experiments should be designed so that power is high.

▨ **TABLE 6.6**

In any hypothesis testing setting four situations can arise. An ideal study is one in which α and β are small and power is high.

Decision	True state	
	H_0 true	H_1 true
Reject H_0	Type I error (probability $= \alpha$)	Correct (probability $=$ power)
Fail to reject H_0	Correct decision	Type II error (probability $= \beta$)

It is not possible to get something for nothing even in a statistical setting. If α is preset at an extremely small value to minimize the chances of making a Type I error, a price is paid. Alpha and beta are interrelated in that as α goes down, β goes up. This in turn implies that power is decreased. To improve power, the sample size chosen must be adjusted to account for the α level chosen.

Suppose that the null value is incorrect and $\mu \neq \mu_0$. Common sense indicates that it is easier to detect a large difference between μ_0 and μ than it is to detect one that is very small. In our example it is easier to detect an average change in cholesterol level of 20 mg/dl than it is to detect a change of only 1 mg/dl. An experiment designed to detect large differences will not require as large a sample as one designed to detect small ones.

Variability also plays a role in the choice of sample size. It is easier to draw accurate conclusions concerning populations that are stable than it is to do so with populations that exhibit high variability. Sample sizes can be smaller in the former case than in the latter.

It should be clear that to choose an appropriate sample size the researcher must consider three things.

1. The size of the test desired (α)
2. The magnitude of the difference between μ_0 and μ that is deemed to be important
3. The variance of the sampled population

Tables have been constructed to allow us to determine the proper sample size for choosing between μ_0 and some alternative value μ_1. Table VII of Appendix B is one such table. To use the table, the subject matter expert, the researcher, must be willing to specify μ_1, the alternative value of μ that is of practical importance. He or she must also specify α and β, thus fixing the power desired. In addition, an estimate of σ, the population standard deviation, must be obtained. Example 6.6.4 illustrates the use of Table VII.

EXAMPLE 6.6.4. Let us test H_0: $\mu \leq 10$ versus H_1: $\mu > 10$. Suppose that it is important that a mean of 12 be detected. We want to design an experiment such that the power for detecting a mean of 12 is 90%. Suppose that we decide to preset α at .05 and that an estimate for the population variance based on a pilot study is $s^2 = 16$. To determine the appropriate sample size we enter Table VII with α, β, and Δ where $\Delta = |\mu_0 - \mu_1|/\hat{\sigma}$. The symbol $\hat{\sigma}$ represents an estimate for the population standard deviation. In this case, $\alpha = .05$, $\beta = .10$, and $\Delta = |10 - 12|/4 = .5$. We are conducting a right-tailed (single-sided) test. Table 6.7 shows a portion of Table VII. The sample size, 36, is found by locating the desired values of α, β, and Δ in the table.

EXAMPLE 6.6.5. Consider the study described in Example 6.6.3. Since we do not want to risk marketing an ineffective drug, let us set α at .01. From a practical standpoint, it is decided that the drug is not worth marketing unless an average decrease in cholesterol level is at least 20 mg/dl. Since a change of this magnitude would be a major contribution to the treatment of high cholesterol, we want very much to be able to detect a difference of this size. Let us design the study so that our power is .95 ($\beta = .05$). It is known that the standard deviation in readings for this age group is 30. (See Exercise 5 of Section 5.4.) To determine the proper sample size, we enter Table VII with $\alpha = .01$, $\beta = .05$, and $\Delta = |0 - 20|/30 = .67$. Notice that $\Delta = .67$ is not listed. Since it is safer to have too large a sample rather than one that is too small, we take a conservative approach by using $n = 41$ ($\Delta = .65$) rather than $n = 35$ ($\Delta = 70$).

The message of this subsection is simple. Unplanned experiments are often poorly conducted experiments. Sample sizes must be chosen carefully, and in general small samples yield small power. From the outset, experiments based on small samples are usually doomed to failure unless the difference between μ_0 and μ is extreme. Small samples simply cannot be expected to detect small but perhaps important differences between μ_0 and μ.

▩ EXERCISES 6.6

1. Consider the data given in Example 6.3.2 as a pilot study. How large a sample is required to estimate the average length of a howling session for the wolf pack to within .1 minute with 99% confidence?

2. How large a sample is needed to estimate the average total protein level among adults to within .5 g/dl with 95% confidence if these values are known to have a range of approximately 2.5 g/dl?

3. A researcher wants to estimate the average weight loss obtained by patients at a residential weight loss clinic during the first week of a controlled diet and exercise regimen. How large a sample is needed to estimate this mean to within .5 pound with 95% confidence? Assume that these data are available from preliminary observations on five individuals:

   3.0   2.7   4.0   5.0   1.2

4. An ad appearing in *American Forests*, April 1990, claims that a new chemical used to prepare a site for pine seedlings will produce 1-year-old pines that have an average height more than 1 foot taller than trees grown on sites prepared using the next best chemical treatment. It is known that X, the first year's growth, usually lies between 0 and 36 inches. How large a sample is needed to test the claim at the $\alpha = .05$ level with power = .90?

5. Consider the experiment of Example 6.5.4. If it is crucial that a mean as high as 7.2 be detected, how large a sample is required to test the given hypothesis at

TABLE 6.7

The test is single-sided with $\alpha = .05$, $\beta = .10$, power $= .90$, and $\Delta = .50$. Hence $n = 36$.

Level of t test

Single-sided test	$\alpha=.005$					$\alpha=.01$					$\alpha=.025$					$\alpha=.05$				
Double-sided test	$\alpha=.01$					$\alpha=.02$					$\alpha=.05$					$\alpha=.1$				
$\beta=$	.01	.05	.1	.2	.5	.01	.05	.1	.2	.5	.01	.05	.1	.2	.5	.01	.05	[.1]	.2	.5
.05																				
.10																				
.15																				122
.20										139					99					70
.25					110					90				128	64			139	101	45
.30				134	78				115	63			119	90	45		122	97	71	32
.35			125	99	58			109	85	47		109	88	67	34		90	72	52	24
.40		115	97	77	45		101	85	66	37	117	84	68	51	26	101	70	55	40	19
.45		92	77	62	37	110	81	68	53	30	93	67	54	41	21	80	55	44	33	15
[.50]	100	75	63	51	30	90	66	55	43	25	76	54	44	34	18	65	45	[36]	27	13
.55	83	63	53	42	26	75	55	46	36	21	63	45	37	28	15	54	38	30	22	11
.60	71	53	45	36	22	63	47	39	31	18	53	38	32	24	13	46	32	26	19	9
.65	61	46	39	31	20	55	41	34	27	16	46	33	27	21	12	39	28	22	17	8
.70	53	40	34	28	17	47	35	30	24	14	40	29	24	19	10	34	24	19	15	8
.75	47	36	30	25	16	42	31	27	21	13	35	26	21	16	9	30	21	17	13	7
.80	41	32	27	22	14	37	28	24	19	12	31	22	19	15	9	27	19	15	12	6
.85	37	29	24	20	13	33	25	21	17	11	28	21	17	13	8	24	17	14	11	6
.90	34	26	22	18	12	29	23	19	16	10	25	19	16	12	7	21	15	13	10	5
.95	31	24	20	17	11	27	21	18	14	9	23	17	14	11	7	19	14	11	9	5
1.00	28	22	19	16	10	25	19	16	13	9	21	16	13	10	6	18	13	11	8	5

Value of $\Delta = \dfrac{\mu - \mu_0}{\sigma}$

245

the $\alpha = .05$ level in such a way that the power of the test is .95? (Use the data of Example 6.5.4 as a pilot study.)

6. It is reported that the average daily nutrient intake in healthy young women is 2300 kcal. The reported standard deviation is 237 kcal. The study is based on a small sample, and hence it is of interest to replicate the study. How large a sample is needed to detect a mean that differs from the reported mean by 100 kcal in either direction with $\alpha = .10$ and power $= .9$? (*Hint:* The test is double-sided.) (Based on information found in Reinhold Tuschl et al., "Energy Expenditure and Everyday Eating Behavior in Healthy Young Women," *American Journal of Clinical Nutrition,* July 1990, pp. 81–86.)

TECHNOLOGY TOOLS

TI83

XV.   Random number generator

The TI83 calculator can be used to generate random integers and can therefore be used to perform the functions of the random digit table discussed in Section 6.1. To use the generator, one must specify the smallest and largest integer desired. We illustrate by demonstrating the selection of 10 random integers selected from the integers 0 to 100.

TI83 Keystroke		Purpose	
1.	MATH ◁	1.	Accesses the probability screen of the calculator
2.	5	2.	Accesses the random integer generator; rand Int (
3.	0 , 100)	3.	Identifies 0 as the lower bound and 100 as the upper bound of the integers to be selected
4.	ENTER	4.	Selects and displays the first random integer
5.	ENTER	5.	Selects and displays the second random integer
6.	Continue to press ENTER until 10 random integers are selected	6.	Selects the remaining random integers

XVI.   *T* confidence interval on μ

The TI83 calculator can construct confidence intervals on μ based on raw data or on knowledge of the values of $\bar{x}$ and s alone. We demonstrate by reproducing the confidence interval found in Example 6.3.2.

TI83 Keystroke	**Purpose**
1. STAT 1	1. Accesses the STAT data editor

2. 1.0
   ENTER
   1.2
   ENTER
   ⋮
   1.8
   ENTER
	2. Enters the raw data

3. STAT
   ◁
   8
	3. Selects the program used to construct a T confidence interval on μ

4. cursor on DATA	4. Indicates that raw data is to be used

5. ▽
   ▽
   ▽
   ▽
   ENTER
	5. Forms a 95% confidence interval on μ

Note that the default confidence level on the calculator is .95. The level can be changed by entering a new level to replace .95.

To construct a confidence interval via information on $\bar{x}$ and s, these steps are used: ($\bar{x}$ and s are those of Example 6.2.3.)

TI83 Keystroke	**Purpose**

1. STAT
   ◁
   8
	1. Selects the program used to construct a T confidence interval on μ

2. cursor to stats ENTER	2. Indicates that values of $\bar{x}$ and s will be supplied rather than raw data
3. ▽ 1.57	3. Enters 1.57 as the value of $\bar{x}$
4. ▽ .26	4. Enters .26 as the value of s
5. ▽ 16	5. Enters 16 as the sample size
6. ▽ .95	6. Enters .95 as the desired confidence level
7. ▽ ENTER	7. Constructs the confidence interval

XVII.   *T* test

The TI83 is programmed to conduct any of the three types of T test on the mean. It can perform the test using either raw data or information on $\bar{x}$ and s. We illustrate by using the data for the two-tailed test of Example 6.5.6. In this case, we shall demonstrate how to allow the calculator to find and draw the P value.

TI83 Keystroke	Purpose
1. STAT 1	1. Accesses the stat data editor
2. 7.23 ENTER 7.32 ENTER $\vdots$ 7.24 ENTER	2. Enters data
3. STAT $\triangleleft$ 2	3. Accesses the one-sample T test screen
4. cursor on data ENTER $\triangledown$	4. Indicates that raw data is to be used
5. 7.25 $\triangledown$ $\triangledown$ $\triangledown$	5. Enters 7.25 as the null value
6. $\triangledown$	6. Indicates that the test is two-tailed
7. $\triangleright$ ENTER	7. Evaluates the test statistic; finds and draws the P value (Notice that there will be some roundoff error in the text value. The calculator value is the more accurate of the two.)

SAS Package

VII. T test

SAS is able to conduct a one-sample T test via the procedure PROC MEANS. This procedure can also be used to find $\bar{x}, s,$ and $s/\sqrt{n}$ which are the necessary components for constructing a confidence interval on the mean. This procedure can only deal with a null value of 0, so to test any other value a transformation must be used. In particular, if $\mu_0 \neq 0$, we form a new variable by subtracting μ_0 from each data point. If the average value of the original variable X is μ_0 then the average value of $X - \mu_0$ will be 0. Thus to test H$_0$: $\mu_X = \mu_0$ we test H$_0$: $\mu_X - \mu_0 = 0$ via PROC MEANS. Example 6.5.6 is used to demonstrate this idea. In this example $\mu_0 = 7.25$.

SAS Code	**Purpose**
OPTIONS LS = 80 PS = 60	Sets printing specifications
NODATE;	
DATA BLOOD;	Names the data set
INPUT X @@;	Names the variable; more than one
	observation can appear per line
TRANSFRM = X − 7.25;	Forms a new variable; if the mean of
	X is 7.25, the mean of TRANSFRM
	is 0
LINES;	Signals that the data follow
	immediately
7.23 7.32 7.25 7.26	Data lines
7.28 7.27 7.29 7.24	
;	Signals the end of the data
PROC MEANS MEAN STD	Asks for $\bar{x}, s, s/\sqrt{n}$ to be
T PRT;	found for all variables; tests
	$H_0: \mu_0 = 0$ for all variables
	and prints the P value of the
	test
TITLE 'TTEST ON THE AVERAGE	Titles the output
PROTEIN LEVEL';	

The output of this program is shown below. These statistics for the variable X are given on the printout:

    ① $\bar{x}$, the average value of X

    ② s, the standard deviation of X

    ③ $s/\sqrt{n}$, the standard error of the mean

Notice that these values agree with those in the text apart from roundoff differences. Statistics for the variable TRANSFRM = $X − 7.25$ are given as follows:

    ④   the average value of TRANSFRM; notice that this average is, as expected, 7.25 less than $\bar{x}$

    ⑤   the standard deviation of TRANSFRM; this is the same as s because subtracting 7.25 from X changes location but does not change variability or dispersion

    ⑥   the standard error of TRANSFRM; this is the same as $s/\sqrt{n}$

The T test of interest is shown at ⑦ with its corresponding P value at ⑧. The observed value of the T statistic differs a bit from the text (text value = 1.756) due to the fact that SAS is retaining seven decimal places in its calculations. In this test and all that follow, SAS automatically conducts a *two-tailed test*. The P value .1334 shown at ⑧ is for the two-tailed alternative H_1: $\mu \neq 7.25$. Since we are conducting such a test, $P = .1334$. This is consistent with the statement in the text that $.10 < P < .20$.

SAS is not set up to construct a *T* type confidence interval automatically. However, as you can see, it will find $\bar{x}$ and $s/\sqrt{n}$ easily. A confidence interval can be found quickly from this information if desired.

Note: If you are conducting a one-tailed *T* test, then the *P* value found by SAS should be divided by 2 to get the correct *P* value for your test. SAS will not think for you. You are responsible for interpreting the printout correctly in the context of your study.

TTEST ON THE AVERAGE TOTAL PROTEIN LEVEL

Variable	Mean	Std Dev	Std Error	T	Prob>|T|
X	7.2675000 ①	0.0291548 ②	0.0103078 ③	705.0510620	0.0001
TRANSFRM	0.0175000 ④	0.0291548 ⑤	0.0103078 ⑥	1.6977494 ⑦	0.1334 ⑧

7

Chi-Squared Distribution and Inferences on the Variance

In this chapter we introduce another important family of continuous random variables. These random variables, called chi-squared, are used in several different statistical settings. Their application in drawing conclusions concerning the population variance is presented here.

■ 7.1

CHI-SQUARED DISTRIBUTION AND
INTERVAL ESTIMATION OF THE POPULATION VARIANCE

It has already been argued that the sample variance S^2 is a logical point estimator for the population variance σ^2. The estimates for σ^2 obtained in repeated samples from the same population fluctuate about the true population variance. Thus far, estimates for σ^2 have been of interest in that they are needed to evaluate the T statistic used to make inferences on the population mean.

On some occasions interest centers not on the mean, but on the variance itself. Thus it is necessary to be able not only to find a point estimate for σ^2, but also to construct a confidence interval on or test a hypothesis concerning this parameter.

> **EXAMPLE 7.1.1.** Copper, a mineral required to some degree by most plants, is classed as a micronutrient. Its concentration in a plant is measured in parts per million and is determined by burning the plant completely and analyzing the ash. The copper concentration varies from species to species. An experiment is run to estimate this variability.

> **EXAMPLE 7.1.2.** The Lhasa apso is a dog of Tibetan ancestry. The breed was introduced in England in 1921 and was first bred for show in 1933. The desired shoulder height in males is 10.5 inches. However, there is a fair amount of natural variability in height. A breeder is attempting to reduce this variability in the animals by selective breeding.

EXAMPLE 7.1.3. In manufacturing a drug, its potency varies from time to time. This variability must not be allowed to become too large. A large variance could result in some batches of the drug being too weak to be effective while others are too strong and potentially dangerous. Periodically tests are run to monitor the variance of the drug being produced.

Each of these three examples calls for an inference to be made concerning a population variance. To construct a confidence interval on σ^2 or to test a hypothesis concerning its value, it is necessary to introduce another family of continuous random variables. The general characteristics of members of this family, called *chi-squared variables* (X^2), are as follows:

1. There are infinitely many chi-squared random variables, each identified by one parameter γ, called *degrees of freedom*. The parameter γ is always a positive integer. The notation X_γ^2 denotes a chi-squared variable with γ degrees of freedom.
2. Each chi-squared variable is continuous.
3. The graph of the density of each chi-squared variable with $\gamma \geq 2$ is an asymmetric curve of the general shape shown in Figure 7.1a; when $\gamma = 1$, the graph assumes the shape shown in Figure 7.1b.
4. Chi-squared variables cannot assume negative values.
5. Parameter γ is both a shape and a location parameter in that

$$E[X_\gamma^2] = \gamma \qquad \text{and} \qquad \text{Var } X_\gamma^2 = 2\gamma$$

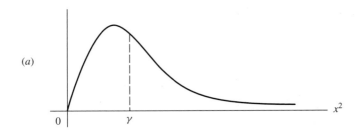

(a)

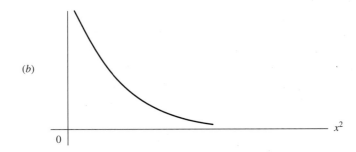

(b)

▨ **FIGURE 7.1**

(a) Typical chi-squared curve with $\gamma \geq 2$. The balance point of the curve is γ, its degrees of freedom. (b) Chi-squared curve with $\gamma = 1$.

That is, the average value of a chi-squared random variable is the same as its degrees of freedom, and its variance is twice its degrees of freedom.

A partial summary of the cumulative distribution function for chi-squared variables with various degrees of freedom is given in Table VIII of Appendix B. In that table, degrees of freedom appear as row headings, probabilities appear as column headings, and points associated with those probabilities are listed in the body of the table.

EXAMPLE 7.1.4. Consider a chi-squared random variable with 10 degrees of freedom. This random variable is denoted by X_{10}^2. Its average value is 10, the same as its degrees of freedom, and its variance is 20, twice its degrees of freedom.

(a) Find $P[X_{10}^2 \leq 2.56]$. To find this probability, look in row 10 of Table VIII. The number 2.56 is found in column .010. Therefore, $P[X_{10}^2 \leq 2.56] = F(2.56) = .01$.
(b) Find $P[X_{10}^2 \geq 16]$. Since 16 is found in column .900 of row 10, $P[X_{10}^2 \leq 16] = .900$. This, in turn, means that $P[X_{10}^2 \geq 16] = 1 - F(16) = 1 - .90 = .1$.
(c) The point with 5% of the area to its right and 95% to its left is shown in Figure 7.2. Its numerical value, found in row 10 and column .95 of the chi-squared table, is 18.3.
(d) The point with 95% of the area to its right and 5% to its left is found in row 10 and column .05. Its numerical value is 3.94.
(e) Find the area under the graph of the X_{10}^2 density between 3.25 and 20.5. This area, which is also equal to $P[3.25 \leq X_{10}^2 \leq 20.5]$, is shown in Figure 7.3a. Since the area to the left of 20.5 is .975 and the area to the left of 3.25 is .025, the area between these values is $.975 - .025 = .950$. (See Figure 7.3b.)

Confidence Interval on σ^2 (Optional)

To construct a confidence interval on σ^2 we need a random variable that involves this parameter in its expression whose distribution is known. If such a random variable can be found, then an algebraic argument similar to that used to construct a confidence

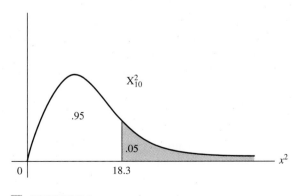

FIGURE 7.2
$P[X_{10}^2 \geq 18.3] = .05$.

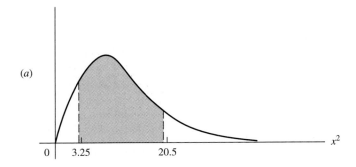

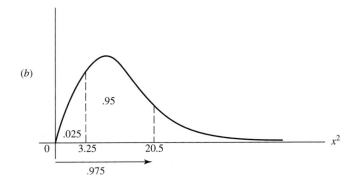

▨ **FIGURE 7.3**
(*a*) Shaded area $= P[3.25 \leq X_{10}^2 \leq 20.5]$.
(*b*) $P[3.25 \leq X_{10}^2 \leq 20.5] = .95$.

interval on μ can be used to find confidence bounds for σ^2. Theorem 7.1.1 provides the needed random variable.

THEOREM 7.1.1. Let $X_1, X_2, X_3, \ldots, X_n$ be a random sample of size n from a distribution that is normal with mean μ and variance σ^2. The random variable $(n-1)S^2/\sigma^2$ is distributed as a chi-squared random variable with $n-1$ degrees of freedom.

Example 7.1.5 illustrates how this theorem is used to create a confidence interval on σ^2.

EXAMPLE 7.1.5. To estimate the variance in the copper concentration in plants found in the New River Valley, a random sample of 16 plants was obtained, the plants were burned, and the ash was analyzed. The following observations on X, the copper concentration (in parts per million), were obtained (assume that X is normally distributed):

5	3	34	18	27	14
8	50	38	43	35	
20	70	25	60	19	

For these data $s^2 = 377.30$. The partition of the X_{15}^2 curve needed to construct a 90% confidence interval on σ^2 is shown in Figure 7.4.

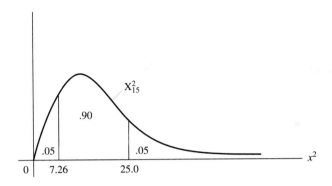

FIGURE 7.4

Partition of X_{15}^2 to obtain a 90% confidence interval on σ^2.

Notice that since the sample is of size 16, the number of degrees of freedom involved is 15, the sample size minus 1. As in the past, a 90% confidence interval is obtained by partitioning the curve so that 90% of the area is in the center with the remaining 10% split into two equal portions. From Figure 7.4, it is clear that

$$P[7.26 \leq X_{15}^2 \leq 25] = .90$$

In this case, the chi-squared random variable is

$$\frac{(n-1)S^2}{\sigma^2} = \frac{15S^2}{\sigma^2}$$

Therefore, we know that

$$P\left[7.26 \leq \frac{15S^2}{\sigma^2} \leq 25\right] = .90$$

Our target is to isolate σ^2 in the middle of the inequality. This is done by first inverting each portion of the inequality and then multiplying by $15S^2$. This results in the following sequence of steps:

$$P\left[7.26 \leq \frac{15S^2}{\sigma^2} \leq 25\right] = .90$$

$$P\left[\frac{1}{25} \leq \frac{\sigma^2}{15S^2} \leq \frac{1}{7.26}\right] = .90$$

$$P\left[\frac{15S^2}{25} \leq \sigma^2 \leq \frac{15S^2}{7.26}\right] = .90$$

The lower confidence bound is

$$\frac{15S^2}{25} = \frac{15(377.30)}{25.0} = 226.38$$

and the upper bound is

$$\frac{15S^2}{7.26} = \frac{15(377.30)}{7.26} = 779.55$$

We are 90% confident that the true variance in the copper concentration of plants in the New River Valley lies between 226.38 and 779.55 inclusive. To find a 90% confidence interval on the population standard deviation σ, we need only take the square root of these numerical bounds. Thus we can report that we are 90% confident that the true population standard deviation lies between $\sqrt{226.38} = 15.04$ and $\sqrt{779.54} = 27.92$ parts per million inclusive.

The technique used in Example 7.1.5 can be generalized to obtain any desired degree of confidence by choosing the points from the chi-squared table appropriately. Notice that since the chi-squared distribution is not symmetric, two distinct points must be read from the table. The point that appears in the lower boundary will be denoted by χ_1^2. It is the larger of the two points read from the table. The point that appears in the upper boundary will be denoted by χ_2^2. The general confidence bounds are given in Theorem 7.1.2.

THEOREM 7.1.2. Confidence interval on σ^2. Let $X_1, X_2, X_3, \ldots, X_n$ be a random sample of size n from a distribution that is normal with mean μ and variance σ^2. The lower and upper bounds, respectively, for a confidence interval on σ^2 are

$$L_1 = \frac{(n-1)S^2}{\chi_1^2} \qquad L_2 = \frac{(n-1)S^2}{\chi_2^2}$$

where the χ^2 points are points from the chi-squared distribution with $n - 1$ degrees of freedom.

As in the case of the T distribution, chi-squared points for large samples can be approximated using the standard normal distribution. The way in which this is done is demonstrated in Exercise 5 at the end of this section. This exercise makes it possible to construct confidence intervals on σ^2 for samples larger than those that can be handled using the chi-squared table. Chi-squared points for large samples can also be obtained from most computer packages and from the TI83 calculator.

■ EXERCISES 7.1

1. Consider the random variable X_9^2.
    (a) Find $P[X_9^2 \leq 2.09]$.
    (b) Find $P[X_9^2 \geq 11.4]$.
    (c) Find $P[14.7 \leq X_9^2 \leq 16.9]$.
    (d) Find the point with area .025 to its right.
    (e) Find the point with area .01 to its left.
    (f) Find points χ_1^2 and χ_2^2 such that the area to the right of χ_2^2 equals the area to the left of χ_1^2 and $P[\chi_1^2 \leq X_9^2 \leq \chi_2^2] = .90$. (*Hint:* Draw a picture of these points.)
2. Consider the random variable X_{15}^2. Find:
    (a) $E[X_{15}^2]$
    (b) Var X_{15}^2
    (c) The point with area .05 to its right
    (d) The point with area .10 to its left

(e) $P[X_{15}^2 \leq 7.26]$

(f) $P[X_{15}^2 \geq 27.5]$

3. During severe winter weather, salt is used for deicing roads. To approximate the amount of salt being introduced into the environment from this source, a study was run in New England. The following observations were obtained on random variable X, the total number of metric tons of salt used on roadways per week in randomly selected counties across the region:

3900	3875	3820	3860	3840
3852	3800	3825	3790	

(a) Find a point estimate for μ.

(b) Find a point estimate for σ^2.

(c) Assume that X is normally distributed. Find a 90% confidence interval on μ.

(d) Find 90% confidence intervals on σ^2 and σ.

4. The typical plant cell has a large amount of cytoplasm bounded by a cell membrane called the plasma membrane. The mean thickness of this membrane varies from species to species. A random sample of 20 species yielded the following observations on X, the thickness of the cell membrane, in angstroms:

80	90	85	82	75	58	70
84	87	81	87	61	73	84
85	70	78	95	77	52	

(a) Find a point estimate for σ^2.

(b) Assume that X is normally distributed. Find 95% confidence intervals on μ, σ^2, and σ.

5. *Normal approximation to χ^2.* Note that the chi-squared table lists values of γ from 1 to 30. Therefore it can be used for sample sizes from 2 to 31. For samples larger than this, chi-squared points can be approximated by the formula

$$\chi_r^2 \doteq \left(\tfrac{1}{2}\right)\left[z_r + \sqrt{2\gamma - 1}\right]^2$$

where the subscript r gives the area desired to the *right* of the point. Remember that γ denotes the degrees of freedom associated with the chi-squared point. For example, for a sample of size 50, the point $\chi_{.025}^2$ is given by

$$\chi_{.025}^2 \doteq \left(\tfrac{1}{2}\right)\left[z_{.025} + \sqrt{2\gamma - 1}\right]^2$$
$$= \left(\tfrac{1}{2}\right)\left[1.96 + \sqrt{2(49) - 1}\right]^2$$
$$\doteq 69.72$$

Approximate each of the points listed in parts a to c.

(a) $\chi_{.05}^2$ and $\chi_{.90}^2$; $\gamma = 79$

(b) $\chi_{.025}^2$ and $\chi_{.975}^2$; $\gamma = 99$

(c) $\chi_{.005}^2$ and $\chi_{.995}^2$; $\gamma = 74$

6. A study of obesity in children under the age of 12 is conducted. A sample of 100 obese children is obtained, and the age of each child at the onset of obesity is ascertained. The sample mean is found to be 4 years with a sample standard deviation of 1.5 years.

(a) Find a 95% confidence interval for the average age at the onset of obesity in children.

(b) Find a 95% confidence interval on the variance in the age at the onset of obesity.

(c) Find a 95% confidence interval on the standard deviation in the age at the onset of obesity.

(Based on information found in Rebecca Unger, Lisa Kreeger, and Katherine Christoffel, "Childhood Obesity," *Clinical Pediatrics,* July 1990, pp. 368–373.)

7. A study is conducted to estimate characteristics of the floodplain of a portion of the Mississippi River. One variable studied is X, the width of the floodplain. A sample of measurements obtained at 61 randomly selected sites yields $\bar{x} = 3400$ m and $s = 100$ m.

(a) Find a 90% confidence interval on the average width of the floodplain in the region.

(b) Find 90% confidence intervals on the variance and standard deviation of X.

(Based on information found in Frederick Swanson and Richard Sparks, "Long Term Ecological Research and the Invisible Place," *Bioscience,* August 1990, pp. 502–508.)

7.2
TESTING HYPOTHESES ON
THE POPULATION VARIANCE (OPTIONAL)

If there is a preconceived theory concerning the magnitude of the variance or standard deviation of a random variable, then it is appropriate to handle the problem as a hypothesis testing problem.

Hypothesis tests on σ^2 take the same three general forms as those on the mean. These are summarized below, with σ_0^2 representing the hypothesized value of the population variance.

I $H_0: \sigma^2 \leq \sigma_0^2$	II $H_0: \sigma^2 \geq \sigma_0^2$	III $H_0: \sigma^2 = \sigma_0^2$
$H_1: \sigma^2 > \sigma_0^2$	$H_1: \sigma^2 < \sigma_0^2$	$H_1: \sigma^2 \neq \sigma_0^2$
Right-tailed test	Left-tailed test	Two-tailed test

The test statistic for testing each of these is

$$\frac{(n-1)S^2}{\sigma_0^2}$$

This statistic, under the assumption that the hypothesized value of σ^2 is correct, follows a chi-squared distribution with $n-1$ degrees of freedom.

In a right-tailed test H_0 is rejected for values of the test statistic that are too large to have occurred by chance; a left-tailed test is conducted by rejecting H_0 for small values of the test statistic. As in the case of T tests, the decision is made based on the calculated P value. Example 7.2.1 illustrates the test and explains the logic behind the rejection rules.

EXAMPLE 7.2.1. The current variance in the height of male Lhasa apsos is .25. A breeder is attempting to reduce this figure. After a period of selective breeding, a random sample of 15 males is to be chosen from among the animals and measured. Since the researcher's contention is taken as the alternative hypothesis, the purpose of the experiment is to test

$$H_0: \sigma^2 \geq .25 \qquad H_1: \sigma^2 < .25$$

The test statistic to be used is

$$\frac{(n-1)S^2}{\sigma_0^2} = \frac{14S^2}{.25}$$

which, if H_0 is true, has a chi-squared distribution with $n - 1 = 14$ degrees of freedom. Since S^2 is an estimator for σ^2, if H_0 is true, we expect the numerical value of S^2 to lie close to .25, the hypothesized value of σ^2. This forces the ratio $S^2/.25$ to lie close to 1 and the value of the test statistic to be close to 14, its expected value. If, however, the alternative is true and the population variance is actually smaller than the hypothesized value of .25, we expect S^2 to have a value smaller than .25. This, in turn, must force the ratio $S^2/.25$ to be smaller than 1, resulting in a value smaller than 14 for the test statistic. Thus it is logical to reject H_0 in favor of H_1 if the observed value of the test statistic is too small to have occurred by chance. When the experiment was run, a sample variance of .21 was obtained. The value of the test statistic is $14(.21)/.25 = 11.76$.

The P value is the probability of observing a value of 11.76 or smaller. This probability is pictured in Figure 7.5. Its value is approximated from row 14 of the chi-squared table. Since the value 11.76 lies between 10.2 (area to the left .25) and 13.3 (area to the left .50), the P value lies between .25 and .50. Since this probability is large, we will not reject H_0.

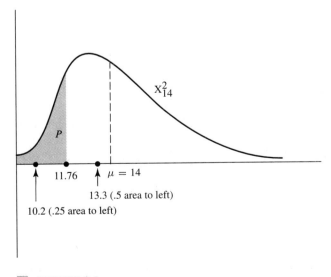

FIGURE 7.5

We do not have sufficient evidence to support the claim that selective breeding has reduced the variability in heights of male Lhasa apsos.

As in the case of T tests, H_0 can be tested using a preset α level if so desired. If this is done, we reject H_0 if the calculated P value is at most equal to α.

Notice that as in the case of T tests, a normality assumption has been made. In the case of the chi-squared statistic, violating this assumption can lead to serious errors. If the population from which the sampling is done appears not to be normal, then another method must be used to test hypotheses on σ^2. One such method is given in [2].

▨ EXERCISES 7.2

1. One variable studied by biologists is the internal body temperature of poikilothermic animals (animals whose body temperature fluctuates with the surroundings). The lethal dose (LD_{50}) for desert lizards is 45°C. It has been observed that most of these animals hide during the heat of a summer day to avoid approaching this lethal dose. An experiment was conducted to study X, the time (in minutes) required for the body temperature of a desert lizard to reach 45°C, starting from its normal body temperature while in the shade. The following observations were obtained:

10.1	12.5	12.2	10.2	12.8	12.1
11.2	11.4	10.7	14.9	13.9	13.3

(a) Find point estimates for μ, σ^2, and σ.
(b) Assume X is normal. On the basis of these data, can it be concluded that the mean time required to reach the lethal dose is less than 13 minutes? Explain your answer on the basis of the P value.
(c) On the basis of these data, can it be concluded that the standard deviation of X is less than 1.5 minutes? Explain your answer on the basis of the P value. *Hint:* Testing

$$H_0: \sigma \geq 1.5 \qquad H_1: \sigma < 1.5$$

is equivalent to testing

$$H_0: \sigma^2 \geq (1.5)^2 \qquad H_1: \sigma^2 < (1.5)^2$$

2. Calcium is normally present in mammalian blood in concentrations of about 6 milligrams per 100 milliliters of whole blood. The normal standard deviation of this variable is 1 milligram of calcium per 100 milliliters of whole blood. Variability larger than this can lead to severe disturbances in blood coagulation. A series of nine tests on a patient revealed a sample mean of 6.2 milligrams of calcium per 100 milliliters of whole blood and a sample standard deviation of 2 milligrams of calcium per 100 milliliters of blood. Is there evidence at the $\alpha = .05$ level that the mean calcium level for this patient is higher than normal? Is there evidence at the $\alpha = .05$ level that the standard deviation of the calcium level is higher than normal?

3. To meet the respiratory needs of warm-water fish, the dissolved oxygen content should average 6.5 parts per million with a standard deviation of no more than

1.2 parts per million. As the water temperature increases, the dissolved oxygen decreases. This can cause fish to suffocate. A study is run on the effects of hot summer weather on a large lake. After a particularly hot period, water samples are taken from 25 randomly selected locations in the lake, and the dissolved oxygen content is determined. A sample mean of 6.3 parts per million and a sample standard deviation of 1.7 resulted.

(a) Is this evidence at the $\alpha = .05$ level that the mean oxygen content in the lake has decreased from the acceptable level of 6.5 parts per million?

(b) Test

$$H_0: \sigma \leq 1.2$$

$$H_1: \sigma > 1.2$$

On the basis of the given data, can H_0 be rejected at the $\alpha = .05$ level?

4. The average growth of mature spruce trees near Whitewater Bay, Alaska, is thought to be 19 inches per year with a standard deviation of .5 inch. Researchers believe that severe drought conditions have led to a decrease in both of these values. A sample of 50 trees yields an average growth of 18.9 inches with a sample standard deviation of .15 inch.

(a) State the research hypothesis concerning the mean growth. Do the data support this theory? Explain based on the P value of your test.

(b) State the research hypothesis concerning the standard deviation. Do the data support this theory? Explain based on the P value of your test.

(c) From a practical point of view do you believe that the difference in mean growth is enough to cause concern?

(Based on information found in Herbert McClean, "Return to Admirality," *American Forests,* August 1989, pp. 21–24.)

8

Inferences on Proportions

In this chapter we discuss inferences on one proportion and the comparison of two proportions. The Central Limit Theorem, studied in Chapter 6, will provide the theoretical justification for the procedures presented here. It will be assumed throughout the discussion that sample sizes are large enough to justify the use of this theorem.

◼ 8.1
POINT ESTIMATION

We begin with a general description of the problem to be considered. There is a population of interest, a particular trait is being studied, and each member of the population can be classified as either having or failing to have the trait. Inferences are to be made on the parameter p, the proportion of the population with the trait. (See Figure 8.1.)

Notice that in this case there is a departure from our usual notational convention of denoting population parameters by Greek letters. There is no convenient and commonly employed Greek symbol for the population proportion. We use the letter p because it is a natural choice to represent a proportion, percentage, or probability.

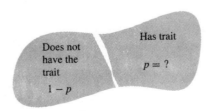

◼ FIGURE 8.1
Population partitioned by the presence of the trait.

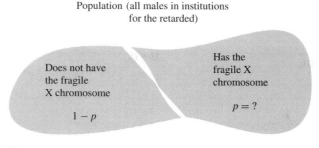

Population (all males in institutions
for the retarded)

Does not have
the fragile
X chromosome

$1 - p$

Has the
fragile X
chromosome

$p = ?$

FIGURE 8.2

Population partitioned by the presence of the fragile
X chromosome.

Example 8.1.1 illustrates a setting in which interest centers on estimating a population proportion.

EXAMPLE 8.1.1. More males than females suffer from some form of mental retardation. One possible explanation for this phenomenon, the fragile X syndrome, has been proposed recently. This inherited defect usually is passed on from mother to son, and it appears as a defect on the X chromosome. A study is run to estimate the proportion of males in institutions for the retarded who have this defect. In this case, the population of interest is males in institutions for the retarded; the trait under study is having the fragile X chromosome. We wish to obtain a point estimate for the proportion p of males in these institutions who have this particular defect. Schematically, this is shown in Figure 8.2.

What is a logical point estimator for p? Common sense indicates that we should draw a random sample from the population of interest, determine the proportion of

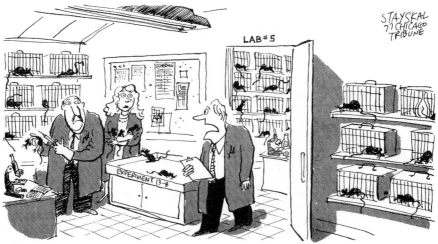

"OH, OH, I JUST DISCOVERED 79% OF MY RATS HAVE CANCER ... AND I DIDN'T INJECT THEM WITH ANYTHING YET!"

objects in the sample with the trait, and use this "sample proportion" as an estimate of the population proportion p. That is, common sense points to

$$\frac{X}{n} = \frac{\text{number of objects in sample with trait}}{\text{sample size}} = \text{sample proportion}$$

as a logical estimator for p.

To emphasize the fact that the sample proportion is an estimator for the population proportion, we shall use "hat" notation. In this notation a hat ($\wedge$) is placed over the parameter to indicate that the statistic given is a point estimator for the parameter. In this case, we indicate that the statistic X/n is an estimator for p by writing

$$\frac{X}{n} = \hat{p}$$

EXAMPLE 8.1.2. A random sample was obtained of 150 males in institutions for the retarded. Of these, 4 were found to have the fragile X chromosome. Based on this sample,

$$\hat{p} = \frac{x}{n} = \frac{4}{150} = .027$$

Note that by multiplying by 100, this proportion can be converted to a percentage (2.7%). If, in fact, this estimate accurately reflects the true percentage of male retardates with this defect, this could mean that the disorder is the second greatest known cause of mental retardation after Down's syndrome.

The sample proportion will be used in the next section to develop confidence intervals on the population proportion. To do so, we must ask, What is the distribution of $\hat{p}$? This question is answered by Theorem 8.1.1. The proof of this theorem is outlined in Exercise 7.

THEOREM 8.1.1. For large sample sizes, the sample proportion

$$\hat{p} = \frac{X}{n} = \frac{\text{number of objects in sample with trait}}{\text{sample size}}$$

is approximately normally distributed. Furthermore, the average value of $\hat{p}$ is p and its variance is $p(1-p)/n$.

EXERCISES 8.1

1. One of the most troublesome forms of venereal disease is caused by the common herpes simplex virus. A recent study tested an ointment containing the sugar 2-deoxy-D-glucose on 36 women with genital herpes infections. Within 4 days, the symptoms were cleared up in 32 of the 36 cases. Find a point estimate for p, the proportion of women for whom this treatment will be effective.

2. A national survey was run to estimate the proportion p of individuals 16 years old and under who smoke regularly. Of 1000 individuals interviewed, 200 smoked regularly. Find a point estimate for p.

TABLE 8.1

Results of a survey of 20 persons seen at a free clinic

Person	Employed?	Person	Employed?
1	Yes $x_1 = 1$	11	No $x_{11} = 0$
2	Yes $x_2 = 1$	12	Yes $x_{12} = 1$
3	No $x_3 = 0$	13	No $x_{13} = 0$
4	No $x_4 = 0$	14	No $x_{14} = 0$
5	No $x_5 = 0$	15	No $x_{15} = 0$
6	No $x_6 = 0$	16	No $x_{16} = 0$
7	No $x_7 = 0$	17	Yes $x_{17} = 1$
8	No $x_8 = 0$	18	Yes $x_{18} = 1$
9	No $x_9 = 0$	19	No $x_{19} = 0$
10	No $x_{10} = 0$	20	Yes $x_{20} = 1$

3. A recent study indicates that acute stress can induce changes in the heart that may lead to death. Evidence was obtained by examining 15 cases in which people died after a physical assault even though the injuries alone were not severe enough to cause death. Of the cases, 11 showed a type of heart-cell death called myofibrillar degeneration. Find a point estimate of p, the proportion of deaths due to myofibrillar degeneration in assault cases.

4. Consider a small pilot study designed to estimate the proportion of patients seen at a free clinic who are currently employed. A sample of 20 individuals is obtained. We code the data by letting $X_i = 1$ if the ith person sampled is employed; $X_i = 0$ otherwise. The data obtained are shown in Table 8.1.
   (a) Find $\sum x_i$.
   (b) Argue that $\sum x_i = x$, the number of persons in the sample that are employed.
   (c) Estimate the proportion of persons in the sample that are employed.

5. Draw a random sample of 30 one-digit numbers from the random number table (Table IV of Appendix B). Let $X_i = 1$ if the ith number drawn is a 5, and let $X_i = 0$ otherwise. Estimate the proportion of 5s in the table.

6. Draw a random sample of size 10 from the trees listed in Table V of Appendix B. Let $X_i = 1$ if the tree sampled has an MDBH greater than 5, and let $X_i = 0$ otherwise.
   (a) Find $\sum x_i$.
   (b) Find the number of trees in the sample with an MDBH greater than 5.
   (c) Estimate the proportion of trees with an MDBH greater than 5.
   (d) Estimate the number of trees listed in the table with an MDBH greater than 5.

7. Define a collection of independent random variables $X_1, X_2, \ldots, X_n$ by letting $X_i = 1$ if the ith member of the sample has the trait of interest and letting $X_i = 0$ otherwise. For example, if the first male sampled in Example 8.1.2 has the fragile X chromosome, then $x_1 = 1$; if this individual does not have this chromosome, then $x_1 = 0$. If the probability of observing the trait is p, then the probability of not observing the trait is $1 - p$. This implies that the density for the discrete random variable X_i is

X_i	0	1
$f(X_i)$	$1 - p$	p

(a) Use the method of Section 4.2 to verify that $E[X_i] = p$, $E[X_i^2] = p$, and Var $X_i = p(1 - p)$.

(b) Argue that X, the number of objects in the sample with the trait, is given by

$$X = \sum_{i=1}^{n} X_i$$

(c) Assume that n is large enough for the Central Limit Theorem to be applicable. Use this theorem to argue that X/n is approximately normally distributed with mean p and variance $p(1 - p)/n$ as claimed in Theorem 8.1.1.

(d) For large samples, what is the approximate distribution of the random variable

$$\frac{\hat{p} - p}{\sqrt{\dfrac{p(1 - p)}{n}}}$$

8. *Capture-recapture method for sampling wildlife populations.* One parameter of interest to foresters is N, the population size of certain species of wild animals. For example, it is important to know the number of bears in the wild in the Great Smoky Mountains so that this population can be protected or controlled. Unfortunately, it is impossible to take a census of this population because of its mobility and the large geographical area involved. Hence N must be approximated statistically. In the capture-recapture method, a number of animals are caught, tagged, and released. They are allowed to disperse. Several days or weeks later, a second sample of animals is obtained. The proportion of tagged animals in this sample is determined. This sample proportion is used as an estimate for the proportion of tagged animals in the population. Let

T = number of animals captured and tagged originally

p = proportion of tagged animals in population $= \dfrac{T}{N}$

C = number of animals caught in second sample

R = number of animals recaptured
   = number of tagged animals in second sample

$\hat{p}$ = proportion of tagged animals in second sample $= \dfrac{R}{C}$

Since $\hat{p}$ estimates p, $\hat{p} \doteq p$. Substituting, we may conclude that

$$\frac{R}{C} \doteq \frac{T}{N}$$

Solving this equation for N, we see that

$$N \doteq \frac{CT}{R}$$

For example, if originally $T = 20$ bears were tagged, $C = 15$ were caught in the second sample, and of these $R = 3$ were tagged, then the estimated number of bears living in the wild is

$$\hat{N} = \frac{CT}{R} = \frac{15(20)}{3} = 100$$

(a) A study is conducted of falcons in northwest Canada. Thirty falcons were tagged, twenty falcons were caught in the second sample, and of these two were tagged. Use this information to estimate N, the number of falcons living free in the area.

(b) In the mid 1930s, the trumpeter swan of North America was in danger of extinction. At this time, Yellowstone Park and an adjacent hot springs area at Red Rock Lakes, Montana, were designated as a refuge. In the late 1960s, a study was conducted of the swans in this area. Fifty swans were captured and tagged. A second sample of 30 swans contained 5 that were tagged. Use this information to estimate the total swan population in this region at this time.

(c) The capture-recapture method is to be used to roughly estimate the number of drug addicts in New York City. For 6 months note is made of the drug addicts arrested for the first time for minor offenses. Then they are released. In this way, 500 addicts are "tagged." During the next year 1800 addicts were arrested for various offenses, and 20 were from the tagged group. Based on this information, estimate the total number of drug addicts in New York City.

8.2

INTERVAL ESTIMATION OF p

We turn now to the problem of confidence interval estimation of p. That is, we would like to extend our point estimate of p to an interval of values so that a confidence level can be reported. To do so, we must find a random variable whose expression involves p and whose probability distribution is known at least approximately. This is easily done.

From Theorem 8.1.1, we know that $\hat{p}$ is approximately normally distributed with mean p and variance $p(1 - p)/n$. Standardization via Theorem 5.3.1 allows us to conclude that the random variable

$$\frac{\hat{p} - p}{\sqrt{p(1 - p)/n}}$$

approximately follows the Z or standard normal distribution.

Recall that to find a confidence interval on the mean, we began with the Z random variable

$$\frac{\bar{X} - \mu}{\sigma/\sqrt{n}}$$

The random variable

$$\frac{\hat{p} - p}{\sqrt{p(1 - p)/n}}$$

has the same algebraic structure. Here $\hat{p}$ plays the role of $\bar{X}$, p corresponds to μ, and $\sqrt{p(1-p)/n}$ is equivalent to $\sigma/\sqrt{n}$. The algebraic argument given in Section 6.4 to obtain the confidence bounds $\bar{X} \pm z\sigma/\sqrt{n}$ could be repeated to obtain these bounds for a confidence interval on p:

$$L_1 = \hat{p} - z\sqrt{\frac{p(1-p)}{n}}$$

$$L_2 = \hat{p} + z\sqrt{\frac{p(1-p)}{n}}$$

However, there is a problem here that has not been encountered before. The bounds L_1 and L_2 must be *statistics*. Unfortunately, this is not the case. As written, L_1 and L_2 both involve the unknown parameter p. This means that we are attempting to use p to estimate p —a seemingly impossible situation! This problem can be overcome in a natural way. Namely, we can estimate $p(1-p)$ by replacing p by its estimator $\hat{p}$. Recall that when the true standard deviation is replaced by an estimator, the distribution changes from Z to T_{n-1}. We will not make this change here because in realistic settings sample sizes for estimating proportions are large. For large samples, t points are approximated by z points. Hence the confidence bounds for p are given by

$$L_1 = \hat{p} - z\sqrt{\frac{\hat{p}(1-\hat{p})}{n}}$$

$$L_2 = \hat{p} + z\sqrt{\frac{\hat{p}(1-\hat{p})}{n}}$$

Example 8.2.1 illustrates the use of this interval.

EXAMPLE 8.2.1. The adult screwworm fly is metallic blue and triple the size of a house-fly. The screwworm lays eggs in wounds of warm-blooded animals and causes severe infection. An experiment was conducted to learn how to control this population. Screwworm pupae were exposed to a radiation dose of 2500 rad in hopes of sterilizing most males. Since the females mate but once, mating with a sterilized male results in sterile eggs. It was found that after radiation, 415 of the 500 matings observed resulted in sterile eggs. The point estimate for the proportion of sterile matings produced by this dosage level is $\hat{p} = \frac{415}{500} = .83$. To construct a 95% confidence interval on p, consider the partition of the standard normal curve in Figure 8.3. A 95% confidence interval on p is given by

$$\hat{p} \pm z\sqrt{\frac{\hat{p}(1-\hat{p})}{n}} = .83 \pm 1.96\sqrt{\frac{.83(.17)}{500}}$$

$$= .83 \pm .03$$

Converting to percentages, we can be approximately 95% confident that the true percentage of sterile matings resulting from this level of radiation is between 80 and 86% inclusive.

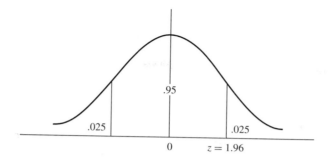

FIGURE 8.3

Partition of Z to obtain a 95% confidence interval on p.

EXERCISES 8.2

1. Use the data of Example 8.1.2 to find a 95% confidence interval on the proportion of males with the fragile X chromosome in institutions for the retarded. Would a 90% confidence interval on this proportion be longer or shorter than the interval just constructed?

2. Use the data of Exercise 2 of Section 8.1 to find a 99% confidence interval on the proportion of individuals 16 years old and under who smoke regularly. If you read an article that claimed that this proportion is .23, would you be surprised? Explain.

3. In running a white cell count, a drop of blood is smeared thinly and evenly on a glass slide, stained with Wright's stain, and examined under a microscope. Of 200 white cells counted, 125 were neutrophils, a white cell produced in the bone marrow whose function, in part, is to take up infective agents in the blood.
   (a) Find a point estimate for p, the proportion of neutrophils found among the white cells of this individual.
   (b) Find a 90% confidence interval on p.
   (c) In a normally healthy individual, the percentage of neutrophils among the white cells is 60 to 70%. Based on the interval obtained in part b, is there clear evidence of a neutrophil imbalance in this individual? Explain.

4. One defense that organisms have against predators is that of being obnoxious, that is, having a disagreeable taste, odor, or spray. One such insect is the walkingstick. Of 50 bluejays that had been sprayed by a walkingstick, 42 remained aloof from the insect for at least 2 weeks. Use this information to find a 94% confidence interval on p, the proportion of bluejays that will avoid further contact with the walkingstick for as long as 2 weeks.

5. In 1987 over 3 million acres were reforested with 2 billion seedlings. A severe drought during the next growing season killed many of these seedlings. A sample of 1000 seedlings is obtained, and it is discovered that 300 are dead. Find a 90% confidence interval on the proportion of dead seedlings. Use this information to estimate the number of dead seedlings in the population. (Based on information found in Howard Burnett, "A Report on Our Stressed-Out Forests," *American Forests,* April 1989, pp. 21–25.)

6. A study of chest pain in children is conducted. It is found that of 137 children who experienced chest pain, 100 have a normal X-ray. Find a 95% confidence interval on the proportion of children who experience chest pain that have a normal chest X-ray. (Based on information found in Steven Selbst, Richard Ruddy, and B. J. Clark, "Chest Pain in Children," *Clinical Pediatrics,* vol. 29, no. 7, July 1990, pp. 374–377.)

7. Consider the study of Exercise 6. Of 191 children with chest pain, 160 exhibit a normal electrocardiogram. Find a 95% confidence interval on the proportion of children with chest pain that will have a normal electrocardiogram.

8. Use the data of Exercise 3 of Section 8.1 to find a 95% confidence interval on the proportion of deaths due to myofibrillar degeneration in assault cases. Is *n* large enough to get a good idea of the value of *p* from this interval?

8.3
SAMPLE SIZE FOR ESTIMATING *p*

As in the past, the question of sample size should be addressed in the planning stages of an experiment. Example 8.3.1 illustrates the problem that can arise in an unplanned study.

> EXAMPLE 8.3.1. The newest development in the treatment of acne is a drug called *cis*-13-retinoic acid. A recent study tested this drug on 14 patients suffering from severe acne. Of the 14 patients tested, 13 showed dramatic clearing of their active lesions. To construct a 99% confidence interval on *p*, the proportion of patients on whom the drug will be effective, the partition of the standard normal curve shown in Figure 8.4 is needed. The confidence interval is given by
>
> $$\hat{p} \pm z\sqrt{\frac{\hat{p}(1-\hat{p})}{n}}$$
>
> where $\hat{p} = \frac{13}{14} = .93$. In this case the confidence bounds are $.93 \pm 2.575\sqrt{.93(.07)/14}$ or $.93 \pm .18$. The lower boundary of this interval is .75; the upper boundary is 1.11. Notice that the proportion of objects in a population cannot exceed 1, or 100%. Thus we take the upper boundary of the interval to be 1.00. We can be 99% confident that the drug will be effective on 75 to 100% of those patients on whom it is used.

There is a point to be made from Example 8.3.1. It is obvious that the interval obtained is not very informative. It is much too long to give the experimenter any clear

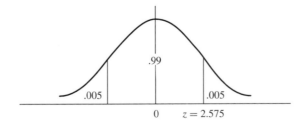

FIGURE 8.4

Partition of Z to obtain a 99% confidence interval on *p*.

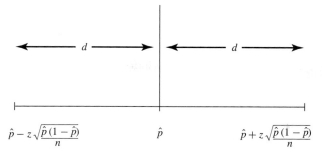

FIGURE 8.5
Confidence interval on p.

indication of the actual value of p. The problem is caused by two factors: the degree of confidence required is very high (99%), and the sample size is too small. Thus we can correct the problem by reducing the level of confidence or increasing the sample size or doing both.

This brings up one other important question. How large a sample should be selected so that $\hat{p}$ lies within a specified distance d of p with a stated degree of confidence? There are two ways to answer this question. The first is applicable when an estimate of p based on some prior experiment is available. This method is illustrated schematically in Figure 8.5.

Since p is expected to lie in the confidence interval, $\hat{p}$ and p should differ from one another by at most d where d is given by

$$d = z\sqrt{\frac{\hat{p}(1 - \hat{p})}{n}}$$

This equation is solved for n as follows:

$$d = z\sqrt{\frac{\hat{p}(1 - \hat{p})}{n}}$$

$$d^2 = z^2\frac{\hat{p}(1 - \hat{p})}{n}$$

$$n = \frac{z^2\hat{p}(1 - \hat{p})}{d^2}$$

Thus we obtain the following formula for finding the sample size needed to estimate p with a stated degree of accuracy and confidence when a prior estimate of p is available:

$$n \doteq \frac{z^2\hat{p}(1 - \hat{p})}{d^2} \quad \text{(prior estimate available)}$$

The use of this formula is illustrated in Example 8.3.2.

EXAMPLE 8.3.2. If we wish to further test the acne-combating drug of Example 8.3.1, how large a sample should we use to estimate p to within $d = .02$ with 90% confidence?

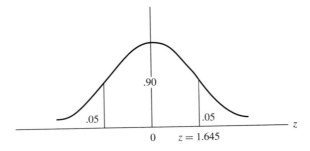

FIGURE 8.6

Point required to obtain a 90% confidence interval on p.

Since a prior estimate $\hat{p} = .93$ is available, the above formula is applicable. The point z called for in the formula is the same point required to construct a 90% confidence interval on p. This point is shown in Figure 8.6. Thus the sample size required is

$$n = \frac{z^2 \hat{p}(1 - \hat{p})}{d^2} = \frac{(1.645)^2(.93)(.07)}{(.02)^2}$$

$$\doteq 441$$

The second method for determining sample size for estimating proportions is based on the fact that the term $\hat{p}(1 - \hat{p})$ can never exceed $\frac{1}{4}$ regardless of the value of $\hat{p}$. This fact can be verified using techniques of calculus. Its proof is outlined in Exercise 7. If no prior estimate of p is available, an appropriate sample size can be found by substituting $\frac{1}{4}$ for $\hat{p}(1 - \hat{p})$ in the previous equation. Thus the formula for finding the sample size required to estimate p with a stated degree of accuracy and confidence when *no* prior estimate of p is available is

$$\boxed{n \doteq \frac{z^2}{4d^2} \quad \text{(no prior estimate available)}}$$

The use of this formula is illustrated in Example 8.3.3.

EXAMPLE 8.3.3. Normal red blood cells in humans are shaped like biconcave disks. Occasionally hemoglobin, a protein that readily combines with oxygen, is imperfectly formed in the cell. One type of imperfect hemoglobin causes the cells to have a caved-in, or "sicklelike," appearance. These "sickle" cells are less efficient carriers of oxygen than normal cells and result in an oxygen deficiency called sickle-cell anemia. This condition has a significant prevalence among blacks. A study is to be run to estimate the percentage of blacks in Virginia with this condition. How large a sample should be chosen to estimate this percentage to within 1 percentage point with 98% confidence? No prior estimate of p is assumed available. The z point required is shown in Figure 8.7. Since 1 percentage point is .01, the desired sample size is

$$n \doteq \frac{z^2}{4d^2} = \frac{(2.33)^2}{4(.01)^2} = 13,573$$

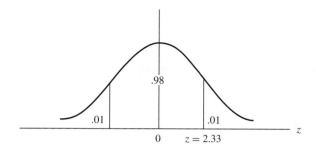

FIGURE 8.7
Point required to obtain a 98% confidence interval on p.

EXERCISES 8.3

1. When the study of Example 8.3.3 was conducted, of the 13,573 blacks sampled, 1085 were found to have sickle-cell anemia. Use this information to find a 98% confidence interval on the percentage of blacks in the state who have the disease.

2. How large a sample would be required to estimate the proportion of deaths due to myofibrillar degeneration in assault cases to within .02 with 95% confidence? (Use the data of Exercise 3 of Section 8.1 to obtain a prior estimate of p.)

3. One problem associated with the use of the supersonic transport (SST) is the sonic boom. In the late 1960s and early 1970s, preliminary tests were run over Oklahoma City, St. Louis, and other areas. After the tests were run, a survey was to be conducted to estimate the percentage of people who felt that they could not live with the sonic booms. How large a sample should have been chosen to estimate the percentage to within 3 percentage points with 94% confidence?

4. The Environmental Protection Agency recently identified 30,000 waste dumping sites in the United States that were considered to be at least potentially dangerous. How large a sample is needed to estimate the percentage of these sites that do pose a serious threat to health to within 2 percentage points with 90% confidence?

5. How large a sample is needed to estimate the proportion of bluejays that will avoid further contact with a walkingstick for as long as 2 weeks to within 3 percentage points with 94% confidence? (*Hint:* Use the data of Exercise 4 of Section 8.2 to obtain an estimate of p.)

6. How many patients must be sampled in order to estimate the proportion of children with chest pain that had a normal chest X-ray to within 4 percentage points with 99% confidence? (*Hint:* Use the data of Exercise 6 of Section 8.2 as a pilot study.)

7. It has been claimed that $p(1 - p) \leq \frac{1}{4}$. Consider the function $g(p) = p(1 - p)$.
   (*a*) Find the derivative of g.
   (*b*) Maximize $g(p)$ by setting $g'(p)$ to 0 and solving for p.
   (*c*) Use the second derivative test to verify that $p = \frac{1}{2}$ in fact maximizes $g(p)$.

◼ 8.4

HYPOTHESIS TESTING ON p

We consider now the problem of testing a hypothesis on a proportion p. This implies that a value for p has been proposed prior to conducting the study. The purpose of the experiment is to gather statistical evidence that either supports or refutes this value. The hypotheses tested can assume any one of the usual three forms, depending on the purpose of the study. Let p_0 denote the hypothesized value of p. Then these forms are as follows:

I H_0: $p \leq p_0$	II H_0: $p \geq p_0$	III H_0: $p = p_0$
H_1: $p > p_0$	H_1: $p < p_0$	H_1: $p \neq p_0$
Right-tailed test	Left-tailed test	Two-tailed test

EXAMPLE 8.4.1. One theory of learning that has caused a great deal of controversy is that of "transfer of training by cannibalism." In one study to gain statistical support for this theory, a group of planarians was trained to avoid electric shock. Then they were ground up and fed to a group of 100 untrained planarians. If no training is transferred to the untrained planarians by this cannibalism, then the probability that an untrained planarian can avoid the shock is assumed to be $\frac{1}{2}$; otherwise, this probability is greater than $\frac{1}{2}$. Since the purpose of the study is to gain suport for the theory, the statement that $p > \frac{1}{2}$ becomes the alternative hypothesis. So we are testing

$$H_0: p \leq \frac{1}{2}$$

$$H_1: p > \frac{1}{2}$$

EXAMPLE 8.4.2. Until recently, p, the death rate from a highly fatal viral infection of the brain, herpes simplex virus encephalitis, has been 70%. A study is run to test the new drug vidarabine for use in treating this disease. Since it is hoped that vidarabine will reduce the death rate, this statement becomes the alternative hypothesis. That is, we are testing

$$H_0: p \geq .70$$

$$H_1: p < .70$$

To test a hypothesis on p, a test statistic must be developed. The statistic should be logical. Furthermore, to find the P value of the test, its probability distribution must be known at least approximately under the assumption that the null hypothesis is true. Again, the test statistic chosen is the same as the random variable used to generate the confidence bounds for p. In particular,

$$\frac{\hat{p} - p_0}{\sqrt{p_0(1 - p_0)/n}}$$

will serve as the test statistic. This statistic is logical in that basically it compares the estimated value of p, namely $\hat{p} = X/n$, with the hypothesized value of p, namely p_0.

If these are close in value, indicating that H_0 is true, then the observed value of the statistic will be close to zero. If $\hat{p}$ and p_0 differ greatly, indicating that H_0 is false, then the observed value of the test statistic will be either a very large positive value or a very large negative value. For large sample sizes, the test statistic is approximately standard normal.

EXAMPLE 8.4.3. The theory of learning by cannibalism is to be confirmed by testing

$$H_0: p \le .5$$

$$H_1: p > .5 \quad \text{(cannibalism increases the probability of avoiding shock)}$$

When the experiment described in Example 8.4.1 was conducted, 57 of the 100 planarians tested did avoid the shock. The observed value of the test statistic is

$$\frac{x/n - p_0}{\sqrt{p_0(1 - p_0)/n}} = \frac{\frac{57}{100} - .5}{\sqrt{.5(.5)/100}} = 1.4$$

Since the test is right-tailed, the P value is given by

$$P = P[Z \ge 1.4]$$

This P value is pictured in Figure 8.8. Its value can be found from the Z table, Table III of Appendix B. In this case,

$$P = P[Z \ge 1.4] = 1 - P[Z \le 1.4]$$

$$= 1 - .9192$$

$$= .0808$$

The method for testing hypotheses on p illustrated here does assume that sample sizes are large enough so that the Central Limit Theorem is applicable. (See Theorem 6.2.2.) As indicated in Section 6.2, samples as small as 25 usually are safe. Remember that power is affected by sample size. It is usually difficult to detect small but perhaps important differences between p and p_0 with small samples. However, there are times, especially in medical settings, when samples by necessity are small. For example, in studying a rare condition, there might be only 8 or 10 known cases. The researcher must do the best he or she can with the available resources. A test based on the binomial distribution that is appropriate with small samples is given in Chapter 13.

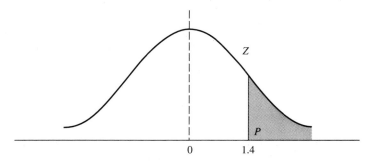

FIGURE 8.8

P value for the right-tailed test of Example 8.4.3. $P = P[Z \ge 1.4] = .0808$.

■ EXERCISES 8.4

1. Opponents of the construction of a dam on the New River claim that a majority of residents living along the river also are opposed to its construction. A survey is conducted to gain support for this point of view.
   (a) Set up the appropriate null and alternative hypotheses.
   (b) Of 500 people surveyed, 270 opposed the construction. Is this sufficient evidence to claim that a majority of residents are opposed? Explain your answer based on the P value of the test. To what type of error are you subject now? Discuss the practical consequences of making such an error.

2. A new type of Japanese beetle trap is being tested. The manufacturer claims that the trap attracts and kills more than 90% of the beetles that come within 30 feet of the trap. An experiment is conducted to gain evidence to support this claim.
   (a) Set up the appropriate null and alternative hypotheses.
   (b) The experiment is conducted by releasing 900 beetles near the trap. If H_0 is true, what is the maximum number that you would expect to see attracted to the trap? Of the 900, in fact, 825 were attracted to the trap and killed. Is this sufficient evidence to support the claim? Explain based on the P value of the test.
   (c) To what type of error are you now subject? Discuss the practical consequences of making such an error.

3. Consider Example 8.4.2. Of 50 subjects on whom vidarabine was tested, 14 died. Find the P value for this test.

4. Among patients with lung cancer, usually 90% or more die within 3 years. As a result of new forms of treatment, it is felt that this rate has been reduced.
   (a) Set up the null and alternative hypotheses needed to support this contention.
   (b) In a recent study of 150 patients diagnosed with lung cancer, 128 died within 3 years. Can H_0 be rejected at the $\alpha = .1$ level? At the $\alpha = .05$ level? Do you think that there is sufficient evidence to claim that the new methods of treatment are more effective than the old? Explain.

5. The current method for treating acute myeloblastic leukemia is to give the patient intensive chemotherapy at the time of diagnosis. Historically this has resulted in a 70% remission rate. In studying a new method of treatment, 50 volunteers are used. How many of the patients would have to go into remission for researchers to claim at the $\alpha = .025$ level that the new method produced a higher remission rate than the old?

6. The severe drought of 1987 affected both the death rate of seedlings and the growth rate of established trees. It is thought that a majority of the trees in the affected areas have a 1987 growth ring that is less than $\frac{1}{2}$ the size of the trees' other growth rings. A sample of 250 trees yields 150 with this characteristic. Do these data support the claim? Explain. (Based on information found in Howard Burnett, "A Report on Our Stressed-Out Forests," *American Forests,* April 1989, pp. 21–25.)

7. It is thought that more than 85% of all children who experience chest pain will nevertheless have a normal echocardiogram. A sample of 139 of these children yields 123 with normal echocardiograms.
   (a) State the research hypothesis.
   (b) Find a point estimate for the proportion of children with chest pain who exhibit normal echocardiograms. Based on this estimate do you think that the research claim will be substantiated upon testing?

(*c*) Test H$_0$: $p \leq .85$ versus H$_1$: $p > .85$. Can H$_0$ be rejected at the $\alpha = .10$ level?

(*d*) Explain any apparent contradiction between the results of parts *b* and *c*.

(Based on information found in Steven Selbst, Richard Ruddy, and B. J. Clark, "Chest Pain in Children," *Clinical Pediatrics,* vol. 29, no. 7, July 1990, pp. 374–377.)

8. *Power.* Suppose that we want to test

$$H_0: p = .5$$

$$H_1: p = .6$$

We agree to reject H$_0$ if the observed value of the Z test statistic exceeds 1.96. Since $P[Z > 1.96] = .025$, we are presetting α at .025. Recall that power is given by

$$\text{Power} = P[\text{reject } H_0 \,|\, H_1 \text{ is true}]$$

In this case,

$$\text{Power} = P[Z > 1.96 \,|\, p = .6]$$

For example, suppose that $n = 20$. What is the power of the test? In this case

$$\text{Power} = P\left[\frac{\hat{p} - .5}{\sqrt{.5(.5)/20}} > 1.96 \,\Big|\, p = .6 \right]$$

We first isolate $\hat{p}$ as follows:

$$\text{Power} = P\left[\hat{p} - .5 > 1.96\sqrt{\frac{.5(.5)}{20}} \,\Big|\, p = .6 \right]$$

$$= P\left[\hat{p} > .5 + 1.96\sqrt{\frac{.5(.5)}{20}} \,\Big|\, p = .6. \right]$$

$$= P[\hat{p} > .72 \,|\, p = .6]$$

If $p = .6$, we can standardize $\hat{p}$ by subtracting its mean of .6 and dividing by its standard deviation, $\sqrt{.6(.4)/20}$. We see that

$$\text{Power} = P\left[\frac{\hat{p} - .6}{\sqrt{.6(.4)/20}} > \frac{.72 - .6}{\sqrt{.6(.4)/20}} \,\Big|\, p = .6. \right]$$

If $p = .6$, the random variable on the left of this inequality follows a standard normal distribution. Hence,

$$\text{Power} = P[Z > 1.09] = 1 - P[Z \leq 1.09]$$

$$= 1 - .8621$$

$$= .1379$$

Notice that a sample of size 20 gives very little chance of detecting the difference between the proportions .5 and .6. To see the effect of sample size on power, find the power of the above test for each of the samples of parts *a* to *c*.

(*a*) $n = 50$

(*b*) $n = 200$

(*c*) $n = 1000$

(*d*) If we changed the test so that $\alpha = .1$, would you expect the power to go up, down, or remain the same? Explain.

▪ 8.5
COMPARING TWO PROPORTIONS: ESTIMATION

The problem of comparing two proportions arises frequently in biological and medical studies. The general situation can be described as follows: There are two populations of interest; the same trait is studied in each population; each member of each population can be classified as either having the trait or failing to have it; and in each population the proportion having the trait is unknown. Inferences are to be made on p_1, p_2, and $p_1 - p_2$, where p_1 and p_2 are the proportions in the first and second populations with the trait, respectively. (See Figure 8.9.)

> **EXAMPLE 8.5.1.** Annually, kidney failure claims the lives of many people. A study is conducted among kidney patients to compare the rate of kidney failure among those treated with the steroid drug prednisone to the rate among those who received a placebo. Here the two populations of interest are kidney patients treated with the drug and those not receiving it. The trait under study in each case is that of suffering kidney failure. (See Figure 8.10.)

The problem of point estimation of the difference between two proportions is solved in the obvious way. We simply estimate p_1 and p_2 individually and then take as our estimate for $p_1 - p_2$ the difference between the two. That is,

$$\widehat{p_1 - p_2} = \hat{p}_1 - \hat{p}_2 = \frac{X_1}{n_1} - \frac{X_2}{n_2}$$

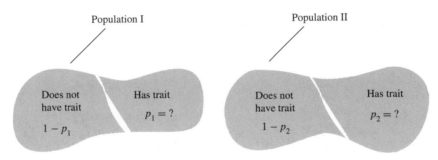

FIGURE 8.9

Comparing two proportions. What is the difference between p_1 and p_2?

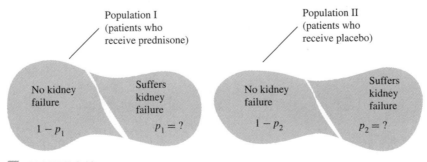

FIGURE 8.10

$p_1 - p_2 = ?$

where n_1 and n_2 are the sizes of the samples drawn from the two populations and X_1 and X_2 are the number of objects, respectively, in the samples with the trait.

EXAMPLE 8.5.2. In studying the use of prednisone in the treatment of kidney patients, 72 subjects at 19 hospitals were used. Among the 34 patients treated with prednisone, only one person developed kidney failure. However, of the 38 who received a placebo, kidney failure developed in 10. Based on this study, $\hat{p}_1 = \frac{1}{34} \doteq .03$ and $\hat{p}_2 = \frac{10}{38} \doteq .26$. The estimated difference between the two population proportions is

$$\widehat{p_1 - p_2} = \hat{p}_1 - \hat{p}_2 = .03 - .26 = -.23$$

Confidence Interval on the Difference in Two Proportions

To extend the point estimator $\hat{p}_1 - \hat{p}_2$ to an interval estimator, we must pause to consider the probability distribution of this random variable. Its approximate distribution is given in Theorem 8.5.1. This theorem can be proved partially using the rules for expected value and variance given in Appendix A. The proof is outlined in Exercise 12 at the end of this section.

THEOREM 8.5.1. For large sample sizes, the estimator $\hat{p}_1 - \hat{p}_2$ is approximately normal with mean $p_1 - p_2$ and variance

$$\frac{p_1(1 - p_1)}{n_1} + \frac{p_2(1 - p_2)}{n_2}$$

To construct a confidence interval on $p_1 - p_2$, we must find a random variable whose expression involves this parameter and whose probability distribution is known at least approximately. This is done easily now. We simply standardize the random variable $\hat{p}_1 - \hat{p}_2$ to conclude that the random variable

$$\frac{(\hat{p}_1 - \hat{p}_2) - (p_1 - p_2)}{\sqrt{p_1(1 - p_1)/n_1 + p_2(1 - p_2)/n_2}}$$

is approximately *standard* normal. Rather than repeat an algebraic argument given previously, let us consider three intervals that have been derived already and note their similarities:

Parameter being estimated	Began derivation with	Distribution	Bounds
μ (σ^2 known)	$\dfrac{\bar{X} - \mu}{\sigma/\sqrt{n}}$	Z	$\bar{X} \pm z\dfrac{\sigma}{\sqrt{n}}$
μ (σ^2 unknown)	$\dfrac{\bar{X} - \mu}{S/\sqrt{n}}$	T	$\bar{X} \pm t\dfrac{S}{\sqrt{n}}$
p	$\dfrac{\hat{p} - p}{\sqrt{p(1 - p)/n}}$	$\sim Z$ (approximately Z)	$\hat{p} \pm z\sqrt{\dfrac{p(1 - p)}{n}}$

The algebraic structure of each of the beginning variables is the same and is of the form

$$\frac{\text{Estimator} - \text{parameter}}{D}$$

where D is the standard deviation or the estimator for the standard deviation of the estimator in the numerator. This is also the algebraic form assumed by the variable

$$\frac{(\hat{p}_1 - \hat{p}_2) - (p_1 - p_2)}{\sqrt{p_1(1 - p_1)/n_1 + p_2(1 - p_2)/n_2}} \sim Z$$

The confidence bounds in the previous cases took the form

$$\text{Estimator} \pm \text{probability point} \times D$$

Applying this notion to the above random variable, we find the proposed confidence bounds for a confidence interval on $p_1 - p_2$ to be

$$(\hat{p}_1 - \hat{p}_2) \pm z\sqrt{\frac{p_1(1 - p_1)}{n_1} + \frac{p_2(1 - p_2)}{n_2}}$$

Once again, there is a slight problem. The proposed bounds are not *statistics*. They include the unknown population proportions p_1 and p_2. As in the one-sample case, this problem can be overcome by replacing the population proportions with their estimators $\hat{p}_1$ and $\hat{p}_1$. The following formula is obtained for finding confidence intervals on the difference between two population proportions:

$$\boxed{(\hat{p}_1 - \hat{p}_2) \pm z\sqrt{\frac{\hat{p}_1(1 - \hat{p}_1)}{n_1} + \frac{\hat{p}_2(1 - \hat{p}_2)}{n_2}}}$$

This formula is illustrated in Example 8.5.3.

EXAMPLE 8.5.3. To construct a 95% confidence interval on the difference in the rate of kidney failure between those receiving prednisone and those not receiving the drug, the partition of the standard normal curve shown in Figure 8.3 is needed. From Example 8.5.2, $n_1 = 34$, $n_2 = 38$, $\hat{p}_1 = .03$, $\hat{p}_2 = .26$, and $\hat{p}_1 - \hat{p}_2 = -.23$. The desired confidence bounds are

$$(\hat{p}_1 - \hat{p}_2) \pm z\sqrt{\frac{\hat{p}_1(1 - \hat{p}_1)}{n_1} + \frac{\hat{p}_2(1 - \hat{p}_2)}{n_2}} = -.23 \pm 1.96\sqrt{\frac{.03(.97)}{34} + \frac{.26(.74)}{38}}$$

$$= -.23 \pm .15$$

We can be 95% confident that the difference in failure rates is between -38% and -8%. Note that zero is not in this interval. This is important since we can interpret this to mean that we are 95% confident that the two rates are, in fact, different. Since both bounds are negative, we can further infer that the failure rate for those on the drug is smaller than that for those not on the drug by at least 8%.

■ **EXERCISES 8.5**

1. The drug Anturane, marketed since 1959 for the treatment of gout, is being studied for use in preventing sudden deaths from a second heart attack among patients who have already suffered a first attack. In the study, 733 patients received Anturane and 742 were given a placebo. After 8 months it was found that of 42

deaths from a second heart attack, 29 had occurred in the placebo group and 13 in the Anturane group. Use these data to estimate the difference in the percentage of sudden deaths among Anturane users and among patients not receiving the drug.

2. An antibiotic called doxycycline is being tested for use in preventing "traveler's diarrhea." The drug was tested on 38 Peace Corps volunteers who were going to Kenya. Half were given doxycycline, and half were given a dummy dose. Of those on doxycycline, 17 were protected from the disorder while only 11 from the other group were protected. Find a point estimate on the difference in the protection rates among those using doxycycline and those not using it.

3. One of the best studied examples of natural selection is that of the peppered moth. Until 1845 all reported species had been light in color, but in that year a black moth was captured at Manchester. Because of industrialization in the area, the trunks of trees, rocks, and even the ground in the region had become blackened by soot. This mutant black form quickly spread. H. B. D. Kettlewell felt that the spread was due in part to the fact that the black color protected the moth from natural predators, in particular birds. Entomologists at the time claimed that they had never seen a bird eat a peppered moth of any color and discounted his idea. In an experiment to study the theory, Kettlewell marked a sample of 100 moths of each color and then released them. He returned at night with light traps and recovered 40% of the black moths but only 19% of the light-colored ones. Assume that the moths not recovered had fallen prey to a predator. Find a point estimate for the difference in the survival rates.

4. Construct a 95% confidence interval on the difference in the percentage of sudden deaths among Anturane users and among patients not on the drug, based on the data of Exercise 1. If a 90% confidence interval were constructed based on the same data, which interval would be longer? Why? Verify your answer. Have you gained evidence to support the statement that the death rate from second attacks is lower among patients on the drug than among patients not on the drug? Explain.

5. Using the data of Exercise 2, construct a 90% confidence interval on the difference in protection rates among those using doxycycline and those not on the drug. Have you gained evidence to support the theory that doxycycline tends to give protection against "traveler's diarrhea"? Explain.

6. Use the data of Exercise 3 to construct a 98% confidence interval on the difference in survival rates among black moths and light-colored moths in the Manchester region. Does the interval lend support to the statement that the black color tends to protect these moths from predators? Explain.

7. A study is conducted of survival rates of adult birds in the tropics and in the temperate zone. Initially 500 adult birds were tagged with leg bands and released in Panama, a tropical region. A year later, 445 were recaptured. If we assume that those not recovered had fallen victim to a predator, the estimated 1-year survival rate for adult birds in the region is $\hat{p}_1 = \frac{445}{500} = .89$. A similar experiment in Illinois, in the temperate zone, resulted in recovery of 252 of the 500 birds for an estimated survival rate of approximately .504. Find a 90% confidence interval on the difference in the 1-year survival rates for the two regions.

8. Use an argument similar to that given in Section 8.3 to show that the common sample size $n = n_1 = n_2$ needed to estimate the difference in proportions to within d

with a stated degree of confidence is given by

$$
n = \begin{cases} \dfrac{z^2[\hat{p}_1(1 - \hat{p}_1) + \hat{p}_2(1 - \hat{p}_2)]}{d^2} & \text{if prior estimates for } p_1 \text{ and } p_2 \text{ are available} \\[2ex] \dfrac{z^2}{2d^2} & \text{if no prior estimates are available} \end{cases}
$$

9. Use the data of Exercise 1 as a pilot study to determine the common sample size required to estimate the difference in the percentage of sudden deaths among Anturane users and among patients not on the drug to within 2 percentage points with 95% confidence. Now do the same but with 90% confidence.

10. Use the data of Exercise 3 as a pilot study to determine the common sample size needed to estimate the difference in survival rates between the two groups of moths to within 3 percentage points with 98% confidence.

11. A study is to be conducted to compare the percentage of intravenous drug users among persons who are HIV positive (at risk of developing AIDS) to the percentage of intravenous drug users among persons who are HIV negative. What common sample size should be chosen to estimate the difference in percentages to within 2 percentage points with 95% confidence? Compare this answer to that obtained in Exercise 9. Is there a practical advantage to having prior estimates of p_1 and p_2 available?

12. It can be shown that the sum or difference of two independent normally distributed random variables is also normally distributed. Since $\hat{p}_1$ and $\hat{p}_2$ are based on random samples independently drawn from separate populations, these approximately normally distributed random variables are independent. Their difference is also normally distributed by the above result.

   (a) Find $E[\hat{p}_1 - \hat{p}_2]$

   (b) Use the rules for variance to find $\text{Var}[\hat{p}_1 - \hat{p}_2]$.

▇ 8.6

COMPARING TWO PROPORTIONS: HYPOTHESIS TESTING

Frequently problems arise in which it is theorized prior to the experiment that one proportion or percentage differs from another by a specified amount. The purpose of the experiment is to gain statistical support for the contention. These hypotheses take any one of the following three forms, where $(p_1 - p_2)_0$ represents the hypothesized value of the difference in proportions:

$$
\begin{array}{ll}
\text{I} \quad H_0: p_1 - p_2 \leq (p_1 - p_2)_0 & \text{II} \quad H_0: p_1 - p_2 \geq (p_1 - p_2)_0 \\
\phantom{\text{I} \quad} H_1: p_1 - p_2 > (p_1 - p_2)_0 & \phantom{\text{II} \quad} H_1: p_1 - p_2 < (p_1 - p_2)_0 \\
\phantom{\text{I} \quad} \text{Right-tailed test} & \phantom{\text{II} \quad} \text{Left-tailed test}
\end{array}
$$

$$
\begin{array}{l}
\text{III} \quad H_0: p_1 - p_2 = (p_1 - p_2)_0 \\
\phantom{\text{III} \quad} H_1: p_1 - p_2 \neq (p_1 - p_2)_0 \\
\phantom{\text{III} \quad} \text{Two-tailed test}
\end{array}
$$

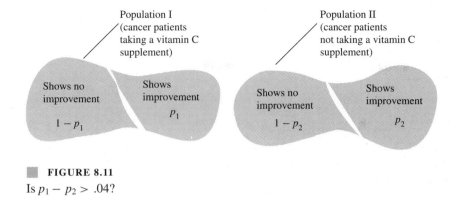

FIGURE 8.11

Is $p_1 - p_2 > .04$?

For instance, consider Example 8.6.1.

EXAMPLE 8.6.1. Proponents of vitamin C claim that it will improve the chances of survival in cancer patients. Further, it is felt that the percentage of patients showing improvement among those who take a vitamin C supplement exceeds that of those who do not take a supplement by more than 4 percentage points. The situation is pictured in Figure 8.11. From the point of view of the proponents of vitamin C, we are testing

$$H_0: p_1 - p_2 \leq .04 \qquad H_1: p_1 - p_2 > .04$$

To test such hypotheses, a test statistic must be found that is logical and whose probability distribution is known at least approximately under the assumption that the null hypothesis is true. To derive such a statistic, consider the random variable

$$\frac{(\hat{p}_1 - \hat{p}_2) - (p_1 - p_2)_0}{\sqrt{p_1(1 - p_1)/n_1 + p_2(1 - p_2)/n_2}}$$

This is the same random variable as that used in Section 8.5 to construct confidence intervals on $p_1 - p_2$. If the null hypothesis is true, then this random variable is approximately standard normal. However, there is one problem. A test statistic must be a statistic! The random variable above is *not* a statistic, for it contains the unknown population proportions p_1 and p_2. The logical way to overcome this problem is to replace p_1 and p_2 with their estimators $\hat{p}_1$ and $\hat{p}_2$, to obtain the approximately standard normal *statistic:*

$$\boxed{\frac{(\hat{p}_1 - \hat{p}_2) - (p_1 - p_2)_0}{\sqrt{\hat{p}_1(1 - \hat{p}_1)/n_1 + \hat{p}_2(1 - \hat{p}_2)/n_2}}}$$

This is a logical choice for a test statistic since it compares the estimated difference in proportions $\hat{p}_1 - \hat{p}_2$ with the hypothesized difference $(p_1 - p_2)_0$. If the hypothesized value is correct, then the estimated difference and the hypothesized difference should be close in value. This forces the numerator above to be close to zero and thus yields a small value for the test statistic. Large positive or large negative values of the test statistic indicate that the null hypothesis is not true and should be rejected in favor of an appropriate alternative.

The use of this statistic is illustrated in Example 8.6.2.

EXAMPLE 8.6.2. A group of 150 patients is used to test the theory that vitamin C is an aid in the treatment of cancer. The hypothesis being tested is

$$H_0: p_1 - p_2 \leq .04$$

$$H_1: p_1 - p_2 > .04$$

Since the inequality in the alternative points to the right, the test is a right-tailed test based on the standard normal distribution.

The 150 patients were divided into two groups of 75. One group received 10 grams of vitamin C per day; the other received a placebo every day. Of those receiving vitamin C, 47 showed some improvement within 4 weeks; of those on the placebo, only 43 showed any improvement. Based on these data, $\hat{p}_1 = \frac{47}{75} \doteq .63$ and $\hat{p}_2 = \frac{43}{75} \doteq .57$. The observed value of the test statistic is

$$\frac{(\hat{p}_1 - \hat{p}_2) - (p_1 - p_2)_0}{\sqrt{\hat{p}_1(1 - \hat{p}_1)/n_1 + \hat{p}_2(1 - \hat{p}_2)/n_2}} = \frac{(.63 - .57) - .04}{\sqrt{(.63)(.37)/75 + (.57)(.43)/75}}$$

$$= .25$$

Since the test is right-tailed,

$$P = P[Z \geq .25] = 1 - P[Z \leq .25]$$

$$= 1 - .5987$$

$$= .4013$$

Since this probability is large, we cannot reject H_0. Practically speaking, this means that there is not sufficient evidence in this study to support the contention that vitamin C helps in treating cancer to the extent claimed.

Testing That the Null Value Is Zero: Pooled Test

Although the hypothesized difference $(p_1 - p_2)_0$ can be any value at all, the most commonly encountered proposed value is zero. In this case, in effect, the hypotheses considered previously compare p_1 with p_2 and take the following form:

I $H_0: p_1 \leq p_2$	II $H_0: p_1 \geq p_2$	III $H_0: p_1 = p_2$
$H_1: p_1 > p_2$	$H_1: p_1 < p_2$	$H_1: p_1 \neq p_2$
Right-tailed test	Left-tailed test	Two-tailed test

Hypotheses of this sort can be tested via the previously developed test statistic with $p_1 - p_2$ set equal to zero. However, an alternative procedure is available. This procedure makes use of the fact that if H_0 is true and $p_1 = p_2$, then $\hat{p}_1$ and $\hat{p}_2$ are both estimators for the same proportion, which we denote by p. We want to combine, or "pool," $\hat{p}_1$ and $\hat{p}_2$ to form an estimator for p. We can simply average $\hat{p}_1$ and $\hat{p}_2$, but in so doing we ignore whatever differences might exist between the two sample sizes involved. To take these differences into account we form an estimator that gives more importance to the sample proportion obtained from the larger sample. That is, we form a "weighted" proportion using sample sizes as weights. Thus, we estimate the common population proportion p by the pooled estimator $\hat{p}$ where $\hat{p}$ is given by

$$\hat{p} = \frac{n_1 \hat{p}_1 + n_2 \hat{p}_2}{n_1 + n_2}$$

Note that $\hat{p}$ is just the total number of objects with the trait of interest in the two samples combined divided by the combined sample sizes.

If we now replace p_1 and p_2 by $\hat{p}$ in the formula given previously we obtain the following test statistic for testing H_0: $p_1 - p_2 = 0$:

$$\frac{(\hat{p}_1 - \hat{p}_2) - 0}{\sqrt{\hat{p}(1-\hat{p})/n_1 + \hat{p}(1-\hat{p})/n_2}}$$

This simplifies to

$$\frac{\hat{p}_1 - \hat{p}_2}{\sqrt{\hat{p}(1-\hat{p})\left(\dfrac{1}{n_1} + \dfrac{1}{n_2}\right)}}$$

EXAMPLE 8.6.3. An important enemy of the snail (*Cepaea nemoralis*) is the song thrush. These birds select snails from snail colonies and take them to nearby rocks. There the birds break open the snails, eat the soft parts, and leave the shells. In a study of natural selection, the proportion of unbanded shells in the rocks was compared to the proportion of unbanded snails in the nearby colony, a bog near Oxford, England. The background in the bog was fairly uniform. It was felt that, because of their ability to blend into the background, the unbanded snails would be better protected from predators than the banded members of the colony. This would result in the proportion of unbanded shells in the rocks being smaller than that of unbanded snails in the colony. The situation is pictured in Figure 8.12.

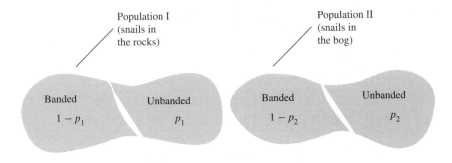

FIGURE 8.12

Is $p_1 < p_2$?

By taking the theory to be supported as the alternative hypothesis, the purpose of the study is to test

$$H_0: p_1 \geq p_2$$

$$H_1: p_1 < p_2 \quad \text{(unbanded snails are protected in bog)}$$

Of 863 broken shells around the rocks, 377 were unbanded. This yields a point estimate for p_1 of $\hat{p}_1 \doteq \frac{377}{863} = .44$. Of 560 individuals collected in the bog, 296 were unbanded, which gives a point estimate for p_2 of $\hat{p}_2 = \frac{296}{560} \doteq .53$.

The pooled estimate for p is

$$\hat{p} = \frac{863(.44) + 560(.53)}{863 + 560} \doteq .47$$

Note that $\hat{p}$ is also given by

$$\hat{p} = \frac{377 + 296}{863 + 560} = \frac{673}{1423} \doteq .47$$

as expected. Thus the observed value of the test statistic is

$$\frac{(\hat{p}_1 - \hat{p}_2)}{\sqrt{\hat{p}(1-\hat{p})\left(\dfrac{1}{n_1} + \dfrac{1}{n_2}\right)}} = \frac{(.44 - .53)}{\sqrt{.47(1-.47)\left(\dfrac{1}{863} + \dfrac{1}{560}\right)}}$$

$$= \frac{-.09}{.0271}$$

$$= -3.321$$

The fact that this value is negative is not surprising. The test is a left-tailed test that calls for the rejection of H_0 for large negative values of the test statistic. Is -3.321 "large"? To answer this question, note from Table III in Appendix B that $P[Z \leq -3.321] = .0005$. Thus the P value for the test is .0005. There are two possible explanations for this small P value:

1. The unbanded snails are not really protected by their coloration. We simply *by chance* observed an event that occurs only about 5 times in every 10,000 trials.
2. The unbanded snails are protected in the bog by their ability to blend into the uniform background.

We prefer the latter explanation!

There is one further point to make: While p_1 and p_2 have been referred to as proportions, and on occasion they have been converted to percentages, they also can be thought of as being probabilities. This is true because they are always numbers between 0 and 1 that, in effect, represent the probability of selecting on a random draw an object from the population having the trait under study.

▄ EXERCISES 8.6

1. Consider the results of Example 8.6.2. To what type of error is the experimenter subject? Discuss the practical consequences of making such an error. Is it correct to contend that it has been shown that vitamin C does not help in treating cancer to the extent claimed? Explain.

2. A study of color in tiger beetles is conducted to gain evidence to support the contention that the proportion of black beetles may vary from locality to locality. A sample of 500 beetles caught in one season near Providence, Rhode Island, yielded 95 black ones. A catch of 112 beetles from Aqueduct, New York, contained 17 black individuals.

   (a) Set up the appropriate two-tailed hypothesis.

   (b) Find a point estimate for the difference between the proportions of black beetles in the two regions. Do you think, based on this estimate, that there is a difference in the two proportions?

   (c) Test the hypothesis of part a. What is the P value of the test? Remember that the test is two-tailed.

3. A study is conducted to detect the effectiveness of mammographies. From 31 cases of breast cancer detected in women in the 40- to 49-year-old age group 6 were found by the use of mammography alone. In older women, 38 of 101 cancers detected were found by mammography alone. Is this evidence at the $\alpha = .05$ level that the probability of detecting cancer by mammography alone is higher with older women than with younger? Explain your answer by setting up and testing the appropriate statistical hypothesis.

4. In a 1970 study, blood tests were run on 759 patients suffering from various infections of the bloodstream. In 46 of these cases, at least two different organisms were isolated from the same blood sample. A similar study of 838 patients conducted in 1975 yielded 109 with two or more organisms present. Based on these samples, can you safely claim that the proportion of such cases has increased by more than 6 percentage points during the 5-year period? Explain your answer by setting up the appropriate hypothesis and finding its P value.

5. In a recent study of knee injuries among football players playing on natural grass, two types of shoes were compared. In 266 players wearing multicleated soccer shoes, 14 knee injuries were incurred. Of 2055 players wearing conventional seven-post football shoes, 162 such injuries were reported. Is this evidence at the $\alpha = .1$ level that the probability of sustaining a knee injury while wearing the football shoe is higher than that of doing so while wearing the soccer shoe? Could the same statement be made at the $\alpha = .05$ level?

6. When a drug company advertises a new drug, a profile of the drug is included. One such profile includes a comparison of side effects of the drug with the side effects of its nearest competitor. The drug in question is used to treat heartburn. These data on the percentage of persons exhibiting the side effect are obtained:

Side effect	Company brand ($n = 465$), %	Competitor ($n = 195$), %
Headache	2.4	2.6
Diarrhea	1.9	.5

   (a) Test for differences in the percentages of patients experiencing headache. (*Hint:* The test is two-tailed.)

   (b) Test for differences in the percentage of patients experiencing diarrhea.

   (Information obtained from an advertisement appearing in *Emergency Medicine,* November 1990, pp. 27–30.)

TECHNOLOGY TOOLS

TI83

XVIII.   Confidence intervals on proportions

The TI83 calculator can find confidence intervals on p or $p_1 - p_2$ using information on the number of objects with the trait of interest and sample sizes. We illustrate in the two sample settings by recreating the confidence interval found in Example 8.5.3. Remember that the calculator will retain more decimal places in its computations than was done in the text. Therefore there will be some slight discrepancies in the final results.

TI83 Keystroke	**Purpose**
1. STAT ◁ ALPHA B	1. Accesses the screen needed to form a confidence interval on $p_1 - p_2$
2. 1 ENTER	2. Enters 1 as the value of x_1
3. 34 ENTER	3. Enters 34 as the value of n_1
4. 10 ENTER	4. Enters 10 as the value of x_2
5. 38 ENTER	5. Enters 38 as the value of n_2
6. .95 ENTER	6. Asks for a 95% confidence interval to be constructed
7. ENTER	7. Calculates and displays the 95% confidence interval on $p_1 - p_2$

Confidence intervals on p are found by changing step 1 to read

STAT
◁
ALPHA
A

XIX.   Hypothesis tests on proportions

The TI83 calculator can test hypotheses on the value of p or compare p_1 to p_2 via the "pooled" proportions test described in Section 8.6. We illustrate using the data of Example 8.6.3.

TI83 Keystroke	**Purpose**
1. STAT ◁ 6	1. Accesses the screen needed to conduct a "pooled" proportions test
2. 377 ENTER	2. Enters 377 as the value of x_1
3. 863 ENTER	3. Enters 863 as the value of n_2
4. 296 ENTER	4. Enters 296 as the value of x_2
5. 560 ENTER	5. Enters 560 as the value of n_2
6. ▷ ENTER	6. Indicates that the test is left-tailed
7. ▽ ENTER	7. Conducts the test; gives the observed values of the test statistic (-3.385657423); gives the P value of the test $(.000355)$; gives the pooled estimate for p $(.4729444835)$

One-sample tests on the value of a proportion can be conducted by replacing step 1 by

STAT
◁
5

9

Comparing Two Means and Two Variances

In this chapter we continue the study of two sample problems by considering methods for comparing the means of two populations. The problem is considered under two different experimental conditions, namely, when the samples drawn are independent and when the data are paired. These terms are explained in depth in the following sections.

9.1
POINT ESTIMATION: INDEPENDENT SAMPLES

The general situation can be described as follows. There are two populations of interest, each with unknown mean; one random sample is drawn from the first population and one from the second in such a way that objects selected from population I have no bearing on the objects selected from population II (such samples are said to be independent); the population means are to be compared by using point estimation. (See Figure 9.1.

EXAMPLE 9.1.1. Until recently, Swedish farmers dusted up to 80% of all grains sown with a fungicide containing methyl mercury. A study is run to compare the mean mercury level in eggs produced in Sweden with that of eggs produced in Germany, where methyl mercury is not used. A random sample of eggs produced in Sweden is selected; a random sample of eggs produced in Germany is chosen. These samples are independent in the sense that the eggs selected in one country in no way affect those selected in the other. The study can be visualized as shown in Figure 9.2.

The logical way to estimate the difference in population means $\mu_1 - \mu_2$ is to estimate each mean individually by using the methods of Chapter 6 and then estimate $\mu_1 - \mu_2$ to be the difference between these individual estimates. That is,

$$\widehat{\mu_1 - \mu_2} = \hat{\mu}_1 - \hat{\mu}_2 = \bar{X}_1 - \bar{X}_2$$

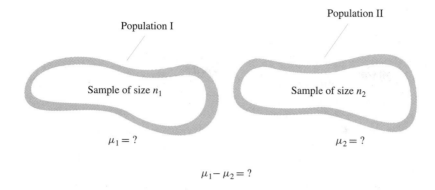

FIGURE 9.1

Independent random samples drawn from two populations.

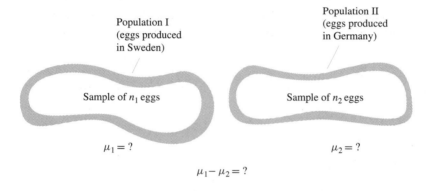

FIGURE 9.2

Two independent random samples of eggs from Germany and Sweden.

where $\bar{X}_1$ is the sample mean based on the sample from population I and $\bar{X}_2$ is the sample mean based on the independent sample drawn from population II.

EXAMPLE 9.1.2. When the study of Example 9.1.1 was conducted, the following data on the mercury levels in eggs were obtained:

Sweden	Germany
$n_1 = 2000$	$n_2 = 2500$
$\bar{x}_1 = .026$ ppm	$\bar{x}_2 = .007$ ppm
$s_1 = .01$	$s_2 = .004$

Based on this information, an estimate for the difference in mean mercury levels in eggs from the two countries is

$$\widehat{\mu_1 - \mu_2} = \hat{\mu}_1 - \hat{\mu}_2 = \bar{x}_1 - \bar{x}_2$$
$$= .026 - .007$$
$$= .019 \text{ ppm}$$

Theorem 9.1.1, which concerns the distribution of the estimator $\bar{X}_1 - \bar{X}_2$, provides the theoretical basis for confidence interval estimation and hypothesis testing on $\mu_1 - \mu_2$. The theorem can be partially verified using the rules of expectation and variance given in Appendix A.

> **THEOREM 9.1.1. Distribution of $\bar{X}_1 - \bar{X}_2$.** Let $\bar{X}_1$ and $\bar{X}_2$ be the sample means based on independent samples of sizes n_1 and n_2, drawn from normal distributions with means μ_1 and μ_2 and variances σ_1^2 and σ_2^2, respectively. Then the random variable $\bar{X}_1 - \bar{X}_2$ is normal with mean $\mu_1 - \mu_2$ and variance $\sigma_1^2/n_1 + \sigma_2^2/n_2$.

As in the one-sample case, because of the Central Limit Theorem it is safe to assume that for large sample sizes $\bar{X}_1 - \bar{X}_2$ is at least approximately normal even if the samples are drawn from populations that are not themselves normal.

EXERCISES 9.1

1. It is generally accepted that sex differences in response to heat stress do exist. A group of 10 men and 8 women were put through a vigorous exercise program that involved the use of the treadmill. The environment was hot, and a minimal amount of water was available to the subjects. The random variable of interest is the percentage of body weight lost. These data resulted:

Men		Women	
2.9	3.7	3.0	3.8
3.5	3.8	2.5	4.1
3.9	4.0	3.7	3.6
3.8	3.6	3.3	4.0
3.6	3.7		

Find a point estimate for the difference in the average percentage of body weight lost between men and women exercising under these conditions.

2. A study is run to compare some of the physical attributes of female Olympic swimmers with those of female Olympic runners. One variable of interest is the total body fat in kilograms. Samples of 12 runners and 10 swimmers were obtained. These data resulted:

Runners		Swimmers	
11.2	7.6	14.1	12.7
10.1	7.3	15.1	13.7
9.4	6.9	11.4	11.9
9.2	5.5	14.3	10.7
8.3	5.0	9.2	8.7
8.2	3.7		

Find a point estimate for the difference in mean total body fat between female Olympic runners and swimmers.

3. A sample of size 20 is to be chosen from a normal distribution with mean 15 and variance 16. An independent sample of size 25 is selected from a normal distribu-

tion with mean 10 and variance 18. What is the mean of the random variable $\bar{X}_1 - \bar{X}_2$? What is its variance? What is its standard deviation? What type of variable $(Z, T, X^2, \ldots)$ is this variable?

$$\frac{(\bar{X}_1 - \bar{X}_2) - 5}{\sqrt{\frac{16}{20} + \frac{18}{25}}}$$

4. A study is conducted to investigate the effect of parking lot water runoff on the density of nearby vegetation. Two areas were studied. One was subject to runoff from a large parking area; the other was not near a parking lot and serves as a control. Each area was subdivided into a number of 2-meter by 20-meter plots. The number of plants found per plot was determined. These data were obtained:

Parking lot drainage area		Control area	
62	64	72	59
76	74	77	64
58	71	60	62
57	59	59	75
79	54	61	69
82	49	64	64
72	53	69	71
77		65	

   (a) Estimate the average number of plants per plot found in each area.
   (b) Estimate the difference in the average number of plants per plot. Subtract in this order: control area minus drainage area.
   (c) It is thought that pollutants from the parking lot will decrease the number of plants found in the drainage area. Does the point estimate found in part b tend to support this idea? Can you be very sure from this point estimate that the idea is correct? If you want to support this idea in such a way that you can report a probability of error, what should you do?
   (Based on a study conducted by Thomas Edward Wilkerson IV, Department of Biology, Radford University, 1993.)
5. A study is conducted to compare the average reading level of patients seen at public community clinics to those seen at university clinics. These data result:

Community clinic	University clinic
$n = 30$	$n = 90$
$\bar{x} = 5.4$ (5th grade, 4th month)	$\bar{x} = 6.8$ (6th grade, 8th month)

   Estimate the difference in the average reading level of patients from these two types of clinics. (Based on information found in Terry Davis et al., "The Gap Between Patient Reading Comprehension and the Readability of Patient Education Materials," *The Journal of Family Practice,* November 1990, pp. 533–537.)
6. Consider the situation described in Exercise 5. If we assume that the reading levels at each clinic vary from 1 to 12, we can use the idea explained in Section 6.6 to approximate each sample standard deviation. In this case, $s_1 = s_2 \doteq range/4 = 2.75$.

(a) Use the information given in Exercise 5 to find a 95% confidence interval on the average reading level of patients seen (1) at the community clinic and (2) at the university clinic.

(b) Written material given to patients at these clinics in analyzed for readability. These average reading levels are obtained for various materials:

Patient consent form	16.1
Diet for a healthy heart	14.8
High blood pressure	8.6
Alcoholics Anonymous's 12 steps	11.3
Pregnancy problems	12.0

Do these data indicate that reading materials given to patients are written on a level that is too high for the intended audience? Explain based on the confidence intervals found in part a.

9.2

COMPARING VARIANCES: F DISTRIBUTION

There are two reasons for wanting to be able to compare population variances. First, many studies have as their primary purpose the comparison of two means. However, there are two statistics used to make this comparison. One is used when the population variances seem to be equal; the other is appropriate when these variances appear to be different. We need a way to compare variances so that the proper statistic for comparing means can be chosen. We shall develop a rule of thumb for this purpose. The second reason for wanting to compare variances is that such a comparison is of special interest to us. We want to be able to draw conclusions about the relationship between the two variances because this relationship is of concern to us in our study. We shall develop an "F test" for making such comparisons.

Rule of Thumb Variance Comparison

Consider a situation in which two independent samples are available. The primary purpose of the study is to compare the means of the two populations from which these samples are drawn.

There are two statistics used to compare the means of two normal populations. This is due to the fact that there are two distinct possibilities.

These are

1. σ_1^2 and σ_2^2 are unknown but are assumed to be equal.
2. σ_1^2 and σ_2^2 are unknown and are not assumed to be equal.

The first task of the researcher is to determine which situation exists in his or her study. This means that we need to develop a procedure by which we can quickly determine whether the evidence tends to point to the fact that σ_1^2 and σ_2^2 are different.

EXAMPLE 9.2.1. A study of prescribing practices is conducted. The purpose is to analyze the prescribing of digoxin, an important and commonly used drug that is potentially toxic. It is known that usually the dosage level for those over age 64 should be lower than that for younger persons. To run the study, independent samples are drawn from each group. The digoxin dosage level is obtained for each patient selected.

Two questions are posed. Each is to be answered statistically, based on information obtained from the samples. The primary question is this: Is $\mu_1 < \mu_2$? However, before this question can be answered, we must consider the question, Is $\sigma_1^2 = \sigma_2^2$?

It is easy to find a logical statistic for comparing variances. Recall that the sample variance S_1^2 is an estimator for σ_1^2 and that the sample variance S_2^2 estimates σ_2^2. Thus to compare σ_1^2 with σ_2^2, we simply compare S_1^2 with S_2^2. This is done not by looking at the difference between the two, but by looking at S_1^2/S_2^2, the ratio of the two. If the two unknown populations are, in fact, equal, then S_1^2 and S_2^2 are both estimating the same thing. In this case, we expect S_1^2 and S_2^2 to be close in value, forcing the ratio S_1^2/S_2^2 to be close to 1. That is, values near 1 support the notion that $\sigma_1^2 = \sigma_2^2$.

To use the rule of thumb to compare population variances, we designate the *larger* of the two sample variances as s_1^2 and the smaller as s_2^2. If the ratio s_1^2/s_2^2 is close to 1, then there is little evidence that σ_1^2 and σ_2^2 are different. However, if s_1^2/s_2^2 is much larger than 1, then we have evidence that the population variances are different. How large must this ratio be for us to be convinced that $\sigma_1^2 \neq \sigma_2^2$? This question is answered by the rule of thumb.

RULE OF THUMB FOR COMPARING σ_1^2 TO σ_2^2. Let s_1^2 and s_2^2 be sample variances based on samples drawn from normal distributions. Assume that $s_1^2 \geq s_2^2$. If $s_1^2/s_2^2 \geq 2$, then assume that $\sigma_1^2 \neq \sigma_2^2$.

This rule of thumb says simply that if the larger sample variance is at least twice as large as the smaller then we shall assume that σ_1^2 and σ_2^2 are not the same. We choose a statistic for comparing means with this in mind.

EXAMPLE 9.2.2. When the digoxin study described in Example 9.2.1 is conducted these data are obtained:

Patients over 64	Patients 64 and under
$n_1 = 41$	$n_2 = 29$
$\bar{x}_1 = .265$ mg/day	$\bar{x}_2 = .268$ mg/day
$s_1 = .102$ mg/day	$s_2 = .068$ mg/day
$s_1^2 = .010404$	$s_2^2 = .004624$

Before comparing μ_1 to μ_2 we compare variances. The larger sample variance is designated as s_1^2. The ratio s_1^2/s_2^2 is given by

$$s_1^2/s_2^2 = .010404/.004624 = 2.25$$

Since the value of this ratio exceeds 2, we conclude that the population variances σ_1^2 and σ_2^2 are different.

This rule of thumb is rather liberal. We do not want to use a statistic to compare means that assumes that $\sigma_1^2 = \sigma_2^2$ if there is even the slightest indication that this assumption is not true. In Exercise 9 you are asked to investigate this rule of thumb mathematically.

F Test for Comparing Variances: *F* Distribution (Optional)

A formal hypothesis test on the relationship between two variances can be performed. This test can be run as a means of choosing the appropriate statistic to compare means, or it can be run because interest centers on the population variances themselves. The test can assume any one of the usual three forms, depending on the purpose of the study. These forms are

I H_0: $\sigma_1^2 \le \sigma_2^2$	II H_0: $\sigma_1^2 \ge \sigma_2^2$	II H_0: $\sigma_1^2 = \sigma_2^2$
H_1: $\sigma_1^2 > \sigma_2^2$	H_1: $\sigma_1^2 < \sigma_2^2$	H_1: $\sigma_1^2 \ne \sigma_2^2$
Right-tailed test	Left-tailed test	Two-tailed test

The test statistic used to test any one of these hypotheses is S_1^2/S_2^2, the same statistic used in the rule of thumb. In this case, S_1^2 does not have to be the larger of the two sample variances. If the null hypothesis is true and the population variances are really equal, then we expect S_1^2 and S_2^2 to be close in value, forcing S_1^2/S_2^2 to be close to 1. If the ratio is close to zero, then we naturally conclude that the population variances are not equal and that, in fact, $\sigma_1^2 < \sigma_2^2$. Conversely, if S_1^2/S_2^2 is much larger than 1, we also conclude that the population variances are different and, in this instance, that $\sigma_1^2 > \sigma_2^2$.

When we use the phrases *close to zero* and *much larger than one,* we are speaking in terms of probabilities. That is, an observed value of the statistic is "close to zero" when it is too *small* to have reasonably occurred by chance if, in fact, the population variances are equal. Similarly, an observed value is "much larger than one" if it is too *large* to have reasonably occurred by chance. To determine the probability of observing various values of the statistic S_1^2/S_2^2, we must know its probability distribution. We show that this statistic follows a distribution previously unencountered. In particular, if the population variances are equal, it follows what is called an *F* distribution. This distribution is defined in terms of a distribution previously studied, namely, the chi-squared distribution. In particular, an *F* random variable can be written as the ratio of two independent chi-squared random variables, each divided by their respective degrees of freedom.

> **DEFINITION 9.2.1. *F* distribution.** Let $X_{\gamma_1}^2$ and $X_{\gamma_2}^2$ be independent chi-squared random variables with γ_1 and γ_2 degrees of freedom, respectively. Then the random variable
>
> $$\frac{X_{\gamma_1}^2/\gamma_1}{X_{\gamma_2}^2/\gamma_2}$$
>
> follows what is called an *F distribution* with γ_1 and γ_2 degrees of freedom.

The important properties of the family of *F* random variables are summarized:

1. There are infinitely many *F* random variables, each identified by two parameters γ_1 and γ_2, called *degrees of freedom*. These parameters are always positive integers; γ_1 is associated with the chi-squared random variable of the numerator of the *F* variable, and γ_2 is associated with the chi-squared variable of the denominator. The notation F_{γ_1, γ_2} denotes an *F* random variable with γ_1 and γ_2 degrees of freedom.

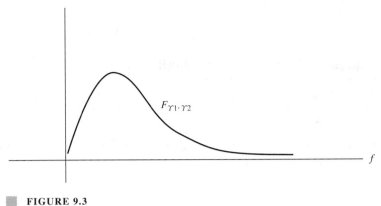

FIGURE 9.3

A typical F density.

2. Each F random variable is continuous.
3. The graph of the density of each F variable is an asymmetric curve of the general shape shown in Figure 9.3.
4. The F variables cannot assume negative values.

A partial summary of the cumulative distribution function for F variables with various degrees of freedom is given in Table IX of Appendix B. There γ_1, the degrees of freedom for the numerator, appears as column headings; γ_2, the degrees of freedom for the denominator, appears as row headings.

Points with areas .01, .025, .05, and .1 to the right can be read directly from the table. Points with these areas to the left can be computed from the table. The technique is demonstrated in Example 9.2.3.

> **EXAMPLE 9.2.3.** Consider $F_{10,15}$, the F random variable with 10 and 15 degrees of freedom.
>
> (a) Find $P[F_{10,15} \leq 2.54]$. Scan the F tables under column 10 and row 15 until you find the value 2.54. This is found in the table labeled $P[F_{\gamma_1,\gamma_2} \leq f] = .95$. Hence $P[F_{10,15} \leq 2.54] = .95$.
>
> (b) Find $P[F_{10,15} \geq 3.06]$. The value 3.06 is found in column 10 and row 15 of the table labeled $P[F_{\gamma_1,\gamma_2} \leq f] = .975$. Hence $P[F_{10,15} \leq 3.06] = .975$. This, in turn, implies that $P[F_{10,15} \geq 3.06] = 1 - .975 = .025$.
>
> (c) The point with area .025 to its right (.975 to the left) is 3.06.
>
> (d) The point with area .05 to its right (.95 to its left) is 2.54.
>
> (e) The point with area .01 to its right (.99 to its left) is 3.80.
>
> (f) What point has area .975 to its right (.025 to the left)? This point is the left-tailed point shown in Figure 9.4. Its value cannot be read directly from Table IX. It is calculated by taking the reciprocal of the corresponding right-tailed point for an F random variable with the degrees of freedom reversed. Consider the $F_{15,10}$ random variable. Notice that we have reversed the degrees of freedom. The point on this curve with .025 area to the right is 3.52. Hence the desired left-tailed point has value $1/3.52 = .28$.
>
> (g) The left-tailed point with area .95 to the right and .05 to the left is
>
> $$\frac{1}{2.85} = .35$$

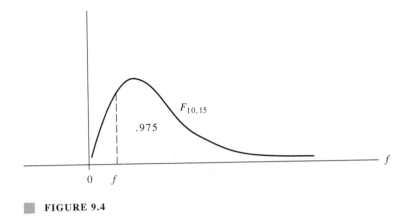

■ FIGURE 9.4

Occasionally the table does not allow for the reading of a desired right-tailed F point. For example, if the numerator has 50 degrees of freedom, the F point is not listed. We can, however, read points for 40 and 60 degrees of freedom. Each of these gives a good approximation of the point desired. We shall take a conservative approach and choose the point that slightly overestimates the point of interest. In most cases, this means that we choose the lower of the two possible degrees of freedom in forming our estimate.

Theorem 9.2.1 provides the statistic needed to test hypotheses on the relationship between two population variances.

THEOREM 9.2.1. Let S_1^2 and S_2^2 be sample variances based on independent random samples of sizes n_1 and n_2 drawn from normal populations with means μ_1 and μ_2 and variances σ_1^2 and σ_2^2, respectively. If $\sigma_1^2 = \sigma_2^2$, then the statistic S_1^2/S_2^2 follows an F distribution with $n_1 - 1$ and $n_2 - 1$ degrees of freedom.

Note that the degrees of freedom associated with the statistic S_1^2/S_2^2 are $n_1 - 1$ and $n_2 - 1$. That is, the number of degrees of freedom for the numerator is 1 less than the size of the sample drawn from population I; that of the denominator is 1 less than the size of the sample drawn from population II. We illustrate the use of the statistic S_1^2/S_2^2 as a test statistic in Example 9.2.4.

EXAMPLE 9.2.4. In the digoxin study of Example 9.2.2, we wish to test

$$H_0: \sigma_1^2 = \sigma_2^2$$
$$H_1: \sigma_1^2 \neq \sigma_2^2$$

These data were obtained:

Patients over age 64	Patients aged 64 and under
$n_1 = 41$	$n_2 = 29$
$\bar{x}_1 = .265$ mg/day	$\bar{x}_2 = .268$ mg/day
$s_1 = .102$ mg/day	$s_2 = .068$ mg/day
$s_1^2 = .010404$	$s_2^2 = .004624$

The test is a two-tailed test. Hypothesis H_0 should be rejected in favor of H_1 if the observed value of the test statistic is too large or too small to have occurred by chance when the population variances are equal. The number of degrees of freedom associated with the test statistic is $n_1 - 1 = 41 - 1 = 40$ and $n_2 - 1 = 29 - 1 = 28$. The observed value of the test statistic is

$$s_1^2/s_2^2 = \frac{.010404}{.004624} = 2.25$$

By scanning the F table with 40 and 28 degrees of freedom we see that $P[F_{40,28} \geq 2.05] = .025$ and that $P[F_{40,28} \geq 2.35] = .01$. Since the observed value of the test statistic lies between 2.05 and 2.35, the P value for a right-tailed test lies between .01 and .025. However, since the test that is being conducted is two-tailed, the P value that is reported is double that of the one-tailed test. That is, for the test as stated,

$$.02 < P < .05$$

Since this probability is small, we reject H_0 and conclude that the two population variances are different. Notice that in this case the F test yields the same conclusion as the rule of thumb.

One important point should be emphasized. We are assuming, once again, that the populations under study are normal. This assumption is necessary for the statistic S_1^2/S_2^2 to have an F distribution. The consequence of violating this assumption is that the P value or α level reported, as the case may be, may not be accurate. However, it has been found that this problem is minimized if the samples are of *equal size*.

The advantage of the rule of thumb over the F test is obvious. It is a quick and easy way to answer the question, Is $\sigma_1^2 = \sigma_2^2$? The advantages of the F test over the rule of thumb are that directional hypotheses can be tested and a P value can be attached to the test.

If the only purpose of comparing variances is to determine an appropriate statistic for comparing means, then we suggest that the rule of thumb be used. If interest centers on the relationship between the two population variances, then the F test should be used.

Both SAS and the TI83 calculator are programmed to conduct the F test for comparing variances.

EXERCISES 9.2

1. A study is conducted of airspeed in various bird species. The brown pelican is to be compared to the American oystercatcher. The birds are clocked flying cross-wind with a wind speed of 5 to 8 mi/h. The following information is obtained (assume normality):

Brown pelican	Oystercatcher
$n_1 = 9$	$n_2 = 12$
$\bar{x}_1 = 26.05$ mi/h	$\bar{x}_2 = 30.19$ mi/h
$s_1 = 6.34$ mi/h	$s_2 = 3.20$ mi/h

Use the rule of thumb to see if there is evidence that $\sigma_1^2 \neq \sigma_2^2$.
2. A study is conducted to compare the average diameter of tree rings for Fraser firs found at an elevation of about 5000 feet for two different years, 1983 and 1988.

These data are obtained:

1983	1988
$n_1 = 10$	$n_2 = 10$
$\bar{x}_1 = .535$ mm	$\bar{x}_2 = .439$ mm
$s_1 = .049$	$s_2 = .055$

Use the rule of thumb to see if there is evidence that $\sigma_1^2 \neq \sigma_2^2$.
(Based on a study conducted by Christopher Cook, Department of Biology, Radford University, 1993.)

3. A study is run to consider the effect of maternal smoking on unborn babies. The study involves a random sample of 3461 nonsmokers and 2238 smokers. All subjects in the study are white women. The variable of interest is the baby's birth weight in grams. Assume that this random variable is normally distributed. The following information is available:

Nonsmokers	Smokers
$n_1 = 3461$	$n_2 = 2238$
$\bar{x}_1 = 3480.1$ g	$\bar{x}_2 = 3256.5$ g
$s_1 = 8.68$ g	$s_2 = 11.02$ g

Based on the rule of thumb, is there sufficient evidence to claim that $\sigma_1^2 \neq \sigma_2^2$?

4. Use Table IX in Appendix B to find each of the following: [In parts d to k the subscript on the f point denotes the area to the right of the point. For example, $f_{.05}(15, 12$ DF) denotes the point associated with the $F_{15,12}$ curve with .05 area to the right and .95 area to the left.]

(a) $P[F_{24,15} \leq 2.29]$ (g) $f_{.1}(50, 9$ DF)
(b) $P[F_{20,3} \leq 14.17]$ (h) $f_{.9}(24, 15$ DF)
(c) $P[F_{\infty,29} \leq 2.03]$ (i) $f_{.95}(40, 30$ DF)
(d) $f_{.05}(15, 12$ DF)   (j) $f_{.975}(20, 20$ DF)
(e) $f_{.01}(30, 5$ DF)   (k) $f_{.99}(20, 35$ DF)
(f) $f_{.1}(40, 9$ DF)

5. In each part of Figure 9.5, find the points a and b indicated.

6. In a study of carbohydrate metabolism, the root growth in peas grown in water at 6°C is to be compared with the growth of plants grown in fructose solution at the same temperature. It is thought that the variance will be larger among plants grown in water. The following information is available (assume normality):

Grown in water	Grown in fructose
$n_1 = 16$	$n_2 = 25$
$\bar{x}_1 = 9.48$ mm/120 h	$\bar{x}_2 = 9.46$ mm/120 h
$s_1 = .53$	$s_2 = .25$

Based on the F test, can it be concluded that $\sigma_1^2 > \sigma_2^2$? What is the approximate P value for the test?

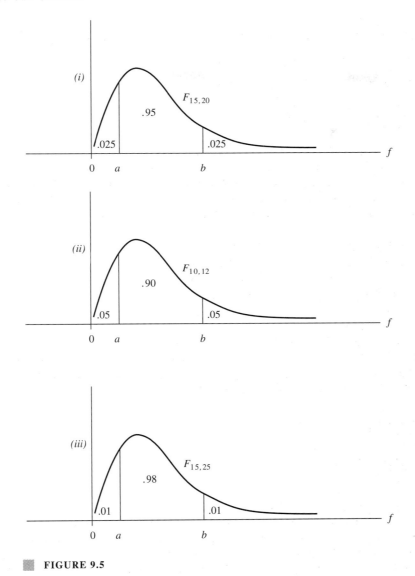

(i)

$F_{15, 20}$

.95

.025

.025

0 *a* *b*

f

(ii)

$F_{10, 12}$

.90

.05

.05

0 *a* *b*

f

(iii)

$F_{15, 25}$

.98

.01

.01

0 *a* *b*

f

FIGURE 9.5

7. Consider the study described in Exercise 1 of Section 9.1. It is thought that the variance for women is larger than that for men. Find s_M^2 and s_W^2, the sample variances
   for the percentage of body weight lost by the men and the women, respectively.
   Find s_W^2 and s_M^2. Based on the F test, can it be concluded at the $\alpha = .05$ level that
   $\sigma_W^2 > \sigma_M^2$? (Assume normality.)
8. Consider the study described in Exercise 2 of Section 9.1. It is thought that the
   variance for swimmers is larger than that for runners, Find s_R^2 and s_S^2, the sample variances for the total body fat for female Olympic runners and swimmers, respectively.

Find s_S^2/s_R^2. Based on the F test, can it be concluded at the $\alpha = .05$ level that $\sigma_S^2 > \sigma_R^2$? (Assume normality.)

9. The rule of thumb is designed in such a way that its results are consistent with those obtained by the F test for moderate- to large-sized samples at the $\alpha = .20$ level; for smaller-sized samples, the rule of thumb is more liberal than the F test in that the rule of thumb will declare variances unequal when the F test will not. Consider the F distribution for $F(f) = .9$. In testing

$$\text{H}_0: \sigma_1^2 = \sigma_2^2$$

this table gives values above which s_1^2/s_2^2 must lie to reject H_0 at the $\alpha = .20$ level.

(a) Consider $F_{15,15}$. If $s_1^2/s_2^2 = 3.00$, will the rule of thumb reject H_0? Will the F test reject H_0?

(b) Consider $F_{10,10}$. If $s_1^2/s_2^2 = 2.0$, will the rule of thumb reject H_0? Will the F test reject H_0?

(c) Give another example in which the rule of thumb and the F test agree.

(d) Give another example in which the rule of thumb rejects H_0 but the F test does not.

(e) Is there any case in which the rule of thumb does not reject H_0 but the F test does? Explain.

9.3

INFERENCES ON $\mu_1 - \mu_2$: POOLED T

Recall that there are two settings in which means comparisons are made. We either proceed as though the population variances, though unknown, are equal, or we assume that they differ in value. We allow the data to guide our decision. Therefore, our approach to comparing means will be as follows:

1. Test $\text{H}_0: \sigma_1^2 = \sigma_2^2$ versus $\text{H}_1: \sigma_1^2 \neq \sigma_2^2$ via the rule of thumb discussed in Section 9.2.
2. If H_0 is not rejected, we will proceed as though the population variances are equal. Population means will be compared using a "pooled" T procedure.
3. If H_0 is rejected, then there is evidence that the population variances are not the same. Population means will be compared using the Smith-Satterthwaite T procedure, which is introduced in Section 9.4.

As in the past, we present techniques for confidence interval estimation and hypothesis testing. We begin by considering these procedures in the setting in which population variances are assumed to be equal.

Interval Estimation of $\mu_1 - \mu_2$

We begin by developing the bounds for a confidence interval on the difference in population means.

> **EXAMPLE 9.3.1.** In a study of angina in rats, 18 animals with a history of angina were randomly split into two groups of 9 each. One group was given a placebo and the other an experimental drug FL113. After controlled exercise on a treadmill, the recovery time of

each rat was determined. It is thought that FL113 will reduce the average recovery time. The following information is available:

Placebo	FL113
$n_1 = 9$	$n_2 = 9$
$\bar{x}_1 = 329$ seconds	$\bar{x}_2 = 283$ seconds
$s_1 = 45$ seconds	$s_2 = 43$ seconds

The ratio $s_1^2/s_2^2 = 45^2/43^2 = 1.09$ is used to compare variances. Since this ratio is less than 2, by the rule of thumb there is little evidence that σ_1^2 and σ_2^2 are different. Therefore, in comparing means, we assume that the population variances, although unknown, are equal. A point estimate for the difference in mean recovery time is $\bar{x}_1 - \bar{x}_2 = 329 - 283 = 46$ seconds.

It is known that $\bar{X}_1 - \bar{X}_2$ is the logical point estimator for $\mu_1 - \mu_2$. To extend this point estimator to a confidence interval, once again we must find a random variable whose expression involves the parameter of interest, in this case $\mu_1 - \mu_2$, whose distribution is known. Such a random variable is provided by Theorem 9.1.1. This theorem states that when normal populations are sampled, the random variable $\bar{X}_1 - \bar{X}_2$ is normal with mean $\mu_1 - \mu_2$ and variance $\sigma_1^2/n_1 + \sigma_2^2/n_2$. By standardizing this variable it can be concluded that the random variable

$$\frac{(\bar{X}_1 - \bar{X}_2) - (\mu_1 - \mu_2)}{\sqrt{\sigma_1^2/n_1 + \sigma_2^2/n_2}}$$

is standard normal.

Since no difference has been detected between σ_1^2 and σ_2^2, these variances are assumed to be equal. Let σ^2 denote this common population variance. That is, let $\sigma_1^2 = \sigma_2^2 = \sigma^2$. Substituting into the above expression, we conclude that

$$\frac{(\bar{X}_1 - \bar{X}_2) - (\mu_1 - \mu_2)}{\sqrt{\sigma^2(1/n_1 + 1/n_2)}}$$

is standard normal. Since σ^2 is unknown, it must be estimated from the data. This is done by a *pooled* sample variance. Note that we already have two estimators for σ^2, namely, S_1^2 and S_2^2. The idea is to pool, or combine, these estimators to form a single estimator for σ^2 in such a way that sample sizes are taken into account. It is natural to want to attach greater importance, or "weight," to the sample variance associated with the larger sample. The pooled variance does exactly this. We define it thus:

DEFINITION 9.3.1. Pooled variance. Let S_1^2 and S_2^2 be sample variances based on independent samples of sizes n_1 and n_2, respectively. The *pooled variance*, denoted S_p^2, is given by

$$S_p^2 = \frac{(n_1 - 1)S_1^2 + (n_2 - 1)S_2^2}{n_1 + n_2 - 2}$$

Note that we weight S_1^2 and S_2^2 by multiplying by $n_1 - 1$ and $n_2 - 1$, respectively. The more natural way to weight is to multiply by the corresponding sample sizes, n_1 and n_2, respectively. We choose to weight in this somewhat odd way so that the random variable $(n_1 + n_2 - 2)S_p^2/\sigma^2$ will follow a chi-squared distribution. This is necessary so that the test statistic that we use to test for equality of means will follow a T distribution.

EXAMPLE 9.3.2. Consider a sample variance $s_1^2 = 24$ based on a sample size 16 and a second sample variance $s_2^2 = 20$ based on a sample size 121. The value of the ratio s_1^2/s_2^2 is $24/20 = 1.20$. Since the rule of thumb does not lead us to believe that σ_1^2 and σ_2^2 are different, s_1^2 and s_2^2 are both estimates for the same variance, σ^2.

The pooled estimate for the common population variance is

$$s_p^2 = \frac{(n_1 - 1)s_1^2 + (n_2 - 1)s_2^2}{n_1 + n_2 - 2}$$

$$= \frac{15(24) + 120(20)}{16 + 121 - 2}$$

$$= \frac{2760}{135} = 20.44$$

Note that this estimate is quite different from 22, the value that would be obtained by ignoring sample sizes and arithmetically averaging s_1^2 and s_2^2.

To obtain a random variable that can be used to construct a confidence interval on $\mu_1 - \mu_2$, we replace the unknown population variance σ^2 in the Z random variable

$$\frac{(\bar{X}_1 - \bar{X}_2) - (\mu_1 - \mu_2)}{\sqrt{\sigma^2(1/n_1 + 1/n_2)}}$$

by the pooled estimator S_p^2, to obtain the random variable

$$\frac{(\bar{X}_1 - \bar{X}_2) - (\mu_1 - \mu_2)}{\sqrt{S_p^2(1/n_1 + 1/n_2)}}$$

As in the one-sample case, replacing the population variance by its estimator does affect the distribution. The former random variable is a Z variable; the latter has a T distribution with $n_1 + n_2 - 2$ degrees of freedom. The algebraic structure of this variable is the same as that encountered previously, namely,

$$\frac{\text{Estimator} - \text{parameter}}{D}$$

where D is the standard deviation of the estimator in the numerator or the estimator for this standard deviation. Therefore, the confidence interval on $\mu_1 - \mu_2$ takes the same general form as most of the intervals encountered previously.

THEOREM 9.3.1. Confidence interval on $\mu_1 - \mu_2$: Pooled variance. Let $\bar{X}_1$ and $\bar{X}_2$ be sample means based on independent random samples drawn from normal distributions with means μ_1 and μ_2, respectively, and common variance σ^2. Let S_p^2 denote the pooled sample variance. The bounds for a confidence interval on $\mu_1 - \mu_2$ are

$$(\bar{X}_1 - \bar{X}_2) \pm t\sqrt{S_p^2\left(\frac{1}{n_1} + \frac{1}{n_2}\right)}$$

where the point t is found relative to the $T_{n_1+n_2-2}$ distribution.

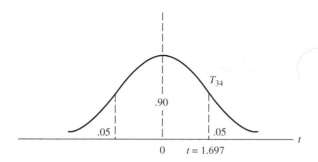

FIGURE 9.6

Partition of the T_{34} curve needed to obtain a 90% confidence interval on $\mu_1 - \mu_2$.

EXAMPLE 9.3.3. In a study of the feeding habits of bats, 25 females and 11 males are tagged and tracked by radio. One variable of interest is X, the distance flown per feeding pass. The experiment yielded the following information (assume normality):

Females	Males
$n_1 = 25$	$n_2 = 11$
$\bar{x}_1 = 205$ meters	$\bar{x}_2 = 135$ meters
$s_1 = 100$ meters	$s_2 = 95$ meters

Note that $s_1^2/s_2^2 = 100^2/95^2 = 1.11$. Since this ratio is less than 2, the rule of thumb does not indicate that the population variances differ. Since no differences can be detected in population variances, we pool s_1^2 and s_2^2 to obtain

$$s_p^2 = \frac{(n_1 - 1)s_1^2 + (n_2 - 1)s_2^2}{n_1 + n_2 - 2}$$

$$= \frac{24(100^2) + 10(95)^2}{25 + 11 - 2} = 9713.24$$

To compare means, let us find a 90% confidence interval on $\mu_1 - \mu_2$. The number of degrees of freedom needed is $n_1 + n_2 - 2 = 25 + 11 - 2 = 34$. The partition of the T_{34} curve needed is shown in Figure 9.6 The bounds for the confidence interval are

$$(\bar{x}_1 - \bar{x}_2) \pm t\sqrt{s_p^2\left(\frac{1}{n_1} + \frac{1}{n_2}\right)} = (205 - 135) \pm 1.697\sqrt{9713.24\left(\frac{1}{25} + \frac{1}{22}\right)}$$

$$= 70 \pm 60.51$$

We can be 90% confident that the difference in mean feeding pass distances between female and male bats is between 9.49 and 130.51 meters. This interval does not contain the number 0 and is positive-valued throughout, an indication that the mean distance for females is higher than that for males. Some biologists have interpreted this to mean that the females are being driven from the closer feeding grounds by the more aggressive males. This theory, however, has not been confirmed.

Pooled T Tests

As in previous instances, the random variable used to derive confidence bounds for a parameter also serves as a test statistic for testing various hypotheses concerning the parameter. In this case, the random variable

$$\boxed{\frac{(\bar{X}_1 - \bar{X}_2) - (\mu_1 - \mu_2)_0}{\sqrt{S_p^2(1/n_1 + 1/n_2)}} = T_{n_1+n_2-2}}$$ (*T* Test on $\mu_1 - \mu_2$: Variances Pooled)

serves as a test statistic for testing any of the usual hypotheses, where $(\mu_1 - \mu_2)_0$ denotes the hypothesized difference in population means. The hypothesized difference can be any value whatever. However, the most commonly encountered hypothesized value is zero. In this case, the purpose is to determine whether the population means differ and, if so, which is the larger. That is, the hypotheses take these forms:

I H_0: $\mu_1 \leq \mu_2$	II H_0: $\mu_1 \geq \mu_2$	III H_0: $\mu_1 = \mu_2$
H_1: $\mu_1 > \mu_2$	H_1: $\mu_1 < \mu_2$	H_1: $\mu_1 \neq \mu_2$
Right-tailed test	Left-tailed test	Two-tailed test

Since the test statistic used to distinguish between H_0 and H_1 uses the pooled estimator for σ^2, the *T* test that is demonstrated in this section is called a *pooled T test*.

EXAMPLE 9.3.4. The summary data for the study of angina in rats of Example 9.3.1 are as follows:

Placebo	FL113
$n_1 = 9$	$n_2 = 9$
$\bar{x}_1 = 329$ seconds	$\bar{x}_2 = 283$ seconds
$s_1 = 45$ seconds	$s_2 = 43$ seconds

The point estimate for the difference in mean recovery time between those on a placebo and those receiving the experimental drug is $\bar{x}_1 - \bar{x}_2 = 46$ seconds. Is this difference great enough for us to conclude that the experimental drug tends to reduce recovery time? To answer this question, we must find the pooled estimate for the common population variance. This estimate is

$$s_p^2 = \frac{(n-1)s_1^2 + (n_2-1)s_2^2}{n_1 + n_2 - 2}$$

$$= \frac{8(45)^2 + 8(43)^2}{9 + 9 - 2}$$

$$= \frac{45^2 + 43^2}{2} = 1937$$

Note that since the sample sizes are the *same,* in this case the pooled estimate is the arithmetic average of the individual estimates s_1^2 and s_2^2. Now we evaluate the test statistic:

$$\frac{(\bar{x}_1 - \bar{x}_2) - (\mu_1 - \mu_2)_0}{\sqrt{s_p^2(1/n_1 + 1/n_2)}} = \frac{46 - 0}{\sqrt{1937(\frac{1}{9} + \frac{1}{9})}}$$

$$= 2.22$$

The number of degrees of freedom associated with the pooled T statistic is $n_1 + n_2 - 2 = 16$. The research theory is that FL113 will reduce the average recovery time ($H_1: \mu_1 > \mu_2$). Since the test is right-tailed,

$$P = P[T_{16} > 2.22]$$

Since the observed value of the test statistic (2.22) lies between 2.120 and 2.583, the P value lies between .01 and .025. We do have evidence to support the contention that the experimental drug is effective in reducing the recovery time in rats with angina.

EXERCISES 9.3

1. (a) Let $s_1^2 = 42$, $s_2^2 = 37$, $n_1 = 10$, $n_2 = 14$. Find s_p^2.
   (b) Let $s_1^2 = 28$, $s_2^2 = 30$, $n_1 = 20$, $n_2 = 20$. Find s_p^2. (Do not use your calculator!)
   (c) Let $s_1^2 = 20$, $s_2^2 = 40$, $n_1 = 10$, $n_2 = 50$. Find s_p^2. Why is s_p^2 closer in value to s_2^2 than to s_1^2?

2. The feeding habits of two species of net-casting spiders are studied. these species, the *Dinopis* and *Menneus,* coexist in eastern Australia. One variable of interest is the size of the prey of each species. The *adult Menneus* is about the same size as the juvenile *Dinopis*. It is known that there exists a difference in prey size between the adult and juvenile *Dinopis* because of their size difference. Is there a difference in mean prey size between adult *Dinopis* and adult *Menneus*? If so, what is the cause? To answer these questions, the following observations were obtained on the size, in millimeters, of the prey of the two species:

Adult *Dinopis*		Adult *Menneus*	
12.9	11.9	10.2	5.3
10.2	7.1	6.9	7.5
7.4	9.9	10.9	10.3
7.0	14.4	11.0	9.2
10.5	11.3	10.1	8.8

   (a) Use the rule of thumb to compare population variances.
   (b) If no differences are detected in population variances, find s_p^2 and then find a 90% confidence interval on $\mu_1 - \mu_2$.
   (c) On the basis of the interval of part b, is there evidence of a difference in mean prey size between the two species? Explain. (Biologists think that any difference detected may be explained by differences in placement and size of the webs built by the two.)

3. Consider the data of Exercise 1 of Section 9.1. Use the rule of thumb to check for differences in population variances. If appropriate, find s_p^2 and a 95% confidence interval on the difference in population means.

4. Consider the data of Exercise 2 of Section 9.1. Assume normality and use the rule of thumb to check for differences in population variances. If appropriate, find s_p^2 and find a 98% confidence interval on the difference in population means. Based

on this interval, do you think that a difference exists between the mean total body fat of female Olympic runners and swimmers? Explain.

5. A study is conducted of two drug treatments for potential use in heart transplants. The purpose of the drugs is to act as an immunosuppressant—to repress the body's natural tendency to reject the transplant. Male ACI rats serve as donors; male Lewis-Brown Norway rats serve as recipients. These rats are known to be poor matches. The variable of interest is X, the survival time in days. The following summary statistics are obtained:

Sodium salicylate alone	Sodium salicylate and azathioprine
$n_1 = 9$	$n_2 = 9$
$\bar{x}_1 = 16$ days	$\bar{x}_2 = 15$ days
$s_1 = 10.1$ days	$s_2 = 10$ days

Use this information to compare population variances. Find a 90% confidence interval on the difference in mean survival times between the two treatments. Interpret this interval in terms of its practical implications.

6. Since elevated cholesterol level is a major risk factor in the development of atherosclerotic heart disease and coronary-artery disease, it is important to determine what levels to expect in various age groups. A study is conducted to compare the cholesterol level in males aged 20 to 29 to females of the same age group. These data are obtained:

Male	Female
$n_1 = 96$	$n_2 = 85$
$\bar{x}_1 = 167.16$ mg/dL	$\bar{x}_2 = 178.12$ mg/dL
$s_1 = 30$ mg/dL	$s_2 = 32$ mg/dL

(a) Check for differences in population variances.
(b) Find a 95% confidence interval on the difference in the average cholesterol levels between these two groups.
(Based on means reported in Marvin Bell and Sharon Joseph, "Community Screening for Hypercholesterolemia," *Journal of Family Practice,* October 1990, pp. 365–368.)

7. In a study of diverticular disease and diet, 23 vegetarians were used. One variable of interest was total dietary fiber. The following information was obtained for two groups, those without the disease and those with it (assume normality):

Without	With
$n_1 = 18$	$n_2 = 5$
$\bar{x}_1 = 42.7$ g	$\bar{x}_2 = 27.7$ g
$s_1 = 9.9$ g	$s_2 = 9.5$ g

Check for differences in population variances. Is there sufficient evidence to claim that the mean total dietary fiber content in the diets of those without the disease is higher than that of those with it? Explain your answer on the basis of the P value of the test.

8. Another variable of interest in the study of angina in rats (see Example 9.3.1) is the oxygen intake, measured in milliliters per minute. The experiment provided the following information:

Placebo	FL113
$n_1 = 9$	$n_2 = 9$
$\bar{x}_1 = 1509$ mL/min	$\bar{x}_2 = 1702$ mL/min
$s_1 = 169$ mL/min	$s_2 = 181$ mL/min

Use this information to compare population variances. Based on this experiment, is there sufficient evidence to claim that the mean oxygen intake of rats on FL113 is higher than that of those taking the placebo? Explain your answer based on the *P* value of the test.

9. In a study of body characteristics of the ring-billed gull, the variable considered is the bill length. The following data are available:

Female	Male
$n_1 = 51$	$n_2 = 41$
$\bar{x}_1 = 59.1$ mm	$\bar{x}_2 = 65.2$ mm
$s_1 = 1.9$ mm	$s_2 = 2.0$ mm

Use this information to check for differences in population variances. Is there evidence to support the contention that the mean bill length in males is longer than in females? Explain your answer on the basis of the *P* value of the test.

10. One variable used to compare the physical attributes of female Olympic swimmers and runners is the circumference of the upper arm, in centimeters, while relaxed. The following data are available:

Swimmers	Runners
$n_1 = 10$	$n_2 = 12$
$\bar{x}_1 = 27.3$ cm	$\bar{x}_2 = 23.5$ cm
$s_1 = 1.9$ cm	$s_2 = 1.7$ cm

Assuming normality, check for differences in population variances. Is there sufficient evidence to claim that the mean circumference of the upper arm is larger in swimmers than in runners? Explain your answer on the basis of the *P* value of the test.

11. It is thought that adolescent boys who smoke begin to smoke at an earlier age than do adolescent female smokers. Do these data support this contention?

Male	Female
$n_1 = 33$	$n_2 = 14$
Average age at onset of smoking	Average age at onset of smoking
$= 11.3$ years	$= 12.6$ years
$s_1^2 = 4$	$s_2^2 = 3.5$

(Means found in Nadu Tuakli, Mindy Smith, and Caryl Heaton, "Smoking in Adolescence: Methods for Health Education and Smoking Cessation," *Journal of Family Practice,* October 1990, pp. 369–373.)

9.4

INFERENCES ON $\mu_1 - \mu_2$: UNEQUAL VARIANCES

If a difference is detected when the population variances are compared, then pooling is inappropriate. It is still possible to compare means by using an approximate T statistic. Again, the desired statistic is found by modifying the Z variable

$$\frac{(\bar{X}_1 - \bar{X}_2) - (\mu_1 - \mu_2)}{\sqrt{\sigma_1^2/n_1 + \sigma_2^2/n_2}}$$

in a logical way. Since now there is evidence that $\sigma_1^2 \neq \sigma_2^2$, each population variance is estimated separately; these estimates are *not* combined. Instead, the population variances in the Z random variable above are replaced by their respective estimators, S_1^2 and S_2^2, to obtain the random variable

$$\boxed{\frac{(\bar{X}_1 - \bar{X}_2) - (\mu_1 - \mu_2)}{\sqrt{S_1^2/n_1 + S_2^2/n_2}}}$$

As in the past, making this change results in a change in distribution from Z to an approximate T. The number of degrees must be estimated from the data. Several methods have been suggested for doing this. Here we demonstrate the Smith-Satterthwaite procedure. According to this procedure, γ, the number of degrees of freedom, is given by

$$\boxed{\gamma \doteq \frac{[S_1^2/n_1 + S_2^2/n_2]^2}{\dfrac{[S_1^2/n_1]^2}{n_1 - 1} + \dfrac{[S_2^2/n_2]^2}{n_2 - 1}}}$$

The value for γ will not necessarily be an integer. If it is not, we round it *down* to the nearest integer. We round down rather than up in order to take a conservative approach. Recall that as the number of degrees of freedom associated with T random variables increases, the corresponding bell-shaped curves become more compact. Practically speaking, this means that, for example, the point associated with the T_{10} curve with 5% of the area to the right (1.812) is a little larger than the point associated with the T_{11} curve with 5% of the area to the right (1.796). As a result of this conservative approach, a confidence interval based on the T_{10} distribution is a little longer than one based on the T_{11} curve. Furthermore, if we can reject a null hypothesis based on the T_{10} distribution, it will also be rejected based on the T_{11} distribution. The converse does not necessarily hold.

Confidence bounds for a confidence interval on $\mu_1 - \mu_2$ when variances are unequal are similar to those encountered earlier. They are

$$\boxed{(\bar{X}_1 - \bar{X}_2) \pm t\sqrt{\frac{S_1^2}{n_1} + \frac{S_2^2}{n_2}}} \qquad \begin{array}{l}\text{(Confidence Interval on} \\ \mu_1 - \mu_2\text{: Variances Different)}\end{array}$$

where t is a point based on the T distribution with γ degrees of freedom. The degrees of freedom are calculated using the Smith-Satterthwaite equation.

The test statistic for testing H_0: $(\mu_1 - \mu_2) = (\mu_1 - \mu_2)_0$ versus any of the usual three alternatives is

$$T_\gamma = \frac{(\bar{X}_1 - \bar{X}_2) - (\mu_1 - \mu_2)_0}{\sqrt{S_1^2/n_1 + S_2^2/n_2}} \qquad \begin{matrix}(T \text{ Test on } \mu_1 - \mu_2: \\ \text{Variances Different})\end{matrix}$$

where γ is calculated using the Smith-Satterthwaite equation. This procedure is illustrated in Example 9.4.1.

EXAMPLE 9.4.1. A study of energy requirements for growth and maintenance of nestling house martins was conducted in Perthshire, Scotland. The following summary statistics were obtained on the normal variable X, the number of kilocalories per gram per hour required per bird:

Incubating adults	Prebreeding adults
$n_1 = 57$	$n_2 = 12$
$\bar{x}_1 = .0167 \text{ kcal/(g)(h)}$	$\bar{x}_2 = .0144 \text{ kcal/(g)(h)}$
$s_1 = .0042 \text{ kcal/(g)(h)}$	$s_2 = .0024 \text{ kcal/(g)(h)}$

Do these data indicate that the average number of kilocalories required for incubating adults is higher than that for prebreeding adults?

The observed value of the statistic S_1^2/S_2^2 is $(.0042)^2/(.0024)^2 = 3.0625$. Since this value exceeds 2, we have evidence that $\sigma_1^2 \neq \sigma_2^2$. We will not pool the sample variances since they do not appear to be estimating a common population variance. The value of the T_γ statistic is

$$\frac{(\bar{x}_1 - \bar{x}_2) - (\mu_1 - \mu_2)_0}{\sqrt{s_1^2/n_1 + s_2^2/n_2}} = \frac{.0167 - .0144}{\sqrt{(.0042)^2/57 + (.0024)^2/12}} = 2.59$$

The number of degrees of freedom associated with this statistic is

$$\gamma \doteq \frac{[s_1^2/n_1 + s_2^2/n_2]^2}{\dfrac{[s_1^2/n_1]^2}{n_1 - 1} + \dfrac{[s_2^2/n_2]^2}{n_2 - 1}}$$

$$= \frac{[(.0042)^2/57 + (.0024)^2/12]^2}{[(.0042)^2/57]^2/56 + [(.0024)^2/12]^2/11} = 27.5$$

Since degrees of freedom must be a positive integer, we round this down to 27. Based on the T_{27} distribution, the probability of obtaining a value of 2.59 or larger is between .01 and .005. That is, the P value for the test of H_0: $\mu_1 \leq \mu_2$ is between .01 and .005. Since this value is very small, we conclude that the mean energy requirement for incubating birds is higher than for prebreeding ones.

Both the TI83 calculator and SAS are programmed to conduct either a pooled T test or the Smith-Satterthwaite T test. When using these tools it is the task of the researcher to decide which of these two tests is appropriate. The technology tools do the computational work for you; they do not interpret the results.

☐ EXERCISES 9.4

1. Consider Example 9.4.1. If one failed to check for equality of variances and mistakenly pooled variances, what would be the observed value of the test statistic? How many degrees of freedom would be used? Would the P value be affected?
2. Strontium 90, a radioactive element produced by nuclear testing, is closely related to calcium. In dairy lands, strontium 90 can make its way into milk via the grasses eaten by dairy cows. Then it becomes concentrated in the bones of those who drink the milk. In 1959 a study was conducted to compare the mean concentration of strontium 90 in the bones of children to that of adults. It was thought that the level in children was higher because the substance was present during their formative years. Is this contention supported by the following data? Explain (assume normality).

Children	Adults
$n_1 = 121$	$n_2 = 61$
$\bar{x}_1 = 2.6$ picocuries per gram	$\bar{x}_2 = .4$ picocurie per gram
$s_1 = 1.2$ picocuries per gram	$s_2 = .11$ picocurie per gram

3. A study is conducted to compare tortoises found on Malabar to those found on Grande-Terre, islands in the Aldabra atoll in the Indian Ocean. One variable of interests is X, the weight of an egg at the time of lay. Randomly selected samples from the two islands yield the following summary data (assume normality):

Grande-Terre	Malabar
$n_1 = 31$	$n_2 = 148$
$\bar{x}_1 = 64.0$ grams	$\bar{x}_2 = 82.7$ grams
$s_1 = 6.5$ grams	$s_2 = 3.6$ grams

Is there evidence that the mean weight of an egg at the time of lay on Malabar is higher than that on Grande-Terre? Explain.

4. A study of red-billed queleas is conducted. The purpose is to compare a colony located near Lake Chad to one located in Botswana. The Lake Chad colony failed because the adults abandoned the nests; the Botswana colony survived. One variable thought to influence the ability of a female to maintain the nest is X, her muscle protein level. One aim of the study is to compare the muscle protein levels of females in the two colonies.

   (*a*) At the beginning of the laying cycle, the following data were collected:

Lake Chad	Botswana
$n_1 = 100$	$n_2 = 100$
$\bar{x}_1 = .99$ gram	$\bar{x}_2 = 1.00$ gram
$s_1 = .01$ gram	$s_2 = .01$ gram

Compare population variances and test for equality of means, using the appropriate T statistic. Relative to this variable, do the populations seem to be identical at the beginning of the laying cycle?

(b) At the end of the laying cycle, the following data were obtained:

Lake Chad	Botswana
$n_1 = 100$	$n_2 = 100$
$\bar{x}_1 = .87$ gram	$\bar{x}_2 = .90$ gram
$s_1 = .02$ gram	$s_2 = .01$ gram

Compare population variances and test for equality of means, using the appropriate T statistic. Relative to this variable, do the populations now seem to be identical?

5. Consider the data of Exercise 3 of Section 9.2. The purpose of the study is to gain evidence to support the contention that the mean weight of newborns is lower among mothers who are smokers than among nonsmokers. Do the data support this contention? Be ready to defend your choice of a test statistic.

6. A study is conducted to investigate the ability of monocytes to kill certain yeast cells found in patients with cirrhosis of the liver. These cells are harmful in that they leave the patient open to recurrent infections of various sorts. Blood samples are taken from 16 cirrhosis patients and 9 healthy controls. The following data are obtained on the percentage of yeast cells killed by monocytes in the culture (assume normality):

Controls	Patients
$n_1 = 9$	$n_2 = 16$
$\bar{x}_1 = 44.22\%$	$\bar{x}_2 = 28.22\%$
$s_1 = 6.17\%$	$s_2 = 4.11\%$

Compare population variances. Based on the results, compare population means, using the appropriate T statistic. Is there sufficient evidence to claim that the mean percentage of yeast cells killed by monocytes among controls is higher than among patients? Explain.

7. A study is conducted to compare the lead concentration in the water in two households. In one household 50/50 lead–tin solder had been used in the water pipes leading to the home; the solder had not been used in the other location. Data are on water samples taken from the kitchen and bathrooms of the homes as soon as the taps were turned on.

Site 1 (50/50 lead–tin solder used)	Site 2
$n_1 = 25$	$n_2 = 25$
$\bar{x}_1 = 390$ ppb	$\bar{x}_2 = 10$ ppb
$s_1 = 217.5$ ppb	$s_2 = 5$ ppb

It is thought that the average lead concentration in the water at site 1 exceeds that of site 2. Test this hypothesis. (Information found in E. Cosgrove et al.,

"Childhood Lead Poisoning," *Journal of Environmental Health,* July 1989, pp. 346–349.)

8. A study is conducted of preoperative cross-matching in elective surgery. The operation studied is elective abdominal hysterectomy. The variable of interest is X, the number of cross-matched units of blood immediately available. The purpose is to compare the mean number of units available in 1990 to that currently available. The following summary data are available:

1990	Current
$n_1 = 25$	$n_2 = 25$
$\bar{x}_1 = 2.73$	$\bar{x}_2 = 1.27$
$s_1 = .65$	$s_2 = 1.0$

After comparing population variances, find a 95% confidence interval on $\mu_1 - \mu_2$. Is there evidence of a decrease in the mean number of units available from 1990 to the current year? Explain.

9. Consider the data of Exercise 1 of Section 9.2. Find a 90% confidence interval on the difference in the mean airspeed of brown pelicans and oystercatchers when flying cross-wind. Based on this interval, is there evidence that a difference in population means exists? Explain.

10. Consider the data of Exercise 6 of Section 9.2. Find a 95% confidence interval on the difference in the mean growth of peas grown in water and those grown in the fructose solution. Based on this interval, is there evidence of any difference in growth rates? Explain.

11. Studies of hazardous wastes are conducted at two locations. Wastes of interest are those generated by households and small businesses. Examples of such wastes are used oil from automobiles, batteries, antifreeze, paint and paint thinner, and solvents. These data are obtained:

Albuquerque	Anchorage
$n_1 = 96,320$	$n_2 = 81,609$
$\bar{x}_1 = 16.59$ pounds per year	$\bar{x}_2 = 22.06$ pounds per year
$s_1^2 = 25$	$s_2^2 = 36$

Find a 95% confidence interval on the difference in the average number of pounds of hazardous waste produced per sampling unit per year. (Based on studies reported in David Wigglesworth, "Hazardous Waste Management at the Local Level," *Journal of Environmental Health,* August 1989, pp. 323–326.)

12. Competition between species plays an important role in the growth of plants. A study is conducted to investigate the effect of competition on the growth of lettuce. Sixty-four lettuce seeds were planted and allowed to grow in an environment in which only lettuce was present. Thirty-five lettuce seeds were planted in an environment in which the plants were in competition with spinach plants. At the conclusion of the study the dry weight in grams of each lettuce plant was obtained. These data result:

Lettuce alone	Lettuce in competition with spinach
$n_1 = 64$	$n_2 = 35$
$\bar{x}_1 = .030$ g	$\bar{x}_2 = .023$ g
$s_1 = .018$ g	$s_2 = .012$ g

Do these data support the theory that the average dry weight of plants grown in competition is less than that grown in the absence of competition? Be ready to defend your choice of test statistic. (Based on a study conducted by Melissa M. Stone, Department of Biology, Radford University, 1996.)

■ 9.5

INFERENCES ON $\mu_1 - \mu_2$: PAIRED T

In many instances problems arise in which two random samples are available but they are *not* independent; rather, each observation in one sample is naturally or by design paired with an observation in the other. Examples of this sort of pairing occur in twin studies in psychology, medicine, and education; in studies involving pre- and posttests in education and physical education; in studies in which two treatments are administered to the same subject; and in many other settings. Consider Example 9.5.1.

EXAMPLE 9.5.1. A study was conducted to investigate the effect of physical training on the serum cholesterol level. Eleven subjects participated in the study. Prior to training, blood samples were taken to determine the cholesterol level of each subject. Then the subjects were put through a training program that centered on daily running and jogging. At the end of the training period, blood samples were taken again and a second reading on the serum cholesterol level was obtained. Thus, two sets of observations on the serum cholesterol level of the subjects are available. The data sets are not independent; they are based on the same subjects taken at different times and so are naturally paired by subject. These data were collected:

Subject	Pretraining level x, mg/dL	Posttraining level y, mg/dL
1	182	198
2	232	210
3	191	194
4	200	220
5	148	138
6	249	220
7	276	219
8	213	161
9	241	210
10	480	313
11	262	226

The purpose is to estimate the difference between the mean cholesterol level before and after training.

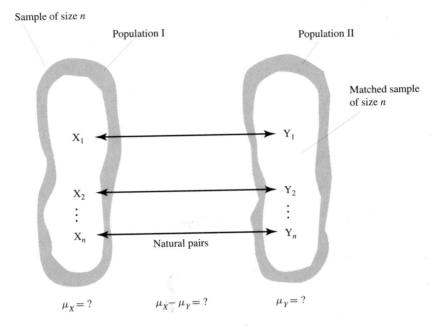

FIGURE 9.7

Paired data.

When pairing such as just illustrated occurs, the methods of Sections 9.3 and 9.4 are no longer applicable. Rather, a procedure for comparing means must take into account the fact that the observations are paired. This is easily done. Consider the generalization of the problem shown in Figure 9.7. Note that associated with this situation is a population of differences $D = X - Y$ and a random sample of differences selected from that population, $D_i = X_i - Y_i$, $i = 1, 2, 3, \ldots, n$. (See Figure 9.8.)

The average value of the difference D is the difference in the average values of X and Y. That is,

$$\mu_D = \mu_X - \mu_Y$$

Therefore, the original question, What is $\mu_X - \mu_Y$? is equivalent to, What is μ_D? We are reduced from the original two-sample problem to the *one*-sample problem of making an inference on the mean of the population of differences. This problem is not new, and it can be handled by using the methods of Chapter 6. In particular, the formula for the confidence bounds on $\mu_X - \mu_Y = \mu_D$ is

$$\bar{D} \pm \frac{t S_d}{\sqrt{n}}$$

(Confidence Interval on the Average Difference)

where $\bar{D}$ and S_d are the sample mean and sample standard deviation of the sample of difference scores, respectively, and t is the appropriate point relative to the T_{n-1} distribution. Use of this formula is illustrated in Example 9.5.2.

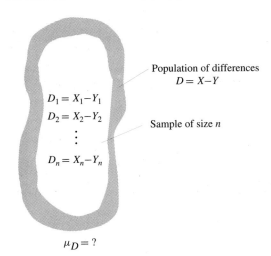

FIGURE 9.8

Paired data generate a population of differences.

Population of differences
$D = X - Y$

Sample of size n

$\mu_D = ?$

EXAMPLE 9.5.2. Consider the data of Example 9.5.1, and form the sample of difference scores by subtracting the second cholesterol reading from the first.

Subject	Pretraining x	Posttraining y	Difference $d = x - y$
1	182	198	−16
2	232	210	22
3	191	194	−3
4	200	220	−20
5	148	138	10
6	249	220	29
7	276	219	57
8	213	161	52
9	241	210	31
10	480	313	167
11	262	226	36

To construct a 90% confidence interval on μ_D, we need to compute the sample mean and the sample standard deviation for the set of difference scores:

For these data,

$$\bar{d} = 33.2 \qquad s_d = 51.1$$

The partition of the $T_{n-1} = T_{10}$ curve needed is shown in Figure 9.9. The desired confidence bounds are

$$\bar{d} \pm t \frac{s_d}{\sqrt{n}} = 33.2 \pm 1.812 \frac{51.1}{\sqrt{11}}$$

$$= 33.2 \pm 27.9$$

We can be 90% confident that the mean difference in serum cholesterol levels is between 5.3 and 61.1 mg/dL. That is, we can be 90% confident that the mean cholesterol level will be reduced by at least 5.3 mg/dL.

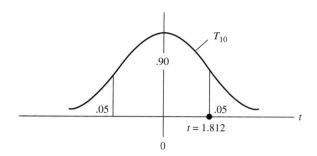

FIGURE 9.9
Partition of the T_{10} curve needed
to obtain a 90% confidence
interval on μ_D.

Paired T Tests

Means can be compared by using the hypothesis testing approach also. The null
hypothesis $\mu_X = \mu_Y$ is equivalent to the hypothesis $\mu_D = 0$. The test statistic for testing
this hypothesis based on the sample of difference scores is

$$\boxed{\frac{\bar{D} - 0}{S_d / \sqrt{n}}} \qquad \text{(Paired } T \text{ Test)}$$

which follows a T distribution with $n - 1$ degrees of freedom if H_0 is true. The use of
this statistic is illustrated in the following example.

> **EXAMPLE 9.5.3.** A study is conducted of tooth emergence in Australian aborigines. The
> purpose is to detect differences, if they exist, in the time of emergence of left- and right-
> side permanent teeth. One tooth studied is the incisor. All subjects are male. The age of the
> subject at the time of emergence of the left incisor and his age at the time of emergence of
> the right incisor are determined. Thus each subject produces a pair of observations. Sum-
> mary statistics for the study are as shown, where the order of subtraction is left-side age
> minus right-side age:
>
> $$n = 17 \qquad \bar{d} = 1.5 \text{ yr} \qquad s_d = 4.7$$
>
> The observed value of the test statistic is
>
> $$\frac{\bar{d} - 0}{s_d / \sqrt{n}} = \frac{1.5}{4.7 / \sqrt{17}} = 1.31$$
>
> Notice that $P[T_{16} \geq 1.31] > .10$. Since no directional preference is indicated, the test is
> two-tailed. The P value for the two-tailed test exceeds .20. There is not enough evidence
> based on this study to claim that there is a difference in the mean time of emergence of left
> and right incisors in male Australian aborigines.

In using these procedures, the assumption is made that the variable $D = X - Y$ is
at least approximately normally distributed.

■ EXERCISES 9.5

1. The effect of physical training on the triglyceride level was also studied by using the 11 subjects of Example 9.5.1. The following pretraining and posttraining readings (in milligrams of triglyceride per 100 milliliters of blood) were obtained:

Subject	Pretraining	Posttraining
1	68	95
2	77	90
3	94	86
4	73	58
5	37	47
6	131	121
7	77	136
8	24	65
9	99	131
10	629	630
11	116	104

Find a 90% confidence interval on the mean change in triglyceride level. Is there evidence that a difference exists? If so, what is the direction of the change?

2. A study was conducted to compare the sodium content in the plasma of young southern fur seals with the level in the milk of these seals. The following observations on the sodium content [in millimoles per liter of milk (or plasma)] were obtained in 10 randomly selected seals:

Subject	Milk	Plasma
1	93	147
2	104	157
3	95	142
4	81.5	141
5	95	142
6	95	147
7	76.5	148
8	80.5	144
9	79.5	144
10	87.0	146

Find a 95% confidence interval on the mean difference in sodium levels in the two body fluids. Is there evidence that a difference exists? If so, what is the direction of the difference?

3. A study is conducted to determine the effect of a home meter for helping diabetics control their blood glucose levels. A random sample of 36 diabetics participate in the study. Blood glucose levels were obtained for each patient before they were taught to use the meter and again after they had utilized the meter for several weeks. A mean sample difference of 2.78 mmol/liter with a sample standard deviation of 6.05 mmol/liter was recorded (subtraction done in the order of "before" minus "after"). Is there sufficient evidence to claim that the monitor is effective in helping

patients to reduce their blood glucose levels? Support your answer based on the P value of the test.

4. It was thought that a program of regular, moderately strenuous exercise could benefit patients who had suffered a previous myocardial infarction Eleven subjects participated in a study to test this contention. Before the program was begun, the working capacity of each person was determined by measuring the time it took to reach a heart rate of 160 beats per minute while walking on a treadmill. After 25 weeks of controlled exercise, the treadmill measurements were repeated and the difference in times for each subject recorded. The following data resulted:

Subject	Pretest	Posttest
1	7.6	14.7
2	9.9	14.1
3	8.6	11.8
4	9.5	16.1
5	8.4	14.7
6	9.2	14.1
7	6.4	13.2
8	9.9	14.9
9	8.7	12.2
10	10.3	13.4
11	8.3	14.0

Do these data support the contention of the investigators? Support your answer based on the P value of the test.

5. Temperature data gathered at 1000 land and sea weather stations across the world yielded an average temperature of 57°F in 1950. In 1988, the average temperature at these stations was 57.6°F. By pairing the 1988 and 1950 readings by station it is estimated that the standard deviation in the difference in readings is $s_d = 4.1$°F. Do these data support the contention that the average temperature in 1988 is higher than in 1950? Explain based on the P value of the appropriate test. (Based on temperatures reported in U.S. Senator Timothy Wirth, "Conservation Is the Key," *Journal of Environmental Health,* Spring 1990, p. 25.)

TECHNOLOGY TOOLS

TI83

The TI83 calculator will perform the F test described in Section 9.2. It will also find both pooled and nonpooled confidence intervals and test hypotheses on the relationship between μ_1 and μ_2 using either the pooled or the Smith-Satterthwaite T test. In finding confidence intervals on running T tests you will be asked whether or not you want to pool variances. You can use either raw data or summary statistics in each case.

XX   *F* test for comparing variances

To illustrate the F test we use the data of Example 9.2.4.

TI83 Keystroke	**Purpose**
1. STAT ◁ ALPHA D	1. Accesses the screen used to conduct the F test
2. cursor to STATS ENTER	2. Indicates that summary statistics rather than raw data will be used to conduct the test
3. ▽ .102	3. Enters .102 as the value of s_1
4. ▽ 41	4. Enters 41 as the value of n_1
5. ▽ .068	5. Enters .068 as the value of s_2
6. ▽ 29	6. Enters 29 as the value of n_2
7. ▽ ENTER	7. Indicates that the test is two-tailed
8. ▽ ENTER	8. Calculates and then displays the value of the F statistic (2.25); displays the P value for the two-tailed test (.0271927299)

XXI   Confidence interval on $\mu_1 - \mu_2$

This procedure is illustrated using the data of Example 9.3.3. In this example, we shall be pooling.

TI83 Keystroke	**Purpose**
1. STAT ◁ 0	1. Accesses the screen needed to form a confidence interval on $\mu_1 - \mu_2$
2. cursor to STATS ENTER	2. Indicates that summary statistics rather than raw data will be used to form the confidence interval
3. ▽ 205	3. Enters 205 as the value of $\bar{x}_1$
4. ▽ 100	4. Enters 100 as the value of s_1
5. ▽ 25	5. Enters 25 as the value of n_1
6. ▽ 135	6. Enters 135 as the value of $\bar{x}_2$
7. ▽ 95	7. Enters 95 as the value of s_2

8.	$\triangledown$	8.	Enters 11 as the value of n_2
	11		
9.	$\triangledown$	9.	Enters .90 as the confidence level
	.90		desired
10.	$\triangledown$	10.	Asks for the variances to be pooled
	$\triangleright$		
	ENTER		
11.	$\triangledown$	11.	Calculates and displays the 90%
	ENTER		confidence interval on $\mu_1 - \mu_2$;
			gives the value of s_p

XXII   Two-sample T test

The data of Example 9.4.1 is used to illustrate the two-sample T test. In this example, pooling is not appropriate.

TI83 Keystroke		**Purpose**	
1.	STAT	1.	Accesses the screen needed
	$\triangleleft$		to conduct a two-sample T test
	4		
2.	cursor to STATS	2.	Indicates that summary statistics
	ENTER		rather than raw data will be used to
			conduct the test
3.	$\triangledown$	3.	Enters .0167 as the value of $\bar{x}_1$
	.0167		
4.	$\triangledown$	4.	Enters .0042 as the value of s_1
	.0042		
5.	$\triangledown$	5.	Enters 57 as the value of n_1
	57		
6.	$\triangledown$	6.	Enters .0144 as the value of $\bar{x}_2$
	.0144		
7.	$\triangledown$	7.	Enters .0024 as the value of s_2
	.0024		
8.	$\triangledown$	8.	Enters 12 as the value of n_2
	12		
9.	$\triangledown$	9.	Indicates that the test is right-tailed
	$\triangleright$		
	$\triangleright$		
	ENTER		
10.	$\triangledown$	10.	Indicates that variances should not be
	ENTER		pooled
11.	$\triangledown$	11.	Calculates the degrees of freedom
	ENTER		(27.51045397); calculates the
			observed value of the test statistic
			(2.588564596); displays the P value
			for the right-tailed test
			(.0076098754)

XXIII   Paired T test

The TI83 calculator can find confidence intervals on the average difference and test hypotheses on the value of μ_D. The technique is illustrated using the data of Example 9.5.2.

TI83 Keystroke	**Purpose**
1. STAT 1	1. Accesses the STAT data editor

2. 182
     ENTER
     232
     ENTER
     $\vdots$
     262
     ENTER
	2. Enters observations on x
	     (pretraining) into column L_1

3   $\triangleright$
     198
     ENTER
     210
     ENTER
     $\vdots$
     226
     ENTER
	3. Enters observations on y
	     (posttraining) into column L_2

4. STAT
     1
     $\triangleright$
     $\triangle$
     2nd
     L_1
     $-$ (subtract)
     2nd
     L_2
     ENTER
	4. Defines L_3 to be $L_1 - L_2$ thus forming
	     a column of difference scores

5. STAT
     $\triangleleft$
     8
	5. Accesses the screen needed to find a
	     confidence interval on μ_D

6. cursor to DATA
     ENTER
	6. Indicates that raw data will be
	     used to conduct the test

7. ∇
     2nd
     L_3
	7. Indicates that a confidence interval
	     is to be found using data in column
	     L_3

8. ∇
     ∇
     ENTER
	8. Indicates that the confidence level is
	     .90

9. ENTER	9. Finds and displays the 90% confidence interval on μ_D

SAS Package

VIII   Two-sample T test

One advantage of running a two-sample T test on the computer is that P values for all pertinent tests are found and reported. The job of the researcher is to interpret the output correctly. We illustrate the idea by considering the data of Exercise 2 of Section 9.3. The SAS code needed to analyze these data is as follows:

SAS Code	**Purpose**
OPTIONS LS=80 PS=60	Sets printing specifications
NODATE;	
DATA SPIDER;	Names data set
INPUT GROUP SIZE;	Names variables
LINES;	Indicates that data
	follows immediately
1 12.9	
1 10.2	Data lines; group 1 is adult
⋮	*Dinopsis* and group 2 is
1 11.3	adult *Menneus*
2 10.2	
2 6.9	
⋮	
2 8.8	
;	Signals the end of the data
PROC TTEST;	Calls for a two-sample T test
CLASS GROUP;	to be run; names the
	variable, GROUP, that
	identifies the two populations
	under study
TITLE 'TESTING FOR EQUALITY	Titles output
OF MEANS AND VARIANCES';	

Notice that in Exercise 2 of Section 9.3 we are comparing the average prey size of the adult *Dinopis* to that of the adult *Menneus*. To decide whether or not to pool variances, the F test or the rule of thumb can be used. The value of s_1^2/s_2^2 with s_1^2 being the larger sample variance is given at ①. Since this value is less than 2, pooling is appropriate. If variances are being compared via the F test, then the P value for the two-tailed test of H_0: $\sigma_1^2 = \sigma_2^2$ is given at ②. Since this P value is large, we have little evidence that $\sigma_1^2 \neq \sigma_2^2$. The F test also indicates that pooling is appropriate. Thus in comparing means a pooled procedure is used. The observed value of the pooled T statistic, its degrees of freedom, and the P value for the two-tailed test of H_0: $\mu_1 = \mu_2$ are given by ③, ④, and ⑤, respectively. If a one-tailed test were being conducted, the researcher would have to realize this fact and divide the reported P value by 2 to obtain the proper P value for the test. The Smith-Satterthwaite T statistic, its degrees of freedom, and the P value for the two-tailed test for equality of means are given by ⑥, ⑦, and $\circled{8}$, respectively. It would be appropriate to use these values to compare means if the rule of thumb or the F test had led us to believe that the population variances were unequal.

TESTING FOR EQUALITY OF MEANS AND VARIANCES
TTEST PROCEDURE

VARIABLE: SIZE

GROUP	N	MEAN	STD DEV	STD ERROR	MINIMUM	MAXIMUM
1	10	10.26000000	2.51360741	0.79487246	7.00000000	14.40000000
2	10	9.02000000	1.89666374	0.59977774	5.30000000	11.00000000

VARIANCES	T	DF	PROB > |T|
	$\circled{6}$	$\circled{7}$	$\circled{8}$
UNEQUAL	1.2453	16.7	0.2302
EQUAL	1.2453	18.0	0.2290
	$\circled{3}$	$\circled{4}$	$\circled{5}$

FOR HO: VARIANCES ARE EQUAL, F' = 1.76 WITH 9 AND 9 DF   PROB > F' = 0.4142
                                         $\circled{1}$ $\circled{2}$

IX Paired T test

The SAS procedure PROC MEANS can be used to run a paired T test. We let SAS from the difference scores and then use PROC MEANS to analyze these differences. The data of Exercise 4 of Section 9.5 are used to illustrate how this is done.

SAS CODE	Purpose
OPTIONS LS=80 PS=60 NODATE;	Sets printing specifications
DATA EXERCISE;	Names the data set
INPUT PRETEST POSTTEST;	Names the variables
D=POSTTEST − PRETEST;	Forms the difference scores
LINES;	Signals that the data follow immediately
7.6 14.7	
9.9 14.1	Data lines
$\vdots$	
8.3 14.0	
;	Signals the end of the data
PROC MEANS MEAN	Asks for $\bar{d}$, s_d to be computed;
STD T PRT;	asks for the T statistic to be computed; finds the P value for testing H$_0$: $\mu_D = 0$ versus H$_1$: $\mu_D \neq 0$
TITLE 'PAIRED T TEST';	Titles output

The output of this program is shown below. Note that $\bar{d}$ is given at ①. The value of s_d is found at ②. The observed value of the test statistic is given at ③, and the P value of the two-tailed test is shown at ④. Since the test that we want is right-tailed, the P value for the test is found by dividing the value shown at ④ by 2. That is, $P = .0001/2 = .00005$.

PAIRED T TEST

Variable	Mean	Std Dev	T	Prob > |T|
PRETEST	8.8000000	1.1392980	25.6177904	0.0001
POSTTEST	13.9272727	1.2345776	37.4148522	0.0001
D	① 5.1272727	② 1.4819520	③ 11.4748922	④ 0.0001

10

k-Sample Procedures:
Introduction to Design

In Chapters 6 and 7 we discuss methods for making inferences on the mean and variance of a single population. Chapter 9 is concerned with methods for comparing the means and variances of two populations. Now we extend the methods of Chapter 9 to include more than two populations. We also introduce some of the elementary aspects of experimental design and *analysis of variance* (ANOVA). The term *experimental design* refers to a broad area of applied statistics that concerns itself with methods for collecting and analyzing data which attempt to maximize the amount and improve the accuracy of the information from a given experiment. The term *analysis of variance* refers to an analytic procedure whereby the total variation in some measured response is subdivided into components that can be attributed to some recognizable source and that can be used to test various hypotheses of interest.

10.1
ONE-WAY CLASSIFICATION, COMPLETELY RANDOM DESIGN WITH FIXED EFFECTS

The first design that we present is the *one-way classification, completely random design with fixed effects*. While describing this design, we introduce some of the general concepts and terminology underlying the areas of experimental design and analysis of variance. We begin by considering two studies that can be analyzed via the analysis of variance technique.

> **EXAMPLE 10.1.1.** A study is run to compare the effectiveness of three comprehensive therapeutic programs for the treatment of mild-to-moderate acne. Three methods are employed:
>
> I. This older method entails twice-daily washing with a polyethylene scrub and an abrasive soap together with the use of 250 mg of tetracycline daily.

    II. This method, currently in use, entails the use of tretinoin cream, avoidance of the sun, twice-daily washing with an emollient soap and water, and utilization of 250 mg of tetracycline twice daily.

    III. This new method entails water avoidance, twice-daily washing with a lipid-free cleanser, and use of tretinoin cream and benzoyl peroxide.

These three treatments are to be compared for effectiveness in reducing the number of acne lesions in patients. Thirty-five patients participate in the study. These patients are randomly split into three subgroups of size 10, 12, and 13. One group is assigned treatment I; another, treatment II; and the third, treatment III. At the end of 16 weeks, the percentage improvement in the number of lesions is noted for each patient.

EXAMPLE 10.1.2. One source of water pollution is industrial and agricultural runoff that is rich in phosphorus. Too much phosphorus can cause a population explosion of plants and microorganisms referred to as *bloom*. In a given region, the phosphorus level in four major lakes is to be determined by drawing and analyzing water samples from each lake. It is thought that one of the lakes is being unduly polluted by the runoff from a nearby industrial plant. It is hoped that by comparing the phosphorus level of this lake with that of others in the area this fact will become evident.

Examples 10.1.1 and 10.1.2 illustrate two commonly encountered experimental situations in which the *one-way classification, completely random design with fixed effects* comes into play. They are described in general as follows:

1. We have a collection of N experimental units and wish to study the effects of k different treatments. These units are randomly divided into k groups of size n_1, $n_2, \ldots, n_k$, and each subgroup receives a different treatment. A response is noted. The k subgroups are viewed as constituting independent random samples of size $n_1, n_2, \ldots, n_k$ drawn from populations with mean responses $\mu_1, \mu_2, \ldots, \mu_k$, respectively. We want to test the null hypothesis that the treatments have the same average effect:

$$H_0: \mu_1 = \mu_2 = \cdots = \mu_k \qquad \text{(no difference in means for the } k \text{ treatments)}$$

$$H_1: \mu_i \neq \mu_j \text{ for some } i \text{ and } j \qquad \text{(at least one mean differs from others)}$$

2. We have k populations, each identified by some common characteristic to be studied in the experiment. Independent random samples of sizes $n_1, n_2, \ldots, n_k$ are selected from each of the k populations, respectively. Each sample receives the same treatment, and any differences observed in the measured responses are attributed to basic differences among the k populations. The hypothesis is

$$H_0: \mu_1 = \mu_2 = \cdots = \mu_k \qquad \text{(no difference in population means)}$$

$$H_1: \mu_i \neq \mu_j \text{ for some } i \text{ and } j \qquad \text{(at least one mean differs from others)}$$

where μ_i denotes the mean response for the ith population.

Although these situations are experimentally somewhat different, they are similar in that each results in k independent random samples drawn from k populations with

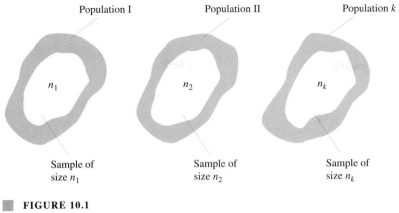

FIGURE 10.1

H_0: $\mu_1 = \mu_2 = \cdots = \mu_k$. (Are the population means equal?)

means $\mu_1, \mu_2, \ldots, \mu_k$, respectively. The purpose of the experiment in each case is to compare population means. This design represents the natural extension of the two-sample unpaired means comparison of Chapter 9 to more than two samples. The situation can be visualized as shown in Figure 10.1.

EXAMPLE 10.1.3. Example 10.1.1 satisfies the first general description. A collection of $N = 35$ patients, each suffering from mild-to-moderate acne, is available for experimentation. There are $k = 3$ treatments to be compared. The patients are randomly divided into three subgroups of sizes $n_1 = 10$, $n_2 = 12$, and $n_3 = 13$. Each subgroup receives a different treatment, and the response noted is the percentage improvement in the number of lesions observed at the end of 16 weeks of treatment. The three subgroups are viewed as constituting independent random samples drawn from the populations of all patients receiving treatments I, II, and III, respectively. Based on the data obtained, we wish to test

H_0: $\mu_1 = \mu_2 = \mu_3$ (no difference in mean
                      response among three treatments)

H_1: $\mu_i \neq \mu_j$ for some i and j (at least one treatment mean
                      differs from others)

EXAMPLE 10.1.4. Example 10.1.2 satisfies the second general description. We are studying $k = 4$ lakes. Each lake constitutes a population. Independent samples are selected from each lake. Each sample receives the same treatment in that each is analyzed for phosphorus by the same method. Any differences in mean phosphorus levels that appear are attributed to the fact that the samples were drawn from different lakes with varying water compositions.

Each example is a *one-way classification, completely random design with fixed effects*. The term *one-way classification* refers to the fact that only one factor is under study in each experiment. The experiment involves k levels of this factor. In Example 10.1.1, the factor of interest is the type of treatment received. No other factors, such as age, skin type, dietary habits, or sex of the patient, are being considered. Three treatments are being studied; thus the factor is being investigated at three levels. In Example 10.1.2, the only factor being considered is the lake involved. No other factors, such as temperature, season, or depth of the lake, are of interest in the study. Since four lakes are involved, four levels of the factor are under study. The term *completely random design* refers to the fact that no attempt has been made to match experimental units across samples. The *k* samples are independent of one another. The term *fixed effects* refers to the fact that the levels of the factor involved are specifically selected by the experimenter because they are of particular interest. They are not randomly selected from a larger group of possible levels. In Example 10.1.1, the purpose of the experiment is to compare the three specific treatments. The treatments are not randomly selected from a large group of acne treatments available. In Example 10.1.2, the four lakes selected for the study are chosen specifically because they are the major lakes in the region. They are not randomly selected from all the lakes in the region.

Data Format and Notation

The data collected in a single-factor experiment are conveniently recorded in the following format:

Data layout for one-way classification

	Factor level			
1	**2**	**3**	. . .	**k**
X_{11}	X_{21}	X_{31}	. . .	X_{k1}
X_{12}	X_{22}	X_{32}	. . .	X_{k2}
X_{13}	X_{23}	X_{33}	. . .	X_{k3}
X_{1n_1}	X_{2n_2}	X_{3n_3}	. . .	X_{kn_k}

Note that n_i is the size of the sample drawn from the ith population and that $N = \sum_{i=1}^{k} n_i$ denotes the total number of responses. Furthermore, X_{ij}, $i = 1, 2, \ldots, k$, $j = 1, 2, \ldots, n_i$, is a random variable denoting the response of the jth experimental unit to the ith level of the factor. In using sample data to compare population means, these statistics are required:

$$T_{i\cdot} = \sum_{j=1}^{n_i} X_{ij} = \text{total of all responses in } i\text{th level, } i = 1, 2, \ldots, k$$

$$\bar{X}_{i\cdot} = \frac{T_{i\cdot}}{n_i} = \text{sample mean for } i\text{th level, } i = 1, 2, \ldots, k$$

$$T_{\cdot\cdot} = \sum_{i=1}^{k} \sum_{j=1}^{n_i} X_{ij} = \sum_{i=1}^{k} T_{i\cdot} = \text{total of all responses}$$

$$\bar{X}_{\cdot\cdot} = \frac{T_{\cdot\cdot}}{N} = \text{sample mean of all responses}$$

$$\sum_{i=1}^{k} \sum_{j=1}^{n_i} X_{ij}^2 = \text{sum of square of each response}$$

In this notation note that the dot indicates the subscript over which summation is being conducted. For example, $T_{1\cdot}$ is the sum of all of the observations in level 1. That is,

$$T_{1\cdot} = X_{11} + X_{12} + X_{13} + \cdots + X_{1n_1}$$

The first subscript is always 1; the second subscript varies from 1 to n_1. The dot in T_1. indicates that the second subscript is the one whose value changes. The evaluation of these statistics is illustrated in Example 10.1.5.

EXAMPLE 10.1.5. When the experiment of Example 10.1.1 was conducted, the following data resulted. Recall that the observed response is the percentage improvement in the number of acne lesions noted per patient at the end of 16 weeks of treatment.

Factor (treatment received) level

I		II		III	
48.6	50.8	68.0	71.9	67.5	61.4
49.4	47.1	67.0	71.5	62.5	67.4
50.1	52.5	70.1	69.9	64.2	65.4
49.8	49.0	64.5	68.9	62.5	63.2
50.6	46.7	68.0	67.8	63.9	61.2
		68.3	68.9	64.8	60.5
				62.3	

Note that $n_1 = 10, n_2 = 12, n_3 = 13$, and $N = \sum_{i=1}^{3} n_i = 10 + 12 + 13 = 35$. The observation 70.1 corresponds to the response of the third experimental unit to the second factor level and thus is the observed value of the random variable X_{23}. The observed values of the other pertinent statistics are

$$T_1. = \sum_{j=1}^{10} X_{1j} = \text{sum of responses to treatment I}$$

$$= 48.6 + 49.4 + 50.1 + \cdots + 46.7 = 494.6$$

$$T_2. = \sum_{j=1}^{12} X_{2j} = \text{sum of responses to treatment II}$$

$$= 68.0 + 67.0 + 70.1 + \cdots + 68.9 = 824.8$$

$$T_3. = \sum_{j=1}^{13} X_{3j} = \text{sum of responses to treatment III}$$

$$= 67.5 + 62.5 + 64.2 + \cdots + 60.5 = 826.8$$

$$\bar{X}_1. = \frac{T_1.}{n_1} = \text{sample mean of responses to treatment I}$$

$$= \frac{494.6}{10} = 49.46$$

$$\bar{X}_2. = \frac{T_2.}{n_2} = \text{sample mean of responses to treatment II}$$

$$= \frac{824.8}{12} = 68.73$$

$$\bar{X}_3. = \frac{T_3.}{n_3} = \text{sample mean of responses to treatment III}$$

$$= \frac{826.8}{13} = 63.60$$

$$T_{..} = \sum_{i=1}^{3} T_{i.} = T_{1.} + T_{2.} + T_{3.} = \text{grand total of all responses}$$

$$= 494.6 + 824.8 + 826.8 = 2146.2$$

$$\bar{X}_{..} = \frac{T_{..}}{N} = \text{sample mean of all responses}$$

$$= \frac{2146.2}{35} = 61.32$$

$$\sum_{i=1}^{3} \sum_{j=1}^{n_i} X_{ij}^2 = (48.6)^2 + (49.4)^2 + (50.1)^2 + \cdots + (60.5)^2$$

$$= 133{,}868.94$$

Testing H_0: $\mu_1 = \mu_2 = \cdots = \mu_k$

To see how these statistics can be used to test the hypothesis that the population means are equal, we must introduce a model for the *one-way classification, completely random design with fixed effects.* A model is a mathematical representation of a typical response that breaks the response into components attributable to various identifiable sources. The following notation is used in writing the model:

$\mu_i =$ theoretical average or expected response
    at ith level, $i = 1, 2, \ldots, k$
  $=$ mean of ith population (unknown constant)

$\mu =$ theoretical average or expected response, ignoring
    factor levels (unknown constant)
  $=$ mean of population that results by combining
    k populations into one

Note that if the levels of the factor have no effect on the response, then the means μ_1, $\mu_2, \ldots, \mu_k$ will all be the same and will equal the grand mean μ; if the factor levels do affect the response, then this will not be the case. Thus the difference between the mean of the ith level and the grand mean $\mu_i - \mu$ indicates the effect, if any, of the ith level of the factor. Furthermore, note that even though each member of the ith population receives the same treatment, the responses obtained will still vary somewhat because of random influences. That is, within each population there is some natural variability about the population mean. For a particular response X_{ij}, this variability is given by the difference $X_{ij} - \mu_i$. This difference is referred to as the *random error.* With these comments in mind, the model for the *one-way classification, completely random design with fixed effects,* can be expressed as follows:

MODEL

$$X_{ij} \equiv \mu + (\mu_i - \mu) + (X_{ij} - \mu_i) \qquad \begin{array}{l} i = 1, 2, \ldots, k \\ j = 1, 2, \ldots, n_i \end{array}$$

This model expresses mathematically the idea that each response can be partitioned into three recognizable components as follows:

| Response of jth experimental unit of ith treatment (X_{ij}) | $\equiv$ overall mean response (μ) | + deviation from overall mean due to fact that unit received ith treatment ($\mu_i - \mu$) | + random deviation from ith population mean due to random influences ($X_{ij} - \mu_i$) |

Figure 10.2 illustrates this idea graphically.

As in the past, to test the null hypothesis, a test statistic must be derived. The statistic should be logical, but more importantly, its probability distribution must be known under the assumption that the null hypothesis is true and the k population means are equal. For this to occur, certain assumptions must be made about the populations from which the samples are drawn. In particular, we assume the following:

MODEL ASSUMPTIONS

1. The k samples represent independent random samples drawn from k specific populations with means $\mu_1, \mu_2, \ldots, \mu_k$, where $\mu_1, \mu_2, \ldots, \mu_k$, are unknown constants.
2. Each of the k populations is normally distributed.
3. Each of the k populations has the *same* variance, σ^2.

Note that these assumptions parallel those made in Chapter 9 relative to the pooled T procedure for comparing two means.

Analysis of variance has been defined as a procedure whereby the total variation in some measured response is subdivided into components that can be attributed to recognizable sources. Since $\mu, \mu_1, \mu_2, \ldots, \mu_k$ are theoretical population means, the

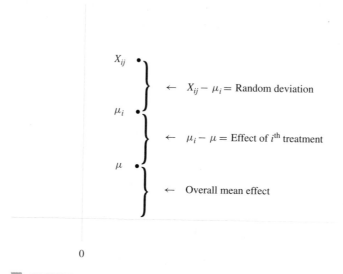

0

FIGURE 10.2

Value of the *ij*th observation is partitional into three components: the overall mean effect μ, the effect of the *i*th treatment $\mu_i - \mu$, and the random or unexplained deviation $X_{ij} - \mu_i$.

model does this in only the theoretical sense. To partition an observation in a practical way, these theoretical means must be replaced by their estimators $\bar{X}_{..}, \bar{X}_{1.}, \bar{X}_{2.}, \ldots, \bar{X}_{k.}$, respectively. By replacing the theoretical means by their estimators in the model, the following identity is obtained:

$$X_{ij} \equiv \bar{X}_{..} + (\bar{X}_{i.} - \bar{X}_{..}) + (X_{ij} - \bar{X}_{i.})$$

Note that $\bar{X}_{..}$ is an estimator for μ, the overall mean of the combined population; $\bar{X}_{i.} - \bar{X}_{..}$ is an estimator for $\mu_i - \mu$, the effect of the *i*th treatment; and $X_{ij} - \bar{X}_{i.}$ is an estimator for $X_{ij} - \mu_i$, the random error. The term $X_{ij} - \bar{X}_{i.}$ is usually called a *residual*. This identity is equivalent to

$$X_{ij} - \bar{X}_{..} \equiv (\bar{X}_{i.} - \bar{X}_{..}) + (X_{ij} - \bar{X}_{i.})$$

If each side of the above identity is squared and then summed over all possible values of *i* and *j*, the following identity, called the *sum-of-squares identity for the one-way classification design*, results.

SUM-OF-SQUARES IDENTITY

$$\sum_{i=1}^{k} \sum_{j=1}^{n_i} (X_{ij} - \bar{X}_{..})^2 \equiv \sum_{i=1}^{k} n_i (\bar{X}_{i.} - \bar{X}_{..})^2 + \sum_{i=1}^{k} \sum_{j=1}^{n_i} (X_{ij} - \bar{X}_{i.})^2$$

The derivation of this identity is a straightforward application of the rules of summation. Note that there are three components in this identity. Each has a practical interpretation that should not be overlooked. In particular,

$$\sum_{i=1}^{k} \sum_{j=1}^{n_i} (X_{ij} - \bar{X}_{..})^2 = \text{sum of squares of deviations of observations from grand mean}$$
$$= \text{measure of total variability in data}$$
$$= \text{total sum of squares} = SS_{\text{Total}}$$

$$\sum_{i=1}^{k} n_i (\bar{X}_{i.} - \bar{X}_{..})^2 = \text{weighted sum of squares of deviations of level or treatment means from grand mean}$$
$$= \text{measure of variability in data attributed to fact that different levels or treatments are used}$$
$$= \text{treatment sum of squares} = SS_{\text{Tr}}$$

$$\sum_{i=1}^{k} \sum_{j=1}^{n_i} (X_{ij} - \bar{X}_{i.})^2 = \text{sum of squares of deviations of observations from treatment mean associated with observation}$$
$$= \text{measure of variability in data attributed to random fluctuation among subjects within same factor level}$$
$$= \text{residual, or error, sum of squares} = SS_E$$

By using this shorthand notation, the sum-of-squares identity can be written

$$SS_{\text{Total}} = SS_{\text{Tr}} + SS_E$$

To test $H_0: \mu_1 = \mu_2 = \cdots = \mu_k$

we need to define two statistics that are functions of SS_{Tr} and SS_E. The first, called the *treatment mean square* MS_{Tr}, is found by dividing SS_{Tr} by $k - 1$; the second, called the *error mean square* MS_E, is found by dividing SS_E by $N - k$. That is, we define

$$MS_{Tr} = \frac{SS_{Tr}}{k - 1} = \text{treatment mean square}$$

$$MS_E = \frac{SS_E}{N - k} = \text{residual mean square}$$

Since each of these mean squares is a statistic, it is also a random variable. As such, it has a probability distribution and a mean, or an expected, value. These expected values are particularly important, for they provide the logical basis for testing for equality of means by the ANOVA procedure. Although the proofs are beyond the scope of this text, it can be shown that

$$E[MS_{Tr}] = \sigma^2 + \sum_{i=1}^{k} \frac{n_i(\mu_i - \mu)^2}{k - 1}$$

and

$$E[MS_E] = \sigma^2$$

How can MS_{Tr} and MS_E be used to test H_0? To answer this question, we need only note that if H_0 is true, then $\mu_1 = \mu_2 = \cdots = \mu_k = \mu$ and hence

$$\sum_{i=1}^{k} \frac{n_i(\mu_i - \mu)^2}{k - 1} = 0$$

If H_0 is not true, this term will be positive. Thus if H_0 is true, we would expect MS_{Tr} and MS_E to be close in value, since both estimate the same parameter, namely σ^2; if H_0 is not true, we would expect MS_{Tr} to be somewhat larger than MS_E. This suggests the ratio

$$\frac{MS_{Tr}}{MS_E}$$

as a logical test statistic. If H_0 is true, its value should lie close to 1; otherwise, it should have a value larger than 1. The ratio can be used as a test statistic since if H_0 is true, it is known to have an F distribution with $k - 1$ and $N - k$ degrees of freedom. The test is always a right-tailed test with rejection of H_0 occurring for values of the statistic

$$\boxed{F_{k-1,N-k} = \frac{MS_{Tr}}{MS_E}}$$ (Test Statistic)

that appear to be *too large* to have occurred by chance.

Computing SS_{Total}, SS_{Tr}, and SS_E directly from the definitions given is awkward. For this reason computational formulas have been developed that are easier to handle and are especially convenient for use with electronic calculators. These formulas are a direct consequence of the rules of summation.

TABLE 10.1

Analysis of variance: One-way classification, completely random design with fixed effects

Source of variation	Degrees of freedom DF	Sum of squares SS	Mean square MS	Expected mean square	F ratio
Treatment, or level	$k-1$	$\sum_{i=1}^{k} \frac{T_{i.}^2}{n_i} - \frac{T_{..}^2}{N}$ (SS_{Tr})	$\frac{SS_{Tr}}{k-1}$	$\sigma^2 + \sum_{i=1}^{k} \frac{n_i(\mu_i - \mu)^2}{k-1}$	$F_{k-1,N-k} = \frac{MS_{Tr}}{MS_E}$
Residual, or error	$N-k$	$SS_{Total} - SS_{Tr}$ (SS_E)	$\frac{SS_E}{N-k}$	σ^2	
Total	$N-1$	$\sum_{i=1}^{k} \sum_{j=1}^{n_i} X_{ij}^2 - \frac{T_{..}^2}{N}$ (SS_{Total})			

COMPUTATIONAL FORMULAS

$$SS_{Total} = \sum_{i=1}^{k} \sum_{j=1}^{n_i} X_{ij}^2 - \frac{T_{..}^2}{N}$$

$$SS_{Tr} = \sum_{i=1}^{k} \frac{T_{i.}^2}{n_i} - \frac{T_{..}^2}{N}$$

$$SS_E = SS_{Total} - SS_{Tr}$$

Everything that has been said here can be summarized conveniently in tabular form. Keep in mind that k denotes the number of treatments or levels of the factor being investigated; n_i, the number of observations selected from the ith population; $T_{i.}$, the sum of the observations for the ith level; N, the total number of observations; and $T_{..}$, the sum of all observations. See Table 10.1. Note that the columns labeled "degrees of freedom" and "sum of squares" are additive. That is, the degrees of freedom for treatments and for error add to $N-1$, the total number of degrees of freedom. Furthermore, $SS_{Tr} + SS_E = SS_{Total}$.

The ANOVA procedure is illustrated in Example 10.1.6.

EXAMPLE 10.1.6. In Example 10.1.5, we began the calculations necessary to test the null hypothesis that the three acne treatments have the same mean effect. In particular, the following values were obtained:

$T_{1.} = 494.6$ $\quad \sum_{i=1}^{3} \sum_{j=1}^{n_i} X_{ij}^2 = 133{,}868.94$ $\quad n_1 = 10$

$T_{2.} = 824.8$ $\qquad\qquad\qquad\qquad\qquad\qquad n_2 = 12$

$T_{3.} = 826.8$ $\qquad\qquad\qquad\qquad\qquad\qquad n_3 = 13$

$T_{..} = 2146.2$ $\qquad\qquad\qquad\qquad\qquad\qquad N = 35$

From these basic statistics we can evaluate SS_{Total}, SS_{Tr}, and SS_E:

$$SS_{Total} = \sum_{i=1}^{3} \sum_{j=1}^{n_i} X_{ij}^2 - \frac{T_{..}^2}{N}$$

$$= 133{,}868.94 - \frac{(2146.2)^2}{35} = 2263.96$$

$$SS_{Tr} = \sum_{i=1}^{3} \frac{T_{i.}^2}{n_i} - \frac{T_{..}^2}{N}$$

$$= \frac{(494.6)^2}{10} + \frac{(824.8)^2}{12} + \frac{(826.8)^2}{13} - \frac{(2146.2)^2}{35} = 2133.66$$

$$SS_E = SS_{Total} - SS_{Tr}$$

$$= 2263.96 - 2133.66 = 130.30$$

The corresponding mean squares are given by

$$MS_{Tr} = \frac{SS_{Tr}}{k-1} = \frac{SS_{Tr}}{2} = \frac{2133.66}{2} = 1066.83$$

$$MS_E = \frac{SS_E}{N-k} = \frac{SS_E}{32} = \frac{130.30}{32} = 4.07$$

The observed value of the test statistic is

$$F_{k-1,N-k} = F_{2,32} = \frac{MS_{Tr}}{MS_E}$$

$$= \frac{1066.83}{4.07} = 262.12$$

Remember that H_0 is to be rejected if this value is significantly larger than 1. This certainly appears to be the case! To be sure, we check the F tables. From these tables, we see that

$$P = P[F_{2,32} > 262.12] < .01$$

Since this P value is small, we do have statistical evidence that the three treatments differ in mean effect. It is customary to summarize the results in an analysis-of-variance (ANOVA) table. The ANOVA table for these data is shown in Table 10.2.

A few comments of a practical nature should be made. We are assuming that the sampled populations are normally distributed and that population variances are equal. Tests are available for checking these assumptions. In Chapter 13 we present the Lilliefors test, a graphical procedure for testing for normality, and Bartlett's test, an analytic procedure used to compare variances. It should also be noted that in the one-way classification model, sample sizes can be unequal. However, there are some distinct advantages to having equal sample sizes. First, the consequences of violating the assumption of equal variances are not serious if the samples are the same size. Thus, in this case, running Bartlett's test or some other test for equal variances, though desirable, is not essential. Second, if H_0 is rejected and the population means are declared

TABLE 10.2
ANOVA for the data of Example 10.1.6

Source	DF	SS	MS	F
Treatment	2	2133.66	1066.83	262.12
Error	32	130.30	4.07	
Total	34	2263.96		

unequal, usually some further tests are desirable. Many of these tests are designed with equal sample sizes in mind.

    In practice, one-way studies are usually run on the computer rather than by hand. In the Technology Tools section at the end of this chapter, we present the TI83 analysis and the SAS program used to conduct such studies.

▎ EXERCISES 10.1

1. Carbon dioxide is known to have a critical effect on microbiological growth. Small amounts of CO_2 stimulate the growth of many organisms, while high concentrations inhibit the growth of most. The latter effect is used commercially when perishable food products are stored. A study is conducted to investigate the effect of CO_2 on the growth rate of *Pseudomonas fragi,* a food spoiler. Carbon dioxide is administered at five different atmospheric pressures. The response noted is the percentage change in cell mass after a 1-hour growing time. Ten cultures are used at each level. The following data are found:

Factor (CO_2 pressure in atmospheres) level

0.0	.083	.29	.50	.86
62.6	50.9	45.5	29.5	24.9
59.6	44.3	41.1	22.8	17.2
64.5	47.5	29.8	19.2	7.8
59.3	49.5	38.3	20.6	10.5
58.6	48.5	40.2	29.2	17.8
64.6	50.4	38.5	24.1	22.1
50.9	35.2	30.2	22.6	22.6
56.2	49.9	27.0	32.7	16.8
52.3	42.6	40.0	24.4	15.9
62.8	41.6	33.9	29.6	8.8

(*a*) We assume fixed effects. What does this imply concerning the atmospheric levels chosen?

(*b*) State the null hypothesis to be tested.

(*c*) Find the values of $T_{i.}$, $\bar{X}_{i.}$, $T_{..}$, $\bar{X}_{..}$, and $\sum_{i=1}^{5} \sum_{j=1}^{10} X_{ij}^2$.

(*d*) Find SS_{Total}, SS_{Tr}, and SS_E.

(*e*) Find MS_{Tr} and MS_E.

(*f*) Evaluate the F statistics used to test H_0.

(*g*) Can H_0 be rejected? Explain based on the P value of the test.

(*h*) What assumptions are you making concerning the five sampled populations?

2. Chlorpropamide/alcohol flushing (CPAF) is a facial flushing experienced by diabetic patients on chlorpropamide after consumption of alcohol. An experiment is run to study the ability of indomethacin to block this reaction. Three groups of diabetics participated in the study: I, diabetics with no complications; II, diabetics with severe retinopathy; and III, diabetics with large-vessel disease. Each patient's facial temperature is taken at the beginning of the experiment, and then 250 mg of chlorpropamide is given. After 12 hours the patient is given 40 mL of sherry and the facial

temperature is noted. The experiment is repeated, with each patient receiving 100 mg of indomethacin 75 minutes before receiving the sherry. Again the change in facial temperature is noted. The following observations are obtained on X, the difference in temperature (temperature after indomethacin is used minus temperature before indomethacin is taken):

Factor (type of diabetic) level

I	II	III
−.23	.32	−.35
−.76	.25	−.13
−.15	.29	.16
−.34	.07	.12
−.54	.10	−.43
−1.90	.18	.49
−2.07	.16	−.30
−1.21	.23	.44

(a) State the null hypothesis to be tested.

(b) Test the null hypothesis by completing the ANOVA table. Assume normality.

(c) Practically speaking, what is the significance of the negative signs associated with some of the observations?

3. A study is run of the sulfur content of five major coal seams in Texas. Core samples are taken at random from each of the seams and analyzed. The data on the percentage of sulfur per plug are shown below. Assuming normality and equal variances, test for equality of means. What conclusions can be drawn from these data?

Factor (coal seam) level

1	2	3	4	5
1.51	1.69	1.56	1.30	.73
1.92	.64	1.22	.75	.80
1.08	.90	1.32	1.26	.90
2.04	1.41	1.39	.69	1.24
2.14	1.01	1.33	.62	.82
1.76	.84	1.54	.90	.72
1.17	1.28	1.04	1.20	.57
	1.59	2.25	.32	1.18
		1.49		.54
				1.30

4. A study is run to determine the effects of a chloralkali plant on fish living in the river that flows past the plant. The variable of interest is the total mercury level in micrograms per gram of body weight per fish in the area. Fish samples are taken from four sites along the river:

   I. 5.5 km above the plant
   II. 3.7 km below the plant
   III. 21 km below the plant
   IV. 133 km below the plant

The following data are found:

Factor (location along river) level

I	II	III	IV
.45	1.64	1.56	.65
.35	1.67	1.55	.59
.32	1.85	1.69	.69
.68	1.57	1.67	.62
.53	1.59	1.60	.70
.34	1.61	1.68	.64
.61	1.53	1.65	.81
.41	1.40	1.59	.58
.51	1.70	1.75	.53
.71	1.48	1.49	.75

Assuming normality, test for equality of means.

5. A study is conducted of several species of birds that are similar in nature and share a common environment. The song of each species has a distinctive set of features that permits recognition. One characteristic under investigation is the length of the song in seconds. Three species are studied: the towhee, the common yellowthroat, and the brown thrasher. The following data are obtained:

Factor (species) level

Towhee	Common yellowthroat	Brown thrasher
1.11	2.17	.42
1.23	1.85	.93
.91	1.99	.77
.95	1.74	.37
.99	1.54	.50
1.08	1.86	.48
1.18	1.87	.68
1.29	2.04	.62
1.12	1.69	.39
.88		.67
1.34		1.03
		.79

Assuming normality and equal variances, test the null hypothesis that the mean song lengths are the same for all three species.

6. A study is conducted to investigate the growth of red oak trees at three different elevations (975 meters, 825 meters, and 675 meters). The variable is the core measurement in centimeters for a 10-year period. These data result:

975 m	825 m	675 m	975 m	825 m	675 m
3.8	5.0	1.8	2.8	3.0	2.3
1.3	2.0	2.3	3.8	1.6	1.1
2.6	2.9	2.0	1.5	1.4	1.1
2.2	3.4	2.2	4.0	3.0	2.6
2.0	3.2	2.4	1.7	1.3	2.1

Based on these data, can it be concluded that there was a difference in the average 10-year growth for these trees at these three elevations? Explain based on the P value of your ANOVA. (Based on a study conducted by Allison Field, Department of Biology, Radford University, 1996.)

▨ 10.2

PAIRED AND MULTIPLE COMPARISONS

Once a one-way classification analysis of variance has been run to compare k population means, we shall be in exactly one of two possible situations:

1. We have been unable to reject H_0. Based on the available data, we have been unable to detect any differences among the k population means. In this case, the analysis of the data is complete.
2. We have been able to reject H_0 and therefore conclude that there are some differences among the k population means. In this case, the analysis of the data has just begun, since it is natural to continue the investigation to try to pinpoint where the differences lie.

There are several methods for detecting differences among population means once the hypothesis of equality has been rejected. Lentner and Bishop [9] present a very good overview of most of these. Here, we discuss two possibilities. These are *Bonferroni T tests* and *Duncan's multiple range test.*

Bonferroni T Tests: Paired Comparisons

Consider a set of k population means. There are $\binom{k}{2} = k(k-1)/2$ possible pairs of means that can be formed. Thus there are $k(k-1)/2$ possible tests of the form

$$H_0: \mu_i = \mu_j$$
$$H_1: \mu_i \neq \mu_j$$

that can be conducted. For example, if we are comparing five means, then $k = 5$ and there are $k(k-1)/2 = 10$ possible tests that can be performed. These are

$H_0: \mu_1 = \mu_2 \qquad H_0: \mu_1 = \mu_3 \qquad H_0: \mu_1 = \mu_4 \qquad H_0: \mu_1 = \mu_5$
$H_1: \mu_1 \neq \mu_2 \qquad H_1: \mu_1 \neq \mu_3 \qquad H_1: \mu_1 \neq \mu_4 \qquad H_1: \mu_1 \neq \mu_5$

$\qquad H_0: \mu_2 = \mu_3 \qquad H_0: \mu_2 = \mu_4 \qquad H_0: \mu_2 = \mu_5$
$\qquad H_1: \mu_2 \neq \mu_3 \qquad H_1: \mu_2 \neq \mu_4 \qquad H_1: \mu_2 \neq \mu_5$

$\qquad H_0: \mu_3 = \mu_4 \qquad H_0: \mu_3 = \mu_5$
$\qquad H_1: \mu_3 \neq \mu_4 \qquad H_1: \mu_3 \neq \mu_5$

$\qquad H_0: \mu_4 = \mu_5$
$\qquad H_1: \mu_4 \neq \mu_5$

Since one of the model assumptions is that the population variances are equal, each of these hypotheses can be tested using a two-tailed pooled T test as described in Chapter 9. In such a test, the test statistic is

$$T_{n_i+n_j-2} = \frac{|\bar{X}_{i\cdot} - \bar{X}_{j\cdot}|}{\sqrt{S_p^2(1/n_i + 1/n_j)}}$$

where S_p^2 is the pooled estimator for σ^2, the common population variance, based on samples drawn from populations i and j. In the setting we are now considering, another estimator of σ^2 is available, namely MS_E. Since this estimator is based on all available data, the T test can be improved by using

$$\boxed{T_{N-k} = \frac{|\bar{X}_{i\cdot} - \bar{X}_{j\cdot}|}{\sqrt{MS_E(1/n_i + 1/n_j)}}}$$

as the test statistic. Performing $k(k-1)/2$ individual T tests by hand is laborious, but it can be done. Many commercial statistical packages include a procedure for conducting Bonferroni T tests based on the above statistic.

This procedure has a serious drawback that must be handled with care. Namely, if all tests are performed at an α level of significance, then the overall probability of making at least one incorrect rejection, denoted by α', is larger than α and its value is usually unknown. However, it can be shown that whenever a set of c tests is conducted each at the α level of significance, then α' is at most $1 - (1 - \alpha)^c$. For example, if $k = 5$, then, as shown previously, there are 10 possible pairs of means that can be compared. If each test is conducted at the $\alpha = .05$ level, then the probability of making at least one incorrect rejection is at most $1 - (1 - .05)^{10} = .40$. It is easy to see that as k increases, the overall probability of error may become unacceptably high. To compensate for this problem, it is suggested that *only those tests of real interest to the researcher be conducted.* As a parallel, consider a physician who orders a series of diagnostic tests to be run on a particular patient. Each test has a predetermined false- positive rate; that is, there is a chance that each test will detect a condition that is in fact not present. If enough tests are conducted, eventually a false-positive result will be obtained. If enough tests are conducted, eventually the patient will be found to have a condition that is in fact not present and an error will be made. The physician should not routinely check for every known disorder, but rather should test only for those conditions which he or she suspects might be the cause of the patient's problem.

To conduct Bonferroni T tests in a responsible way, we choose some reasonably small target upper bound b for the probability of making at least one incorrect rejection. We then conduct each T test at the b/c level of significance where c denotes the actual number of tests run. For example, if we want α' to be at most .10 and we run all possible tests for $k = 5$ groups, we would conduct each of our paired comparisons at the $\alpha = .10/10 = .01$ level of significance. Example 10.2.1 illustrates the procedure.

EXAMPLE 10.2.1. A chemical engineer is studying a newly developed polymer to be used in removing toxic wastes from water. Experiments are conducted at five different temperatures. The response noted is the percentage of impurities removed by the treatment. These data are obtained:

Temperature

I	II	III	IV	V
40	36	49	47	55
45	42	51	49	60
42	38	53	51	62
48	39	53	52	63
50	37	52	50	59
51	40	50	51	61

The ANOVA table for these data is given in Table 10.3. Notice that the hypothesis H_0: $\mu_1 = \mu_2 = \mu_3 = \mu_4 = \mu_5$ can be rejected with $P < .01$. Suppose that we want to run all 10 paired comparisons and that we want the probability of making at least one incorrect rejection to be at most .10. To achieve this goal, each T test must be conducted at the $b/c = .10/10 = .01$ level. The test statistic for the two-tailed test is

$$T_{N-k} = \frac{|\bar{X}_{i\cdot} - \bar{X}_{j\cdot}|}{\sqrt{MS_E(1/n_i + 1/n_j)}}$$

Since sample sizes are each equal to 6, in this case the T statistic is of the form

$$T_{25} = \frac{|\bar{X}_{i\cdot} - \bar{X}_{j\cdot}|}{\sqrt{7.63\left(\frac{1}{6} + \frac{1}{6}\right)}}$$

where $MS_E = 7.63$ is obtained from the ANOVA given in Table 10.3. From the T table, it can be seen that

$$P[T_{25} \geq 2.787] = .005$$

Hence for the P value of the two-tailed T test to be at most .01, the observed value of the test statistic must be at least 2.787. This point is called the *critical point* for an $\alpha = .01$ level test. It is critical in the sense that points on or above this value lead to the rejection of H_0 whenever α has been preset at .01. Notice that for

$$\frac{|\bar{X}_{i\cdot} - \bar{X}_{j\cdot}|}{\sqrt{7.63\left(\frac{1}{6} + \frac{1}{6}\right)}}$$

TABLE 10.3
ANOVA for the data of Example 10.2.1

Source	DF	SS	MS	F
Treatment	4	1458.13	364.53	47.78
Error	25	190.67	7.63	
Total	29	1648.80		

to equal or exceed 2.787, the absolute difference $|\bar{X}_{i.} - \bar{X}_{j.}|$ must equal or exceed

$$2.787\sqrt{7.63\left(\tfrac{1}{6} + \tfrac{1}{6}\right)} = 4.44$$

To conduct each test, we need only compare the absolute differences between the respective sample means to this value. If $|\bar{X}_{i.} - \bar{X}_{j.}| \geq 4.44$, then we reject H_0: $\mu_i = \mu_j$ and conclude that the two population means μ_i and μ_j are different. For example, to test H_0: $\mu_1 = \mu_2$ we find $\bar{X}_{1.}$ and $\bar{X}_{2.}$. In this case, $\bar{X}_{1.} = 46.0$ and $\bar{X}_{2.} = 38.7$. The difference $|\bar{X}_{1.} - \bar{X}_{2.}|$ is 7.3. Since $7.3 > 4.44$, we can conclude that $\mu_1 \neq \mu_2$. The other nine pairs of means can be compared in a similar way.

Notice that the magnitude of the difference between $\bar{X}_{i.}$ and $\bar{X}_{j.}$ that is necessary to declare μ_i and μ_j to be different depends on n_i and n_j. If all sample sizes are the same, as in Example 10.2.1, then a single critical difference can be used to conduct all paired comparisons. However, if sample sizes are not the same, then a separate critical difference must be found for each test.

Duncan's Multiple Range Test

Duncan's multiple range test was presented by D. B. Duncan. It is one of the oldest methods for comparing means currently in use and is referred to in the literature quite often. For this reason you should be familiar with its use. Unlike the Bonferroni T tests discussed earlier, an attempt is made to account for the position of a pair of means in the list of ordered sample means. For example, assume that we have a collection of five sample means $\bar{X}_{1.}$, $\bar{X}_{2.}$, $\bar{X}_{3.}$, $\bar{X}_{4.}$, and $\bar{X}_{5.}$ ordered from smallest to largest. The statistic $|\bar{X}_{1.} - \bar{X}_{5.}|$ is used to test H_0: $\mu_1 = \mu_5$. The Bonferroni procedure compares these population means via a T test that does not take into account the fact that the sample means $\bar{X}_{1.}$ and $\bar{X}_{5.}$ are the extremes in a set of five means; Duncan's procedure does recognize this fact and makes an adjustment for it. The adjustment entails changing critical points so that sample means that lie side by side are not required to exhibit as much difference as those that are separated in order to declare the corresponding population means to be "significantly different." The test was originally designed for use with samples of equal size. However, the test has been extended by C. Y. Kramer to include samples of unequal size. We illustrate first the procedure for *equal* sample sizes.

EXAMPLE 10.2.2. Water samples from each of four lakes are analyzed for phosphorus. The phosphorus level is given in parts per million (ppm). The following summary statistics, based on 20 randomly selected samples from each lake, are obtained:

$$T_{1.} = .40 \qquad\qquad T_{4.} = 1.00$$
$$T_{2.} = .20 \qquad\qquad T_{..} = 1.62$$
$$T_{3.} = .02 \qquad \sum\sum X_{ij}^2 = .2880$$

The ANOVA for the experiment is given in Table 10.4. We shall use the $F_{3,60}$ distribution to approximate that of the $F_{3,76}$ distribution. From the F table, we see that

$$P[F_{3,60} \geq 3.34] = .025$$

TABLE 10.4

ANOVA for the data of Example 10.2.2.
The null hypothesis of equality of means
can be rejected with .025 < P < .05

Source	DF	SS	MS	F
Treatment	3	.0272	.0091	3.0333
Error	76	.2280	.0030	
Total	79	.2552		

and

$$P[F_{3,60} \geq 2.76] = .05$$

Since 3.0333, the observed value of our F statistic, lies between 2.76 and 3.34, the P value of the test for equality of means lies between .025 and .05. This P value is small, so we reject $H_0: \mu_1 = \mu_2 = \mu_3 = \mu_4$ and conclude that there are differences in the mean phosphorus levels in the four lakes. Just what these differences are remains to be seen.

Duncan's multiple range test is designed to detect differences in population means by comparing sample means. This is done by dividing the k sample means, and therefore the k population means, into subgroups so that means within subgroups are not considered to be significantly different. The test is performed as follows:

1. Linearly order the k sample means.
2. Consider any subset of p sample means $2 \leq p \leq k$. For the means of any of the corresponding populations to be considered different, the range of the means in the subgroup (largest to smallest) must exceed a specific value, called the *shortest significant range SSR_p*.
3. The shortest significant range is calculated by means of Table X in Appendix B and the following formula:

$$SSR_p = r_p \sqrt{\frac{MS_E}{n}}$$

where r_p = least significant studentized range obtained from Table X
  MS_E = error mean square from ANOVA
  n = common sample size
  γ = degrees of freedom for MS_E

4. Results are summarized by underlining any subset of adjacent means that are not considered to be significantly different at the α level selected.

The procedure is illustrated by continuing the analysis of the data of Example 10.2.2.

EXAMPLE 10.2.3. The estimated mean phosphorus levels for the four lakes are

$$\bar{x}_{1.} = \frac{T_{1.}}{20} = \frac{.40}{20} = .02 \text{ ppm}$$

$$\bar{x}_{2.} = \frac{T_{2.}}{20} = \frac{.20}{20} = .01 \text{ ppm}$$

$$\bar{x}_{3.} = \frac{T_{3.}}{20} = \frac{.02}{20} = .001 \text{ ppm}$$

$$\bar{x}_{4.} = \frac{T_{4.}}{20} = \frac{1.00}{20} = .05 \text{ ppm}$$

In linear order, these are

$\bar{x}_{3.}$	$\bar{x}_{2.}$	$\bar{x}_{1.}$	$\bar{x}_{4.}$
.001	.01	.02	.05

Next we construct a chart giving the values of SSR_p for $\alpha = .05$. The chart is based on $\gamma = 60$ degrees of freedom, since this value is closest to the 76 value required for the Duncan test. Note that $MS_E = .0030$ is obtained from the ANOVA of Example 10.2.2, the value of r_p reported is given in Table X of Appendix B, and $SSR_p = r_p\sqrt{MS_E/20}$.

p	2	3	4
r_p	2.829	2.976	3.073
SSR_p	.0346	.0364	.0376

The differences in population means are detected by comparing the largest sample mean with the smallest, the largest with the next smallest, and so forth. Thus potentially we need to consider pairs of sample means in the order

1. $\bar{x}_{4.} - \bar{x}_{3.}$ 4. $\bar{x}_{1.} - \bar{x}_{3.}$
2. $\bar{x}_{4.} - \bar{x}_{2.}$ 5. $\bar{x}_{1.} - \bar{x}_{2.}$
3. $\bar{x}_{4.} - \bar{x}_{1.}$ 6. $\bar{x}_{2.} - \bar{x}_{3.}$

However, when sample sizes are equal, once a group of means has been found to be not significantly different, no further test will declare them to differ. Thus, in practice, it may not be necessary to perform all the comparisons indicated. The needed comparisons are shown in Table 10.5.

No further comparisons need be made at this point since no differences have been detected among the mean phosphorus levels of lakes 1, 2, and 3. In summary, we may conclude that $\mu_4 \neq \mu_3$ and $\mu_4 \neq \mu_2$. No other differences have been detected.

TABLE 10.5

Difference d	Number in subgroup p	SSR_p (from chart)	Is $d > SSR_p$?	Groupings
$\bar{x}_{4.} - \bar{x}_{3.} = .0490$	4	.0376	Yes	$\bar{x}_{3.}\ \bar{x}_{2.}\ \bar{x}_{1.}\ \bar{x}_{4.}$
$\bar{x}_{4.} - \bar{x}_{2.} = .04$	3	.0364	Yes	$\bar{x}_{3.}\ \bar{x}_{2.}\ \bar{x}_{1.}\ \bar{x}_{4.}$
$\bar{x}_{4.} - \bar{x}_{1.} = .03$	2	.0346	No	$\bar{x}_{3.}\ \bar{x}_{2.}\ \underline{\bar{x}_{1.}\ \bar{x}_{4.}}$
$\bar{x}_{1.} - \bar{x}_{3.} = .019$	3	.0364	No	$\underline{\bar{x}_{3.}\ \bar{x}_{2.}\ \bar{x}_{1.}}\ \bar{x}_{4.}$

C. Y. Kramer in 1956 extended Duncan's multiple range test to include unequal sample sizes. The test is performed in a manner similar to Duncan's original procedure with two variations. In particular, the shortest significant range for the adjusted test, denoted SSR_p', is given by

$$\boxed{SSR_p' = r_p\sqrt{MS_E}}$$

where r_p = least significant studentized range obtained from Table X
$\quad MS_E$ = error mean square from ANOVA

In addition, the test statistic for comparing two population means μ_i and μ_j is

$$\boxed{|\bar{x}_{i.} - \bar{x}_{j.}|\sqrt{\frac{2n_in_j}{n_i + n_j}}}$$

This test statistic reflects the sample sizes, and the means μ_i and μ_j are considered different if and only if the observed value of the statistic exceeds SSR_p'. The procedure is illustrated in Example 10.2.4.

> **EXAMPLE 10.2.4.** In Example 10.1.6, it was concluded that the three acne treatments under study did differ in mean effect. To pinpoint the differences, we use Duncan's multiple range test. Since the sample sizes are not equal, Kramer's adjustment is appropriate. From previous results it is known that

$$n_1 = 10 \qquad \bar{x}_{1.} = 49.46 \qquad MS_E = 4.07$$
$$n_2 = 12 \qquad \bar{x}_{2.} = 68.73 \qquad \sqrt{MS_E} \doteq 2.02$$
$$n_3 = 13 \qquad \bar{x}_{3.} = 63.60$$

In linear order, the sample means are

$\bar{x}_{1.}$	$\bar{x}_{3.}$	$\bar{x}_{2.}$
49.46	63.60	68.73

Using Table X of Appendix B with $\alpha = .01$ and $\gamma = 30$ degrees of freedom (as an approximation to $\gamma = 32$ degrees of freedom) and the formula $SSR_p' = r_p\sqrt{MS_E}$, we obtain the following adjusted values for the shortest significant range:

p	2	3
r_p	3.889	4.506
SSR_p'	7.85	9.10

To compare μ_2 to μ_1, we evaluate the test statistic thusly:

$$|\bar{x}_{2.} - \bar{x}_{1.}|\sqrt{\frac{2n_1n_2}{n_1 + n_2}} = |68.73 - 49.46|\sqrt{\frac{2 \cdot 10 \cdot 12}{10 + 12}}$$
$$= 63.65$$

Since this value exceeds $SSR'_3 = 9.10$, we can conclude that $\mu_1 \neq \mu_2$. The statistic

$$|\bar{x}_{2.} - \bar{x}_{3.}|\sqrt{\frac{2n_2 n_3}{n_2 + n_3}} = |68.73 - 63.60|\sqrt{\frac{2 \cdot 12 \cdot 13}{12 + 13}}$$

$$= 18.12$$

is used to compare μ_2 with μ_3. Since this value exceeds $SSR'_2 = 7.85$, we can conclude that $\mu_2 \neq \mu_3$. The last comparison is μ_3 with μ_1. The necessary statistic is

$$|\bar{x}_{3.} - \bar{x}_{1.}|\sqrt{\frac{2n_3 n_1}{n_3 + n_1}} = |63.60 - 49.46|\sqrt{\frac{2 \cdot 13 \cdot 10}{13 + 10}}$$

$$= 47.54$$

Since this value also exceeds SSR'_2, we conclude that $\mu_1 \neq \mu_3$. Summarizing these results, we have

Old	New	Current
$\bar{x}_{1.}$	$\bar{x}_{3.}$	$\bar{x}_{2.}$

That is, at the $\alpha = .01$ level we may conclude that each of the means is significantly different from each of the others.

Recall that if sample sizes are equal, we might not have to make all the possible comparisons. When sample sizes are equal, whenever the most extreme pair of means is found to be not significantly different, then all means within the subgroup are assumed to be equal with no further testing required. This is not true with unequal sample sizes. In this case *all* the comparisons must be made.

A Note on Computing

As you can see, the computations needed to complete an analysis of variance (ANOVA) are extensive. Commercial computer packages are available to do the initial analysis, and most include the ability to request paired and multiple comparisons. Hence, the primary job of the researcher is to recognize an experimental setting that calls for a one-way analysis of variance and to have the ability to interpret the resulting printout correctly.

In Example 10.2.5 we present the output of a SAS program used to analyze the data of Example 10.2.1. Bonferroni *T* tests and Duncan's multiple range test are both run for illustrative purposes. In practice, one or the other would be used but not both. The SAS code used to produce this output is given in the Technology Tools section at the end of this chapter.

> **EXAMPLE 10.2.5.** The SAS printout for the analysis of the data of Example 10.2.1 follows. Notice that the source that SAS labels as "Model" is our "Treatment" source. Otherwise the SAS output agrees with that obtained by hand and shown in Table 10.3 (apart from some roundoff differences). Notice that the Duncan procedure finds no difference between the mean percent of impurities removed by polymers 3 and 4 as these polymers are both labeled B on the printout. All other polymers differ from these and from one another. The results of the Bonferroni test differ slightly from those obtained using the Duncan procedure.

The Bonferroni test detects no difference between the mean responses for polymers 4 and 1 as both are labeled C on the printout. The difference in interpretation between the two tests is due to the fact that the Bonferroni test is very conservative. To obtain an overall probability of making at least one incorrect rejection of .05, each of the 10 possible paired comparisons is being conducted at the $.05/10 = .005$ level.

```
                                  SAS
                   Analysis-of-Variance Procedure
Dependent Variable:        PERCENT
                                    Sum of          Mean
Source                     DF       Squares         Square    F Value        Pr>F
Model                       4    1458.133333     364.533333    47.80         .0001
Error                      25     190.666667       7.626667
Corrected Total            29    1648.800000
                     R-Squares            C.V.    Root MSE            PERCENT Mean
                     0.884360         5.613094    2.761642           49.2000000
Source                     DF      Anova SS    Mean Square    F Value        Pr>F
TEMP                        4    1458.133333     364.533333    47.80         .0001
```

```
              SAS                                            SAS
   Analysis-of-Variance Procedure                Analysis-of-Variance Procedure
Duncan's Multiple Range Test for variable:     Bonferroni (Dunn) T tests for variable:
             PERCENT                                       PERCENT
NOTE: This test controls the type I comparisonwise    NOTE: This test controls the type I ex-
   error rate, not the experimentwise error rate.     perimentwise error rate, but generally has a
   Alpha = 0.05  DF = 25  MSE = 7.626667               higher type II error rate than REGWQ.
Number of Means      2     3     4     5               Alpha = 0.05  DF = 25  MSE = 7.62667
Critical Range    3.281 3.447 3.562 3.632        Minimum Significant Difference = 4.908
Means with the same letter are not significantly  Means with the same letter are not significantly
            different.                                     different.
   Duncan Grouping   Mean  N  TEMP            Bon Grouping     Mean  N  TEMP
             A       60.000 6   5                     A       60.000 6   5
             B       51.333 6   3                     B       51.333 6   3
             B                                        B
             B       50.000 6   4            C        B       50.000 6   4
             C       46.000 6   1            C
             D       38.667 6   7            C                46.000 6   1
                                                     D       38.667 6   2
```


▨ EXERCISES 10.2

1. Consider the data of Example 10.2.1.
   (*a*) Verify that

$$T_{1.} = 276 \qquad \bar{X}_{1.} = 46.0 \qquad \sum_{i=1}^{5}\sum_{j=1}^{6} X_{ij}^2 = 74,268$$

$$T_{2.} = 232 \qquad \bar{X}_{2.} = 38.7$$

$$T_{3.} = 308 \qquad \bar{X}_{3.} = 51.3$$

$$T_{4.} = 300 \qquad \bar{X}_{4.} = 50.0$$

$$T_{5.} = 360 \qquad \bar{X}_{5.} = 60.0$$
$$T_{..} = 1476 \qquad \bar{X}_{..} = 49.2$$

(b) Verify the ANOVA given in Table 10.3.

(c) Test the other nine hypothesis of the form H_0: $\mu_i = \mu_j$ versus H_1: $\mu_i \neq \mu_j$. Report your results schematically by ordering the sample means from smallest to largest and underlining pairs that are not significantly different.

2. In each case, determine the number of paired comparisons possible.
   (a) $k = 3$
   (b) $k = 6$
   (c) $k = 10$

3. Let $\alpha = .05$ and assume that all possible paired comparisons are to be made. For each value of k given in Exercise 2, find an upper bound for α', the overall probability of making at least one incorrect rejection. In each case, what α level should be used to guarantee that $\alpha' \leq .10$?

4. Scientists concerned with treatment of tar sand wastewater studied three treatment methods for the removal of organic carbon. (Based on W. R. Pirie, *Statistical Planning and Analysis for Treatments of Tar Sand Wastewater*, Technical Information Center, Office of Scientific and Technological Information, United States Department of Energy.) The three treatment methods used were air flotation (AF), foam separation (FS), and ferric-chloride coagulation (FCC). The organic carbon material measurements for the three treatments yielded the following data:

AF	FS	FCC
34.6	38.8	26.7
35.1	39.0	26.7
35.3	40.1	27.0
35.8	40.9	27.1
36.1	41.0	27.5
36.5	43.2	28.1
36.8	44.9	28.1
37.2	46.9	28.7
37.4	51.6	30.7
37.7	53.6	31.2

(a) Test H_0: $\mu_1 = \mu_2 = \mu_3$ at the $\alpha = .10$ level.

(b) If H_0 is rejected, use Bonferroni T tests to pinpoint differences in population means. Let α' be at most .06.

5. It was known that a toxic material was dumped in a river leading into a large saltwater commercial fishing area. Civil engineers studied the way the water carried the toxic material by measuring the amount of the material (in parts per million) found in oysters harvested at three different locations, ranging from the estuary out into the bay where the majority of commercial fishing was carried out. The resulting data are given on below.

(a) Test for differences in the average parts per million of toxic material found in oysters harvested at the three sites.

(b) If H_0: $\mu_1 = \mu_2 = \mu_3$ is rejected, use Bonferroni T tests to pinpoint differences that exist. Let α' be at most .15.

Site 1 (estuary)	Site 2 (far bay)	Site 3 (near bay)
15	19	22
26	15	26
20	10	24
20	26	26
29	11	15
28	20	17
21	13	24
26	15	
	18	

6. Continue the analysis of the data of Exercise 1 of Section 10.1 by applying Duncan's multiple range test with $\alpha = .01$.

7. Continue the analysis of the data of Exercise 2 of Section 10.1 by applying Duncan's multiple range test with $\alpha = .01$.

8. Continue the analysis of the data of Exercise 3 of Section 10.1 by applying Duncan's multiple range test with Kramer's adjustment with $\alpha = .01$.

9. Continue the analysis of the data of Exercise 4 of Section 10.1 by applying Duncan's multiple range test with $\alpha = .01$.

10. Continue the analysis of the data of Exercise 5 of Section 10.1 by applying Duncan's multiple range test with Kramer's adjustment.

11. A study is conducted among blue-collar workers in trades in which workers are routinely exposed to asbestos. An asbestosis screening program was conducted, and a later survey divided the sample obtained into three groups, those who quit smoking, those who reduced their smoking level, and those who maintained their smoking level after the screening program. These data are obtained on the alveolar carbon monoxide (CO_a) level of the three groups.

Quit	Reduced	Continued
36	34	28
40	5	2
19	47	51
25	37	33
43	46	28
54		29
		30

(a) Test for equality of means.

(b) If the null hypothesis of equal means is rejected, pinpoint the differences that exist by conducting appropriate Bonferroni T tests. Maintain an overall α level of at most .15.

(Based on means found in Kaye Kilburn and Raphael Warshaw, "Effects of Individually Motivating Smoking Cessation in Male Blue Collar Workers," *American Journal of Public Health,* November 1990, pp. 1334–1337.)

■ **10.3**
RANDOM EFFECTS (OPTIONAL)

The model presented in Section 10.1 is called the *fixed-effects model.* Recall that this implies that the factor levels, or "treatments," are selected specifically by the experimenter because they are of particular interest. The purpose of the experiment is to make inferences about the means of the particular populations from which the samples are drawn. No other populations are of interest. If, however, we want to make a broad generalization concerning a larger set of populations, and not just the *k* populations from which we sample, then the model is called a *random-effects model.* In this case, the *k* sampled populations are considered to be a random sample of populations drawn from the larger set. The hypothesis of interest is not that $\mu_1 = \mu_2 = \cdots = \mu_k$. Rather, we want to determine whether some variability exists among the population means of the larger set. Consider Example 10.3.1.

> **EXAMPLE 10.3.1.** Bacteriological media in use in hospital laboratories are obtained from different manufacturers. It is suspected that the quality of the media varies from manufacturer to manufacturer. To test this theory, a list of manufacturers of a particular medium is compiled, the names of three are randomly selected from the list, and samples of the media from these three sources are tested. The tests are conducted by placing 2 drops of a measured suspension of a standard organism, *Escherichia coli,* on the plate, allowing the culture to grow for 24 hours, and then determining the number of colonies (in thousands) of the organism present at the end of this period. The purpose is not to compare these particular three manufacturers—they were chosen at random and constitute only a sample of all manufacturers of the media. Rather, we wish statistical support for the general statement that the quality of the media differs among manufacturers.

Mathematically, the random-effects model can be written as follows:

MODEL

$$X_{ij} \equiv \mu + T_i + E_{ij} \qquad \begin{array}{l} i = 1, 2, \ldots, k \\ j = 1, 2, \ldots, n_i \end{array}$$

where μ = overall mean effect

$T_i = \mu_i - \mu$ (μ_i is mean *i*th population selected for study)

$E_{ij} = X_{ij} - \mu_i$ = residual, or random, error

We assume the following:

MODEL ASSUMPTIONS

1. The *k* samples represent independent random samples drawn from *k* populations randomly selected from a larger set of populations.
2. Each of the populations in the larger set is normal, and thus each of the *k* sampled populations is also normal.
3. Each of the populations in the larger set has the same variance, σ^2, and thus each of the *k* sampled populations also has variance σ^2.
4. Variables $T_1, T_2, \ldots, T_k$ are independent normal random variables, each with mean 0 and common variance σ_{Tr}^2.

The model itself and the first three model assumptions are similar to those of the fixed-effects model. However, one important difference between the two is expressed mathematically as model assumption 4. In the fixed-effects model, the treatments, or levels, used in the experiment are purposely chosen by the experimenter because they are of particular interest. If the experiment were replicated (repeated), the same treatments would be used. That is, the same populations would be sampled each time, and the k treatment effects $\mu_i - \mu$ would not vary. This implies that in the fixed-effects model, the k terms $\mu_i - \mu$ are considered *unknown constants*. In the random-effects model, this is not the case. Since the first step in a random-effects experiment is to randomly select k populations for study, those actually chosen will vary from replication to replication. Thus in the random-effects model, the k terms $T_i = \mu_i - \mu$ are not constants, but are, in fact, *random variables* whose values for a given replication depend on the choice of the k populations to be studied. These variables are assumed to be independent normal random variables with mean 0 and common variance σ_{Tr}^2.

If the population means in the larger set are equal, then the treatment effects $T_i = \mu_i - \mu$ will not vary. That is, σ_{Tr}^2 will be zero. Thus in the random-effects model, the hypothesis of equal means is tested by considering

$$H_0: \sigma_{\text{Tr}}^2 = 0 \quad \text{(no variability in treatment effects)}$$

$$H_1: \sigma_{\text{Tr}}^2 \neq 0$$

Even though theoretically the random-effects model differs from the fixed-effects one, the data are handled in exactly the same way. The only change necessary in the analysis-of-variance table occurs in the column of the expected mean square. For this model $E[MS_{\text{Tr}}]$ is changed to read

$$E[MS_{\text{Tr}}] = \sigma^2 + n_0 \sigma_{\text{Tr}}^2$$

where

$$n_0 = \frac{N - \sum_{i=1}^{k} n_i^2 / N}{k - 1}$$

The analysis of variance is summarized in Table 10.6. Again note that if H_0 is true ($\sigma_{\text{Tr}}^2 = 0$), we would expect MS_{Tr} and MS_E to be close in value, since both estimate the same parameter, σ^2. If H_0 is not true, we would expect MS_{Tr} to be larger than MS_E, thus

TABLE 10.6

Analysis of variance: One-way classification, completely random design with random effects

Source of variation	Degrees of freedom DF	Sum of squares SS	Mean square MS	Expected mean square	F ratio
Treatment, or level	$k - 1$	$\sum_{i=1}^{k} \dfrac{T_{i.}^2}{n_i} - \dfrac{T_{..}^2}{N}$	$\dfrac{SS_{\text{Tr}}}{k - 1}$	$\sigma^2 + n_0 \sigma_{\text{Tr}}^2$	$\dfrac{MS_{\text{Tr}}}{MS_E}$
Residual, or error	$N - k$	$SS_{\text{Total}} - SS_{\text{Tr}}$	$\dfrac{SS_E}{N - k}$	σ^2	
Total	$N - 1$	$\sum_{i=1}^{k} \sum_{j=1}^{n_i} X_{ij}^2 - \dfrac{T_{..}^2}{N}$			

■ **TABLE 10.7**

ANOVA for the data of Example 10.3.2.
The hypothesis H_0: $\sigma_{Tr}^2 = 0$ is rejected
with .05 < P < .10

Source	DF	SS	MS	F
Treatment	2	110.6	55.3	3
Error	27	497.7	18.43	
Total	29	608.3		

forcing the *F* ratio to be larger than 1. Thus the test is to reject H_0 for observed values of the $F_{k-1,\ N-k}$ statistic that are too large to have occurred by chance.

> **EXAMPLE 10.3.2.** In the experiment of Example 10.3.1, three manufacturers of bacteriological media are randomly chosen. Samples of size 10 are drawn from the stock of each and tested. The following summary data result:
>
> $$T_{1.} = 527 \qquad T_{3.} = 480$$
> $$T_{2.} = 502 \qquad T_{..} = 1509$$
> $$\sum_{i=1}^{3} \sum_{j=1}^{10} X_{ij}^2 = 76{,}511$$
>
> The ANOVA for these data is shown in Table 10.7. Notice that $P[F_{2,27} > 3.35] = .05$ and $P[F_{2,27} > 2.51] = .10$. Since 3, the observed value of the test statistic, lies between 2.51 and 3.35, the *P* value lies between .05 and .10. We can reject H_0: $\sigma_{Tr}^2 = 0$ and conclude that there is evidence of variability in quality among manufacturers.
>
> In the random-effects model, no further tests are necessary even if H_0 is rejected. The purpose of the experiment is to make a general statement concerning the populations from which the *k* sampled populations are drawn. This has been done.

■ **EXERCISES 10.3**

1. A study is run of the behavior of the male great titmouse. The purpose is to determine whether there is a difference in the mean height (in meters) at which the bird performs various activities. A list of 10 of the most important activities is compiled. Four—singing, feeding, preening, and resting—are randomly chosen for monitoring. These data, based on 20 observations each, result:

Singing	Feeding	Preening	Resting
$T_{1.} = 186$	$T_{2.} = 44$	$T_{3.} = 120$	$T_{4.} = 70$

   $$\sum_{i=1}^{4} \sum_{j=1}^{20} X_{ij}^2 = 7915.8$$

   On the basis of these data, can it be concluded that activities are performed at different heights? Explain your answer using the ANOVA and the *P* value involved.
2. Which model, fixed effects or random effects, is more likely to be found? Explain.

▪ 10.4

RANDOMIZED COMPLETE BLOCKS

The procedure presented in this section is an extension of the paired T procedure for comparing the means of two normal populations presented in Chapter 9. Recall that the purpose of pairing is to minimize the effect of some extraneous variable, a variable not under study in the experiment, by pairing experimental units that are similar with respect to this variable. Each member of the pair receives a different treatment, and any differences in response are attributed to treatment effects since the effect of the extraneous variable has been neutralized by pairing. This pairing is illustrated in Figure 10.3.

When we want to compare the means of k populations in the presence of an extraneous variable, a procedure known as *blocking* is used. A *block* is a collection of k, rather than two, experimental units that are as nearly alike as possible relative to the extraneous variable. Each treatment is randomly assigned to one unit within each block. Since once again the effect of the extraneous variable has been neutralized among treatments by matching like experimental units, any differences in response are attributed to treatment effects. The blocking procedure is illustrated in Figure 10.4.

The design presented here is called the *randomized complete block* design with fixed effects. The work *block* refers to the fact that experimental units have been matched relative to some extraneous variable; *randomized* refers to the fact that treatments are randomly assigned within blocks; and to say that the design is *complete* implies that each treatment is used exactly once within each block. The term *fixed effects* applies to both blocks and treatments. That is, it is assumed that neither blocks nor treatments are randomly chosen. Any inferences made apply to only the k treatments and the b blocks actually used. The null hypothesis of interest is

$$H_0: \ \mu_{1.} = \mu_{2.} = \cdots = \mu_k.$$

where $\mu_{i.}$ denotes the mean of the ith treatment.

EXAMPLE 10.4.1. An experiment is conducted to compare the energy requirements of three physical activities: running, walking, and bicycle riding. The variable of interest is X,

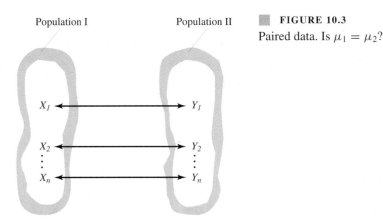

Population I Population II

FIGURE 10.3
Paired data. Is $\mu_1 = \mu_2$?

$X_1 \longleftrightarrow Y_1$

$X_2 \longleftrightarrow Y_2$

$X_n \longleftrightarrow Y_n$

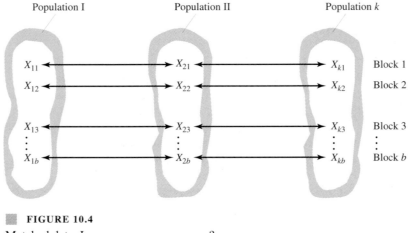

■ FIGURE 10.4
Matched data. Is $\mu_{1.} = \mu_{2.} = \cdots = \mu_{k.}$?

the number of kilocalories expended per kilometer traveled. Since it is thought that metabolic differences among individuals may affect the number of kilocalories required for a given activity, we want to control this extraneous variable. To do so, eight subjects are selected. Each is asked to run, walk, and bicycle a measured distance, and the number of kilocalories expended per kilometer is determined for each subject during each activity. The activities are run in random order with time for recovery between activities. Each individual serves as a block. Each activity is monitored exactly once for each individual, and thus the design is complete. Any differences in the mean number of kilocalories expended will be attributed to differences among the activities themselves, since the effect of individual differences among subjects has been neutralized by blocking. The null hypothesis of interest is

$$H_0: \mu_{1.} = \mu_{2.} = \mu_{3.}$$

where $\mu_{1.}, \mu_{2.}, \mu_{3.}$ denote the mean number of kilocalories expended per kilometer while running, walking, and bicycle riding, respectively.

Data Format and Notation

The data collected in a randomized complete block design are conveniently recorded in the following format:

Data layout of randomized complete block design

Block	Treatment				
	1	**2**	**3**	$\cdots$	**k**
1	X_{11}	X_{21}	X_{31}	$\cdots$	X_{k1}
2	X_{12}	X_{22}	X_{32}	$\cdots$	X_{k2}
3	X_{13}	X_{23}	X_{33}	$\cdots$	X_{k3}
$\vdots$					
b	X_{1b}	X_{2b}	X_{3b}	$\cdots$	X_{kb}

Note that b denotes the number of blocks used in the experiment and the number of observations per treatment; k denotes the number of treatments being investigated and the number of observations per block; $N = kb$ denotes the total number of responses. Variable X_{ij}, $i = 1, 2, \ldots, k$ and $j = 1, 2, \ldots, b$, is a random variable denoting the response to the ith treatment in the jth block. In using sample data to compare population means, these sample statistics are required:

$$T_{i.} = \sum_{j=1}^{b} X_{ij} = \text{total of all responses to } i\text{th treatment}, i = 1, 2, \ldots, k$$

$$\bar{X}_{i.} = \frac{T_{i.}}{b} = \text{sample mean for } i\text{th treatment}, i = 1, 2, \ldots, k$$

$$T_{.j} = \sum_{i=1}^{k} X_{ij} = \text{total of all responses in } j\text{th block}, j = 1, 2, \ldots, b$$

$$\bar{X}_{.j} = \frac{T_{.j}}{k} = \text{sample mean for } j\text{th block}, j = 1, 2, \ldots, b$$

$$T_{..} = \sum_{i=1}^{k} \sum_{j=1}^{b} X_{ij} = \sum_{i=1}^{k} T_{i.} = \sum_{j=1}^{b} T_{.j} = \text{total of all responses}$$

$$\bar{X}_{..} = \frac{T_{..}}{N} = \text{sample mean for all responses}$$

$$\sum_{i=1}^{k} \sum_{j=1}^{b} X_{ij}^2 = \text{sum of squares of each response}$$

The evaluation of these statistics is illustrated in Example 10.4.2.

EXAMPLE 10.4.2. When the experiment of Example 10.4.1 was conducted, the data shown in Table 10.8 on the number of kilocalories expended per kilometer by each subject

▨ **TABLE 10.8***

Block	Treatment 1 (running)	Treatment 2 (walking)	Treatment 3 (bicycling)	Block total	Block mean
1	1.4	1.1	.7	3.2 $(T_{.1})$	1.07 $(\bar{X}_{.1})$
2	1.5	1.2	.8	3.5 $(T_{.2})$	1.17 $(\bar{X}_{.2})$
3	1.8	1.3	.7	3.8 $(T_{.3})$	1.27 $(\bar{X}_{.3})$
4	1.7	1.3	.8	3.8 $(T_{.4})$	1.27 $(\bar{X}_{.4})$
5	1.6	.7	.1	2.4 $(T_{.5})$	.8 $(\bar{X}_{.5})$
6	1.5	1.2	.7	3.4 $(T_{.6})$	1.13 $(\bar{X}_{.6})$
7	1.7	1.1	.4	3.2 $(T_{.7})$	1.07 $(\bar{X}_{.7})$
8	2.0	1.3	.6	3.9 $(T_{.8})$	1.30 $(\bar{X}_{.8})$
Treatment total	13.2 $(T_{1.})$	9.2 $(T_{2.})$	4.8 $(T_{3.})$	27.2 $(T_{..})$	
Treatment mean	1.65 $(\bar{X}_{1.})$	1.15 $(\bar{X}_{2.})$	.6 $(\bar{X}_{3.})$	1.13 $(\bar{X}_{..})$	

*For these data, $\sum_{i=1}^{3} \sum_{j=1}^{8} X_{ij}^2 = 36.18$.

in each of the three activities resulted. Sample treatment totals and means, block totals and means, and the grand total and mean are given in the margins of the table.

Testing H_0: $\mu_1. = \mu_2. = \cdots = \mu_k.$

To write the model for the randomized complete block design with fixed effects, the following notation is needed:

$$\mu = \text{overall mean effect}$$
$$\mu_i. = \text{mean of } i\text{th treatment}, i = 1, 2, \ldots, k$$
$$\mu_{.j} = j\text{th block mean}, j = 1, 2, \ldots, b$$
$$\mu_{ij} = \text{mean for } i\text{th treatment and } j\text{th block}$$
$$\tau_i = \mu_i. - \mu = \text{effect due to fact that experimental}$$
$$\text{unit received } i\text{th treatment}$$
$$\beta_j = \mu_{.j} - \mu = \text{effect due to fact that experimental}$$
$$\text{unit is in } j\text{th block}$$
$$E_{ij} = X_{ij} - \mu_{ij} = \text{residual, or random, error}$$

Using this notation, we can express the model thus:

MODEL

$$X_{ij} = \mu + \tau_i + \beta_j + E_{ij} \qquad \begin{array}{l} i = 1, 2, \ldots, k \\ j = 1, 2, \ldots, b \end{array}$$

This model expresses symbolically the notion that each observation can be partitioned into four recognizable components: an overall mean effect μ, a treatment effect τ_i, a block effect β_j, and a random deviation attributed to unexplained sources E_{ij}. We make the following assumptions:

MODEL ASSUMPTIONS

1. The $k \cdot b$ observations constitute independent random samples, each of size 1, from $k \cdot b$ populations with means $\mu_{ij}, i = 1, 2, \ldots, k$ and $j = 1, 2, \ldots, b$.
2. Each of the $k \cdot b$ populations is normal.
3. Each of the $k \cdot b$ populations has the same variance, σ^2.
4. Block and treatment effects are additive; that is, there is no interaction between blocks and treatments.

Assumptions 1 through 3 are identical to those made in the one-way classification model except that $k \cdot b$, rather than k, populations are under consideration. The fourth assumption is new and needs to be examined more closely. Briefly, to say that block and treatment effects are additive means that the treatments behave consistently across blocks and that the blocks behave consistently across treatments. Mathematically, this means that the difference in the mean values for any two treatments is the same in every block, and the difference in the means for any two blocks is the same for each treatment. If this is not the case, then we say that there is interaction between blocks and treatments. Some numerical examples will help clarify this concept.

EXAMPLE 10.4.3. Three programs have been developed to help patients who have suffered their first heart attacks to adjust physically and psychologically to their condition.

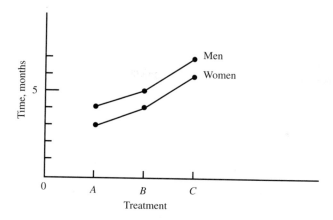

FIGURE 10.5

No interaction: line segments are parallel.

The variable of interest is the time in months needed for the patient to return to an active life. Since it is thought that men and women may react differently to illness, this variable is controlled by blocking. Thus we are dealing with $k \cdot b = 3 \cdot 2 = 6$ normal populations, each assumed to have the same variance. Assume that the means for these six populations are thus:

Block	Treatment		
	A	B	C
Men	$\mu_{11} = 4$	$\mu_{21} = 5$	$\mu_{31} = 7$
Women	$\mu_{12} = 3$	$\mu_{22} = 4$	$\mu_{32} = 6$

Note that the mean for treatment A is 1 less than that for B and 3 less than that for C in each block; the mean for treatment B is 2 less than that for C in each block. That is, the treatments behave consistently across blocks. Similarly, the mean for block 1 (men) always exceeds the mean for block 2 (women) by 1, regardless of the treatment involved. That is, the blocks behave consistently across treatments. When this occurs, we say that block and treatment effects are additive, or that there is *no* interaction between treatments and blocks. This idea is illustrated graphically in Figure 10.5.

Figure 10.5 graphs the treatment means shown in the preceding table. When no interaction exists, the line segments joining any two means will be parallel across blocks. Practically speaking, this means that it is possible to make general statements concerning the treatments without having to specify the block involved. For example, it is correct to say that treatment A is superior to treatments B and C in that it has the shortest mean recovery time.

EXAMPLE 10.4.4. Consider Example 10.4.3 with these population means:

Block	Treatment		
	A	B	C
Men	$\mu_{11} = 4$	$\mu_{21} = 7$	$\mu_{31} = 9$
Women	$\mu_{12} = 3$	$\mu_{22} = 6$	$\mu_{32} = 2$

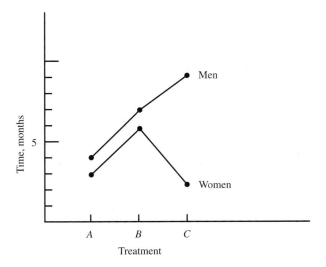

■ **FIGURE 10.6**

Interaction exists: line segments are not parallel.

This table is not additive. To see this, note that the mean of treatment *A* is 5 less than that of treatment *C* in block 1 (men), but 1 more than that of *C* in block 2. That is, the treatments behave differently in various blocks. In this case, we say that the blocks and treatments interact.

The graph for this table is shown in Figure 10.6. Since not all the line segments are parallel, there is interaction between blocks and treatments. Practically speaking, this means that we must be very careful when making statements concerning the treatments because the block involved is also important. For example, it is no longer correct to say that treatment *A* is superior to treatments *B* and *C* because it has the shortest mean recovery time. This statement is true for block 1 (men), but not for block 2 (women).

To derive the sum-of-squares identity for this model, we note that it can be shown that additivity implies that $\mu_{ij} = \mu + (\mu_{i\cdot} - \mu) + (\mu_{\cdot j} - \mu)$. Thus the theoretical model can be written in the form

$$X_{ij} - \mu \equiv (\mu_{i\cdot} - \mu) + (\mu_{\cdot j} - \mu) + \{X_{ij} - [\mu + (\mu_{i\cdot} - \mu) + (\mu_{\cdot j} - \mu)]\}$$

Replacing each of the theoretical means μ, $\mu_{i\cdot}$, $\mu_{\cdot j}$ by their estimators $\bar{X}_{\cdot\cdot}$, $\bar{X}_{i\cdot}$, $\bar{X}_{\cdot j}$, respectively, we obtain the following identity:

$$X_{ij} - \bar{X}_{\cdot\cdot} \equiv (\bar{X}_{i\cdot} - \bar{X}_{\cdot\cdot}) + (\bar{X}_{\cdot j} - \bar{X}_{\cdot\cdot}) + \{\bar{X}_{ij} - [\bar{X}_{\cdot\cdot} + (\bar{X}_{i\cdot} - \bar{X}_{\cdot\cdot}) + (\bar{X}_{\cdot j} - \bar{X}_{\cdot\cdot})]\}$$

If each side of this identity is squared and then summed over all possible values of *i* and *j*, the following sum-of-squares identity for the randomized complete block design results.

SUM-OF-SQUARES IDENTITY

$$\sum_{i=1}^{k}\sum_{j=1}^{b}(X_{ij} - \bar{X}_{\cdot\cdot})^2 = \sum_{i=1}^{k}\sum_{j=1}^{b}(X_{i\cdot} - \bar{X}_{\cdot\cdot})^2 + \sum_{i=1}^{k}\sum_{j=1}^{b}(X_{\cdot j} - \bar{X}_{\cdot\cdot})^2$$

$$+ \sum_{i=1}^{k}\sum_{j=1}^{b}(X_{ij} - \bar{X}_{i\cdot} - \bar{X}_{\cdot j} + \bar{X}_{\cdot\cdot})^2$$

The practical interpretation for each component is similar to that of the one-way classification model. In particular,

$$\sum_{i=1}^{k} \sum_{j=1}^{b} (X_{ij} - \bar{X}_{..})^2 = \text{measure of total variability in data}$$
$$= SS_{\text{Total}}$$

$$\sum_{i=1}^{k} \sum_{j=1}^{b} (\bar{X}_{i.} - \bar{X}_{..})^2 = \text{measure of variability in data}$$
$$\text{attributable to use of}$$
$$\text{different treatments}$$
$$= \text{treatment sum of squares}$$
$$= SS_{\text{Tr}}$$

$$\sum_{i=1}^{k} \sum_{j=1}^{b} (\bar{X}_{.j} - \bar{X}_{..})^2 = \text{measure of variability in data}$$
$$\text{attributable to use of}$$
$$\text{different blocks}$$
$$= \text{block sum of squares}$$
$$= SS_{\text{Blocks}}$$

$$\sum_{i=1}^{k} \sum_{j=1}^{b} (X_{ij} - \bar{X}_{i.} - \bar{X}_{.j} + \bar{X}_{..})^2 = \text{measure of variability in data}$$
$$\text{due to random factors}$$
$$= \text{residual, or error, sum of squares}$$
$$= SS_E$$

Using this notation, we can write the sum-of-squares identity as

$$SS_{\text{Total}} = SS_{\text{Tr}} + SS_{\text{Blocks}} + SS_E$$

The null hypothesis

$$H_0: \quad \mu_{1.} = \mu_{2.} = \cdots = \mu_{k.} \quad \text{(no difference in treatment means)}$$

can be tested by using these mean squares.

$$MS_{\text{Tr}} = \frac{SS_{\text{Tr}}}{k-1} = \text{treatment mean square}$$

$$MS_{\text{Blocks}} = \frac{SS_{\text{Blocks}}}{b-1} = \text{block mean square}$$

$$MS_E = \frac{SS_E}{(k-1)(b-1)} = \text{error mean square}$$

The expected values for the treatment and error mean squares are

$$E[MS_{\text{Tr}}] = \sigma^2 + \frac{b}{k-1} \sum_{i=1}^{k} (\mu_{i.} - \mu)^2$$

$$E[MS_E] = \sigma^2$$

To test H_0, the hypothesis of equal treatment means, the ratio

$$\boxed{\frac{MS_{\text{Tr}}}{MS_E} = F_{k-1,(k-1)(b-1)}}$$
(Test Statistic)

▨ **TABLE 10.9**

Analysis of variance: Randomized complete block design with fixed effects

Source of variation	Degrees of freedom	Sum of squares	Mean square	Expected mean square	*F* ratio
Treatment	$k - 1$	$\sum_{i=1}^{k} \dfrac{T_{i \cdot}^2}{b} - \dfrac{T_{\cdot \cdot}^2}{N}$	$\dfrac{SS_{\text{Tr}}}{k-1}$	$\sigma^2 + \dfrac{b}{k-1} \sum_{i=1}^{k} (\mu_i - \mu)^2$	$\dfrac{MS_{\text{Tr}}}{MS_E}$
Block	$b - 1$	$\sum_{j=1}^{b} \dfrac{T_{\cdot j}^2}{k} - \dfrac{T_{\cdot \cdot}^2}{N}$	$\dfrac{SS_{\text{Blocks}}}{b-1}$		
Error	$(k-1)(b-1)$	$SS_{\text{Total}} - SS_{\text{Tr}} - SS_{\text{Blocks}}$	$\dfrac{SS_E}{(k-1)(b-1)}$	σ^2	
Total	$kb - 1$	$\sum_{i=1}^{k} \sum_{j=1}^{b} X_{ij}^2 - \dfrac{T_{\cdot \cdot}^2}{N}$			

is used. If H_0 is true, this ratio should assume a value close to 1 since in this case $\sum_{i=1}^{k} (\mu_{i \cdot} - \mu)^2 = 0$ and MS_{Tr} and MS_E are each estimating σ^2. If H_0 is not true, then the value of this statistic should be larger than 1. The computational formulas used to evaluate these statistics are similar to those of the one-way classification model and are given in Table 10.9.

EXAMPLE 10.4.5. The following summary data from Example 10.4.2 are needed to continue to analysis of the energy requirements of running, walking, and bicycling:

$$k = 3 \qquad T_{\cdot 1} = 3.2 \qquad T_{\cdot 6} = 3.4$$
$$b = 8 \qquad T_{\cdot 2} = 3.5 \qquad T_{\cdot 7} = 3.2$$
$$N = 24 \qquad T_{\cdot 3} = 3.8 \qquad T_{\cdot 8} = 3.9$$
$$T_{\cdot \cdot} = 27.2 \qquad T_{\cdot 4} = 3.8$$
$$T_{\cdot 5} = 2.4$$

$$\sum_{i=1}^{3} \sum_{j=1}^{8} X_{ij}^2 = 36.18$$

$$T_{1 \cdot} = 13.2 \quad \text{(running)}$$
$$T_{2 \cdot} = 9.2 \quad \text{(walking)}$$
$$T_{3 \cdot} = 4.8 \quad \text{(bicycling)}$$

The ANOVA is shown in Table 10.10. Notice that $P = P[F_{2,14} \geq 78.75] < .01$. Since this probability is small, we can reject

$$H_0: \mu_{1 \cdot} = \mu_{2 \cdot} = \mu_{3 \cdot} \quad \text{(no difference in mean energy requirements)}$$

and conclude that there are differences in the energy requirements for the three activities.

If blocks are randomly chosen, as would probably be the case in Example 10.4.1, then the model is said to be mixed. The block effect in the model is considered to be a random variable and is written as B_j rather than β_j. The analysis of the data is not affected.

TABLE 10.10

ANOVA for the data of Example 10.4.5

Source	DF	SS	MS	F
Treatment	2	4.41	2.205	$78.75(F_{2,14})$
Block	7	.55	.079	
Error	14	.39	.028	
Total	23	5.35		

Effectiveness of Blocking

Since blocking is designed to control the effect of an extraneous variable, the natural question to ask is, Was blocking successful? If so, then SS_{Blocks} should account for a substantial portion of the total sum of squares. This, in turn, reduces SS_E, thereby increasing the value of the F ratio used to test for equality of treatment means and making it more likely that H_0 will be rejected. The power of the test will be improved. Note that the number of degrees of freedom for error in the one-way classification design is $N - k$; in the randomized complete block design it is smaller than this, namely, $(k - 1)(b - 1) = (N - k) - (b - 1)$. In Table IX of Appendix B, observe that as the number of degrees of freedom associated with the denominator of an F ratio decreases, the tabled F value increases. The implication of this is that if blocking is done unnecessarily, we pay a price for this mistake. Namely, the number of degrees of freedom for error decreases, the critical point for testing H_0 increases in size, and it becomes harder to reject H_0. The power of the test will become smaller. It is clear that blocking can help when appropriate but that indiscriminate blocking should be avoided.

When an experiment is being conducted for the first time, intuition, based on knowledge of the subject matter, is the only guide for deciding whether to block. Once the initial experiment is conducted, an assessment of the effectiveness of blocking can be done so that future studies can be designed efficiently. It seems reasonable to suggest that if block means are equal, then blocking is unnecessary; otherwise, blocking is useful. However, there is no known valid way to test the null hypothesis of equal block means. One approach used to investigate the effectiveness of blocking is to estimate the relative efficiency (RE) of the randomized complete block design as compared to the completely randomized design given in Section 10.1. The theoretical development of the notion of relative efficiency is beyond the scope of this text but can be found in [9] and [11]. Relative efficiency is a positive number that can be interpreted as the ratio of the number of observations per treatment needed for the two designs to be equivalent. For example, if $RE = 3$, then the completely randomized design requires three times as many observations as the randomized complete block design to produce a test with the same characteristics; blocking is desirable in this case. If $RE = .5$, then blocking is not desirable since the completely randomized design can accomplish the same thing as the randomized block design using half as many observations. If $RE = 1$, then the designs are equivalent when the sample sizes are identical.

Can we estimate the relative efficiency quickly from our original analysis of variance? Fortunately, there is an easy way to do so. It has been found [10] that there is a linear relationship between $\widehat{RE}$ and the ratio

$$\frac{MS_{\text{Blocks}}}{MS_E}$$

where $\qquad MS_{\text{Blocks}} = \text{block mean square} = \dfrac{SS_{\text{Blocks}}}{b-1}$

This relationship is given by

$$\widehat{RE} = c + (1-c)\frac{MS_{\text{Blocks}}}{MS_E}$$

where $c = b(k-1)/(bk-1)$. It is easy to show that

$$\widehat{RE} = 1 \text{ if and only if } MS_{\text{Blocks}}/MS_E = 1$$
$$\widehat{RE} < 1 \text{ if and only if } MS_{\text{Blocks}}/MS_E < 1$$
$$\widehat{RE} > 1 \text{ if and only if } MS_{\text{Blocks}}/MS_E > 1$$

Thus, to make a judgment about whether blocking in a particular experiment helped or hurt, we can use the information available from our ANOVA to find the value of MS_{Blocks}/MS_E. We then estimate the relative efficiency and decide from practical considerations, such as the time, cost, and effort required to block, whether blocking is worthwhile. As experience is gained, it will become unnecessary to actually compute $\widehat{RE}$. One need only consider the observed value of MS_{Blocks}/MS_E. Values considerably larger than 1 indicate that blocking was beneficial; values near 1 indicate that blocking neither helped nor hurt; values somewhat less than 1 indicate that blocking was not helpful. In the last case, a completely randomized design is preferable in future studies.

It should be noted that some texts include a "test" for blocks based on the statistic MS_{Blocks}/MS_E. However, because of the manner in which randomization is achieved in the randomized complete block design, the test is improper.

As an example, let us continue the analysis of the data given in Example 10.4.5.

EXAMPLE 10.4.6. From the analysis-of-variance table, Table 10.10, we see that

$$MS_{\text{Blocks}} = .079 \quad \text{and} \quad MS_E = .028$$

For these data, $b = 8, k = 3$, and

$$c = \frac{b(k-1)}{bk-1}$$
$$= \frac{8(2)}{23}$$
$$= .696$$

The estimated relative efficiency is

$$\widehat{RE} = c + (1 - c)\frac{MS_{\text{Blocks}}}{MS_E}$$

$$= .696 + .304\frac{.079}{.028}$$

$$= 1.55$$

Since $\widehat{RE} > 1$, it appears that blocking was beneficial in this case. The completely randomized design would require 1.55 as many observations as the randomized complete block design to produce a test of equal power. Notice also that in this case

$$\frac{MS_{\text{Blocks}}}{MS_E} = \frac{.079}{.028} = 2.82$$

exceeds 1, an indication that blocking is useful.

Paired and Multiple Comparisons

As in the one-way classification completely randomized design, paired comparisons can be made by performing $\binom{k}{2}$ Bonferroni-type T tests with α carefully chosen so that α' is kept under control. In this case, the T tests conducted are paired T tests. Keep in mind the fact that this method is feasible only when k is rather small. This is due to the fact that large values of k force α to be *extremely* small, resulting in a test with very little power.

A Duncan multiple range test is available also. The test is conducted as described in Section 10.2 with

$$\boxed{SSR_p = r_p\sqrt{\frac{MS_E}{b}}}$$

Note that, in this design, sample sizes are equal.

A Note on Computing

Most commercial computer packages include a technique for analyzing a randomized complete block design. In Example 10.4.7 we discuss the interpretation of the SAS printout obtained for the data of Example 10.4.5. The code used to produce this printout is given in the Technology Tools section at the end of this chapter.

EXAMPLE 10.4.7. The SAS printout (following) does not look exactly like the ANOVA table that was produced by hand. However, the values obtained by hand are found on the printout apart from roundoff differences. Numbers of interest are

① Degrees of freedom for treatment   ⑥ Error sum of squares
② Degrees of freedom for blocks   ⑦ Mean square error
③ Degrees of freedom for error   ⑧ Block sum of squares
④ Degrees of freedom total   ⑨ Treatment sum of squares
⑤ Total sum of squares

ANOVA for the data of Example 10.4.7

SAS

General Linear Models Procedure

Dependent Variable: KILOCAL

Source	DF	Sum of Squares	Mean Square	F Value	Pr>F
Model	9	4.96666667	.55185185	19.98	.0001
Error	14 ③	.38666667 ⑥	.02761905 ⑦		
Corrected Total	23 ④	5.35333333 ⑤			

R-Square	C.V.	Root MSE	KILOCAL Mean
0.927771	14.66381	0.166190	1.13333333

Source	DF	Type I SS	Mean Square	F Value	Pr>F
BLOCK	7 ②	0.55333333 ⑧	0.07904762	2.86 ⑫	.0446
TRTMENT	2 ①	4.41333333 ⑨	2.20666667	79.90 ⑩	.0001 ⑪

Source	DF	Type III SS	Mean Square	F Value	Pr>F
BLOCK	7	.55333333	.07904762	2.86	.0446
TRTMENT	2	4.41333333	2.20666667	79.90	.0001

SAS

General Linear Models Procedure

Duncan's   Multiple   Range   Test for variable:

KILOCAL

NOTE: This test control the type I comparison-wise error rate, not the experimentwise error rate

Alpha = .05   DF = 14   MSE = 0.027619

Number of Means	2	3
Critical Range	0.178	0.187

Means with the same letter are not significantly different.

Duncan Grouping	Mean	N	TRTMENT
A	1.6500	8	1
⑬ B	1.1500	8	2
C	0.6000	8	3

SAS

General Linear Models Procedure

Bonferroni   (Dunn)   T   tests for variable:

KILOCAL

NOTE: This test controls the type I experimentwise error rate, but generally has a higher type II error rate than REGWQ.

Alpha = .05   DF = 14   MSE = 0.027619

Critical Value of T = 2.72

Minimum Significant Difference=0.2258

Means with the same letter are not significantly different.

Bon Grouping	Mean	N	TRTMENT
A	1.6500	8	1
⑭ B	1.1500	8	2
C	0.6000	8	3

Notice that the F ratio used to test H_0: $\mu_1. = \mu_2. = \mu_3.$ is shown at ⑩ and its P value is given at ⑪. The block mean square used in estimating relative efficiency is shown at ⑫. The results of Duncan's multiple range test are given at ⑬. Notice that no means are identical. The Bonferroni T test results agree with the Duncan results and are shown at ⑭.

■ EXERCISES 10.4

Note: If possible, these problems should be worked using a computer.

1. For each table of population means, decide whether there is interaction between blocks and treatments.

(a)

Block	Treatment			
	A	B	C	D
1	1	3	4	0
2	4	6	7	3
3	2	4	5	1

(b)

Block	Treatment			
	A	B	C	D
1	1	3	0	0
2	4	6	5	3
3	2	4	5	1

(c)

Block	Treatment			
	A	B	C	D
1	1	3	4	0
2	4	5	7	3
3	2	4	5	1

2. The Sitka spruce is economically the most important forest tree in the United Kingdom. However, it exhibits poor natural regeneration as a result of the infrequency of good seed years. There is a definite need to increase seed production. Four hormone treatments are proposed. Since different trees have various natural reproductive characteristics, the effect of tree differences is controlled by blocking. Ten trees are used in the experiment. Four similar branches are selected within each tree. Each branch receives exactly one of the four treatments, with treatments being randomly assigned to branches. Thus each tree constitutes a complete block. The measured response is the number of seeds produced per branch. Assume that this variable, though discrete, is approximately normally distributed. The data are shown in Table 10.11.

   (a) Complete Table 10.11 by computing sample treatment totals and means, block totals and means, and the grand total and grand mean.

   (b) Test the null hypothesis of equal treatment means.

3. Explain the meaning of each of these relative efficiencies in assessing the effectiveness of blocking.

   (a) $RE = 2$

   (b) $RE = 10$

   (c) $RE = .25$

▨ **TABLE 10.11**

Block (tree)	Treatment				Block total	Block mean
	A	**B**	**C**	**D**		
1	89	59	20	51		
2	87	56	15	47		
3	84	52	14	45		
4	92	67	26	56		
5	95	70	28	60		
6	90	62	22	53		
7	89	60	19	51		
8	88	56	17	50		
9	82	50	14	45		
10	94	63	24	53		
Treatment total						
Treatment mean						

(*d*) $RE = .10$

(*e*) $RE = 1$

4. Estimate the relative efficiency for the data of Exercise 2. Does it appear that blocking was useful? Explain.

5. A study is conducted of the effect of light on the growth of ferns. Since plants grow at various rates at different ages, this variable is controlled by blocking. Four young plants (plants grown in the dark for 4 days) and four older plants (plants grown in the dark for 12 days) are utilized in the study, thus producing two blocks each of size 4. Four different light treatments are investigated. Each treatment is randomly assigned to one plant in each block. The treatments consist of exposing-each plant to a single dose of light, returning it to the dark, and measuring the cross-sectional area of the fern tip 24 hours after the light is administered. These data resulted (cross-sectional area is given in square micrometers):

Block (age)	Treatment (wavelength of light)			
	420 nm	**460 nm**	**600 nm**	**720 nm**
Young	1017.6	929.0	939.8	1081.5
Old	854.7	689.9	841.5	797.4

(*a*) Find the sample treatment, block, and grand totals and means.

(*b*) Test the null hypothesis of equal treatment means.

(*c*) Estimate the relative efficiency and comment on the effectiveness of blocking.

6. Use Duncan's multiple range test with $\alpha = .01$ to complete the analysis of the data of Example 10.4.5. Use $\alpha = .01$.

7. Use Duncan's multiple range test to complete the analysis of the data of Exercise 2.

8. A study of the effect of deer season on the habits of deer is conducted. Four paths known to be used by deer are selected. The average number of footprints found per

week on a specified section of each path is determined before deer season begins, during deer season, and after the season ends. Paths are treated as blocks, and these data are obtained:

Path	Before	During	After
1	62.5	57.0	49.0
2	46.5	53.3	50.0
3	45.0	59.3	37.0
4	24.0	35.7	50.0

(a) Test H$_0$: $\mu_{1.} = \mu_{2.} = \mu_{3..}$.

(b) If differences are found in part a, use Bonferroni T tests with an overall α level of at most .15 to pinpoint the differences that exist.

(c) Estimate the relative efficiency and comment on the effectiveness of blocking. (Based on a study conducted by Daniel Brown, Department of Biology, Radford University and the Radford University Consulting Service, October 1990.)

9. A study is conducted to ascertain the effect of ankle taping on the ankle flexibility of runners. Flexibility is measured before taping, after taping, and after running with the ankles taped. One group of subjects was taped using a standard method of taping; the other was taped using a reinforced taping technique. Subjects are treated as blocks. Higher scores represent more flexibility. These data are obtained:

Block (subject)	Treatment (standard taping) Before taping	After taping	After running	Block (subject)	Treatment (standard taping) Before taping	After taping	After running
1	2.5	1.0	4.0	9	12.0	2.5	0.5
2	9.0	1.0	6.5	10	3.5	7.5	3.5
3	6.0	3.0	2.0	11	0.5	1.0	1.0
4	2.5	0.5	1.5	12	6.0	4.0	5.5
5	6.0	4.5	4.5	13	0.0	4.5	1.0
6	3.5	0.0	3.5	14	5.0	2.0	7.5
7	7.5	5.5	3.5	15	0.5	0.5	1.0
8	4.0	2.0	0.0	16	5.5	−0.5	0.5

Block (subject)	Treatment (reinforced taping) Before taping	After taping	After running	Block (subject)	Treatment (reinforced taping) Before taping	After taping	After running
1	6.5	2.5	4.5	9	−3.5	−3.5	0.0
2	4.5	2.5	6.0	10	2.5	2.0	−0.5
3	5.5	4.0	3.0	11	3.0	1.5	1.0
4	5.0	4.0	7.0	12	7.5	8.5	6.5
5	2.0	4.5	4.0	13	9.5	1.0	0.5
6	5.0	2.5	1.5	14	6.0	3.5	2.0
7	10.0	4.0	3.0	15	−0.5	0.5	0.5
8	8.5	0.0	10.5	16	5.5	−0.5	5.0

Analyze each of these data sets and comment on similarities or differences that you find between standard and reinforced taping. (Based on a study conducted by Jay Cantebury, Department of Physical Education, Radford University, 1997.)

10.5
FACTORIAL EXPERIMENTS

In many experiments, two or more variables are being actively investigated. Neither variable is considered extraneous; each is of equal concern. When this occurs, the experiment is called a *factorial experiment,* to emphasize the fact that interest is centered on the effect of two or more factors on a measured response. We present here the *two-way classification, completely random design with fixed effects.* Thus we deal with a model in which two factors, *A* and *B*, are studied with the levels of each factor being purposely, rather than randomly, selected by the experimenter. No matching of like experimental units is done.

EXAMPLE 10.5.1. The *Mirogrex terrae-sanctae* is a commercial sardine-like fish found in the Sea of Galilee. A study is conducted to determine the effect of light and temperature on the gonadosomatic index (GSI), which is a measure of the growth of the ovary. Two photoperiods—14 hours of light, 10 hours of dark and 9 hours of light, 15 hours of dark—and two temperature levels—16 and 27°C—are used. In this way, the experimenter can simulate both summer and winter conditions in the region. This is a factorial experiment with two factors, light and temperature, each being investigated at two levels.

Data Format and Notation

The data collected in a two-way classification design are conveniently recorded in the following format:

Data layout of two-way classification

Factor B	Factor A level				
	1	**2**	**3**	$\cdots$	a
1	X_{111}	X_{211}	X_{311}	$\cdots$	X_{a11}
	X_{112}	X_{212}	X_{312}	$\cdots$	X_{a12}
	X_{11n}	X_{21n}	X_{31n}	$\cdots$	X_{a1n}
2	X_{121}	X_{221}	X_{321}	$\cdots$	X_{a21}
	X_{122}	X_{222}	X_{322}	$\cdots$	X_{a22}
	X_{12n}	X_{22n}	X_{32n}	$\cdots$	X_{a2n}
$\vdots$					
b	X_{1b1}	X_{2b1}	X_{3b1}	$\cdots$	X_{ab1}
	X_{1b2}	X_{2b2}	X_{3b2}	$\cdots$	X_{ab2}
	X_{1bn}	X_{2bn}	X_{3bn}	$\cdots$	X_{abn}

Note that a denotes the number of levels of factor A used in the experiment, b denotes the number of levels of factor b, and $a \cdot b$ is the total number of treatment combinations, where a treatment combination is a level of factor A applied in conjunction with a level of B. We assume that there are n observations for each treatment combination. Thus the total number of responses is $N = a \cdot b \cdot n$. The variable X_{ijk}, $i = 1, 2, \ldots, a$, $j = 1, 2, \ldots, b$, $k = 1, 2, \ldots, n$, is a random variable denoting the response of the kth experimental unit to the ith level of factor A and the jth level of factor B. These sample statistics are needed in analyzing the data. Recall that the dot indicates the subscript over which summation is being conducted.

$$T_{ij\cdot} = \sum_{k=1}^{n} X_{ijk} = \text{total of all responses to } i\text{th level of factor } A \text{ and } j\text{th}$$
$$\text{level of factor } B$$
$$= \text{total of all responses to the } (i - j)\text{th treatment combination}$$

$$\bar{X}_{ij\cdot} = \frac{T_{ij\cdot}}{n} = \text{sample mean for } (i - j)\text{th treatment combination}$$

$$T_{i\cdot\cdot} = \sum_{j=1}^{b} T_{ij\cdot} = \text{total of all responses to } i\text{th level, } i = 1, 2, \ldots, a, \text{ of}$$
$$\text{factor } A$$

$$\bar{X}_{i\cdot\cdot} = \frac{T_{i\cdot\cdot}}{bn} = \text{sample means for } i\text{th level of factor } A$$

$$T_{\cdot j\cdot} = \sum_{i=1}^{a} T_{ij\cdot} = \text{total of all responses to } j\text{th level, } j = 1, 2, \ldots, b, \text{ of}$$
$$\text{factor } B$$

$$\bar{X}_{\cdot j\cdot} = \frac{T_{\cdot j\cdot}}{an} = \text{sample mean for } j\text{th level of factor } B$$

$$T_{\cdots} = \sum_{i=1}^{a} T_{i\cdot\cdot} = \sum_{j=1}^{b} T_{\cdot j\cdot} = \sum_{i=1}^{a}\sum_{j=1}^{b} T_{ij\cdot} = \text{total of all responses}$$

$$\bar{X}_{\cdots} = \frac{T_{\cdots}}{abn} \text{ sample mean for all responses}$$

$$\sum_{i=1}^{a}\sum_{j=1}^{b}\sum_{k=1}^{n} X_{ijk}^2 = \text{sum of squares of each response}$$

These statistics are evaluated in Example 10.5.2.

EXAMPLE 10.5.2. The experiment of Example 10.5.1 was conducted by collecting 20 females in June. Then this group was randomly divided into four subgroups, each of size 5. Each subgroup received one of the four possible treatment combinations. At the end of 3 months, the GSI for each fish was determined. These data resulted:

Factor B (temperature)	Factor A (photoperiod) 9 hours	Factor A (photoperiod) 14 hours	Total (factor *B*)
27°C	(Unnatural) .90 1.06 .98 1.29 1.12 $T_{11.} = 5.35$ $\bar{X}_{11.} = 1.07$	(Simulated summer) .83 .67 .57 .47 .66 $T_{21.} = 3.2$ $\bar{X}_{21.} = .64$	$T_{.1.} = T_{11.} + T_{21.}$ $= 8.55$ $\bar{X}_{.1.} = .855$
16°C	(Simulated winter) 1.30 2.88 2.42 2.66 2.94 $T_{12.} = 12.20$ $\bar{X}_{12.} = 2.44$	(Unnatural) 1.01 1.52 1.02 1.32 1.63 $T_{22.} = 6.5$ $\bar{X}_{22.} = 1.3$	$T_{.2.} = T_{12.} + T_{22.}$ $= 18.7$ $\bar{X}_{.2.} = 1.87$
Total (factor *A*)	$T_{1..} = T_{11.} + T_{12.}$ $= 17.55$ $\bar{X}_{1..} = 1.755$	$T_{2..} = T_{21.} + T_{22.}$ $= 9.7$ $\bar{X}_{2..} = .97$	$T_{...} = 27.25$ (grand total) $\bar{X}_{...} = 1.363$

For these data, $a = 2$, $b = 2$, $n = 5$, and $N = a \cdot b \cdot n = 20$. Also

$$\sum_{i=1}^{2}\sum_{j=1}^{2}\sum_{k=1}^{5} X_{ijk}^2 = 48.26$$

The following notation is needed to write the model for the design:

μ = overall mean effect

$\mu_{i..}$ = mean for *i*th level of factor *A*, $i = 1, 2, \ldots, a$

$\mu_{.j.}$ = mean for *j*th level of factor *B*, $j = 1, 2, \ldots, b$

$\mu_{ij.}$ = mean for $(i - j)$th treatment combination

$\alpha_i = \mu_{i..} - \mu$ = effect due to fact that experimental unit was in *i*th level of factor *A*

$\beta_j = \mu_{.j.} - \mu$ = effect due to fact that experimental unit was in *j*th level of factor *B*

$(\alpha\beta)_{ij} = \mu_{ij} - \mu_{i..} - \mu_{.j.} + \mu$ = effect of interaction between *i*th level of factor *A* and *j*th level of factor *B*

$E_{ijk} = X_{ijk} - \mu_{ij}$ = residual, or random, error

Using this notation, we can express the model as follows:

MODEL

$$X_{ijk} \equiv \mu + \alpha_i + \beta_j + (\alpha\beta)_{ij} + E_{ijk} \quad \begin{matrix} i = 1, 2, \ldots, a \\ j = 1, 2, \ldots, b \\ k = 1, 2, \ldots, n \end{matrix}$$

This model expresses symbolically the idea that each observation can be partitioned into five components: an overall mean effect (μ), an effect due to factor A (α_i), an effect due to factor B (β_j), an effect due to interaction ($\alpha\beta$)$_{ij}$, and a random deviation due to unexplained sources (E_{ijk}). We make the following assumptions:

MODEL ASSUMPTIONS

1. The observations for each treatment combination constitute independent random samples, each of size n, from $a \cdot b$ populations with means μ_{ij}, $i = 1, 2, \ldots, a$, $j = 1, 2, \ldots, b$.
2. Each of the $a \cdot b$ populations is normal.
3. Each of the $a \cdot b$ populations has the same variance, σ^2.

The sum-of-squares identity obtained by replacing each of the theoretical means μ, $\mu_{i.}$, $\mu_{.j}$, μ_{ij} by their estimators $\bar{X}_{...}$, $\bar{X}_{i..}$, $\bar{X}_{.j.}$, $\bar{X}_{ij.}$, respectively, squaring, and summing over i, j, and k is as follows:

SUM-OF-SQUARES IDENTITY

$$SS_{\text{Total}} = SS_A + SS_B + SS_{AB} + SS_E$$

In this identity,

$$SS_{\text{Total}} = \sum_{i=1}^{a}\sum_{j=1}^{b}\sum_{k=1}^{n}(X_{ijk} - \bar{X}_{...})^2 = \text{measure of total variability in data}$$

$$SS_A = \sum_{i=1}^{a}\sum_{j=1}^{b}\sum_{k=1}^{n}(\bar{X}_{i..} - \bar{X}_{...})^2 = \begin{array}{l}\text{measure of variability in} \\ \text{data attributable to use of} \\ \text{different levels of factor } A\end{array}$$

$$SS_B = \sum_{i=1}^{a}\sum_{j=1}^{b}\sum_{k=1}^{n}(\bar{X}_{.j.} - \bar{X}_{...})^2 = \begin{array}{l}\text{measure of variability in data attributable} \\ \text{to use of different levels of factor } B\end{array}$$

$$SS_{AB} = \sum_{i=1}^{a}\sum_{j=1}^{b}\sum_{k=1}^{n}(\bar{X}_{ij.} - \bar{X}_{i..} - \bar{X}_{.j.} + \bar{X}_{...})^2 = \begin{array}{l}\text{measure of variability} \\ \text{in data due to} \\ \text{interaction between} \\ \text{levels of factor } A \text{ and } B\end{array}$$

$$SS_E = \sum_{i=1}^{a}\sum_{j=1}^{b}\sum_{k=1}^{n}(X_{ijk} - \bar{X}_{ij.})^2 = \begin{array}{l}\text{measure of variability in data} \\ \text{due to random, or unexplained,} \\ \text{sources}\end{array}$$

Testing Main Effects and Interaction

The first null hypothesis to be tested is the null hypothesis of no interaction. Mathematically, this hypothesis is

$$H_0: (\alpha\beta)_{ij} = 0 \qquad i = 1, 2, \ldots, a; \qquad j = 1, 2, \ldots, b$$

If this hypothesis is not rejected, then the analysis is continued by testing the null hypothesis of no difference among levels of factor A,

$$H_0': \mu_{1..} = \mu_{2..} = \cdots = \mu_{a..}$$

and the null hypothesis of no difference among levels of factor B,

$$H_0'': \mu_{.1.} = \mu_{.2.} = \cdots = \mu_{.b.}$$

However, if the null hypothesis of no interaction is rejected, then we do not test H_0' and H_0''. In this case, since the levels of factor A do not behave consistently across the levels of factor B, and vice versa, we test for differences among levels of factor A for each of the b levels of factor B individually. This is done by running b individual one-way classification analyses. We test these hypotheses:

$$H_0: \mu_{1j.} = \mu_{2j.} = \cdots = \mu_{aj.} \qquad j = 1, 2, \ldots, b$$

The computational formulas used to compute SS_A, SS_B, and SS_{Total}, are similar to those of previous models:

$$SS_A = \sum_{i=1}^{a} \frac{T_{i..}^2}{bn} - \frac{T_{...}^2}{abn}$$

$$SS_B = \sum_{j=1}^{b} \frac{T_{.j.}^2}{an} - \frac{T_{...}^2}{abn}$$

$$SS_{\text{Total}} = \sum_{i=1}^{a} \sum_{j=1}^{b} \sum_{k=1}^{n} X_{ijk}^2 - \frac{T_{...}^2}{abn}$$

The interaction sum of squares is found by first computing what is called the treatment sum of squares. This is the usual treatment sum of squares that would be obtained if the $a \cdot b$ treatment combinations were analyzed as a one-way classification design. That is,

$$SS_{\text{Tr}} = \sum_{i=1}^{a} \sum_{j=1}^{b} \frac{T_{ij.}^2}{n} - \frac{T_{...}^2}{abn}$$

It can be shown that $SS_{\text{Tr}} = SS_A + SS_B + SS_{AB}$. This allows us to compute the interaction sum of squares by subtraction:

$$SS_{AB} = SS_{\text{Tr}} - SS_A - SS_B$$

The error sum of squares can also be obtained by subtraction:

$$SS_E = SS_{\text{Total}} - SS_{\text{Tr}}$$

The analysis-of-variance table for this design is given in Table 10.12.

The first F ratio to consider in any experiment is

$$\boxed{F_{(a-1)(b-1), ab(n-1)} = \frac{MS_{AB}}{MS_E}} \qquad \text{(Test Statistic)}$$

This ratio is used to test the null hypothesis of no interaction. If this hypothesis is not

▧ **TABLE 10.12**

Analysis of variance: Two-way classification, completely random design with fixed effects

Source of variation	Degrees of freedom	Sum of squares	Mean square	Expected mean square	F ratio
Treatment	$ab - 1$	$\displaystyle\sum_{i=1}^{a}\sum_{j=1}^{b}\frac{T_{ij.}^2}{n} - \frac{T_{...}^2}{abn}$	$\dfrac{SS_{Tr}}{ab-1}$	$\sigma^2 + n\displaystyle\sum_{i=1}^{a}\sum_{j=1}^{b}\frac{(\mu_{ij.}-\mu_{...})^2}{ab-1}$	$\dfrac{MS_{Tr}}{MS_E}$
A	$a - 1$	$\displaystyle\sum_{i=1}^{a}\frac{T_{i..}^2}{bn} - \frac{T_{...}^2}{abn}$	$\dfrac{SS_A}{a-1}$	$\sigma^2 + nb\displaystyle\sum_{i=1}^{a}\frac{(\mu_{j..}-\mu_{...})^2}{a-1}$	$\dfrac{MS_A}{MS_E}$
B	$b - 1$	$\displaystyle\sum_{j=1}^{b}\frac{T_{.j.}^2}{an} - \frac{T_{...}^2}{abn}$	$\dfrac{SS_B}{b-1}$	$\sigma^2 + na\displaystyle\sum_{j=1}^{b}\frac{(\mu_{.j.}-\mu_{...})^2}{b-1}$	$\dfrac{MS_B}{MS_E}$
AB	$(a-1)(b-1)$	$SS_{Tr} - SS_A - SS_B$	$\dfrac{SS_{AB}}{(a-1)(b-1)}$	$\sigma^2 + n\displaystyle\sum_{i=1}^{a}\sum_{j=1}^{b}\frac{(\alpha\beta)_{ij}^2}{(a-1)(b-1)}$	$\dfrac{MS_{AB}}{MS_E}$
Error	$ab(n-1)$	$SS_{Total} - SS_{Tr}$	$\dfrac{SS_E}{ab(n-1)}$	σ^2	
Total	$abn - 1$	$\displaystyle\sum_{i=1}^{a}\sum_{j=1}^{b}\sum_{k=1}^{n} X_{ijk}^2 - \frac{T_{...}^2}{abn}$			

rejected, then the F statistics

$$\boxed{F_{a-1,ab(n-1)} = \frac{MS_A}{MS_E}}\qquad \text{(Test Statistic)}$$

and

$$\boxed{F_{b-1,ab(n-1)} = \frac{MS_B}{MS_E}}\qquad \text{(Test Statistic)}$$

are used to test the null hypotheses of no difference among the means of levels of factors A and B, respectively.

These tests are called tests for "main effects." If the null hypothesis of no interaction is rejected, we do not test for main effects. Rather, b one-way analyses are run to detect differences among levels of factor A at each level of factor B individually. In each case, rejection occurs for values of the F ratio that are too large to have occurred by chance.

We illustrate these ideas by completing the analysis of the data of Example 10.5.2.

EXAMPLE 10.5.3. The following totals were obtained in Example 10.5.2:

$T_{11.} = 5.35 \qquad T_{22.} = 6.5 \qquad T_{.1.} = 8.55$
$T_{21.} = 3.2 \qquad T_{1..} = 17.55 \qquad T_{.2.} = 18.7$
$T_{12.} = 12.20 \qquad T_{2..} = 9.7 \qquad T_{...} = 27.25$

$$\sum_{i=1}^{2}\sum_{j=1}^{2}\sum_{k=1}^{5} X_{ijk}^2 = 48.26$$

TABLE 10.13

ANOVA for the data of example 10.5.3

Source	DF	SS	MS	F
Treatment	3	8.86	2.95	21.07
A	1	3.08	3.08	22.0
B	1	5.15	5.15	36.79
AB	1	.63	.63	4.5*
Error	16	2.27	.14	
Total	19	11.13		

These totals are used to obtain the needed sums of squares:

$$SS_{\text{Tr}} = \frac{(5.35)^2}{5} + \frac{(3.2)^2}{5} + \frac{(12.20)^2}{5} + \frac{(6.5)^2}{5} - \frac{(27.25)^2}{20} = 8.86$$

$$SS_A = \frac{(17.55)^2}{10} + \frac{(9.7)^2}{10} - \frac{(27.25)^2}{20} = 3.08$$

$$SS_B = \frac{(8.55)^2}{10} + \frac{(18.7)^2}{10} - \frac{(27.25)^2}{20} = 5.15$$

$$SS_{AB} = SS_{\text{Tr}} - SS_A - SS_B = 8.86 - 3.08 - 5.15 = .63$$

$$SS_{\text{Total}} = 48.26 - \frac{(27.25)^2}{20} = 11.13$$

$$SS_E = SS_{\text{Total}} - SS_{\text{Tr}} = 11.13 - 8.86 = 2.27$$

The ANOVA is given in Table 10.13.

We look first at the F ratio used to test for interaction (* in the table). The P value for this statistic is

$$P = P[F_{1,16} \geq 4.5] \doteq .05$$

Since this probability is small, we reject the null hypothesis of no interaction and conclude that there is interaction between the light cycle used and the temperature.

The nature of this interaction can be seen in Figure 10.7. Notice that the line segments joining the sample means for the two levels of factor B are not parallel. While there is a decline in GSI as one moves from 9 to 14 hours of light in each case, the decline is more rapid at 16°C than at 27°C. There is an inconsistency in behavior at the two temperatures. To complete the analysis, we conduct two one-way analyses. In particular, we compare the mean GSI at 9 hours light to that at 14 hours light first at 16°C then at 27°C. The results of these tests are shown in Tables 10.14 and 10.15, respectively. Notice that in each case the null hypothesis of equality of means can be rejected with $P < .01$. Thus, at each temperature it can be concluded that there is a difference in the mean GSI between the two photoperiods.

Notice that in this design cell sizes are equal. There are n observations taken at each treatment combination. This is *essential* in order for the analysis just presented to be valid. If cell sizes are not the same, the design is said to be unbalanced. Such

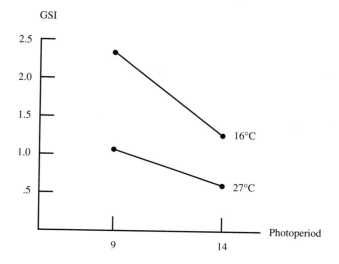

FIGURE 10.7

Line segments are not parallel, indicating an interaction between temperature and photoperiod.

TABLE 10.14

One-way analysis of variance used to compare the mean GSI at 9 hours light to that at 14 hours light when the temperature is 16°C

Source	DF	SS	MS	F
Treatment	1	3.249	3.249	12.306
Error	8	2.1122	.264025	
Total	9	5.3612		

TABLE 10.15

One-way analysis of variance used to compare the mean GSI at 9 hours light to that at 14 hours light when the temperature is 27°C

Source	DF	SS	MS	F
Treatment	1	.46225	.46225	23.228
Error	8	.1592	.0199	
Total	9	.62145		

designs are tricky to handle. If you encounter this situation in a research project, the help of a statistician should be sought in analyzing your data.

Multiple and Paired Comparisons

If the null hypothesis of no interaction is not rejected in a two-way analysis of variance, then interest centers on the main effects. If differences are found among the levels of factor A or B, then Bonferroni T tests or Duncan's multiple range test can be used to pinpoint the differences. Bonferroni tests are pooled T tests which utilize MS_E as the estimator for σ^2.

To pinpoint differences among the levels of factor A, using Duncan's test,

$$SSR_p = r_p \sqrt{\frac{MS_E}{bn}}$$

To determine what differences exist among levels of factor B,

$$SSR_p = r_p \sqrt{\frac{MS_E}{an}}$$

A Note on Computing

As you can see, completely analyzing a two-way analysis of variance by hand is time-consuming. This is especially true for large data sets. In practice, data of this sort are analyzed by computer. Example 10.5.4 illustrates the computer analysis of the data of Example 10.5.3. See the Technology Tools section of the end of this chapter for the SAS code used to produce this output.

EXAMPLE 10.5.4. The two-way analysis-of-variance table for the data of Example 10.5.3 is given in Table 10.16. The table is not in the same format as Table 10.13, but the values given there can be found. In particular, these values of interest are

   ① Degrees of freedom for treatments (cells)
   ② Treatment sum of squares
   ③ Treatment mean square
   ④ Total degrees of freedom
   ⑤ Sum-of-squares total
   ⑥ Degrees of freedom for error
   ⑦ Error sum of squares
   ⑧ Error mean square
   ⑨ Degrees of freedom for interaction
   ⑩ Interaction sum of squares

TABLE 10.16

Two-way analysis of variance for the data of Example 10.5.3. Notice that interaction is present. The analysis is completed by referring to Tables 10.17 and 10.18.

```
                                        SAS
                         General Linear Models Procedure

Dependent
 Variable: GSI
                                  Sum of           Mean
Source              DF           Squares          Square      F Value      Pr>F
Model               3 ①      8.86237500 ②    2.95412500 ③     20.81       .0001
Error              16 ⑥      2.27140000 ⑦     .14196250 ⑧
Corrected Total    19 ④     11.13377500 ⑤

            R-Square            C.V.          Root MSE              GSI Mean
            .795990           27.65351        .376779             1.36250000

Source              DF        Type I SS      Mean Square    F Value       Pr>F
PHOTOPRD            1         3.08112500      3.08112500      21.70       0.0003
TEMP               1         5.15112500      5.15112500      36.29       0.0001
PHOTOPRD*TEMP      1         0.63012500      0.63012500       4.44       0.0513

Source              DF       Type III SS     Mean Square    F Value       Pr>F
PHOTOPRD           1 ⑲     3.08112500 ⑳   3.08112500 ㉑    21.70 ㉒   0.0023 ㉓
TEMP              1 ⑭     5.15112500 ⑮   5.15112500 ⑯    36.29 ⑰   0.0001 ⑱
PHOTOPRD*TEMP     1 ⑨     0.63012500 ⑩   0.63012500 ⑪     4.44 ⑫   0.0513 ⑬
```

⑪ Interaction mean squares

⑫ F ratio used to test the null hypothesis of no interaction

⑬ P value for the test for interaction

⑭ Degrees of freedom for factor B

⑮ Sum of squares for factor B

⑯ Mean square for factor B

⑰ F ratio used to test for overall differences among levels of factor B

⑱ P value for the test on B main effects

⑲ Degrees of freedom for factor A

⑳ Sum of squares for factor A

㉑ Mean square for factor A

㉒ F value used to test for overall differences among levels of factor A

㉓ P value for the test on A main effects

Notice that in this case, we first test for interaction. Since interaction is present, we do not bother with the tests for main effects. Rather, we continue by interpreting the one-way ANOVA given in Tables 10.17 and 10.18. From Table 10.17, we see that there is a difference in mean GSI levels between the two photoperiods ($P = .008$) at 16°C. Table 10.18 shows that there is also a difference in mean GSI levels between the two photoperiods at 27°C ($P = .0013$).

■ **TABLE 10.17**

One-way analysis of variance used to compare photoperiods when the temperature is 16°C

SAS

Analysis-of-Variance Procedure

Dependent
 Variable: GSI

Source	DF	Sum of Squares	Mean Square	F Value	Pr>F
Model	1	3.24900000	3.24900000	12.31	0.0080
Error	8	2.11220000	0.26402500		
Corrected Total	9	5.36120000			

	R-Square	C.V.	Root MSE		GSI Mean
	0.606021	27.47773	0.513834		1.87000000

Source	DF	Anova SS	Mean Square	F Value	Pr>F
PHOTOPRD	1	3.24900000	3.24900000	12.31	0.0080

■ **TABLE 10.18**

One-way analysis of variance used to compare photoperiods when the temperature is 27°C

SAS

Analysis-of-Variance Procedure

Dependent Variable: GSI

Source	DF	Sum of Squares	Mean Square	F Value	Pr>F
Model	1	0.46225000	0.46225000	23.23	0.0013
Error	8	0.15920000	0.01990000		
Corrected Total	9	0.62145000			

	R-Square	C.V.	Root MSE		GSI Mean
	0.743825	16.49911	0.141067		0.85500000

Source	DF	Anova SS	Mean Square	F Value	Pr>F
PHOTOPRD	1	0.4622500	0.46225000	23.23	0.0013

■ **EXERCISES 10.5**

Note: If possible, these problems should be worked using a computer.

1. A study is conducted to determine the effect of water level and type of plant on the overall stem length of pea plants. Three water levels and two plant types are used. Eighteen leafless plants are available for study. These plants are randomly divided into three subgroups, and then water levels are randomly assigned to the groups. A

similar procedure is followed with 18 conventional plants. These data resulted (stem length is given in centimeters):

Factor B	Factor A (water level)			Total (factor B)
(plant type)	Low	Medium	High	
Leafless	69.0	96.1	121.0	1788
	71.3	102.3	122.9	
	73.2	107.5	123.1	
	75.1	103.6	125.7	
	74.4	100.7	125.2	
	75.0 (438)	101.8 (612)	120.1 (738)	
Conventional	71.1	81.0	101.1	1578
	69.2	85.8	103.2	
	70.4	86.0	106.1	
	73.2	87.5	109.7	
	71.2	88.1	109.0	
	70.9 (426)	87.6 (516)	106.9 (636)	
Total (factor A)	864	1128	1374	3366

(a) Verify the totals given.

(b) For these data,

$$\sum_{i=1}^{3}\sum_{j=1}^{2}\sum_{k=1}^{6} X_{ijk}^{2} = 327{,}431.42$$

Use this to find SS_{Total}.

(c) Find SS_{Tr}. Use this and SS_{Total} to find SS_E.

(d) Find SS_A and SS_B. Use these and SS_{Tr} to find SS_{AB}.

(e) Find the ANOVA table, and use it to test the appropriate hypotheses.

(f) If appropriate, continue the analysis, using Duncan's multiple range test.

2. A study is run of the effect of photoperiod and genotype on the latent period of infection of barley mildew isolate AB3. Fifty leaves of each of four genotypes are obtained and randomly split into five subgroups, each of size 10. Each group is infected and then is exposed to a different photoperiod. The response noted is the number of days until the appearance of visible symptoms. The following treatment and level *totals* are found:

Factor B	Factor A (photoperiod: hours darkness per 24-h cycle)					Total
(genotype)	0	2	4	8	16	(factor B)
Armelle	630	610	560	570	590	2,960
Golden Promise	640	630	600	620	620	3,110
Emir	640	630	650	620	580	3,120
Vacla	660	660	620	610	630	3,180
Total (factor A)	2,570	2,530	2,430	2,420	2,420	12,370

(*a*) For these data,

$$\sum_{i=1}^{5}\sum_{j=1}^{4}\sum_{k=1}^{10} X_{ijk}^2 = 773{,}377.2$$

Use this to find SS_{Total}.
(*b*) Find SS_{Tr}. Use this and SS_{Total} to find SS_E.
(*c*) Find SS_A and SS_B. Use these and SS_{Tr} to find SS_{AB}.
(*d*) Find the ANOVA table, and test the appropriate hypotheses.
(*e*) Where appropriate, continue the analysis using Duncan's multiple range test with $\alpha = .05$.

3. A study is run of the capsular solubility in biological fluids of two of the most commonly encapsulated enzyme preparations. The purpose is to determine the effect of capsule type and biological fluid on the time until dissolution of the capsule. Two biological fluids, gastric and duodenal juices, and two capsule types, *C* and *V*, are used. Thus two factors are involved, each being studied at two levels. To conduct the study, 10 empty capsules of each type are obtained and randomly divided into two subgroups, each of size 5. One group is dissolved in gastric juices; the other, in duodenal juices. The response noted is the time at which the first air bubbles are released through perforations in the capsules. These data resulted (time is in minutes):

Factor B (capsule type)	Factor A (fluid type)		Total (factor B)
	Gastric	Duodenal	
C	39.5	31.2	430.5
	45.7	33.5	
	49.8	36.7	
	50.2	42.0	
	63.8 (249)	38.1 (181.5)	
V	47.4	44.0	428.5
	43.5	41.2	
	39.8	47.3	
	36.1	45.3	
	41.2 (208)	42.7 (220.5)	
Total (factor A)	457	402	859

(*a*) Verify the totals given.
(*b*) For these data,

$$\sum_{i=1}^{2}\sum_{j=1}^{2}\sum_{k=1}^{5} X_{ijk}^2 = 37{,}847.26$$

Use this value to find SS_{Total}.
(*c*) Find SS_{Tr}. Use this and SS_{Total} to find SS_E.
(*d*) Find SS_A and SS_B. Use these and SS_{Tr} to find SS_{AB}.
(*e*) Sketch a graph of the sample means for the levels of factor *A* for each level of factor *B*. Does this lead you to suspect the presence of interaction? Explain.
(*f*) Complete the analysis of the data by finding the ANOVA table and testing the appropriate hypotheses.

4. Cotinine is a major metabolite of nicotine. It is currently considered to be the best indicator of tobacco smoke exposure. A study is conducted to detect possible racial differences in cotinine level in young adults. These data are obtained on the cotinine level in milligrams per milliliter:

	White	Black
Male	210	245
	300	347
	150	125
	325	250
(1085)	100	260 (1227)
Female	177	252
	300	152
	106	315
	150	267
(893)	160	275 (1261)

(a) Construct a two-way analysis-of-variance table for these data and use it to test the null hypothesis of no interaction.

(b) If no interaction is found, test for main effects.

(c) If interaction is detected, construct a diagram similar to that shown in Figure 10.6 to investigate the nature of the interaction.

(d) If interaction is detected, compare the mean cotinine level between whites and blacks for females via a one-way analysis of variance. Do the same for males.

(Based on means reported in Lynne Wagenknecht et al., "Racial Differences in Serum Cotinine Levels Among Smokers in the Coronary Artery Risk Development in Young Adults Study," *American Journal of Public Health,* September 1990, pp. 1053–1056.)

5. A study of the effect of wastewater plant discharge water on freshwater ecology is conducted. Two sampling sites are used in the study. One site is upstream from the point at which the plant introduces effluents into the stream; the other is downstream. Samples are taken over a 3-week period. These data are obtained on the number of diatoms found:

	Week		
Site	**1**	**2**	**3**
Up	689	831	558
	756	916	423
Down	204	56	34
	229	73	78

(a) Construct a two-way analysis-of-variance table for these data.

(b) Test for interaction and continue the analysis in an appropriate way depending on the results of this test.

(c) Use Bonferroni T tests with each T test conducted at the $\alpha = .01$ level to pinpoint any differences that exist. What is the maximum overall probability of making at least one incorrect rejection?

(Based on a study by Joseph Hutton, Department of Biology and the Statistical Consulting Service, Radford University, October 1990.)

6. Consider the experiment described in Exercise 5. The printout of Table 10.19 is the analysis for the number of spirochetes found. Interpret the printout.

7. Consider the experiment described in Exercise 5. The printout of Table 10.20 is the analysis for the number of protists found. Interpret the printout.

TABLE 10.19

Analysis of variance for Exercise 6

SAS

SPECIES = spirochetes

Analysis-of-Variance Procedure

Dependent Variable:
COUNT

Source	DF	Sum of Squares	Mean Square	F Value	Pr>F
Model	5	518.7500000	103.7500000	.40	.8321
Error	6	1549.5000000	258.2500000		
Corrected Total	11	2068.2500000			

	R-Square	C.V.	Root MSE	COUNT Mean
	0.250816	64.92993	16.07016	24.7500000

Source	DF	Anova SS	Mean Square	F Value	Pr>F
SITE	1	90.7500000	90.7500000	0.35	0.5750
WEEK	2	84.5000000	42.2500000	0.16	0.8527
SITE*WEEK	2	343.5000000	171.7500000	0.67	0.5484

TABLE 10.20

Analysis of variance for Exercise 7

SAS

SPECIES = protists

Analysis-of-Variance Procedure

Dependent Variable:
COUNT

Source	DF	Sum of Squares	Mean Squares	F Value	Pr>F
Model	5	84,670.00000	16,934.00000	65.93	.0001
Error	6	1,541.00000	256.83333		
Corrected Total	11	86,211.00000			

	R-Square	C.V.	Root MSE	COUNT Mean
	0.982125	16.10655	16.02602	99.5000000

Source	DF	Anova SS	Mean Square	F Value	Pr>F
SITE	1	83,333.33333	83,333.33333	324.46	.0001
WEEK	2	738.50000	369.25000	1.44	.3090
SITE*WEEK	2	598.16667	299.08333	1.16	.3738

TECHNOLOGY TOOLS

TI83

XXIV   One-way ANOVA

The TI83 will conduct the F test needed to test H$_0$: $\mu_1 = \mu_2 = \cdots = \mu_k$. The steps needed to conduct the test are illustrated using the data of Example 10.2.1. Data will be entered in the first five columns of the data editor.

TI83 Keystroke	Purpose
1. STAT 1	1. Accesses the stat data editor
2. 40 ENTER 45 ENTER $\vdots$ 51 ENTER	2. Enters data for temperature I into column L1
3. $\triangleright$ 36 ENTER 42 ENTER $\vdots$ 40 ENTER	3. Enters data for temperature II into column L2
4. $\triangleright$ 49 ENTER 51 ENTER $\vdots$ 50 ENTER	4. Enters data for temperature III into column L3
5. $\triangleright$ 47 ENTER 49 ENTER $\vdots$ 51 ENTER	5. Enters data for temperature IV into column L4

6.	▷ 55 ENTER 60 ENTER ⋮ 61 ENTER	6.	Enters data for temperature V into column L5
7.	STAT ◁ ALPHA F	7.	Accesses the screen needed to conduct a one-way ANOVA ANOVA (
8.	2nd L1 , 2nd L2 , 2nd L3 , 2nd L4 , 2nd L5)	8.	Indicates that the data for the analysis are found in columns L1 through L5
9.	ENTER	9.	Displays the ANOVA; reproduces the information found in Table 10.3

SAS Package

X   One-way ANOVA with multiple comparisons

The SAS code used to produce the output shown in Example 10.2.5 is given below.

SAS Code	Purpose
OPTIONS LS $=$ 80 PS $=$ 60 NODATE;	Sets printing specifications
DATA TOXIC;	Names data set
INPUT TEMP PERCENT;	Names variables
LINES;	Signals that the data follow immediately
1 40	

1	45	
⋮		
1	51	
2	36	
2	42	Data lines
⋮		
2	40	
⋮		
5	55	
5	60	
⋮		
5	61	

SAS Code	Purpose
;	Signals the end of the data
PROC ANOVA;	Calls for the analysis of
CLASSES TEMP;	variance procedure; indicates
MODEL PERCENT = TEMP;	that the data are grouped by
	temperature
MEANS TEMP/DUNCAN	Asks for both Duncan
BON;	and Bonferroni multiple
	comparisons to be run

XI   Randomized complete blocks

The SAS code used to produce the output shown in Example 10.4.7 is given below.

SAS Code	Purpose
OPTIONS LS = 80 PS = 60 NODATE;	Sets printing specifications
DATA EXERCISE;	Names the data set
INPUT BLOCK TRTMENT KILOCAL;	Names the variables
LINES;	Indicates that the data follow immediately

1	1	1.4	
2	1	1.5	
3	1	1.8	
⋮			
8	1	2.0	
1	2	1.1	
2	2	1.2	Data lines
3	2	1.3	
⋮			
8	2	1.3	
1	3	.7	

2	3	.8
3	3	.7
⋮		
8	3	.6

SAS code	Purpose
;	Indicates the end of the data
PROC GLM;	Calls for the analysis to be conducted via the general linear models procedure
CLASSES TRTMENT BLOCK;	Indicates that the data are grouped by block and treatment
MODEL KILOCAL = TRTMENT BLOCK;	
MEANS TRTMENT/DUNCAN BON;	Asks for multiple comparisons on the average kilocalorie to be conducted via both the Duncan and Bonferroni techniques

XII Two-way ANOVA

The SAS code used to produce the output given in Example 10.5.4 is given below.

SAS code	Purpose
OPTIONS LS = 80 PS = 60 NODATE;	Sets printing specifications
DATA MIROGREX;	Names the data set
INPUT PHOTPRD TEMP GSI;	Names variables
LINES;	Signals that data follow

1	1	.9	
1	1	1.06	
⋮			
1	1	1.12	
1	2	.83	
1	2	.67	Data lines
⋮			
1	2	.66	
2	1	1.3	
2	1	2.88	
⋮			
2	1	2.94	
2	2	1.01	
2	2	1.52	
⋮			
2	2	1.63	

;	Signals end of data
PROC GLM;	Calls for the data to be
CLASSES PHOTOPRD TEMP;	analyzed via the general linear models procedure; indicates that data are grouped by photoperiod and temperature
MODEL GSI=PHOTOPRD TEMP PHOTOPRD*TEMP;	Indicates that the response variable (on the left) is GSI; indicates that the factors are photoperiod and temperature; includes an interaction term PHOTOPRD*TEMP

The following code can be added to the above program to produce a graph that gives a visual notion of the possible interaction between temperature and photoperiod. The graph, of course, uses sample means as estimates of the population means in question.

PROC SORT; BY PHOTOPRD TEMP;	Sorts data by photoperiod and temperature
PROC MEANS; BY PHOTOPRD TEMP;	Calculates the sample means for each of the four treatment combinations
OUTPUT OUT=NEW MGSI=MEAN;	Outputs the four sample means into a data set called NEW; calls the means MGSI
PROC PLOT;	Plots the means for each temperature
PLOT MGSI*PHOTOPRD=TEMP;	and photoperiod
TITLE'LOOKING FOR INTERACTION;	Titles output

Regression and Correlation

In this chapter we discuss two types of problems. The first, called *regression,* entails developing an equation by which the average value of a particular random variable of interest can be estimated or predicted based on knowledge of the values assumed by one or more other variables. The second, called *correlation,* involves measuring the strength of the linear relationship between two random variables. We begin with a brief introduction to the topic of regression.

■ 11.1
INTRODUCTION TO SIMPLE LINEAR REGRESSION

In a regression problem, we are primarily interested in a single random variable Y. It is assumed that the value taken on by this random variable depends on or is influenced by the values taken on by one or more other variables. The random variable Y is called the *dependent variable* or the *response;* the variables that influence Y are called *independent variables, predictor variables,* or *regressors.* In making estimates or predictions, the regressors are not treated as random variables. Rather, they are entities that can assume different values but whose values at the time when the prediction is to be made are not determined by chance. To illustrate, suppose that we want to develop an equation to describe the temperature of the water off the continental shelf. Since the temperature depends in part on the depth of the water, two variables are involved. These are X, the water depth, and Y, the water temperature. We are not interested in making inferences on the depth of the water. Rather, we want to describe the behavior of the water temperature under the assumption that the depth of the water is known precisely in advance. The water temperature is the response; the water depth is the only regressor being considered.

To illustrate the notation that will be used, notice that even if the depth of the water is fixed at some value x, the water temperature will still vary because of other random influences. For example, if several temperature measurements are taken at various places each at a depth of $x = 1000$ feet, the measurements will vary in value. For this reason, we must admit that for a given x we are really dealing with a "conditional" random variable, which we denote by $Y|x$ (Y given that $X = x$). This conditional random variable has a mean denoted by $\mu_{Y|x}$. It is obvious that the average temperature of ocean water depends in part on the depth of water; we do not expect the average temperature at $x = 1000$ feet to be the same as that at $x = 5000$ feet. That is, it is reasonable to assume that $\mu_{Y|x}$ is a function of x. We call the graph of this function the *curve of regression of Y on X*. The idea is pictured in Figure 11.1.

Our immediate problem is to estimate the form of $\mu_{Y|x}$ based on data obtained at some selected values $x_1, x_2, x_3, \ldots, x_n$ of the predictor variable X. The actual values used to develop the model are not overly important. If a functional relationship exists, it should become apparent regardless of which X values are used to discover it. However, to be of practical use, these values should represent a fairly wide range of possible values of the independent variable X. Sometimes the values used can be preselected. For example, in studying the relationship between water temperature and water depth, we might know that our model is to be used to predict water temperature for depths from 1000 to 5000 feet. We can choose to measure water temperatures at any depths that we wish within this range. For example, we might take measurements at 1000-foot increments. In this way we preset our X values at $x_1 = 1000$, $x_2 = 2000$, $x_3 = 3000$, $x_4 = 4000$, and $x_5 = 5000$ feet. When the X values used to develop the regression equation are preselected, the study is said to be *controlled*. Sometimes the X values used to develop the equation are chosen via some random mechanism. For example, in studying the effect of air quality on the pH of rainwater, we will be forced to select a sample of days, record the air quality reading for the day, and measure the pH of the rainwater. In this case, the values of X used to develop the

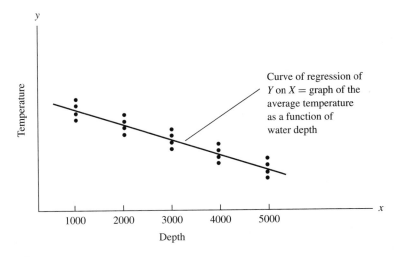

FIGURE 11.1

For a given water depth, the water temperature varies about some unknown average value $\mu_{Y|x}$. The curve joining these mean values is called the curve of regression of Y on X.

regression equation are not preselected by the researcher. They do represent a set of typical X values. Studies of this sort are called *observational studies*. The next two examples further illustrate these types of studies.

> **EXAMPLE 11.1.1.** A physician wants to predict the concentration of a particular drug in the bloodstream 5 minutes after its administration (Y) based on knowledge of the size of the initial dose (X). In this case, the random variable Y is the dependent variable; X is the independent variable. In a laboratory experiment, the values assumed by X are selected by the experimenter. For example, we might choose to experiment with doses of .05, .10, .20, and .30 ml. Since the choice of experimental doses is in the hands of the researcher, this is a controlled study.

> **EXAMPLE 11.1.2.** An ecologist wishes to predict the change in water temperature that occurs at a point 1 mile below an industrial plant after the introduction of hot wastewater into the stream (Y). The prediction is to be based on the amount of water released (X). The response is the change in water temperature; the single regressor is the amount of water released. Since the amount of hot water released varies depending on the level of activity in the plant, the researcher does not control the values of the regressor used to develop the prediction equation. Rather, the values are simply measured at the time of the release of the water. This is an example of an observational study.

Regardless of whether the study is controlled or observational, the purpose of a regression study is the same—to find a reasonable prediction or regression equation. Typical regression curves are shown in Figure 11.2. Note that these curves are theoretical. They are the graphs of the theoretical mean for the dependent variable Y for given values of the independent variable X. They serve as *ideal* prediction curves. Usually we do not know the exact equations for these curves. Our problem is to estimate them from observed data on X and Y. When the graph of $\mu_{Y|x}$ is a straight line (Figure 11.2*b*), we say that the regression of Y on X is *linear*. Otherwise, the regression is said to be *nonlinear* (Figure 11.2*a* and *c*). The term *linear regression* is defined more precisely as follows:

> **DEFINITION 11.1.1. Linear regression.** A curve of regression of Y on X is said to be a *linear regression* if and only if

$$\mu_{Y|x} = \alpha + \beta x$$

for α and β real numbers, $\beta \neq 0$.

The parameter α in the above equation is its y intercept. It is the point at which the straight line crosses the vertical or y axis. The parameter β is the slope of the line. If $\beta > 0$, the line tilts upward as we move from left to right; if $\beta < 0$, the line tilts downward; and if $\beta = 0$, the line is horizontal. For example, since the straight line shown in Figure 11.1 tilts downward from left to right, its slope is negative. The practical implication of this is that as the depth of the water increases, the temperature decreases. In many cases, the algebraic sign of the slope can be anticipated based on knowledge of the subject matter alone.

The title of this section is *introduction to simple linear regression*. This phrase implies three things: *Regression* implies that the purpose of the experiment is prediction. *Simple* means that we will attempt to derive an equation by which the average

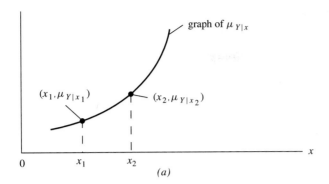

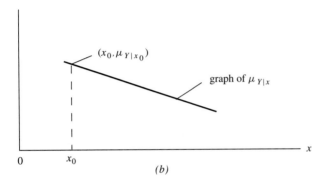

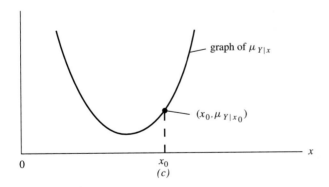

■ **FIGURE 11.2**
(*a*) Nonlinear curve of regression; (*b*) linear curve of regression; (*c*) nonlinear curve of regression.

value of a dependent variable Y can be predicted, based on knowledge of the value assumed by *one* independent variable X. If more than one independent variable were used to predict the average value of Y, then we would use the term *multiple regression*. The word *linear* implies that the prediction equation derived will take the form of a straight line.

In regression analysis, the first job is to determine whether it is reasonable to assume that the curve of regression of Y on X is a straight line. One way to help determine this is to plot a graph of the observed pairs (x, y). Such a graph is called a *scattergram*.

The points usually do not lie exactly in a straight line. However, if linear regression is applicable, then they should exhibit a noticeable linear trend. The next two examples illustrate the use of scattergrams in detecting linear trends.

EXAMPLE 11.1.3. An experiment is conducted to study the relationship between the shell height X and shell length Y (each measured in millimeters) in *Patelloida pygmaea,* a limpet found attached to rocks and shells along sheltered shores in the Indo-Pacific area. These data result:

x	y	x	y	x	y	x	y
.9	3.1	1.9	5.0	2.1	5.6	2.3	5.8
1.5	3.6	1.9	5.3	2.1	5.7	2.3	6.2
1.6	4.3	1.9	5.7	2.1	5.8	2.3	6.3
1.7	4.7	2.0	4.4	2.2	5.2	2.3	6.4
1.7	5.5	2.0	5.2	2.2	5.3	2.4	6.4
1.8	5.7	2.0	5.3	2.2	5.6	2.4	6.3
1.8	5.2	2.1	5.4	2.2	5.8	2.7	6.3

The scattergram shown in Figure 11.3 is obtained by plotting the values of the independent variable X along the horizontal axis and those of the dependent variable Y along the vertical axis. Even though these points do not lie on a single straight line, there is a definite linear trend to the data. The trend is what we are seeking. It identifies the problem as one in which simple linear regression is applicable. It is reasonable to assume that the graph of $\mu_{Y|x}$ is a straight line. We can visualize the theoretical line of regression of Y and X as shown in Figure 11.4. Our problem is to use the data to estimate the values of α and β, thereby estimating the theoretical line of regression of Y on X.

EXAMPLE 11.1.4. In a study of predation, a predator, the *Didinium nasutum,* is introduced to a medium containing its natural prey, the *Paramecium caudatum.*

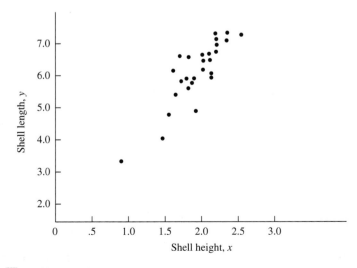

FIGURE 11.3

Scattergram of shell height versus shell length exhibits a linear trend.

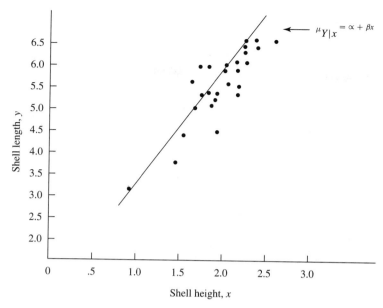

FIGURE 11.4

Theoretical linear curve of regression and ideal curve for predicting shell length based on shell height.

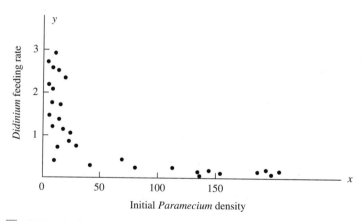

FIGURE 11.5

Scattergram of initial *Paramecium* density versus *Didinium* feeding rate—no linear trend is evident.

The purpose is to predict the average feeding rate of the *Didinium* (Y), based on knowledge of the initial density of the *Paramecium* in the medium (X). The scattergram of the data obtained is shown in Figure 11.5. Clearly, the points do *not* exhibit a linear trend. In this case, it is inappropriate to assume that the graph of $\mu_{Y|x}$ is linear. A more reasonable choice is a hyperbolic curve shown in Figure 11.6. We would *not* use the techniques of simple linear regression to estimate $\mu_{Y|x}$.

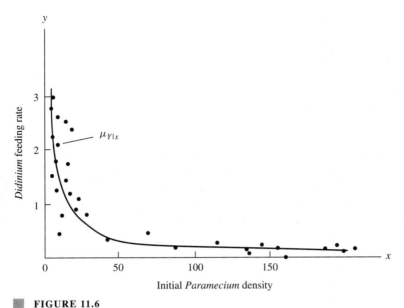

FIGURE 11.6

Theoretical nonlinear curve of regression and ideal curve for predicting
Didinium feeding rate based on initial *Paramecium* density.

Plots of the sort shown in Figures 11.3 and 11.5 are easily obtained using the TI83
or other graphing calculators. They can also be produced by SAS or other computer
packages. Plotting a scattergram should always be the first step in any simple linear regression study.

Our problem in Example 11.1.3 is to estimate mathematically the equation for
$\mu_{Y|x}$ based on the observed data. Note that several straight lines that pass through
some of the data points can be drawn through the scattergram; others can be drawn that
are "close" to most of the data points. Which of these lines should we choose as our
estimate for $\mu_{Y|x}$? Which of the lines best "fits" the data? These questions are an-
swered in Section 11.2.

EXERCISES 11.1

1. Consider the following observations on a dependent random variable Y and an
   independent variable X:

x	y	x	y
1.0	3.0	3.0	7.0
1.1	3.2	3.0	7.1
1.5	4.1	3.1	7.4
1.7	4.2	3.2	6.0
2.0	5.0	3.5	8.1
2.5	6.2	3.6	8.0
3.0	7.3	4.0	9.0

   Plot the scattergram for these data. Does linear regression appear to be applicable?

2. Consider the following observations on the dependent random variable Y, the attention span of a child in minutes, and X, the child's IQ.

x	y	x	y	x	y	x	y
75	2.0	95	5.2	110	7.2	130	3.8
80	3.0	100	5.5	115	6.8	135	2.9
85	4.5	105	6.0	115	6.4	140	2.0
85	4.7	110	6.5	120	5.5		
90	5.0	110	6.7	125	4.2		

Plot the scattergram for these data. Does linear regression appear to be applicable?

3. An experiment is run to study the relationship between the incubation stage (number of days since the eggs were laid) and the mean incubation spell (mean number of minutes of uninterrupted nesting) in the gull-billed tern. The purpose is to derive an equation by which the mean incubation spell Y can be predicted, based on knowledge of the stage of incubation X. By using time-lapse photography, these data are obtained:

x	y	x	y	x	y
.25	30	4	18	12	38
.50	18	5	26	18	55
.50	25	6	21	19	35
1.0	21	7	52	20	30
1.0	22	8	62	20	50
1.0	40	9	45	20	155
1.5	19	10	39	21	35
2	10	10	120	21	38
2.5	55	11	18		
3	23	11	50		

Plot the scattergram for these data. Does linear regression appear to be applicable?

4. A study is conducted to investigate the relationship between the moisture level in soil and the death rate in earthworms. The death rate, Y, is the proportion of worms dying after a 2-week period; the moisture level, x, is measured in milliliters of water per cubic centimeter of soil. These data are obtained:

x	y	x	y
0	.5	.632	0
0	.4	.947	.1
0	.5	.947	.2
.316	.2	.947	.1
.316	.3	1.26	.6
.316	.3	1.26	.5
.632	0	1.26	.4
.632	.1		

Plot a scattergram for these data. Do the data form a linear trend? What sort of curve might be used to describe the trend exhibited by these data? (Based on a study conducted by Jeffrey A. Hollar, Department of Biology, Radford University, 1996.)

■ 11.2
METHOD OF LEAST SQUARES

Recall that in simple linear regression we assume that the graph of the mean of the dependent variable Y for given values of the independent variable X is a straight line. That is, we assume

$$\mu_{Y|x} = \alpha + \beta x$$

where α and β are unknown parameters whose values are to be estimated. The method employed to estimate α and β is called the *method of least squares*. The procedure is illustrated in Example 11.2.1.

EXAMPLE 11.2.1. A study is conducted of photoperiodism in waterfowl. The purpose is to develop an equation by which the average length of the breeding season can be predicted based on knowledge of the photoperiod (number of hours of light per day) under which breeding was initiated. These data are obtained by observing the behavior of 11 *Aythya* (diving ducks):

x (hours of light per day)	y (days in breeding season)
12.8	110
13.9	54
14.1	98
14.7	50
15.0	67
15.1	58
16.0	52
16.5	50
16.6	43
17.2	15
17.9	28

The scattergram for these data together with an imagined theoretical line of regression is shown in Figure 11.7. To estimate the theoretical line of regression, we must estimate α, the y intercept of the line, and β, its slope. The estimates for these parameters are denoted a and b, respectively. Thus the estimated line of regression is given by

$$\hat{\mu}_{Y|x} = a + bx$$

The reasoning behind the method of least squares is quite simple. From the many straight lines that can be drawn through the scattergram, we wish to pick the one that "best fits" the data. The fit is "best" in the sense that the values of a and b chosen will be those that minimize the sum of the squares of the distances between the data points and the estimated regression line. In this way, we are picking the straight line that comes as close as it can to all data points simultaneously.

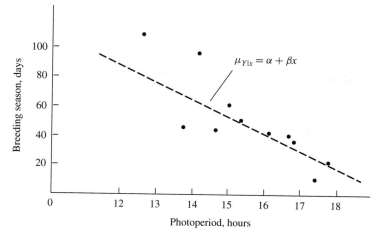

FIGURE 11.7

Theoretical line of regression and ideal curve for predicting the average
length of the breeding season based on the photoperiod.

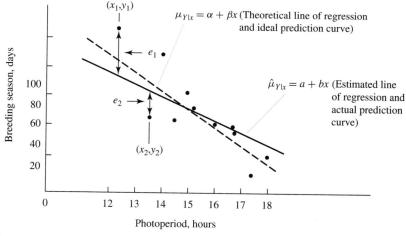

FIGURE 11.8

The actual prediction curve minimizes the sum of the squares of the distances e_i where
e_i is the vertical distance from the data point (x_i, y_i) to the estimated line of regression.

The distance between a data point and the estimated line of regression is called a *residual*. The residuals are denoted by $e_1, e_2, e_3, \ldots, e_n$. They are pictured in Figure 11.8. Using
this notation,

$$e_1 = \text{difference between first data point and}$$
$$\text{estimated regression line}$$
$$= y_1 - (a + bx_1)$$
$$e_2 = y_2 - (a + bx_2)$$
$$e_3 = y_3 - (a + bx_3)$$
$$\vdots$$
$$e_{11} = y_{11} - (a + bx_{11})$$

The sum of the squares of these differences is

$$\sum_{i=1}^{11} e_i^2 = \sum_{i=1}^{11} [y_i - (a + bx_i)]^2$$

This sum, denoted by SS_E, is a function of both a and b. That is, its value depends on the numerical values chosen for the slope and intercept of the estimated line of regression. We want to choose a and b so that SS_E will be as small as possible. Calculus techniques can be used to show that this occurs whenever these equations are satisfied:

$$\sum_{i=1}^{11} y_i = 11a + b\sum_{i=1}^{11} x_i$$

$$\sum_{i=1}^{11} x_i y_i = a\sum_{i=1}^{11} x_i + b\sum_{i=1}^{11} x_i^2$$

These equations are called the *normal equations*. They can be solved for a and b to obtain

$$\hat{\beta} = b = \frac{11\sum_{i=1}^{11} x_i y_i - \sum_{i=1}^{11} x_i \sum_{i=1}^{11} y_i}{11\sum_{i=1}^{11} x_i^2 - \left[\sum_{i=1}^{11} x_i\right]^2}$$

$$\hat{\alpha} = a = \bar{y} - b\bar{x}$$

Thus to evaluate a and b for this data set, we need only calculate four quantities:

$$\sum_{i=1}^{11} x_i \quad \sum_{i=1}^{11} x_i^2 \quad \sum_{i=1}^{11} y_i \quad \sum_{i=1}^{11} x_i y_i$$

For these data, these quantities are

$$\sum_{i=1}^{11} x_i = 169.8 \qquad \sum_{i=1}^{11} y_i = 625$$

$$\sum_{i=1}^{11} x_i^2 = 2645.02 \qquad \sum_{i=1}^{11} x_i y_i = 9286.2$$

Thus

$$\hat{\beta} = b = \frac{11(9286.2) - 169.8(625)}{11(2645.02) - (169.8)^2} = -15.11$$

$$\hat{\alpha} = a = \frac{625}{11} - (-15.11)\frac{(169.8)}{(11)} = 290.06$$

The estimated line of regression and actual prediction equation based on these data is

$$\hat{\mu}_{Y|x} = 290.06 - 15.11x$$

To predict the average length of the breeding season when the photoperiod under which breeding is initiated is 14.5 hours, we substitute $x = 14.5$ into the above equation. Thus our predicted value is

$$\hat{\mu}_{Y|x} = 290.06 - 15.11(14.5) = 70.97 \text{ days}$$

The normal equations and the estimates for α and β given in Example 11.2.1 are generalized by replacing the number 11, the sample size for the given set, by n, the sample size for a general data set. Thus the normal equations for the simple linear regression model are

$$\sum_{i=1}^{n} y_i = na + b \sum_{i=1}^{n} x_i$$

$$\sum_{i=1}^{n} x_i y_i = a \sum_{i=1}^{n} x_i + b \sum_{i=1}^{n} x_i^2$$

(Normal equations)

The general formulas for $\hat{\alpha}$ and $\hat{\beta}$ are

$$\hat{\alpha} = a = \bar{y} - b\bar{x}$$

$$\hat{\beta} = b = \frac{n \sum_{i=1}^{n} x_i y_i - \sum_{i=1}^{n} x_i \sum_{i=1}^{n} y_i}{n \sum_{i=1}^{n} x_i^2 - \left[\sum_{i=1}^{n} x_i\right]^2}$$

(Estimates for α and β)

A word of caution must be added. A given data set gives evidence of linearity only over those values of X covered by the data set. For values of X beyond those covered, there is no evidence of linearity. Thus it is dangerous to use an estimated regression line to predict values of Y corresponding to values of X lying far beyond the range of the X values covered by the data set. We illustrate this point in Example 11.2.2.

EXAMPLE 11.2.2. The following data are obtained on the fastest mile-run times Y (in seconds) of world-class runners from 1954 to 1972:

X (year)	Y (time of run)
54	239.4 (Bannister breaks 4-min mile)
54	238.0
56	238.1
56	238.5
58	234.5
58	236.2
60	235.3
60	234.8
62	235.1
62	234.4
64	234.1
64	234.9
66	231.3 (Ryun)
66	232.7
68	231.4
68	231.8
70	232.0
70	231.9
72	231.4
72	231.5

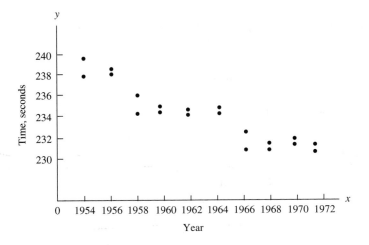

■ **FIGURE 11.9**

Scattergram of year versus time for the mile run for world-class runners.

The scattergram for these data is shown in Figure 11.9. There does appear to be a linear trend. To fit a regression line to the data, these quantities are needed:

$$\sum_{i=1}^{20} x_i = 1260 \qquad \sum_{i=1}^{20} y_i = 4687.3$$

$$\sum_{i=1}^{20} x_i^2 = 80{,}040 \qquad \sum_{i=1}^{20} x_i y_i = 295{,}024.2$$

$$\bar{x} = 63 \qquad \bar{y} = 234.37$$

$$\hat{\beta} = b = \frac{n\sum xy - \sum x \sum y}{n \sum x^2 - \left(\sum x\right)^2} = \frac{20(295{,}024.2) - (1260)(4687.3)}{20(80{,}040) - 1260^2}$$

$$= -.42$$

$$\hat{\alpha} = a = \bar{y} - b\bar{x} = 234.37 - (-.42)(63) = 260.83$$

The estimated regression line is

$$\hat{\mu}_{Y|x} = 260.83 - .42x$$

The line can be used safely to estimate the average time for world-class mile runners from 1954 to 1972, the years covered by the data set. The danger lies in using this equation to predict mile-run times much beyond 1972, because there is no evidence from the data set that a linear trend continues indefinitely. In particular, suppose that we erroneously assume that the linear trend continues, and so we try to predict the average run time for runners in the year 2521. For the year 2521, $x = 621$. Thus the predicted average value of Y is

$$\hat{\mu}_{Y|x} = 260.83 - .42(621) = .01 \text{ second}$$

The value is inconceivable as a possible average time for running 1 mile! The problem arises because at some point beyond 1972, the linear trend ceases and the times level off at some reasonable value.

Estimating an Individual Response

By writing the estimated line of regression as

$$\hat{\mu}_{Y|x} = a + bx$$

we are emphasizing the fact that the points on the line represent the estimated *average* response when the predictor variable assumes the value x. The line can also be used to predict the response itself. Common sense tells us that a logical choice for the predicted value of Y for a given value x is its estimated average value when $X = x$. For example, if we are asked to predict the ocean water temperature at a particular point where the depth is 1000 feet, a logical choice for this prediction is the estimated average temperature at this depth. If asked to predict the length of the breeding season for a particular diving duck that initiated breeding when the photoperiod was 14.5 hours, our best estimate is the estimated average length under these conditions. In Example 11.2.1, this estimated average was found to be 70.97 days. Thus it is correct to write

$$\hat{y} = \hat{\mu}_{Y|x} = 290.066 - 15.11(14.5) = 70.97$$

Be careful when you read the results of a regression study. The equation obtained is the equation for the average value of Y as a function of x. It is used to estimate both the average response and an individual response when the regressor assumes the value x.

We have provided a logical way to estimate α and β and thus fit a straight line to any data set. We also have seen that a scattergram gives some indication of whether linear regression is applicable. However, one important question still must be answered: Does *linear* regression really make sense, or would some other type of curve actually fit the data more closely and thus provide a better prediction equation? This question cannot be ignored. We address it in Section 11.4.

A Note on Computing

Simple linear regression is a very useful statistical technique. For this reason, many handheld calculators are programmed to do regression analysis by merely entering the (x, y) pairs. You should check your calculator manual to see if your calculator has this capability. The Technology Tools section at the end of this chapter demonstrates how to use the TI83 calculator to estimate a line of regression.

Regression analysis for large data sets is routinely done by computer. Example 11.2.3 discusses the computer analysis of the data of Example 11.2.1. The SAS code used to create the printout given is provided in the Technology Tools section of this chapter.

> **EXAMPLE 11.2.3.** To begin a computer analysis of a data set, we first ask the computer to plot a scattergram of the data. If simple linear regression is appropriate, the scattergram should exhibit a visible linear trend. Figure 11.10 shows the SAS-generated scattergram for the data of Example 11.2.1. The response, the length of the breeding season, is graphed on the vertical axis; the regressor, the photoperiod, is graphed on the horizontal axis. There

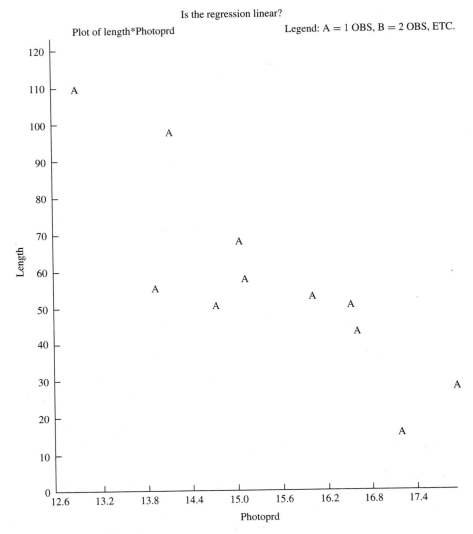

Note: 1 OBS had missing values

FIGURE 11.10

Scattergram for the data of Example 11.2.1. The data exhibit a downward linear trend.

is a visible downward linear trend indicating that as the number of hours of light per day increases, the length of the breeding season decreases. The slope of the estimated regression line will be negative. Figure 11.11 gives the output of the program used to estimate the intercept and slope of the regression line. These are given by ① and ②, respectively. Notice that the estimated slope is negative as expected. The estimated line of regression is

$$\hat{\mu}_{Y|x} = 290.07044608 - 15.11057071x$$

This agrees, apart from roundoff differences, with the equation found earlier. The estimated average length of the breeding season when breeding is initiated during 14.5 hours of light is shown at ③.

IS THE REGRESSION LINEAR?
GENERAL LINEAR MODELS PROCEDURE

DEPENDENT VARIABLE: LENGTH

SOURCE	DF	SUM OF SQUARES	MEAN SQUARES	F VALUE
MODEL	1	5462.88341888	5462.88341888	23.86
ERROR	9	2060.75294475	228.97254942	PR > F
CORRECTED TOTAL	10	7523.63636364		0.0009

R-SQUARE	C.V.	STD DEV	LENGTH MEAN
0.726096	26.6320	15.13183893	56.81818182

SOURCE	DF	TYPE I SS	F VALUE	PR > F
PHOTOPRD	1	5462.88341888	23.86	0.0009

SOURCE	DF	TYPE IV SS	F VALUE	PR > F
PHOTOPRD	1	5462.88341888	23.86	0.0009

PARAMETER	ESTIMATE	T FOR H0: PARAMETER = 0	PR > |T|	STD ERROR OF ESTIMATE
INTERCEPT	290.07044608 ①	6.05	0.0002	47.97110790
PHOTOPRD	-15.11057071 ②	-4.88	0.0009	3.09358185

IS THE REGRESSION LINEAR?

OBS	PHOTOPRD	LENGTH	PREDICT
1	12.8	110	96.6551
2	13.9	54	80.0335
3	14.1	98	77.0114
4	14.7	50	67.9451
5	15.0	67	63.4119
6	15.1	58	61.9008
7	16.0	52	48.3013
8	16.5	50	40.7460
9	16.6	43	39.2350
10	17.2	15	30.1686
11	17.9	28	19.5912
12	14.5		70.9672 ③

FIGURE 11.11

Output of a SAS program used to estimate the line of regression and approximate the average length of the breeding season when breeding is initiated when there are 14.5 hours of light per day.

EXERCISES 11.2

Note: Even though formulas for a and b have been given in this section, these problems should be worked using a computer or a statistical calculator when possible.

1. For the data of Exercise 1 of Section 11.1 find $\sum x, \sum x^2, \sum y, \sum xy, \bar{x}, \bar{y}$. Use these quantities to estimate α and β. Write the equation for the estimated line of

regression, and use it to predict the average value of Y when $x = 3.7$ and also the value of Y itself when $x = 3.7$.

2. Use the regression equation obtained in Example 11.2.1 to predict the length of the breeding season if breeding is initiated when there are 14 hours of light per day. Can this equation be used safely to estimate the length of the breeding season if breeding is initiated when there are 10 hours of light per day? Explain.

3. A numerical index of the degree of illness of patients suffering from Crohn's disease has been developed. The index requires that a diary be kept by the patient and includes information on eight clinical variables. The index, although useful, is cumbersome in practice. A new index has been devised that is easier to use. It is felt that the values obtained with the newer index can be utilized to predict the value that would have been obtained by using the older, proven index. One hundred six patients were evaluated by using both indices. The X values range from .5 to 14.0. The scattergram for the data exhibits a linear trend. For these data,

$$\sum x = 366.1 \qquad \sum y = 12{,}623$$

$$\sum x^2 = 2435.63 \qquad \bar{y} = 119.08$$

$$\bar{x} = 3.45 \qquad \sum xy = 75{,}989.6$$

Use this information to estimate α, β, and $\mu_{Y|x}$. What is the predicted rating on the old index for a patient whose rating on the new index is 5.5? Can we safely predict the rating on the old index for a patient who is rated at $x = 16$ on the new index? Explain.

4. A study is run to develop an equation by which the concentration of estrone in saliva can be used to predict the concentration of this steroid in free plasma. These data are obtained on 14 healthy males:

x (concentration of estrone in saliva, pg/ml)	y (concentration of estrone in free plasma, pg/ml)
7.4	30.0
7.5	25.0
8.5	31.5
9.0	27.5
9.0	39.5
11.0	38.0
13.0	43.0
14.0	49.0
14.5	55.0
16.0	48.5
17.0	51.0
18.0	64.5
20.0	63.0
23.0	68.0

(a) Sketch a scattergram for these data.

(b) Find $\sum x$, $\sum x^2$, $\sum y$, $\sum xy$.

(c) Estimate α, β, $\mu_{Y|x}$.

(d) Use the estimated line of regression to predict the estrone level in the free plasma in a male whose saliva estrone level is 17.5 pg/ml.

5. Use the data of Example 11.1.3.

   (a) Find $\sum x$, $\sum x^2$, $\sum y$, $\sum xy$.

   (b) Estimate α, β, $\mu_{Y|x}$.

   (c) Use the estimated line of regression to predict the shell length of a limpet whose shell height is 2.25 millimeters.

6. Measuring the ability of a person to blow out a candle is a crude way to assess maximum respiratory velocities. A candle test is conducted by holding a lighted candle perpendicular to a wooden board placed on an adjustable bedside tray so that the flame height is the same as the height of the subject's mouth. The candle is placed 5 centimeters from the subject, and he or she is given three attempts to blow it out. If the subject is successful, the candle is moved back 5 centimeters and the experiment is repeated. A resting period is allowed between trials. The predictor variable is X, the farthest distance at which the candle can be extinguished. Responses are

$$FVC = \text{forced vital capacity}$$

$$FEV_1 = \text{forced expiratory volume in 1 second}$$

$$PEFR = \text{peak expiration flow rate}$$

$$FET = \text{forced expiratory time}$$

These estimated regression equations are obtained:

$$\widehat{FVC} = .04039x + .9606$$

$$\widehat{FEV_1} = .037659x + .4983$$

$$\widehat{PEFR} = 4.3379x + 195.5$$

$$\widehat{FET} = -.071331x + 9.5591$$

(a) What is the estimated average response for each of these variables for patients for whom the maximum distance at which the candle can be extinguished is 10 centimeters?

(b) A patient is seen, and it is determined that the maximum distance at which she can extinguish the candle is 10 centimeters. What are the predicted values of each response for this patient?

(c) If these lines were graphed, which line would tilt upward at the sharpest angle?

(d) If these lines were graphed, which line would tilt downward?

(Regression equations found in Bayur Teklu et al., "The Match Test Revisited—Blowing Out a Candle as a Screening Test for Airflow Obstruction," *Journal of Family Practice,* November 1990, pp. 557–562.)

7. A study is conducted to investigate the effect of the decomposition of pine needles on the pH of soil. Various amounts of pine needles were added to topsoil and allowed

to decompose. The pH of the resultant soil was determined. These data result:

Pine needles (g per 170 g of soil)	pH	Pine needles (g per 170 g of soil)	pH
5	7.50	15	6.75
5	7.30	15	6.73
5	7.00	15	6.70
5	6.95	15	6.68
5	6.88	15	6.70
10	6.85	20	6.55
10	6.83	20	6.65
10	6.80	20	6.63
10	6.78	20	6.62
10	6.80	20	6.60

(a) Plot a scattergram of these data.
(b) If linear regression appears to be appropriate, estimate the line of regression.
(c) Based on your estimated regression equation, what is the estimated average pH of soil samples subjected to 18 g of pine needles? What is the estimated pH of a single soil sample subjected to 18 g of pine needles?
(Based on a study by Amy Payne, Department of Biology, Radford University, 1996.)

8. A study is conducted of the effect of light intensity on the rate of photosynthesis of spinach leaves. The study is conducted by using leaf disks in which holes have been punched. The leaves are then submerged in water. Light intensity is measured in foot-candles; rate of photosynthesis is measured by noting the time in seconds that it takes for half of the leaves to float. A quick rising of leaves indicates a high rate of photosynthesis. These data result:

Intensity (ft-c)	Time of rise (seconds)	Intensity (ft-c)	Time of rise (seconds)
400	4500	800	2200
400	4450	800	2000
400	4200	800	1800
400	3900	800	1500
400	3700	800	1400
600	3100	1000	1200
600	2800	1000	1000
600	2750	1000	980
600	2600	1000	990
600	2500	1000	995

(a) Plot a scattergram for these data.
(b) If appropriate, estimate the line of regression.
(c) Based on your estimated line of regression, estimate the average rate of photosynthesis for all samples subjected to an intensity of 650 foot-candles. Estimate the rate of photosynthesis for a single sample subjected to an intensity of 650 foot-candles.
(Based on a study by Shane Bryant, Department of Biology, Radford University, 1996.)

11.3

INTRODUCTION TO CORRELATION

Recall that statistical regression analysis deals with the relationship between a variable X and the mean of a random variable Y. We are not interested in drawing conclusions about X as this variable is of interest only in that it helps estimate the mean response $\mu_{Y|x}$ or predict an individual response $Y|x$. In the regression setting, the predictor variable X is *not* random, whereas the response Y is a random variable. We have been particularly concerned with situations in which the relationship between x and $\mu_{Y|x}$ is linear. Our attention has been focused on estimating the line

$$\mu_{Y|x} = \alpha + \beta x$$

so that the equation obtained can be used to estimate future and average responses for given values of X.

In correlation analysis, both X and Y are random variables and they are of equal interest. We want to determine whether or not there is a linear association between these two random variables. Hence we are seeking to answer the question, Is

$$Y = \alpha + \beta X$$

for some parameters α and β where $\beta \neq 0$? To answer this question, we will develop a parameter that measures the strength of the linear association that exists between X and Y.

The most often used measure of linear association between two random variables is ρ, the Pearson product-moment coefficient of correlation. This parameter is defined in terms of the covariance between X and Y, where the covariance is a measure of the manner in which X and Y vary together. We define covariance as follows:

DEFINITION 11.3.1. Covariance. Let X and Y be random variables with means μ_X and μ_Y, respectively. The *covariance* between X and Y, denoted by Cov (X, Y), is given by

$$\text{Cov } (X, Y) = E[(X - \mu_X)(Y - \mu_Y)] = E[XY] - E[X]E[Y]$$

Note that if small values of X tend to be associated with small values of Y and large values of X with large values of Y, then $X - \mu_X$ and $Y - \mu_Y$ will tend to have the same algebraic sign. This implies that $(X - \mu_X)(Y - \mu_Y)$ will tend to be positive, yielding a positive covariance. If the reverse is true and small values of X tend to be associated with large values of Y and vice versa, then $X - \mu_X$ and $Y - \mu_Y$ will tend to have opposite algebraic signs. This results in a tendency for $(X - \mu_X)(Y - \mu_Y)$ to be negative, yielding a negative covariance.

It is evident that we can tell something about the association between X and Y from the algebraic sign of the covariance. However, this parameter is unbounded. It can assume any real value, and its magnitude is meaningless. To correct this problem, we divide the covariance by $\sqrt{(\text{Var } X)(\text{Var } Y)}$ to form the Pearson coefficient of correlation given in Definition 11.3.2.

DEFINITION 11.3.2. Pearson correlation coefficient. Let X and Y be random variables with means μ_X and μ_Y and variances σ_X^2 and σ_Y^2, respectively. The *correlation* ρ

between X and Y is

$$\rho = \frac{\mathrm{Cov}\,(X,\,Y)}{\sqrt{(\mathrm{Var}\,X)(\mathrm{Var}\,Y)}}$$

Although the proof is beyond the scope of this text, it can be shown that ρ lies between -1 and $+1$ inclusive. If $\rho = 1$, then we say that there is *perfect positive correlation* between X and Y. Large values of X are associated with large values of Y, and small values of X are paired with small values of Y. In this case, (x, y) points will lie in a straight line sloping upward as shown in Figure 11.12a. If $\rho = -1$, then we say that there is *perfect negative correlation* between X and Y. Here large values of X are paired with small values of Y, and small values of X are matched with large values of Y. Points will lie in a straight line sloping downward as pictured in Figure 11.12b. If $\rho = 0$, we say that X and Y are *uncorrelated*. This means only that there is no *linear* association between X and Y. It does not mean that X and Y are unrelated. However, it does imply that if a relationship exists between these two random variables, it is not a straight-line relationship. Figure 11.12c and d illustrates two settings in which $\rho = 0$. In part c there is no obvious relationship between X and Y; in part d there is an apparent relationship, but it is not linear.

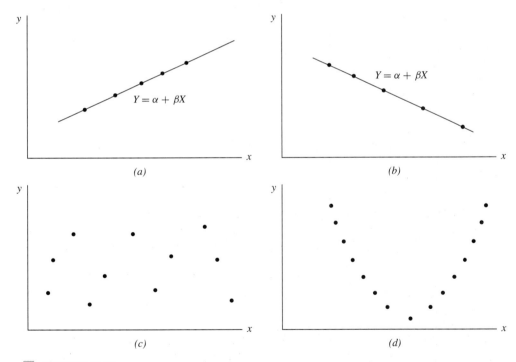

FIGURE 11.12

(a) Perfect positive correlation: $\rho = 1$, $\beta > 0$, all points lie on a straight line with positive slope; (b) perfect positive correlation: $\rho = 1$, $\beta < 0$, all points lie on a straight line with negative slope; (c) uncorrelated: $\rho = 0$, points are randomly scattered; (d) uncorrelated: $\rho = 0$, points indicate a relationship between X and Y, but the relationship is not linear.

EXAMPLE 11.3.1. Consider the random variable X, the height of an adult male, and Y, his weight. Since taller people tend to weigh more than shorter ones, we would expect X and Y to be positively correlated.

EXAMPLE 11.3.2. Let X denote altitude and Y the diversity index of the tree cover. Since the number of species of trees that can survive at high altitudes is rather small, as the altitude increases, the number of different species found should decrease. Hence large values of X should be paired with small values of Y and vice versa. The correlation between these two random variables should be negative.

Estimating ρ

Keep in mind that Cov (X, Y) and ρ are *theoretical* parameters. Neither can be calculated without knowledge of the probability distribution of the pair of variables (X, Y). The statistical problem is to estimate their values from a data set. Since Cov (X, Y) can be expressed as the difference in the theoretical means $E[XY]$ and $E[X]E[Y]$, it can be estimated easily by replacing each theoretical mean by its corresponding sample mean. Thus we estimate

$$E[XY] \quad \text{by} \quad \frac{\sum_{i=1}^{n} x_i y_i}{n}$$

$$E[X] \quad \text{by} \quad \frac{\sum_{i=1}^{n} x_i}{n}$$

$$E[Y] \quad \text{by} \quad \frac{\sum_{i=1}^{n} y_i}{n}$$

By substituting, the estimated covariance becomes

$$\widehat{\text{Cov}(X, Y)} = \sum_{i=1}^{n} \frac{x_i y_i}{n} - \sum_{i=1}^{n} \frac{x_i}{n} \sum_{i=1}^{n} \frac{y_i}{n}$$

$$= \frac{n \sum_{i=1}^{n} x_i y_i - \sum_{i=1}^{n} x_i \sum_{i=1}^{n} y_i}{n^2}$$

Similarly, since Var $X = E[X^2] - (E[X])^2$,

$$\widehat{\text{Var } X} = \frac{\sum_{i=1}^{n} x_i^2}{n} - \left[\sum_{i=1}^{n} \frac{x_i}{n} \right]^2$$

$$= \frac{n \sum_{i=1}^{n} x_i^2 - \left[\sum_{i=1}^{n} x_i \right]^2}{n^2}$$

Combining these results, we get a logical estimate for the correlation coefficient ρ:

$$\hat{\rho} = \frac{\dfrac{n \sum\limits_{i=1}^{n} x_i y_i - \sum\limits_{i=1}^{n} x_i \sum\limits_{i=1}^{n} y_i}{n^2}}{\sqrt{\left[\dfrac{n \sum\limits_{i=1}^{n} x_i^2 - \left[\sum\limits_{i=1}^{n} x_i\right]^2}{n^2}\right]\left[\dfrac{n \sum\limits_{i=1}^{n} y_i^2 - \left[\sum\limits_{i=1}^{n} y_i\right]^2}{n^2}\right]}}$$

The n^2 terms cancel to produce the expression for $\hat{\rho}$ given in Definition 11.3.3.

DEFINITION 11.3.3. Estimate for ρ. The *estimate for* ρ, the Pearson coefficient of correlation, denoted by r, is

$$\hat{\rho} = r = \frac{n \sum xy - \sum x \sum y}{\sqrt{\left[n \sum x^2 - \left(\sum x\right)^2\right]\left[n \sum y^2 - \left(\sum y\right)^2\right]}}$$

Example 11.3.3 illustrates the computation of r.

EXAMPLE 11.3.3. Researchers are investigating the correlation between obesity and an individual's response to pain. Obesity is measured as the percentage over ideal weight (X). Response to pain is measured by using the threshold of the nociceptive flexion reflex (Y), which is a measure of the pricking pain sensation in an individual. Note that both X and Y are random variables. We want to estimate ρ, the correlation coefficient for these variables. These data are obtained:

x (percentage overweight)	y (threshold of nociceptive flexion reflex)
89	2
90	3
75	4
30	4.5
51	5.5
75	7
62	9
45	13
90	15
20	14

The scattergram for these data is shown in Figure 11.13. There appears to be some tendency for small values of X to be associated with large values of Y, and vice versa. However, the tendency is not strong as evidenced by points (30,4.5), for which a small value of X is paired with a small value of Y, and (20,14), for which the reverse is true. Based on these comments, we would expect r, the estimate for ρ, to be negative; but we would not expect it to be very close to -1. That is, we would expect X and Y to be *slightly* negatively correlated. To verify these observations, let us estimate ρ, using Definition 11.3.3. These

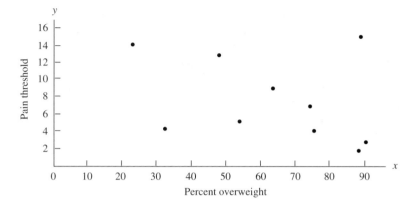

FIGURE 11.13

Scattergram of percentage overweight versus threshold of nociceptive flexion reflex, indicating a slight negative correlation.

sample statistics are needed:

$$\sum x = 627 \qquad \sum y = 77 \qquad \sum xy = 4461.5$$

$$\sum x^2 = 45{,}141 \qquad \sum y^2 = 799.5$$

$$\hat{\rho} = r = \frac{n \sum xy - \sum x \sum y}{\sqrt{\left[n \sum x^2 - \left(\sum x\right)^2\right]\left[n \sum y^2 - \left(\sum y\right)^2\right]}}$$

$$= \frac{10(4461.5) - 627(77)}{\sqrt{[10(45{,}141) - 627^2][10(799.5) - 77^2]}}$$

$$= -.33$$

A word of caution is in order. We have provided a logical point estimator for ρ and a very rough notion as to how to interpret the estimated value. There is still a problem to be solved. Since we are estimating ρ from a data set, it is unlikely that $\hat{\rho}$ will ever assume the easily interpreted values of 1, −1, or 0. We are almost always faced with the problem of interpreting a value such as that obtained in Example 11.3.3 (−.33), which is not clearly close to any of the extreme values 1, −1, or 0.

Figure 11.14 gives a suggested scale for interpreting r. According to the scale, the correlation −.33 is described as "weak" negative correlation. The scale will be justi-fied in Section 11.4. In reading the scale, correlations that equal one of the cutoff points listed will be assumed to lie in the upper classification. For example, a correlation of .5 will be considered a moderate positive correlation, whereas a correlation of −.9 is considered to be a strong negative correlation. The scale given here is not "the law"; it is only a suggested interpretation. Correlation coefficients are somewhat subject mat-ter dependent. In carefully controlled laboratory experiments in biology or chemistry,

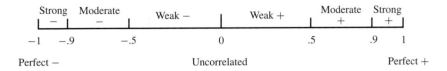

■ **FIGURE 11.14**
Interpretation of the estimated Pearson correlation coefficient r.

correlation coefficients might be expected to be quite high. However, in experiments on human subjects or in observational studies in the field, lower correlation coefficients are typically seen. These lower values might still be deemed to be highly informative by the subject matter expert.

A Note on Computing

Calculating r by hand is tedious, which is why many handheld calculators are programmed to calculate r. You are urged to use a calculator to do the arithmetic computation of Definition 11.3.3. The Technology Tools section at the end of this chapter discusses the procedure for doing so using the TI83 calculator and SAS. The code used to produce Figure 11.15 is given there.

Computer packages that calculate r usually routinely include a test of

$$H_0: \rho = 0 \quad (X \text{ and } Y \text{ are uncorrelated})$$

$$H_1: \rho \neq 0 \quad (\text{there is a correlation between } X \text{ and } Y)$$

One should view this test with caution. It tests only to see if X and Y are at all correlated. It in no way tests to see if the correlation that exists is of any practical importance. For a large data set, a correlation of .05 might test out to be nonzero. However, as we have seen, this correlation is considered to be weak. Just how weak it is will be

ARE PAIN AND OBESITY CORRELATED

VARIABLE	N	MEAN	STD DEV	SUM	MINIMUM	MAXIMUM
PERCENT	10	62.70000000	25.44733123	627.0000000	20.00000000	90.00000000
PAIN	10	7.70000000	4.79119563	77.0000000	2.00000000	15.00000000

CORRELATION COEFFICIENTS/PROB > |R| UNDER H0:RHO = 0/N = 10

	PERCENT	PAIN
PERCENT	1.00000	-0.33391 ①
	0.0000	0.3457 ②
PAIN	-0.33391	1.00000
	0.3457	0.0000

■ **FIGURE 11.15**
SAS printout for finding the correlation coefficient for the data of Example 11.3.3. The null hypothesis of no correlation is not rejected.

explained in the next section. You will see research papers which report that certain correlations are "statistically significant." Keep in mind the fact that this usually means that the correlation test was performed and H_0 was rejected. The correlation is not zero. However, you must judge for yourself from a subject matter standpoint whether or not the correlation is of any practical use. The printout shown in Figure 11.15 gives the SAS output for the program used to find the correlation coefficient for the data of Example 11.3.3. The correlation coefficient, $-.33391$, is shown at ①. The P value for the test

$$H_0: \rho = 0 \quad (X \text{ and } Y \text{ are uncorrelated})$$

$$H_1: \rho \neq 0 \quad (\text{there is a correlation between } X \text{ and } Y)$$

is shown at ②. Since this P value (.3457) is high, we will not reject H_0. The weak negative correlation is not large enough to be able to conclude that there is in fact any linear association between the pain threshold and the percentage overweight.

◼ EXERCISES 11.3

1. Consider the following observations on the random variables X and Y:

x	y
2.0	5.0
2.5	5.5
3.0	6.2
3.5	6.4
4.0	7.0

   (*a*) Plot a scattergram for these data.
   (*b*) On the basis of the scattergram, do you expect r, the estimated correlation coefficient, to be close to 1, -1, or 0?
   (*c*) Find $\sum x, \sum x^2, \sum y, \sum y^2, \sum xy$.
   (*d*) Find r and classify it according to the scale given in Figure 11.14.
2. Consider the following observations on the random variables X and Y:

x	y
2.0	7.2
2.5	7.0
3.0	6.5
3.5	6.0
4.0	5.3

   (*a*) Plot a scattergram for these data.
   (*b*) On the basis of the scattergram, do you expect r to be close to 1, -1, or 0?
   (*c*) Find $\sum x, \sum x^2, \sum y, \sum y^2, \sum xy$.
   (*d*) Determine r and classify it according to the scale given in Figure 11.14.

3. Consider the following observations on the random variables X and Y:

x	y
2.0	4.0
2.1	4.4
2.5	6.3
3.0	9.0
3.5	6.2
3.9	4.3
4.0	4.0

(a) Plot a scattergram for these data.
(b) On the basis of the scattergram, do you expect r to be close to 1, -1, or 0?
(c) Find $\sum x, \sum x^2, \sum y, \sum y^2, \sum xy$.
(d) Calculate r.

4. A study is conducted to estimate the correlation between the random variables X, an individual's score on an obesity index, and Y, the individual's resting metabolic rate. On the obesity index, a high score indicates a high degree of obesity; the metabolic rate is measured in milliliters of oxygen consumed per minute. Each variable is measured on 43 subjects. These sample statistics result:

$$\sum x = 1482.5 \qquad \sum y = 10,719 \qquad \sum xy = 379,207.5$$

$$\sum x^2 = 53,515.25 \qquad \sum y^2 = 2,736,063$$

Find r.

5. In studying the effect of sewage effluent on a lake, measurements are taken of the nitrate concentration of the water. An older manual method has been used to monitor this variable. A new automated method has been devised. If a high positive correlation can be shown between the measurements taken by using the two methods, then the automated method will be put into routine use. These data are obtained (units are micrograms of nitrate per liter of water):

x (manual)	y (automated)
25	30
40	80
120	150
75	80
150	200
300	350
270	240
400	320
450	470
575	583

(a) Find $\sum x, \sum x^2, \sum y, \sum y^2, \sum xy$.

(b) Estimate ρ.

(c) Would you advise putting the automated method into use? Explain.

6. A study is conducted to assess the accuracy with which mothers can judge the food intake of their children. Reports were obtained from the mothers and from an outside observer who spent time in the home watching the food preparation and the eating habits of the child. These correlations between the mother's report and that of the observer are found:

Food	r	Food	r
Fat, g	.52	Calcium, mg	.28
Saturated fat, g	.38	Phosphorus, mg	−.10
Monounsaturated fat, g	.41	Iron, mg	.82
Polyunsaturated fat, g	.58	Vitamin A, IU	.66
Cholesterol, mg	.65	Thiamine, mg	.68
Protein, g	.50	Riboflavin, mg	.52
Carbohydrates, g	.48	Niacin, mg	.72
Sodium, mg	.27	Vitamin C, mg	.50
Potassium, mg	.54	Calories	.71

(a) Explain in a practical sense the significance of the negative correlation for phosphorus.

(b) Categorize each correlation using the scale given in Figure 11.14.

(Correlation reported in Charles Basch et al., "Validation of Mothers' Reports of Dietary Intake by Four to Seven Year-Old Children," *American Journal of Public Health,* November 1990, pp. 1314–1317.)

7. A study is conducted to investigate depression in adolescents. Among the factors considered are worry and satisfaction with the immediate environment. High scores indicate high levels of depression, worry, or satisfaction. These statements are made:

"Depression is positively correlated with worry, $r = .3, P < .001$."

"Depression is negatively correlated with satisfaction, $r = .36, P < .001$."

"Satisfaction and worry scores are negatively correlated, $r = −.16, P < .02$."

(a) Construct scattergrams to illustrate what you would expect the data to look like in each case.

(b) A friend who does not know anything about statistics asks you to interpret these statements in a practical sense. What would you say?

(c) Notice that each statement is accompanied by a P value. State the null and alternative hypotheses involved.

(Statements found in Lirio Covey and Debbie Tam, "Depressive Mood, The Single Parent Home and Adolescent Cigarette Smoking," *American Journal of Public Health,* November 1990, pp. 1330–1333.)

11.4

EVALUATING THE STRENGTH
OF THE LINEAR RELATIONSHIP (OPTIONAL)

As we pointed out in Section 11.2, the method of least squares can be used to fit a straight line to *any* data set. However, the utility of this line as a predictor of future values of the dependent variable *Y* depends entirely on *whether the assumption of linearity is appropriate*. For this reason we need an analytic method for determining how well a straight line fits the data points. We present two methods here. The first employs a statistic called the coefficient of determination; the second uses an analysis-of-variance technique to discover whether the variability in *Y* is well explained by a linear relationship with *X*.

Coefficient of Determination

The estimated coefficient of determination is a statistic used to assess the strength of the linear relationship that exists between *X* and *Y* in either a regression or a correlation setting. It has an easily understood interpretation, and it will allow us to justify the scale used to interpret *r* given in the last section.

Since this coefficient is associated with both regression and correlation analysis, it provides a link between the two procedures. To define this statistic, we must determine the relationship between *r*, the estimated correlation coefficient, and *b*, the estimated slope of the least-squares regression line. We use the following notation:

$$S_{xy} = \sum (x - \bar{x})(y - \bar{y})$$

$$= \frac{n \sum xy - \sum x \sum y}{n} = \text{measure of covariance between } X \text{ and } Y$$

$$S_{xx} = \sum (x - \bar{x})^2$$

$$= \frac{n \sum x^2 - \left(\sum x \right)^2}{n} = \text{measure of variability in } X$$

$$S_{yy} = \sum (y - \bar{y})^2$$

$$= \frac{n \sum y^2 - \left(\sum y \right)^2}{n} = \text{measure of variability in } Y$$

Using this notation, we can express *b* and *r* as

$$b = \frac{n \sum xy - \sum x \sum y}{n \sum x^2 - \left(\sum x \right)^2} = \frac{S_{xy}}{S_{xx}}$$

$$r = \frac{n \sum xy - \sum x \sum y}{\sqrt{[n \sum x^2 - (\sum x)^2][n \sum y^2 - (\sum y)^2]}} = \frac{S_{xy}}{\sqrt{S_{xx} S_{yy}}}$$

Note that

$$b \frac{\sqrt{S_{xx}}}{\sqrt{S_{yy}}} = \frac{S_{xy}}{S_{xx}} \frac{\sqrt{S_{xx}}}{\sqrt{S_{yy}}} = \frac{S_{xy}}{\sqrt{S_{xx} S_{yy}}} = r$$

Thus the equation relating b and r is

$$r = b \frac{\sqrt{S_{xx}}}{\sqrt{S_{yy}}}$$

The practical implication of this relationship is that b and r always have the *same* algebraic sign. Thus a positive correlation implies a regression line with positive slope (a line that rises from left to right); a negative correlation implies a regression line with negative slope (a line that falls from left to right).

Let us now reconsider the sum of squares SS_E that is being minimized in the least-squares procedure:

$$SS_E = \sum_{i=1}^{n} e_i^2 = \sum_{i=1}^{n} [y_i - (a + bx_i)]^2$$

This sum measures the variability of the data points y_i about the estimated regression line $a + bx_i$. If the line closely fits the data points, then SS_E will be small; otherwise, it will be large.

A rather tricky algebraic argument involving the use of the rules of summation given in Appendix A can be used to show that

$$SS_E = S_{yy} - bS_{xy}$$

The argument is given in its entirety in [11]. Dividing each side of the equation by S_{yy}, we obtain

$$\frac{SS_E}{S_{yy}} = 1 - b \frac{S_{xy}}{S_{yy}}$$

Substituting S_{xy}/S_{xx} into this equation for b, we have

$$\frac{SS_E}{S_{yy}} = 1 - \frac{S_{xy}^2}{S_{xx} S_{yy}}$$

Since $r = S_{xy}/\sqrt{S_{xx} S_{yy}}$, we conclude that

$$\frac{SS_E}{S_{yy}} = 1 - r^2$$

or that

$$r^2 = 1 - \frac{SS_E}{S_{yy}} = \frac{S_{yy} - SS_E}{S_{yy}}$$

Since S_{yy} measures the total variation in Y and SS_E measures the random variation of Y about the regression line, $S_{yy} - SS_E$ is a measure of the variation in Y that is not random.

That is, $S_{yy} - SS_E$ is a measure of the variability in Y that can be attributed to a linear association with X.

The statistic r^2 is called the *coefficient of determination*. Thus, in a practical sense,

$$r^2 = \frac{\text{variation in } Y \text{ due to linearity}}{\text{total variation in } Y}$$

If we multiply r^2 by 100, we obtain the percentage of the variation in Y that can be attributed to a linear relationship between X and Y. Thus if r^2 is large, we may conclude that there is a strong linear association between X and Y.

The coefficient of determination can be used to justify the correlation scale given in Figure 11.14. Any correlation that lies strictly between $-.5$ and $.5$ is deemed weak because r^2 for these values is less than $.25$. For these values less than 25% of the variation in Y is attributed to a linear association with X; more than 75% of the variation in Y is unexplained. Moderate correlation coefficients have r^2 values that are at least $.25$ but less than $.81$. To call a correlation strong, we want its absolute value to be at least $.9$. In this case the percent of variation in Y explained by its linear association with X is substantial in that it is 81% or more. Example 11.4.1 illustrates the use of the coefficient of determination.

> **EXAMPLE 11.4.1.** Let us reexamine the relationship between X, the percentage over ideal weight, and Y, an individual's threshold of pain. In Example 11.3.3, we found that $r = -.33$ and interpreted this to indicate a weak negative correlation between the two variables. To get a better idea of the strength of the linear relationship, we compute r^2, the coefficient of determination. The value of this statistic is $r^2 = (-.33)^2 = .1089$. Multiplying by 100, we conclude that only 10.89% of the variation in Y is attributed to a linear association with X. Since this percentage is small, clearly a correlation of $-.33$ is not really very strong. It does not indicate a strong tendency for obese individuals to exhibit a low threshold of pain, and vice versa.

Analysis of Variance

An analysis-of-variance technique is available for testing whether a straight line explains a significant amount of the observed variability in Y. As in any analysis-of-variance procedure, the idea is to partition the total variability in Y, S_{yy}, into components that can be attributed to recognizable sources. This can be done easily since we already established that SS_E, the random variability about the estimated regression line, can be written in the form

$$SS_E = SS_{yy} - bS_{xy}$$

Solving this equation for S_{yy}, we see that

$$S_{yy} = bS_{xy} + SS_E$$

The second component on the right, SS_E, is called the *error,* or *residual, sum of squares;* it is a measure of the variability in Y that is random or unexplained. The first component on the right, bS_{xy}, the *regression sum of squares*, measures the variability in Y attributable to the linear association between X and Y. The regression sum of squares is denoted SS_R. Thus we have partitioned S_{yy} into two components:

$$S_{yy} \qquad = \qquad SS_R \qquad + \qquad SS_E$$

(total variability   (variability in Y (unexplained, or
in Y)   due to regression   random, variation)
on X)

Logically, if the assumption of linear regression is valid, then SS_R should account for most of the variability in Y, with only a small portion being random or unexplained. Thus we should be able to use the relative sizes of SS_R and SS_E in some way to decide whether the assumption of linear regression is reasonable.

This can be done by making some further assumptions concerning the dependent variable Y. Assume that we are dealing with k specific values of the independent variable $x_1, x_2, x_3, \ldots, x_k$. This implies that we are dealing with k random variables $Y|x_1$, $Y|x_2, Y|x_3, \ldots, Y|x_k$. We assume that these variables are independent normal random variables, each with the same variance, σ^2. If linear regression is valid, then the means of these variables lie on the straight line $\mu_{Y|x} = \alpha + \beta x$. This idea is illustrated in Figure 11.16.

Now assume that a random sample of size n_i, $i = 1, 2, \ldots, k$, is selected from each distribution. Let Y_{ij} denote the jth element of the random sample from the distribution of $Y|x_i$. The variable Y_{ij} is a random variable with mean $\alpha + \beta x_i$ and variance σ^2. Its observed value is not expected to lie exactly at the mean value, but is expected to deviate from this value by some random amount, E_{ij}. Thus we may write the following expression, which serves as the model for simple linear regression:

MODEL

$$Y_{ij} = \alpha + \beta x_i + E_{ij} \qquad \begin{aligned} i &= 1, 2, \ldots, k \\ j &= 1, 2, \ldots, n_i \end{aligned}$$

$$\begin{bmatrix} \text{observed value} \\ \text{of } Y \text{ for} \\ \text{particular value} \\ \text{of } X \end{bmatrix} = \begin{bmatrix} \text{mean value of } Y \\ \text{for that value} \\ \text{of } X \end{bmatrix} + \begin{bmatrix} \text{random} \\ \text{deviation} \\ \text{from mean} \end{bmatrix}$$

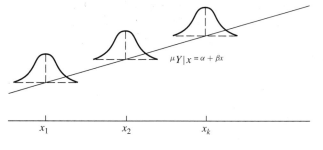

FIGURE 11.16
Each random variable $Y|x_i$ is normally distributed with the same variance.

$\mu_{Y|x} = \alpha + \beta x$

$x_1 \qquad x_2 \qquad x_k$

The assumptions made concerning Y imply these model assumptions:

MODEL ASSUMPTIONS. The random deviations E_{ij} are independent normal random variables, each with mean 0 and variance σ^2.

With these assumptions it is possible to formulate the desired null and alternative hypothesis mathematically and test the null hypothesis by using SS_R and SS_E. We wish to test

H_0: variation in Y not explained by linear model

H_1: significant portion of variation in Y explained by linear model

Note that if $\beta = 0$, the model becomes $Y_{ij} = \alpha + E_{ij}$. That is, if $\beta = 0$, then *all* the variability in Y is assumed to be random; if $\beta \neq 0$, then at least a portion of the variability is assumed to be due to the linear regression of Y on X. Thus the null hypothesis of no linear regression can be expressed in the form H_0: $\beta = 0$. So we are interested in testing

H_0: $\beta = 0$ (no linear regression)

H_1: $\beta \neq 0$

The test statistic for testing this hypothesis utilizes two statistics that are functions of SS_R and SS_E. The first, called the *regression mean square MS_R*, is found by dividing SS_R by 1. The second, the *error mean square MS_E*, is found by dividing SS_E by $n - 2$, where $n = \sum_{i=1}^{k} n_i$ denotes the overall sample size. That is, we define

$$MS_R = \frac{SS_R}{1} \qquad MS_E = \frac{SS_E}{n-2}$$

So if H_0 is true, then the statistic

$$\boxed{\frac{MS_R}{MS_E}}$$

follows an F distribution with 1 and $n - 2$ degrees of freedom. Furthermore, if H_0 is true, then the observed value of this statistic should lie close to 1; otherwise, its value should be inflated. Thus the null hypothesis of no linear regression is rejected if the observed value of the F ratio is too *large* to have reasonably occurred by chance.

Everything that has been said can be summarized conveniently in the analysis-of-variance table given in Table 11.1. The table includes the formulas needed to compute S_{yy}, the total sum of squares, and SS_R, the regression sum of squares. The error sum of squares SS_E is obtained by subtracting SS_R from S_{yy}. Recall that

$$S_{xy} = \frac{n \sum xy - \sum x \sum y}{n} \qquad S_{xx} = \frac{n \sum x^2 - \left(\sum x \right)^2}{n}$$

$$S_{yy} = \frac{n \sum y^2 - \left(\sum y \right)^2}{n} \qquad b = \frac{S_{xy}}{S_{xx}}$$

In Example 11.4.2 we continue the analysis of the data of Example 11.1.3.

TABLE 11.1

ANOVA used to test $H_0: \beta = 0$ (no linear regression)

	Analysis of variance: simple linear regression			
Source of variation	**Degrees of freedom DF**	**Sum of squares SS**	**Mean square MS**	**F ratio**
Regression (model)	1	bS_{xy}	$\dfrac{SS_R}{1}$	$F_{1,n-2} = \dfrac{MS_R}{MS_E}$
Error	$n-2$	$S_{yy} - bS_{xy}$	$\dfrac{SS_E}{n-2}$	
Total	$n-1$	S_{yy}		

EXAMPLE 11.4.2. In Example 11.1.3, the variables of interest are X and Y, the shell height and length, respectively, in the limpet *Patelloida pygmaea*. The scattergram indicates that the assumption of linear regression is valid. We now test that assumption statistically, instead of relying solely on the visual pattern of the data. These quantities are needed:

$$\sum x = 56.6 \qquad \sum y = 151.1 \qquad \sum xy = 311.96$$

$$\sum x^2 = 117.68 \qquad \sum y^2 = 832.85 \qquad S_{xy} = 6.52$$

$$S_{xx} = 3.27 \qquad S_{yy} = 17.45 \qquad N = 28$$

From these quantities we may conclude that

$$\hat{\alpha} = a = 1.36 \qquad r = .8638$$
$$\hat{\beta} = b = 1.99 \qquad r^2 = .7461$$

Since $r^2 = .7461$, we may conclude that 74.61% of the variation in Y can be attributed to a linear association with X. Is this percentage high enough to conclude that a significant amount of the variability in Y is explained by the linear model?

To answer this question, we test

$$H_0: \beta = 0 \quad \text{(no linear regression)}$$

$$H_1: \beta \neq 0$$

using the analysis-of-variance technique. The ANOVA for these data is shown in Table 11.2. Based on the $F_{1,26}$ distribution H_0 can be rejected with $P < .01$. We can conclude that, as expected, the assumption of linear regression is valid. Practically speaking, this means that predictions based on the estimated regression line

$$\hat{\mu}_{Y|x} = 1.36 + 1.99x$$

should be acceptable. Note that when the null hypothesis of no linear regression is rejected, we have concluded that a significant portion of the variability in Y has been explained by the linear model. This does not mean that the linear model is necessarily the best model to use; it does mean that it is at least reasonable.

TABLE 11.2

ANOVA for the data of Example 11.4.2. The null hypothesis of no linear regression is rejected with $P < .01$.

Source	DF	SS	MS	F
Regression	1	$bS_{xy} = 12.97$	12.97	$\dfrac{12.97}{.17} = 76.29$
Error	26	$17.45 - 12.97 = 4.48$	$\dfrac{4.48}{26} = .17$	
Total	27	$S_{yy} = 17.45$		

A Note on Computing

It is now possible to explain more of the printout shown in Figure 11.11. In Example 11.2.3 we noticed from the scattergram that there appears to be a linear trend in the data. The estimated line of regression is seen to be

$$\hat{\mu}_{Y|x} = 290.07044608 - 15.11057071x$$

The r^2 value for these data, .726096, is shown on the printout under R-SQUARE. Thus 72.6096% of the variation in the length of the breeding season is associated with X, the photoperiod. The analysis of variance used to test $H_0: \beta = 0$ is given in the upper portion of Figure 11.11. The source that we labeled regression is called MODEL by SAS. From the printout we see that the observed value of the F statistic used to test H_0 is 23.86 and its P value is .0009. Since P is small, we can reject H_0 and conclude that linear regression is appropriate.

EXERCISES 11.4

1. A study of body characteristics and performance is conducted among master- and first-class Olympic weight lifters. Two variables studied are X, the subject's body weight, and Y, his best reported clean and jerk lift. These data (in pounds) are obtained:

x	y	x	y
134	185	190	336
138	238	190	339
154	260	205	341
178	290	205	358
176	312	206	359

(a) Plot a scattergram for these data. Based on the scattergram, do you expect b to be positive or negative?

(b) Find $\sum x, \sum x^2, \sum y, \sum y^2, \sum xy$ and r.

(c) Find and interpret the coefficient of determination.

(d) Test the appropriateness of the linear regression model. If it is appropriate, find the estimated line of regression of Y on X and use this to estimate the best clean and jerk lift for a weight lifter who weighs 200 pounds.

2. A study of the body's ability to absorb iron and lead is conducted by using radioactive tracer techniques. Ten subjects participate in the study. Each is given an identical oral dose of iron (ferrous sulfate) and lead (lead-203 chloride). After 12 days, the amount of each compound retained in the system is measured, and from this the percentage absorbed by the body is determined. These data result:

x (percentage iron absorbed)	y (percentage lead absorbed)
17	8
22	17
35	18
43	25
80	58
85	59
91	41
92	30
96	43
100	58

(a) Plot a scattergram for these data. Based on the scattergram, do you expect b to be positive or negative?

(b) Find $\sum x, \sum x^2, \sum y, \sum y^2, \sum xy$ and r.

(c) Find and interpret the coefficient of determination.

(d) Test the appropriateness of the linear regression model. If it is appropriate, estimate the true regression line and use it to predict the percentage of iron absorbed by an individual whose system absorbs 15% of the lead ingested.

3. Verify the analysis-of-variance table given in Figure 11.11.

4. (a) Find and interpret the coefficient of determination for the data of Exercise 4 of Section 11.2.

(b) Test the appropriateness of the linear regression model, using the data of Exercise 4 of Section 11.2. Do you think that the prediction given in part d of Exercise 4 of Section 11.2 is likely to be a good estimate for y?

5. Use the data of Exercise 5 of Section 11.3 to find the coefficient of determination for variables X, the nitrate reading taken by an older manual technique, and Y, the reading taken by a new automated method. On the basis of this value, do you think that the new method will well reflect the readings that would have been obtained with the older technique?

6. Consider the correlations given in Exercise 6 of Section 11.3.

(a) Find the coefficient of determination for each food type.

(b) What is the maximum percentage of variation in Y (the mother's report) that is explained by its linear association with X (the observer's report)?

(c) Based on the r^2 value, do you think that the negative correlation associated with phosphorus is of any practical importance? Explain.

7. Consider Exercise 7 of Section 11.3. Find the coefficient of determination for each correlation given.
8. Consider the regression equations given in Exercise 6 of Section 11.2. The values of r for the equation are .805 (FVC), .836 (FEV_1), .825 (PEFR), and $-.689$ (FET). In each case, what percentage of variation in response is linked to the linear association with X, the farthest distance at which the candle can be extinguished?

11.5
CONFIDENCE INTERVAL ESTIMATION (OPTIONAL)

At this time we can find point estimates for α, β, $\mu_{Y|x}$, and $Y|x$, the value of Y for a specified value of X. As in the past, it is natural to want to extend these point estimates to interval estimates so that confidence levels can be reported. With the model assumptions that have been made, this can be done. Consider Example 11.5.1.

EXAMPLE 11.5.1. Although dissolved silicon in seawater is not required by all primary producers, studies have linked the depletion of this substance with decreased productivity. A study is conducted to gain further insight into the behavior of dissolved silicon. The two variables studied are X, the distance in kilometers from shore, and Y, the silicon concentration in micrograms per liter (μg/liter). These measurements, taken over the northwest African shelf, are to be analyzed. (Note that X, the independent variable, is *not* random. Measurements are taken at six preselected distances from shore with four measurements taken at each distance.)

x	y	x	y	x	y
5	6.1	25	3.7	42	3.4
5	6.2	25	3.7	42	3.6
5	6.1	25	3.8	42	3.5
5	6.0	25	3.9	42	3.2
15	5.2	32	3.9	55	3.7
15	5.0	32	3.8	55	3.9
15	4.9	32	3.9	55	3.6
15	5.1	32	3.7	55	3.8

The scattergram for these data is shown in Figure 11.17. There does appear to be a downward linear trend. Therefore, we anticipate a negative slope for the estimated line of regression. We first test the appropriateness of the linear regression model. For these data,

$$\sum x = 696 \qquad \sum y = 103.7 \qquad \sum xy = 2692.5$$

$$\sum x^2 = 26{,}752 \qquad \sum y^2 = 469.81 \qquad S_{xy} = -314.8$$

$$\bar{x} = 29 \qquad \bar{y} = 4.32 \qquad b = \frac{S_{xy}}{S_{xx}} = -.048$$

$$S_{xx} = 6568 \qquad S_{yy} = 21.74 \qquad a = \bar{y} - b\bar{x} = 5.71$$

The analysis-of-variance table is shown in Table 11.3. From the F table we see that $P[F_{1,22} \geq 7.95] = .01$. Since 50.37, the observed F ratio, exceeds this point, $P < .01$. This

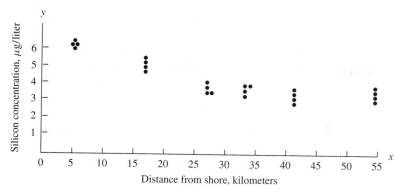

FIGURE 11.17

Scattergram of distance from the shore versus silicon concentration in waters over the northwest African shelf.

P value is small, so we can reject $H_0: \beta = 0$ in favor of $H_1: \beta \neq 0$ and conclude that the assumption of linearity is warranted. We now have *point* estimates for α and β, namely, $\hat{\alpha} = a = 5.71$ and $\hat{\beta} = b = -.048$.

Assume that we are particularly interested in the silicon concentration at a distance of 10 kilometers from shore. Two questions can be asked: What is the *mean* concentration at this distance? and If a *single* water sample is drawn at this distance, what will be the silicon concentration for this sample? These questions already can be answered by using point estimation. In particular, we are being asked to estimate $\mu_{Y|x=10}$ and $Y|x = 10$. Each of these estimates is the same, namely,

$$\hat{\mu}_{Y|x} = \hat{y} = a + bx$$

$$= 5.71 - .048x = 5.23 \ \mu g/liter$$

Our problem now is to extend each of these point estimates to interval estimates so that a confidence level can be reported.

The derivations of the confidence intervals on α, β, $\mu_{Y|x}$, and $Y|x$ are beyond the scope of this text. However, the pattern involved in each case is the same as that seen earlier. Namely, we create the confidence interval by adding a specified amount to the point estimate to obtain an upper bound for the confidence interval; the lower bound is found by subtracting this value from the point estimate. The amount to be added and

TABLE 11.3

ANOVA for the data of Example 11.5.1. The null hypothesis of no linear regression can be rejected with $P < .01$

Source	DF	SS	MS	F
Regression	1	15.11	15.11	50.37
Error	22	6.63	.30	
Total	23	21.74		

subtracted depends on the confidence desired and the estimated standard deviation of the point estimator for the entity involved. In this setting, σ^2 is estimated by $MS_E = SS_E/(n-2)$. To simplify the notation in the work to come, we denote the estimator for σ by S. In this case $S = \sqrt{MS_E}$.

Confidence intervals for the intercept and slope of the regression line are

$$\boxed{a \pm \frac{tS\sqrt{\sum x^2}}{\sqrt{nS_{xx}}}}$$ (Confidence interval on α, the intercept of the true line of regression)

$$\boxed{b \pm \frac{tS}{\sqrt{S_{xx}}}}$$ (Confidence interval on β, the slope of the true line of regression)

In each case, the t point involved is a point associated with the T_{n-2} distribution whose value depends on the confidence desired. Example 11.5.2 continues the analysis of the data of Example 11.5.1 by constructing 95% confidence intervals on the slope and intercept of the true line of regression.

EXAMPLE 11.5.2. To construct a 95% confidence interval on α based on the data of Example 11.5.1, we need only substitute the appropriate values into the formula

$$a \pm t\frac{S\sqrt{\sum x^2}}{\sqrt{nS_{xx}}}$$

For the data given,

$$\sum x^2 = 26{,}752 \qquad n = 24 \qquad a = 5.71$$

$$S_{xx} = 6568 \qquad S = \sqrt{\frac{SS_E}{n-2}} = \sqrt{.30} = .5477$$

The t point needed is shown in Figure 11.18. Its value, 2.074, is found from the table of the T distribution with $n - 2 = 22$ degrees of freedom. The confidence interval is therefore

$$5.71 \pm 2.074\,\frac{\sqrt{.3}\sqrt{26{,}752}}{\sqrt{24(6568)}} = 5.71 \pm .47$$

That is, we can be 95% confident that the intercept of the regression line lies between 5.24 and 6.18.

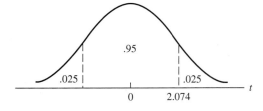

FIGURE 11.18

The T point needed to construct a 95% confidence interval on α, the intercept of the regression line for the data of Example 11.5.1.

A 95% confidence interval on β is found by substituting the values $t = 2.074$, $S = \sqrt{.3}$, $S_{xx} = 6568$, and $b = -.048$ into

$$b \pm t \frac{S}{\sqrt{S_{xx}}}$$

The resulting confidence interval is

$$-.048 \pm 2.074 \frac{\sqrt{.3}}{\sqrt{6568}} = -.048 \pm .014$$

We can be 95% confident that the slope of the regression line lies between $-.062$ and $-.034$. Note that the analysis-of-variance procedure already has indicated that $\beta \neq 0$. Thus it should not be surprising that the confidence interval on β does *not* contain the number 0.

Recall that the estimated regression line can be used to obtain a point estimate for the average response for a given value of X, $\mu_{Y|x}$, or for an individual response, $Y|x$. The two point estimates are identical. However, their interval estimates are not identical. Since it is much harder to predict individual behavior than it is group behavior, it is much harder to trap $Y|x$ than it is to trap $\mu_{Y|x}$. An interval intended to capture $Y|x$ must be wider than one whose purpose is to trap $\mu_{Y|x}$. To distinguish these very similar intervals, we will refer to the interval used to trap $\mu_{Y|x}$ as a confidence interval; an interval constructed to capture $Y|x$ will be called a *prediction interval*. These formulas are used:

$$\hat{\mu}_{Y|x} \pm tS\sqrt{\frac{1}{n} + \frac{(x - \bar{x})^2}{S_{xx}}}$$ (Confidence interval on the average response when $X = x$)

$$\hat{y} \pm tS\sqrt{1 + \frac{1}{n} + \frac{(x - \bar{x})^2}{S_{xx}}}$$ (Prediction interval on the individual response when $X = x$)

In each case the t point involved is found relative to the T_{n-2} distribution. These formulas are illustrated in Example 11.5.3.

EXAMPLE 11.5.3. A 95% confidence interval on the mean silicon concentration drawn 10 kilometers from shore is found by substituting the values $t = 2.074$, $S = \sqrt{.3}$, $n = 24$, $x = 10$, $\bar{x} = 29$, $S_{xx} = 6568$, and $\hat{\mu}_{Y|x} = 5.23$ into

$$\hat{\mu}_{Y|x} \pm tS\sqrt{\frac{1}{n} + \frac{(x - \bar{x})^2}{S_{xx}}}$$

The resulting confidence interval is

$$5.23 \pm 2.074\sqrt{.3}\sqrt{\frac{1}{24} + \frac{(10 - 29)^2}{6568}} = 5.23 \pm .35$$

We can be 95% confident that the *mean* silicon concentration for samples drawn at this distance is between 4.88 and 5.58 μg/liter.

A 95% prediction interval on the silicon concentration for a single water sample drawn 10 kilometers from shore is found by substituting the values $t = 2.074$, $S = \sqrt{.3}$, $n = 24$, $x = 10$, $\bar{x} = 29$, $S_{xx} = 6568$, and $\hat{y} = 5.23$ into

$$\hat{y} \pm tS\sqrt{1 + \frac{1}{n} + \frac{(x - \bar{x})^2}{S_{xx}}}$$

The resulting interval is

$$5.23 \pm 2.074\sqrt{.3}\sqrt{1 + \frac{1}{24} + \frac{(10 - 29)^2}{6568}} = 5.23 \pm 1.19$$

We can be 95% confident that the silicon concentration for the next sample taken 10 kilometers from shore will be between 4.04 and 6.42 μg/liter. As expected, the prediction interval for $Y|x = 10$ is wider than the confidence interval for $\mu_{Y|x=10}$.

▨ EXERCISES 11.5

1. These data are obtained on X, the latitude of the natural breeding range, and Y, the length of the breeding season in days, of 11 species of diving ducks:

x	y	x	y
29	112	53	42
42	98	54	50
45	58	55	18
45	68	60	51
50	28	65	49
50	46		

   (a) Plot a scattergram for these data. Based on the scattergram, do you think that linear regression is applicable?
   (b) Use the analysis-of-variance procedure to test the appropriateness of the linear model.
   (c) Find point estimates for α and β.
   (d) Find 95% confidence intervals on α and β.
   (e) Find a point estimate for the mean length of the breeding season for birds whose natural breeding range is at a latitude of 35 degrees. Find a 95% confidence interval on this parameter.
   (f) Find a point estimate for the length of the breeding season for a single bird whose natural breeding range is at a latitude of 35 degrees. Find a 95% prediction interval on this value.
2. Teaching diabetics to measure their own blood glucose has been of great benefit. A new technique that is less expensive than the current procedure is under investigation. The technique uses a glucose oxidase stick. The stick develops two colors simultaneously, and these colors are matched by eye to a chart that gives the glucose level. If this procedure can be shown to be accurate, it can be put into widespread use. The data shown in the table are obtained on X, the blood glucose level as measured by a diabetic patient using the new glucose oxidase stick, and Y, the patient's

blood glucose level as measured in a laboratory test. (Data are given millimoles per liter.) For these data,

$$\sum x = 295 \qquad \sum y = 303.5 \qquad \sum xy = 3073.55 \qquad S_{xx} = 915.335$$

$$\sum x^2 = 3090.96 \qquad \sum y^2 = 3120.59 \qquad S_{xy} = 835.2375 \qquad S = 1.21$$

$$\bar{x} = 7.375 \qquad \bar{y} = 7.5875 \qquad S_{yy} = 817.78375$$

x	y	x	y	x	y	x	y
1.3	2.4	3.2	4.4	7.0	7.7	15.0	14.9
2.0	3.0	3.6	4.3	8.0	8.0	15.0	13.8
2.4	2.3	3.7	4.3	8.0	10.0	17.5	17.6
2.6	3.0	3.7	5.0	10.0	10.0	18.7	17.5
2.5	2.2	3.8	4.4	10.2	9.5	6.0	6.0
2.6	2.4	4.4	4.5	10.2	11.2	8.7	8.8
2.7	2.5	4.3	5.0	12.5	11.0	5.6	5.7
3.0	3.8	5.0	4.5	11.3	13.0	9.1	9.0
3.7	2.5	5.0	6.2	13.0	13.1	16.2	12.5
3.7	3.5	6.3	6.2	14.5	13.8	9.0	14.0

(a) Plot a scattergram for the data. Does linear regression appear to be appropriate?

(b) Find and interpret the coefficient of determination.

(c) Use the analysis-of-variance procedure to test the appropriateness of the linear model.

(d) Find point estimates for α and β.

(e) Find 90% confidence intervals on α and β.

(f) Find a point estimate for the laboratory-reported glucose level of a patient who reports the level to be 4.0 mmol/liter. Find a 90% prediction interval on this value.

▩ 11.6

MULTIPLE REGRESSION (OPTIONAL)

As mentioned earlier, when more than one regressor is used to estimate the mean response, the problem is one of multiple regression. The model for multiple linear regression assumes the form

$$\mu_{Y \mid x_1, x_2, x_3, \ldots, x_k} = \beta_0 + \beta_1 x_1 + \beta_2 x_2 + \cdots + \beta_k x_k$$

Here Y is the response, and $\mu_{Y \mid x_1, x_2, x_3, \ldots, x_k}$ is the mean response. It is assumed that its value depends on the values assumed by the regressors $x_1, x_2, \ldots, x_k$. The term β_0 represents an unknown intercept, and $\beta_1, \beta_2, \ldots, \beta_k$ represent unknown coefficients. Notice that if $k = 1$, this model coincides with the model for simple linear regression given in Section 11.2.

EXAMPLE 11.6.1. It is known that in mammals the toxicity of various types of drugs, pesticides, and chemical carcinogens can be altered by inducing liver enzyme activity. A study to investigate this sort of phenomenon in chickens was reported in M. Ehrich, C. Larson, and J. Arnold, "Organophosphate Detoxification Related by Induced Hepatic Microsomal Enzymes in Chickens," *American Journal of Veterinary Research,* vol. 45, 1983. Regression analysis was used to study the relationships between induced enzyme activity and detoxification of the insecticide malathion. Butylated hydroxytoluene (BHT) was the enzyme inducer used. Five enzyme activities were used as regressors, and the response was the percentage of detoxification of malathion. The multiple linear regression model expresses the idea that the average percentage of detoxification of malathion is dependent upon the level of each of five enzymes. Mathematically we write

$$\mu_{Y \mid x_1, x_2, x_3, x_4, x_5} = \beta_0 + \beta_1 x_1 + \beta_2 x_2 + \beta_3 x_3 + \beta_4 x_4 + \beta_5 x_5$$

As with simple linear regression, our problem is to use the method of least squares to estimate the parameters β_0, β_1, β_2, . . . , β_k. We want to find the values of these parameters that minimize the sum of squares of the residuals where a residual is the difference between the observed data point and the value of the response predicted by the estimated regression equation. In the case of simple linear regression we were able to derive some simple equations for estimating the slope and intercept, thereby estimating the regression equation. This is not possible here. There are no simple algebraic expressions that can be evaluated to estimate β_0, β_1, β_2, . . . , β_k when $k > 1$. The mathematics required to obtain these estimates is matrix algebra, and estimates are obtained easily only by using a computer. Once estimates have been obtained, the regression equation is used for the same purpose as in the case of simple linear regression. Namely, it can be used to estimate the average response for various values of the regressors or to predict an individual response for these values. Example 11.6.2 illustrates the idea.

EXAMPLE 11.6.2. When the study described in Example 11.6.1 was run, this equation was obtained with the help of a computer:

$$\hat{\mu}_{Y \mid x_1, x_2, x_3, x_4, x_5} = 54.079 + .097x_1 + .034x_2 + .522x_3 - 2.655x_4 + 2.559x_5$$

Suppose we want to estimate the average percentage of detoxification when $x_1 = 350$, $x_2 = 270$, $x_3 = 100$, $x_4 = 85$, and $x_5 = 102$. This is done by substituting these values into the above equation. We obtain

$$\hat{\mu}_{Y \mid x_1, x_2, x_3, x_4, x_5} = 54.079 + .097(350) + .034(270) + .522(100)$$

$$-2.655(85) + 2.559(102)$$

$$= 184.752$$

This is also the predicted percentage of detoxification for an individual chicken at these levels of the five enzymes. Notice the impact of the algebraic sign of the coefficients on the response. A positive coefficient implies that an increase in the enzyme level tends to increase the percentage of detoxification; a negative sign means the opposite. Here in all cases except enzyme 4, as the enzyme level increases, the detoxification percentage increases. With enzyme 4, raising the level tends to inhibit detoxification.

An r^2 value also accompanies a multiple regression study. It has the same meaning here as in the case of simple linear regression. Namely, r^2 gives the percentage of variation in response that is explained by the linear association with the regressors x_1,

$x_2, \ldots, x_k$. In Example 11.6.2 r^2 was found to be .976. This value is very high. We can say that 97.6% of the variation in response can be explained by the linear association between the response and the five enzyme levels.

Multiple regression is a very complex topic. Typically, when a multiple regression study arises, the researcher tries to pinpoint all the variables that he or she believes are important factors in explaining the response. These regressors are chosen not by the statistician but by the subject matter expert, the researcher. An experiment is then conducted that involves taking measurements on all the regressors and on the response. Once this has been done, some detective work takes place. The researcher together with the statistician must decide which of the proposed regressors do the best job of explaining the response. Should all the regressors be used as was done in Example 11.6.1, or would some subset of regressors work just as well or even better? The aim is to find the best set of regressors. There are several criteria used to decide which set is best. Of these, r^2 and MS_E are familiar to you. It is desirable for the final model to have a high r^2 value; we want it to explain a high percentage of the observed variation in response. Since MS_E is a measure of the unexplained variation in response, the final model should have a small error mean square. However, it is known that as more and more regressors are added to the model, r^2 always increases. Does this mean that "more is better"? The answer to this question is *no*. There are other criteria which are much better indicators of the predictive ability of a regression equation than either r^2 or MS_E. These criteria are affected by adding regressors to the model that are not necessary. The predictive ability of the model can actually be hurt by including unimportant regressors. Thus, to pick the best model we must consider all the criteria and make a value judgment. We want to pick the smallest set of regressors that yields a reasonably small MS_E, an acceptably high r^2, and has good predictive value as measured by the other criteria. There are many texts that discuss these ideas in detail. If you have a research project that you recognize as being one of multiple regression, we suggest that you refer to [12] and that you immediately consult a statistician for help in designing your experiment and in analyzing your data.

▨ EXERCISES 11.6

1. Use the regression equation given in Example 11.6.1 to estimate the mean response when $x_1 = 233$, $x_2 = 260$, $x_3 = 82$, $x_4 = 80$, $x_5 = 88$. Estimate the percentage of detoxification for an individual chicken at these enzyme levels.
2. In deriving the regression equation given in Example 11.6.1, the observed response when $x_1 = 233$, $x_2 = 260$, $x_3 = 82$, $x_4 = 80$, $x_5 = 88$ was 152. Use the estimate found in Exercise 1 to find the residual at this point.
3. Consider the regression equation given in Example 11.6.1. Suppose that we keep the enzyme levels for enzymes 1, 2, 3, and 5 as stated in Exercise 1 but we change x_4 from 80 to 81. What effect does this have on the estimated mean response?
4. Use the idea suggested in Exercise 3 to make a general statement concerning the interpretation of the coefficients $b_1, b_2, \ldots, b_k$ in a multiple regression equation.
5. A study of the mechanical compaction of sandstone in Alaska is conducted. The purpose of the study is to determine factors that affect porosity. The regression

equation obtained is

$$\widehat{GF} = 90 + .23P - .72M + .0018\,d$$

where GF = measure of porosity

d = burial depth of material, meters

P = percentage of ductile grains (grains that can be drawn out or hammered thin)

M = matrix content (the matrix is the natural material in which the sandstone is found)

Large values of GF indicate a high degree of compaction and less porosity.

(a) The reported r^2 is .73. Explain what this means.

(b) Consider two samples with identical values for P and M. Sample 2 is to be taken at a depth that is 1 meter deeper than sample 1. What is the estimated difference in GF between the two samples? What would this difference be if sample 2 were taken 10 meters deeper than sample 1?

(c) Consider two samples with identical values for P and d. If the matrix value for sample 2 exceeds that of sample 1 by 20, what is the estimated difference in GF between the two samples?

(Equation found in Richard Smosna, "Compaction Law for Cretaceous Sandstones of Alaska's North Slope," *Journal of Sedimentary Petrology*, July 1989, pp. 572–583.)

6. The regression equation of Exercise 5 has three regressors. There are seven regression equations that can be written that entail the use of one or more of these regressors. Write these seven equations.

7. How many regression equations can be written that entail the use of one or more of the regressors mentioned in Example 11.6.1?

8. In each case, use your knowledge of the subject matter to suggest regressors that might be used to estimate the mean response for the response listed.

(a) Y = weight loss achieved over a 6-month weight reduction regimen

(b) Y = size of the growth ring for one growing season of a randomly selected tree

(c) Y = weight of a newborn baby

(d) Y = height of an adult human being

(e) Y = time required for a patient to fully recover from a broken hip

(f) Y = cholesterol level in a healthy adult

(g) Y = vertical leap of a college basketball player

(h) Y = speed of a bird in flight

TECHNOLOGY TOOLS

TI83

XXV   Scattergrams

Scattergrams can be drawn easily using the TI83 calculator. To illustrate the method we use the data of Example 11.1.3 and reproduce Figure 11.3.

TI83 Keystroke		**Purpose**	
1.	STAT 1	1.	Accesses the stat data editor
2.	.9 ENTER 1.5 ENTER ⋮ 2.7 ENTER	2.	Enters values of x into column L1
3.	▷ 3.1 ENTER 3.6 ENTER ⋮ 6.3 ENTER	3.	Enters values of y into column L2
4.	WINDOW	4.	Accesses window to set graphing specifications
5.	0 ENTER	5.	Sets minimum value of x to 0, a value slightly below the smallest x value
6.	3 ENTER	6.	Sets maximum value of x to 3, a value slightly above the largest value of x
7.	▽ 0 ENTER	7.	Sets minimum value of y to 0
8.	7 ENTER	8.	Sets maximum value of y to 7
9.	2nd $Y =$ ENTER cursor to on ENTER ▽ ▽ ▽ ▽ ▷ ▷ ENTER GRAPH	9.	Draws the scattergram

| 10. TRACE | 10. Allows you to move through the graph from point to point via right and left cursors |

XXVI   Simple linear regression

The data of Example 11.2.1 are used to illustrate how to use the TI83 to produce a scattergram, fit a straight line to the data via the method of least squares, graph the regression line on the scattergram, and then use the estimated regression line to make predictions.

TI83 Keystroke	**Purpose**
1. STAT 1	1. Accesses the stat data editor
2. 12.8 ENTER 13.9 ENTER ⋮ 17.9 ENTER	2. Enters x data into column L1
3. ▷ 110 ENTER 54 ENTER ⋮ 28 ENTER	3. Enters y data into column L2
4. WINDOW 10 ENTER	4. Sets 10 as the minimum value of x
5. 20 ENTER	5. Sets 20 as the maximum value of x
6. ▽ 10 ENTER	6. Sets 10 as the minimum value of y
7. 120 ENTER	7. Sets 120 as the maximum value of y
8. STAT ▷ 8 ENTER	8. Requests that a line of the form $y = a + bx$ be estimated from the data; the case of $a = 290.0704461$ and $b = -15.11057071$ is shown
9. 2nd	9. Draws the scattergram

$Y =$
ENTER
cursor to ON
ENTER
$\triangledown$
ENTER
$\triangledown$
ENTER
$\triangledown$
$\triangledown$
$\triangleright$
$\triangleright$
ENTER
GRAPH

10. $Y =$	10. Inserts estimated line of
VARS	regression onto scattergram
5	
$\triangleright$	
$\triangleright$	
1	
GRAPH	
11. VARS	11. Estimates the average length
$\triangleright$	of the breeding season when
4	$x = 14.5$
1	
1	
ENTER	
2nd	
TRACE	
1	
14.5	
ENTER	

XXVII   Correlation

To illustrate the use of the TI83 to calculate r, we use the data of Example 11.3.3.

TI83 Keystroke	Purpose
1. STAT	1. Accesses the stat data editor
1	
2. 89	2. Enters x data into column L1
ENTER	
90	
ENTER	
⋮	
20	
ENTER	

3. ▷   3. Enters *y* data into column L2
    2
    ENTER
    3
    ENTER
    ⋮
    14
    ENTER
4. STAT   4. Calculates and displays the
    ▷   value of r ($-.339079882$)
    8
    ENTER
    VARS
    5
    ▷
    ▷
    7
    ENTER

SAS Package

XIII   Scattergrams

The data of Example 11.1.3 is used to illustrate the SAS code needed to draw a scattergram.

SAS Code	Purpose
OPTIONS LS = 80 PS = 60 NODATE;	Sets printing specifications
DATA LIMPET;	Names data set
INPUT X Y;	Names variables
LINES;	Indicates that data follow immediately
.9 3.1	
1.5 3.6	
1.6 4.3	Data lines
⋮	
2.7 6.3	
;	Signals end of data
PROC PLOT;	Plots data with *Y* as the
PLOT Y*X;	horizontal axis
TITLE 'IS REGRESSION LINEAR?';	Titles output

The plot produced by this code is shown at the facing page.

```
                              Is Regression Linear?
                     Plot of Y*X.  Ledgend: A = 1 obs, B = 2obs, etc.
    Y  |
       |
       |
  6.4 +                                                      A   A
  6.3 +                                                      A   A           A
  6.2 +                                                      A
  6.1 +
  6.0 +
  5.9 +
  5.8 +                                           A   A   A
  5.7 +                              A   A         A
  5.6 +                                            A   A
  5.5 +                       A
  5.4 +                                            A
  5.3 +                          A   A         A
  5.2 +                       A         A         A
  5.1 +
  5.0 +                          A
  4.9 +
  4.8 +
  4.7 +                    A
  4.6 +
  4.5 +
  4.4 +                             A
  4.3 +                 A
  4.2 +
  4.1 +
  4.0 +
  3.9 +
  3.8 +
  3.7 +
  3.6 +              A
  3.5 +
  3.4 +
  3.3 +
  3.2 +
  3.1 +  A
       |
       |
      --+---+---+---+---+---+---+---+---+---+---+---+---+---+---+---+---+---+---+-
        0.9 1.0 1.1 1.2 1.3 1.4 1.5 1.6 1.7 1.8 1.9 2.0 2.1 2.2 2.3 2.4 2.5 2.6 2.7

                                         X
```

XIV Simple linear regression

In this example we present the SAS code used to produce the output shown in Example 11.2.3.

SAS Code	**Purpose**
OPTIONS LS = 80 PS = 60	Sets printing specifications

SAS Code	Purpose
NODATE;	
DATA DUCKS;	Names data set
INPUT PHOTOPRD LENGTH;	Names variables
LINES;	Signals that data
	follow immediately
12.8 110	
13.9 54	
⋮	
17.9 28	Data lines
14.5 .	Allows SAS to predict Y
	when $x = 14.5$
;	Signals end of data
PROC PLOT;	Produces scattergram
PLOT LENGTH*PHOTOPRD;	shown in Figure 11.10
TITLE 'IS REGRESSION LINEAR?';	Titles output
PROC GLM;	Produces regression analysis;
MODEL LENGTH = PHOTOPRD/P;	response variable is to the left
	of the equals sign in the model
	statement and regressor is to the
	right; P allows SAS to make
	predictions based on the
	estimated regression equation

XV Correlation

The SAS code used to produce Figure 11.15 is given here. The data are that of Example 11.3.3

SAS Code	Purpose
OPTIONS LS = 80 PS = 60	Sets printing specifications
NODATE;	
DATA OBESITY;	Names data set
INPUT PERCENT PAIN;	Names variables
LINES;	Indicates that data
	follow immediately
89 2	
90 3	
⋮	Data Lines
20 14	
;	Signals end of data
PROC CORR;	Calls for the correlation
	procedure
TITLE 'ARE PAIN AND	Titles output
OBESITY CORRELATED?';	

12

Categorical Data

In this chapter we are concerned with the analysis of data characterized by the fact that each observation in the data set can be classified as falling into exactly one of several mutually exclusive "cells," or categories. Interest centers on the number of observations falling into each category. The statistical problem is to determine whether the observed category frequencies tend to support or refute a stated hypothesis.

We are concerned with a problem that arises frequently in practice. Namely, we want to develop a test that will allow us to determine whether or not there is an association between two variables. The test is used to answer such questions as, Is there an association between smoking and hypertension? between obesity and depression? between intravenous drug use and AIDS? Since questions of this type arise frequently, the test discussed in this chapter is cited often in the literature. We begin by considering the case in which each of the two variables is studied at exactly two levels.

12.1

2 × 2 CONTINGENCY TABLES

Webster's dictionary defines the term *contingency* to mean "the quality or state of having a close connection or relationship." The term *contingency table* refers to the fact that the tables constructed are used to test for an association or relationship between two variables. In this section we study 2 × 2 contingency tables. These tables arise when each of the two variables is studied at two levels. The tables have two rows and two columns which result in four cells or categories. Each observation in the data set falls into exactly one cell. The data analysis is based on an examination of the number of observations falling into each category. We illustrate this idea in Example 12.1.1.

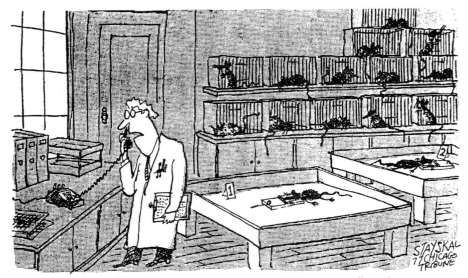

"Hello, FDA? I'd like to report research that directly
links cheese with death in rats."

EXAMPLE 12.1.1. In a study of a new hepatitis vaccine, 1083 male volunteers are used. Five hundred forty-nine are randomly chosen and vaccinated with the new drug. The remaining 534 are not vaccinated. After a time it is found that 70 of the 534 unvaccinated volunteers contracted hepatitis, whereas only 11 of the 549 vaccinated had done so. We are dealing with two characteristics, the vaccination status and the health status of each subject. Each volunteer either was vaccinated or was not vaccinated. Similarly, each either did contract hepatitis or did not. Thus these two characteristics define four categories:

Vaccinated and contracted hepatitis
Not vaccinated and contracted hepatitis
Vaccinated and did not contract hepatitis
Not vaccinated and did not contract hepatitis

Each volunteer falls into exactly one category.

Since we are concerned with the number of observations falling into each cell, we need a notational convention for these cell frequencies. We also need a notational convention to indicate the number of observations falling into each level of each of the two classification variables. We use the following:

$$n_{11} = \text{number of observations falling into cell}$$
$$\text{in row 1 and column 1}$$

$$n_{12} = \text{number of observations falling into cell}$$
$$\text{in row 1 and column 2}$$

$$n_{21} = \text{number of observations falling into cell}$$
$$\text{in row 2 and column 1}$$

n_{22} = number of observations falling into cell
   in row 2 and column 2

$n_{1.} = n_{11} + n_{12}$ = number of observations in row 1

$n_{2.} = n_{21} + n_{22}$ = number of observations in row 2

$n_{.1} = n_{11} + n_{21}$ = number of observations in column 1

$n_{.2} = n_{12} + n_{22}$ = number of observations in column 2

n = total number of observations

This notational convention is illustrated in Example 12.1.2.

EXAMPLE 12.1.2. Table 12.1 summarizes the data of Example 12.1.1 with the appropriate notation indicated. Note that $n_{.1}$ and $n_{.2}$ are column totals that appear along the margins of the 2 × 2 table. They are called *marginal* column totals. Similarly, $n_{1.}$ and $n_{2.}$ are *marginal* row totals.

The general null hypothesis to be tested by a 2 × 2 contingency table is that there is "no association" between the two classification variables. The alternative is that there is an association. The exact form of the null hypothesis depends on the design of the experiment. We study two different experimental settings that lead to 2 × 2 contingency tables:

1. All marginal totals are free to vary.
2. One set of marginal totals is fixed by the researcher; the other is free to vary.

In case 1, the test of no association is called a *test of independence;* in case 2 it is called a *test of homogeneity.* We begin by considering the first experimental setting.

Test of Independence

In a test of independence the only number under direct control of the researcher is the overall sample size. A sample of size n is drawn from the population and each object is classified according to the two variables under study. Cell frequencies as well as

TABLE 12.1

The 2 × 2 contingency table for the data of Example 12.1.1

Hepatitis	Vaccinated		
	Yes	No	
Yes	$11 = n_{11}$	$70 = n_{12}$	$81 = n_{1.}$
No	$538 = n_{21}$	$464 = n_{22}$	$1002 = n_{2.}$
	$549 = n_{.1}$	$534 = n_{.2}$	$1083 = n$

TABLE 12.2

A 2 × 2 contingency table used to test for an association between weight and early success in school. Only the overall sample size is fixed in advance

Successful	Overweight		
	Yes	No	
Yes			$n_1. = ?$ (random)
No			$n_2. = ?$ (random)
	$n._1 = ?$ (random)	$n._2 = ?$ (random)	$n = 500$ (fixed)

column and row totals are not known in advance. An example of a study of this type is given in Example 12.1.3.

> **EXAMPLE 12.1.3.** A study is run to determine whether there is any apparent association between a child's weight and early success in school, as judged by a school psychologist. A random sample is selected consisting of 500 students in grades 1 to 3. Each child is classified according to two criteria, weight and success in school. The 2 × 2 contingency table generated is shown in Table 12.2. In this design, the only fixed quantity is n, the total sample size. Both the row and column marginal totals are free to vary; neither set is fixed by the investigator prior to the experiment.

To derive a test statistic in a test of independence, let us denote the two variables under study by A and B. When both sets of marginal totals are random, the null hypothesis of no association is stated in the form

$$H_0: A \text{ and } B \text{ are independent}$$

The alternative is that there is an association between A and B or that A and B are not independent. Independence means that knowledge of the classification level of an object relative to characteristic A has no bearing on its level relative to characteristic B. For instance, in Example 12.1.3, the null hypothesis is that being overweight is independent of early success in school; knowing that a child is overweight does not help predict success in school. To express this idea mathematically, we use the table of probabilities given in Table 12.3.

We saw in Chapter 3 that for two events to be independent the probability that both occur must equal the product of the probabilities that each event occurs individually. Note that p_{11} denotes the proportion of objects with both A and B, $p._1$ denotes the proportion with characteristic A, and $p_1.$ denotes the proportion with characteristic B. The above definition of independence implies that for A and B to be independent,

$$P[A \text{ and } B] = P[A]P[B]$$

TABLE 12.3

Table of proportions associated with a 2 × 2 contingency table in which all marginal totals are random

Has characteristic B	Has characteristic A		
	Yes	No	
Yes	p_{11}	p_{12}	$p_{1 \cdot}$
No	p_{21}	p_{22}	$p_{2 \cdot}$
	$p_{\cdot 1}$	$p_{\cdot 2}$	1

or

$$p_{11} = p_{\cdot 1} p_{1 \cdot}$$

This relationship must hold for each cell. Hence mathematically the null hypothesis of independence is expressed as

$$H_0: p_{ij} = p_{i \cdot} p_{\cdot j} \qquad \begin{array}{c} i = 1, 2 \\ j = 1, 2 \end{array}$$

The alternative is that $p_{ij} \neq p_{i \cdot} p_{\cdot j}$ for some i and j. This formulation of H_0 is helpful in understanding the logic behind the test statistic. In practice we shall simply write

$$H_0: A \text{ and } B \text{ are independent}$$

when stating the null hypothesis when marginal totals are random.

The test statistic for testing H_0 is based on a simple idea. We compare the observed number of observations in each cell to the number of observations that are expected to fall into the cell if H_0 is true. If these numbers match fairly well, then there is no reason to reject H_0; if there is a wide discrepancy between the observed and expected values, then we take this as evidence that H_0 is not true. Let E_{ij} denote the expected number of observations in cell ij under the assumption that A and B are independent. Since p_{ij} is the theoretical proportion (or percentage) of observations in cell ij, the expected number is found by multiplying this proportion by the total number of observations. That is,

$$E_{ij} = n p_{ij}$$

The proportions p_{11}, p_{12}, p_{21}, and p_{22} are unknown and must be estimated from the data under the assumption that the null hypothesis is true.

How can this be done? Quite simply! Note, for instance, that if H_0 is true and characteristics A and B are independent, then

$$p_{11} = p_{1 \cdot} p_{\cdot 1}$$

Since $p_{1 \cdot}$ is the probability of an observation's falling into row 1, it is logical to estimate p_1. by

$$\hat{p}_{1.} = \frac{\text{number of elements in row 1}}{\text{sample size}} = \frac{n_{1.}}{n}$$

Similarly, since $p_{.1}$ is the probability of an observation's falling into column 1, we estimate $p_{.1}$ by

$$\hat{p}_{.1} = \frac{\text{number of elements in column 1}}{\text{sample size}} = \frac{n_{.1}}{n}$$

Thus

$$\hat{p}_{11} = \hat{p}_{1.}\hat{p}_{.1} = \frac{n_{1.}}{n}\frac{n_{.1}}{n}$$

This, in turn, implies that

$$\hat{E}_{11} = \hat{p}_{11}n = \frac{n_{1.}}{n}\frac{n_{.1}}{n}n$$

Notice that

$$\hat{E}_{11} = \frac{n_{1.}n_{.1}}{n} = \frac{\left(\begin{array}{c}\text{marginal}\\\text{row total}\end{array}\right)\left(\begin{array}{c}\text{marginal}\\\text{column total}\end{array}\right)}{\text{sample size}}$$

A similar argument holds for other cell expectations.

Thus we conclude that for each i and j,

$$\boxed{\hat{E}_{ij} = \frac{n_{i.}n_{.j}}{n} = \frac{\left(\begin{array}{c}\text{marginal}\\\text{row total}\end{array}\right)\left(\begin{array}{c}\text{marginal}\\\text{column total}\end{array}\right)}{\text{sample size}}}$$

The calculation of expected cell frequencies is illustrated in the next example.

EXAMPLE 12.1.4. When the experiment of Example 12.1.3 is run, the data in Table 12.4 are found.

TABLE 12.4

Data used to test for an association between obesity and early success in school

Successful	Overweight		
	Yes	No	
Yes	$n_{11} = 162$	$n_{12} = 263$	$n_{1.} = 425$
No	$n_{21} = 38$	$n_{22} = 37$	$n_{2.} = 75$
	$n_{.1} = 200$	$n_{.2} = 300$	$n = 500$

▓ **TABLE 12.5**

Data used to test for an association between obesity and early success in school. Expected cell frequencies are shown in parentheses

Successful	Overweight		
	Yes	No	
Yes	162 (170)	263 (255)	425
No	38 (30)	37 (45)	75
	200	300	500

The expected cell frequencies under H_0 are

$$\hat{E}_{11} = \frac{n_1.n_1}{n} = \frac{425(200)}{500} = 170$$

$$\hat{E}_{12} = \frac{n_1.n_2}{n} = \frac{425(300)}{500} = 255$$

$$\hat{E}_{21} = \frac{n_2.n_1}{n} = \frac{75(200)}{500} = 30$$

$$\hat{E}_{22} = \frac{n_2.n_2}{n} = \frac{75(300)}{500} = 45$$

We summarize the situation in Table 12.5. Note that there are some differences between what is expected if H_0 is true (listed in parentheses) and what is actually observed. The question is, Are the differences too large to have occurred strictly by chance?

To answer the question just posed we need a test statistic whose probability distribution is known under the assumption that H_0 is true. The test statistic required is

$$X_1^2 = \sum_{\text{all cells}} \frac{(n_{ij} - \hat{E}_{ij})^2}{\hat{E}_{ij}}$$

Notice that the numerator of this statistic compares the observed cell frequencies to the expected cell frequencies by finding the difference between the two for each cell. The differences are squared so that negative differences will not counterbalance positive ones upon addition. If there is a good match, the differences will be small, the numerator will be small, and the observed value of the test statistic will be small. In this case H_0 is not rejected. If there are large discrepancies between the observed and expected frequencies, then the differences will be large, the numerator will be large, and the observed value of the test statistic will be large. In this case H_0 is rejected. Since the P value of the test is found via the chi-squared distribution with one degree of freedom and the test is based on assessing how well the observed frequencies match or fit the ones expected under H_0, this test is called a *chi-squared goodness of fit test.* The test is illustrated by completing the analysis of the data of Example 12.1.3.

EXAMPLE 12.1.5. Consider the observed and estimated expected frequencies given in Table 12.5. The observed value of the test statistic is

$$\sum_{\text{all cells}} \frac{(n_{ij} - \hat{E}_{ij})^2}{\hat{E}_{ij}} = \frac{(162 - 170)^2}{170} + \frac{(263 - 255)^2}{255} + \frac{(38 - 30)^2}{30} + \frac{(37 - 45)^2}{45}$$

$$= 4.18$$

The P value of the test is

$$P = P[X_1^2 \geq 4.18]$$

From the chi-squared table, we see that

$$P[X_1^2 \geq 3.84] = .05 \quad \text{and} \quad P[X_1^2 \geq 5.02] = .025$$

Since 4.18 lies between 3.84 and 5.02, the P value lies between .025 and .05. The P value is small. We can reject H_0 and conclude that obesity and early success in school are not independent.

Chi-squared goodness of fit tests require a large sample to be valid. This naturally brings up the question, How large is large? There are various opinions as to the answer to this question. However, it is usually felt that n should be large enough that no expected frequency is less than 1 and no more than 20% are less than 5. In the case of a 2×2 table, this guideline is met only if no cell frequencies are less than 5. If this guideline is not met, then a small sample test called Fisher's exact test [2] can be used to test for independence.

Test of Homogeneity

We now consider the second experimental setting, one in which one set of marginal totals is fixed by the researcher while the other set is random. This setting occurs when there are two populations under study. We are interested in a particular trait, and we want to answer the question, Is the proportion of objects with the trait the same in both populations? If there is no association between the trait and the population to which an individual belongs, then the proportion with the trait should be the same in each case; if there is an association, then the proportions should differ. Example 12.1.6 is an example of this sort of problem.

EXAMPLE 12.1.6. A large number of people living in a particular section of a community have been exposed over the last 10 years to radioactivity from an atomic waste storage dump. A study is run to find out whether there is any apparent association between this exposure and the development of a specific blood disorder. To conduct the experiment, random samples are chosen of 300 persons from the community who have been exposed to the hazard and 320 persons not so exposed. We are dealing with samples drawn from two populations, those exposed to radioactivity from the dump and those not exposed from this source. Each subject is screened to determine whether he or she has the blood disorder. This experiment generates a 2×2 table of the form shown in Table 12.6. Note that the marginal row totals are fixed at 300 and 320, since these sample sizes are predetermined by

▨ **TABLE 12.6**

A 2 × 2 contingency table with row totals, which represent random samples drawn from two populations, fixed by the researcher

Exposed to radioactivity	Has disorder		
	Yes	No	
Yes			$n_{1.} = 300$ (fixed prior to experiment)
No			$n_{2.} = 320$ (fixed prior to experiment)
	$n_{.1} = ?$ (random)	$n_{.2} = ?$ (random)	$n = 620$

the investigator. The marginal column totals are free to vary; that is, they are random variables whose numerical values are known only at the conclusion of the experiment.

If there is no association between exposure and development of the disorder, then the proportion of persons with the disorder should be the same in each population. If there is an association, then these proportions should differ.

The proportions shown in Table 12.7 are used to express the null hypothesis and to understand the test statistic used to test H_0. The null hypothesis of no association between population (variable B) and trait (variable A) is

$$\boxed{H_0: p_{11} = p_{21}}$$

Notice that if H_0 is true, it is also the case that $p_{12} = p_{22}$. In example 12.1.6 this null hypothesis assumes the form

H_0: proportion of persons with disease among those exposed to radioactivity = proportion of persons with disease among those not exposed

▨ **TABLE 12.7**

Table of proportions associated with a 2 × 2 contingency table in which row totals are fixed

Population	Has trait		
	Yes	No	
1	p_{11}	$p_{12} = 1 - p_{11}$	$n_{1.}$ (fixed)
2	p_{21}	$p_{22} = 1 - p_{21}$	$n_{2.}$ (fixed)
	$n_{.1}$ (random)	$n_{.2}$ (random)	n

In practice, we can state the null hypothesis as

> H₀: proportion with the trait is the same in each population

H_0: proportion with the trait is the same in each population

The test being conducted is a test of homogeneity. The word *homogeneous* means "alike in nature." We are testing to see if the two sampled populations are alike in the sense that the proportion of objects with the trait is the same in each population.

To understand the logic behind the calculation of expectations notice that the expected number of observations in the sample from population 1 with the trait is found by multiplying the sample size of population 1 by the theoretical probability of having the trait. That is, $E_{11} = n_1 . p_{11}$. Similarly $E_{21} = n_2 . p_{21}$. Thus to estimate E_{11} and E_{21} from the contingency table, we need only find a logical way to estimate p_{11} and p_{21}. This is not hard to do. If H_0 is true, $p_{11} = p_{21}$. We denote this common population proportion by p. Furthermore, if the proportion of objects with the trait is the same for both populations, then the overall proportion of objects in the two populations combined will also be p. A logical estimator for the overall proportion of objects with the trait is

$$\hat{p} = \frac{\text{number of objects in column 1}}{\text{overall sample size}}$$

$$= \frac{n_{.1}}{n}$$

Since we are assuming that $p_{11} = p_{21} = p$, we can also use $\hat{p}$ as an estimator for p_{11} and p_{21}. Substitution yields these estimated cell frequencies under H_0:

$$\hat{E}_{11} = n_1 . \hat{p}_{11} = n_1 . \frac{n_{.1}}{n}$$

$$= \frac{\left(\begin{array}{c}\text{marginal}\\ \text{row total}\end{array}\right)\left(\begin{array}{c}\text{marginal}\\ \text{column total}\end{array}\right)}{\text{sample size}}$$

$$\hat{E}_{21} = n_2 . \hat{p}_{21} = n_2 . \frac{n_{.1}}{n}$$

$$= \frac{\left(\begin{array}{c}\text{marginal}\\ \text{row total}\end{array}\right)\left(\begin{array}{c}\text{marginal}\\ \text{column total}\end{array}\right)}{\text{sample size}}$$

The same pattern holds for finding $\hat{E}_{12}$ and $\hat{E}_{22}$. Notice that these expectations are exactly the same as those used in the test of independence. From this point on, the test of homogeneity is identical to that of independence.

EXAMPLE 12.1.7. Table 12.8 gives the observed and expected frequencies (in parentheses) for the experiment described in Example 12.1.6. The observed value of the test

TABLE 12.8

Data used to test for an association between the populations of those exposed to radioactivity and those not similarly exposed

Exposed to radioactivity	Has disorder		
	Yes	**No**	
Yes	52 (48.39)	248 (251.61)	300 (fixed)
No	48 (51.61)	272 (268.39)	320 (fixed)
	100	520	620

statistic is

$$\sum_{\text{all cells}} \frac{(n_{ij} - \hat{E}_{ij})^2}{\hat{E}_{ij}} = .62$$

Since $P = P[X_1^2 \geq .62] > .10$, we cannot reject H_0. There is no evidence of an association between the blood disease and exposure to this source of radioactivity.

EXERCISES 12.1

1. Use the data of Example 12.1.1 to determine whether contracting hepatitis is independent of receiving the hepatitis vaccine.
2. A study is run of a new flu vaccine. A random sample of 900 individuals is chosen, and each is classified according to whether the flu had been contracted during the last year and whether each person had been inoculated. The information shown in Table 12.9 is obtained.

TABLE 12.9

Inoculated	Contracted flu	
	Yes	**No**
Yes	150	200
No	300	250

(a) Are any of the marginal totals fixed?
(b) Set up the appropriate null hypothesis to test for association between variables.
(c) Find the expected frequency for each cell.
(d) Can H_0 be rejected? What is the P value of the test?

3. In a study to determine the association, if any, between maternal rubella and congenital cataracts, a sample is selected of 20 children with the defect and 25 children of similar background and age who do not have the defect. The mother of each child is interviewed to determine whether she had rubella while carrying the child. Data are shown in Table 12.10.

▨ **TABLE 12.10**

| Has congenital | Mother had rubella | |
cataract	Yes	No
Yes	14	6
No	10	15

(a) Are any of the marginal totals fixed?
(b) Set up the appropriate null hypothesis to test for association between variables.
(c) Find the expected frequency for each cell.
(d) Test the null hypothesis.

4. It has long been thought that peptic ulcers are caused by both genetic and environmental factors. A recent study considered the association between the pepsinogen 1 level in the blood and the presence of peptic ulcers; 14 patients who had duodenal ulcers were compared with 49 individuals who did not. The pepsinogen 1 level in the blood of each was determined and classified as high or low. Data obtained are shown in Table 12.11.

▨ **TABLE 12.11**

| Ulcer | Pepsinogen level | | |
	High	Low	
Present	12		14
Absent		31	49

(a) Complete the table.
(b) Set up the appropriate null hypothesis to test for association between variables.
(c) Find the expected number of observations for each cell.
(d) Test the null hypothesis.

5. A small pilot study is run to determine the association between the occurrence of leukemia and a history of allergy. A sample of 19 leukemia patients and 17 controls is selected, and their history of allergy is determined. The results are shown in Table 12.12.

TABLE 12.12

	History of allergy	No history of allergy	
Control	5	12	
Patient	17	2	

(a) Are any of the marginal totals fixed?

(b) Set up the appropriate null hypothesis to test for association between classification variables.

(c) Find the expected frequency for each cell.

(d) Is there evidence of an association between history of allergy and leukemia? Explain your answer based on the P value of the test.

6. A study of the association between hospital type and death in hospital after high-risk surgery during the month of July is conducted. One hundred thirty-nine high-risk surgery patients at major teaching hospitals were selected for study; 528 such patients seen at other types of hospitals were chosen. Of those seen at major teaching hospitals, 32 died; 62 died in the sample drawn from other hospitals.

(a) Construct a 2×2 contingency table to display these data.

(b) Test the null hypothesis of no association. Is the test a test of independence or of homogeneity?

(c) Estimate the probability of in-hospital death among such patients at each of the two types of hospitals during July.

(d) The title of the article from which the data are drawn is "It's Not OK to Get Sick in July." Do you agree? Explain. (Mark Blumberg, "It's Not OK to Get Sick in July," *Journal of the American Medical Association,* August 1, 1990, p. 573.)

7. A sample of 245 patients under the age of 19 seen at an allergy clinic is selected. Each patient is classified by age and by whether or not he or she is allergic to eggs. Of 133 patients over the age of 3, 30 were allergic to eggs; 32 of the 112 patients who were 3 or under exhibited this allergy.

(a) Construct a 2×2 contingency table to display these data.

(b) Test the null hypothesis of no association between age and allergy to eggs. Is this a test of independence or of homogeneity?

(Based on information found in Allan Bock and F. M. Atkins, "Patterns of Food Hypersensitivity During Sixteen Years of Double-Blind, Placebo-Controlled Food Challenges," *The Journal of Pediatrics,* October 1990, pp. 561–567.)

8. The tat protein is a protein released from HIV-1–infected cells. A study is conducted to test for an association between the presence of tat antibodies and Kaposi's sarcoma in AIDS patients. The serum of each of 297 HIV-1 seropositive patients is assayed at the time of or within 1 month of the diagnosis of AIDS. Each sample is classified as being one from a patient with Kaposi's sarcoma or not; it is also classified as containing tat antibodies or not. Of the 78 sarcoma patient samples 10 showed antibodies for tat; 21 of the 219 patients without sarcoma had tat antibodies.

(a) Construct a 2×2 contingency table to display these data.

(b) Test for an association between the presence of the antibody and the presence of Kaposi's sarcoma. Is this a test of independence or homogeneity?

(Based on figures reported in Peter Reiss and Joseph Lange, "Kaposi's Sarcoma and AIDS," *Nature*, August 30, 1990, p. 801.)

9. In a 2×2 contingency table the test of homogeneity is a comparison of two proportions. Recall that a Z test to compare two proportions was developed in Chapter 8. It can be proved that the chi-squared statistic developed here is the square of the pooled Z statistic of Chapter 8. To verify this, analyze the data of Example 12.1.7 via the Z method of Chapter 8. Now square the z value that you obtain and verify that z^2 is the same as the χ^2 value found in Example 12.1.7.

■ 12.2
$r \times c$ CONTINGENCY TABLES

In this section we extend the methods of Section 12.1 to situations in which the number of rows or columns in the contingency table is greater than 2. The purpose of the experiment is as before, namely, to test for association between classification variables by comparing observed cell frequencies with those expected if there is no association. Two classification variables, A and B, are used. We assume that there are c levels relative to variable A and r levels relative to B. Thus the contingency table generated has r rows, c columns, and rc cells, or categories. The notation used is shown in Table 12.13. Note that

$$n_{ij} = \text{observed frequency in } (ij)\text{th cell}$$

$$n_{i.} = \text{marginal row total for } i\text{th row, } i = 1, 2, \ldots, r$$

$$n_{.j} = \text{marginal column total } j\text{th column, } j = 1, 2, \ldots, c$$

We illustrate the use of this notation in Example 12.2.1.

■ **TABLE 12.13**
Table of frequencies associated with an $r \times c$ contingency table. The table has r rows and c columns.

Variable	Variable A					
B	1	2	3	$\cdots$	c	
1	n_{11}	n_{12}	n_{13}	$\cdots$	n_{1c}	$n_{1.}$
2	n_{21}	n_{22}	n_{23}	$\cdots$	n_{2c}	$n_{2.}$
$\vdots$	$\cdots$	$\cdots$	$\cdots$	$\cdots$	$\cdots$	$\cdots$
r	n_{r1}	n_{r2}	n_{r3}	$\cdots$	n_{rc}	$n_{r.}$
	$n_{.1}$	$n_{.2}$	$n_{.3}$	$\cdots$	$n_{.c}$	n

TABLE 12.14

The 2 × 4 contingency table displaying the data of Example 12.2.1

	Blood type				
	0	**A**	**B**	**AB**	
Patients	$n_{11} = 698$	$n_{12} = 472$	$n_{13} = 102$	$n_{14} = 29$	$n_{1.} = 1301$ (fixed)
Controls	$n_{21} = 2892$	$n_{22} = 2625$	$n_{23} = 570$	$n_{24} = 226$	$n_{2.} = 6313$ (fixed)
	$n_{.1} = 3590$	$n_{.2} = 3097$	$n_{.3} = 672$	$n_{.4} = 255$	$n = 7614$

EXAMPLE 12.2.1. A study is run to determine whether there is an association between blood type and duodenal ulcers. A sample of 1301 patients and 6313 controls is selected, and the blood type of each is determined. Among the patients, 698 have type O blood, 472 have type A, 102 have type B, and the rest have type AB. Among controls the figures are 2892, 2625, 570, and 226, respectively. These data are conveniently displayed as a 2 × 4 (two rows and four columns) contingency table, as shown in Table 12.14.

Once again there are two commonly encountered experimental settings. These are

1. All marginal totals are free to vary.
2. One set of marginal totals is fixed by the researcher; the other is free to vary.

As in the case of 2 × 2 tables, setting 1 calls for a test of independence, whereas setting 2 leads to a test of homogeneity. Table 12.15 shows the theoretical proportions associated with an $r \times c$ contingency table. This table allows us to express the null hypothesis of no association symbolically. If all marginal totals are random, then the null hypothesis of no association between classification variables is expressed as

$$\boxed{\text{H}_0\text{: } A \text{ and } B \text{ are independent}}$$

TABLE 12.15

Proportions associated with an $r \times c$ contingency table. In this notation the first subscript gives the row number and the second gives the column number.

Variable B	Variable A				
	1	**2**	**3**	$\cdots$	c
1	p_{11}	p_{12}	p_{13}	$\cdots$	p_{1c}
2	p_{21}	p_{22}	p_{23}	$\cdots$	p_{2c}
3	p_{31}	p_{32}	p_{33}	$\cdots$	p_{3c}
$\vdots$	$\cdots$	$\cdots$	$\cdots$	$\cdots$	$\cdots$
r	p_{r1}	p_{r2}	p_{r3}	$\cdots$	p_{rc}

Statistically, this is expressed in the form

$$H_0: \quad p_{ij} = p_{i \cdot} p_{\cdot j} \qquad \begin{aligned} i &= 1, 2, \ldots, r \\ j &= 1, 2, \ldots, c \end{aligned}$$

As in the case of the 2×2 table, this expresses the idea that if A and B are independent, then the probability of falling into cell $i - j$, p_{ij}, is the probability of falling into row i, $p_{i \cdot}$, multiplied by the probability of falling into column j, $p_{\cdot j}$. If $r = c = 2$, this reduces to the form presented in Section 12.1.

If row totals are fixed, the null hypothesis of no association is expressed as

> H_0: the percentage split among levels of variable A is the same in each population

Statistically this hypothesis is expressed in terms of the proportions shown in Table 12.15. It takes the form

$$H_0: \begin{cases} p_{11} = p_{21} = \cdots = p_{r1} & \text{(proportions in column 1 are identical)} \\ p_{12} = p_{22} = \cdots = p_{r2} & \text{(proportions in column 2 are identical)} \\ \quad \vdots & \\ p_{1c} = p_{2c} = \cdots = p_{rc} & \text{(proportions in column } c \text{ are identical)} \end{cases}$$

Again if $r = c = 2$, this reduces to the form given in Section 12.1.

The test statistic for testing the null hypothesis of no association, regardless of the design, is

$$X^2_{(r-1)(c-1)} = \sum_{\text{all cells}} \frac{(n_{ij} - \hat{E}_{ij})^2}{\hat{E}_{ij}}$$

where $\hat{E}_{ij}$ is the estimated expected frequency in the (ij)th cell. As before,

$$\hat{E}_{ij} = \frac{(\text{marginal row total})(\text{marginal column total})}{\text{sample size}}$$

Notice that the number of degrees of freedom associated with this chi-squared statistic is $(r-1)(c-1)$ where r is the number of rows in the table and c is the number of columns. In a 2×2 table the number of degrees of freedom is $(2-1)(2-1) = 1$ as claimed in Section 12.1.

The test is to reject H_0 for values of the test statistic too large to have occurred by chance. The test is applicable for sample sizes large enough that no expected frequency is less than 1 and no more than 20% are less than 5. We illustrate this procedure in Example 12.2.2.

EXAMPLE 12.2.2. When the data of Example 12.2.1 are analyzed, the observed and expected frequencies shown in Table 12.16 result. The observed value of the test statistic is

$$\frac{(698 - 613.42)^2}{613.42} + \frac{(2892 - 2976.58)^2}{2976.58} + \cdots + \frac{(226 - 221.43)^2}{211.43} = 29.12$$

The number of degrees of freedom involved is

$$(r - 1)(c - 1) = (2 - 1)(4 - 1) = 3$$

From the chi-squared table it can be seen that

$$P = [X_3^2 \geq 29.12] < .005$$

The null hypothesis of no association between blood type and the presence of duodenal ulcers can be rejected. In this study the researcher fixed the number of patients at 1301 and the number of controls at 6313. Hence the test of no association is a test of homogeneity. We are testing to see if there is a difference in the blood type distribution between patients and controls. This hypothesis can be expressed symbolically as

$$H_0: \begin{cases} p_{11} = p_{21} & \text{(percentage of type O among patients} \\ & = \text{percentage of type O among controls)} \\ p_{12} = p_{22} & \text{(percentage of type A among patients} \\ & = \text{percentage of type A among controls)} \\ p_{13} = p_{23} & \text{(percentage of type B among patients} \\ & = \text{percentage of type B among controls)} \\ p_{14} = p_{24} & \text{(percentage of type AB among patients} \\ & = \text{percentage of type AB among controls)} \end{cases}$$

TABLE 12.16

Data used to test for an association between blood type and the presence of duodenal ulcer. Row totals are under control of the researcher.

	Blood type				
	O	A	B	AB	
Patients	698 (613.42)	472 (529.18)	102 (114.82)	29 (43.57)	1301 (fixed)
Controls	2892 (2976.58)	2625 (2567.82)	570 (557.18)	226 (211.43)	6313 (fixed)
	3590	3097	672	255	7614

Since H_0 is rejected, we conclude that there are some differences in these percentages. To get an intuitive idea of what differences exist between patients and controls, note that the estimated probability of a patient's falling into blood group O is given by

$$\frac{\text{Number of patients in group O}}{\text{Number of patients}} = \frac{698}{1301} = .54$$

Similarly, the estimated probability of a control's falling into group O is

$$\frac{\text{Number of controls in group O}}{\text{Number of controls}} = \frac{2892}{6313} = .46$$

It appears that the proportion of persons with type O blood is not the same among patients as among controls. That is,

$$p_{11} \neq p_{21}$$

EXERCISES 12.2

1. Consider the data of Example 12.2.2. Estimate the proportion of patients falling into blood group A and the proportion of controls falling into this group. Do the same for blood groups B and AB. Comment on the results.
2. To convince the public to use safety equipment in automobiles, a random sample of 1000 accidents is chosen from the records. Each accident is classified according to type of safety restraint used by the occupants and severity of injuries received. Data are given in Table 12.17.

TABLE 12.17

Data used to test for an association between the type of safety restraint used and the severity of injuries received in a sample of automobile accidents

	Type of restraint			
Extent of injury	Seat belt only	Seat belt and harness	None	
None	75	60	65	
Minor	160	115	175	
Major	100	65	135	
Death	15	10	25	
				1000

(a) Are any marginal totals fixed by the researcher?
(b) Is the test of no association a test for independence or a test of homogeneity?
(c) State and test H_0. What is the P value of the test?
(d) Estimate the probability of death occurring when no restraint is used, the seat belt and harness are used, and only the seat belt is used. Comment on the practical implications of your findings.

3. A study is run to investigate the association between flower color and fragrance in wild azaleas. Two hundred randomly selected, blooming plants are observed in the wild. Each is classified as to color, and the presence or absence of fragrance is noted. The data are shown in Table 12.18.

TABLE 12.18

Data used to test for an association between color and fragrance in azaleas

Fragrance	Flower color		
	White	Pink	Orange
Yes	12	60	58
No	50	10	10

(a) Are any marginal totals fixed by the researcher?

(b) Is the test of no association a test for independence or a test of homogeneity?

(c) State the appropriate null hypothesis.

(d) Can H_0 be rejected? What is the P value of the test? What practical conclusion can be drawn from these data?

4. In a study of goiter, random samples of specified size are selected from 10 states. The persons chosen are examined for goiter, and the number of cases found is recorded. Data obtained are shown in Table 12.19.

TABLE 12.19

Data used to test for an association between location and presence of goiter

	Goiter test		
	Positive	Negative	
California	36		500
Kentucky	17		350
Louisiana	12		300
Massachusetts	1		300
Michigan	4		350
New York	14		500
South Carolina	7		200
Texas	27		500
Washington	2		200
West Virginia	4		200
			3400

(a) Is the test of no association between location and goiter a test for independence or a test of homogeneity?

(b) State the null hypothesis of interest.

(c) Test H_0.

(d) Estimate the probability of a randomly selected individual from California having goiter. Estimate the probability of a randomly selected individual from Massachusetts having goiter.

5. A study is conducted to consider the association between the sulfur dioxide level in the air and the mean number of chloroplasts per leaf cell of trees in the area. A sample is chosen of 10 areas known to have a high sulfur dioxide concentration, 10 known to have a normal level of sulfur dioxide, and 10 known to have a low sulfur dioxide concentration. Twenty trees are randomly selected from each level, and the mean number of chloroplasts per leaf cell is determined for each tree. On this basis, each tree is classified as having a low, normal, or high chloroplast count. Data obtained are given in Table 12.20.

TABLE 12.20

Data used to test for an association between chloroplast level and sulfur dioxide exposure

SO$_2$ level	Chloroplast level			
	High	Normal	Low	
High	3	4	13	20
Normal	5	10	5	20
Low	7	11	2	20

(a) State the appropriate null hypothesis.

(b) Test the null hypothesis.

(c) Estimate the probability that a randomly selected tree will have a low chloroplast level, given that it is from an area with a high sulfur dioxide concentration. Estimate the probability that a randomly selected tree from an area of normal sulfur dioxide concentration will have a low chloroplast level. Estimate this probability for a randomly selected tree growing in an area of low sulfur dioxide concentration. Comment on the practical implications of these estimates.

6. A study was conducted to ascertain factors that influence a physician's decision to transfuse a patient. A sample of 49 attending physicians was selected. Each physician was asked a question concerning the frequency with which an unnecessary transfusion was given because another physician suggested it. The same question was asked of a sample of 71 residents. The data shown in Table 12.21 resulted.

(a) Test the null hypothesis of no association.

(b) Is this a test of independence or of homogeneity?

(c) Estimate the probability that an attending physician will never order an unnecessary transfusion; that a resident will never do so.

■ **TABLE 12.21**

Data used to test for no association between physician type and tendency to authorize an unnecessary transfusion

Type physician	Frequency of unnecessary transfusion					
	Very frequent (1 per week)	Frequent (1 per 2 weeks)	Occasionally (1 per month)	Rarely (1 per 2 months)	Never	
Attending	1	1	3	31	13	49
Resident	2	13	28	23	5	71

(Data found in Susanne Salem-Schatz, Jerry Avorn, and Stephen Soumerai, "Influence of Clinical Knowledge, Organizational Context, and Practice Style on Transfusion Decision Making," *Journal of the American Medical Association,* July 25, 1990, pp. 476–483.)

7. A study is conducted to investigate the effect of the presence of a large industrial plant on the invertebrate population in a river that passes through the plant. Samples were taken upstream and downstream of the plants. These data are obtained:

	Species						
	A	**B**	**C**	**D**	**E**	**F**	**G**
Upstream	37	12	6	18	7	6	0
Downstream	9	3	7	0	0	6	3

Test for an association between stream site and type of species found. Comment on the applicability of the chi-squared test to these data. (Based on a study by Lawrence Scott Cook, Department of Biology, Radford University, 1994.)

TECHNOLOGY TOOLS

TI83

XXVIII   Testing for an association between two variables

The TI83 can test for an association between two variables. To do so, the $r \times c$ contingency table is entered into a matrix; the calculator will construct the table of expected cell frequencies and will then run the X^2 test of association. To illustrate, we use the data of Example 12.2.1.

T183 Keystroke		Purpose
1.	MATRIX ▷ ▷ ENTER	1.	Accesses the screen needed to enter the contingency table data

2.	2 ENTER 4 ENTER	2.	Indicates that the table is a 2×4 table
3.	698 ENTER 472 ENTER 102 ENTER 29 ENTER	3.	Enters the data from row 1 of Table 12.16
4.	2892 ENTER 2625 ENTER 570 ENTER 226 ENTER	4.	Enters the data from row 2 of Table 12.16
5.	STAT ◁ ALPHA C ▽ ▽ ENTER	5.	Conducts and displays the results of the X^2 test of association
6.	MATRIX ▽ ENTER ENTER	6.	Displays the table of expected cell frequencies

SAS Package

XVI Testing for an association between two variables

SAS can test for an association between two variables using either raw data or information on observed frequencies from a previously generated contingency table. We illustrate the latter using the data of Example 12.2.1.

SAS Code	Purpose
OPTIONS LS = 80 PS = 60 NO DATE;	Sets printing specifications
DATA ULCER;	Names data set
INPUT ROW COLUMN OBSERVED;	Names variables

LINES;	Indicates that data follow immediately

```
1    1    698
1    2    472
1    3    102
1    4    29
2    1    2892
2    2    2625
2    3    570
2    4    226
;
```

	Data lines

;	Signals end of data

PROC FREQ;
TABLES ROW* COLUMN/   Conducts the X^2 test; displays the
    NOCOL NOPERCENT   row percentages for each row;
    EXPECTED CHISQ;   displays the expected cell
    WEIGHT = OBSERVED;   frequencies

The output of this program is given below.

```
                        The SAS System
                   TABLE OF ROW BY COLUMN

        ROW         COLUMN

        Frequency|
        Expected |
        Row Pct  |      1|       2|      3|       4|  Total
        ---------+-------+--------+-------+--------+
            1    |  698  |  472   |  102  |   29   |  1301
                 | 613.42| 529.18 | 114.82| 43.572 |
                 | 53.65 | 36.28  |  7.84 |  2.23  |
        ---------+-------+--------+-------+--------+
            2    | 2892  | 2625   |  570  |  226   |  6313
                 | 2976.6| 2567.8 | 557.18| 211.43 |
                 | 45.81 | 41.58  |  9.03 |  3.58  |
        ---------+-------+--------+-------+--------+
        Total      3590    3097      672     255      7614
```

```
              STATISTICS FOR TABLE OF ROW BY COLUMN

    Statistic                        DF     Value      Prob
    ----------------------------------------------------------
    Chi-Square                        3     29.122 ①   0.000 ②
    Likelihood Ratio Chi-Square       3     29.559      0.000
    Mantel-Haenszel Chi-Square        1     25.002      0.000
    Phi Coefficient                          0.062
    Contingency Coefficient                  0.062
    Cramer's V                               0.062

    Sample Size = 7614
```

Note that the expected cell frequencies differ slightly from those given in the text due to roundoff differences. The observed value of the χ^2 test statistic is given at ①. Its P value, shown at ②, is for all practical purposes 0.

13

Some Additional Procedures and Distribution-Free Alternatives

In this chapter we present some additional procedures which you might find occasion to use. Included in the chapter are alternatives to some of the tests presented in earlier chapters.

Recall that most of the statistical procedures introduced thus far have an underlying assumption of normality. That is, we assume that the samples are drawn from distributions that are normal, or at least approximately so. For many years after the discovery of the normal curve, practitioners felt that virtually every random variable was at least approximately normally distributed. Then as more and more data became available, it became evident that this was not true. However, the statistical tools developed by Fisher, Pearson, and "Student," which presuppose normality, were so appealing to researchers in a wide variety of fields that they were eager to adopt them. To laypeople unable to follow the mathematical derivations of these techniques, the normality "assumption" was thought to be unimportant, a law of nature, or at best satisfied due to some sophisticated mathematical magic. The situation is best described by the words of Lippman in a remark to Poincare (1912) [2]:

> Everyone believes in it (normal law of errors) however, said Monsieur Lippman to me one day, for the experimenters fancy that it is a theorem in mathematics and the mathematicians that it is an experimental fact.

Thus far, we have done only a rough check of the normality assumption using the stem-and-leaf diagram or the histogram. If these diagrams assume a definite bell shape, then the normality assumption is probably reasonable. However, if there is a doubt in your mind concerning its validity, then you should test to see if there is statistical evidence that the data are drawn from a nonnormal distribution. Several methods are available for doing so. Here we consider a graphical method that is especially useful when sample sizes are small.

▨ 13.1
TESTING FOR NORMALITY: THE LILLIEFORS TEST

The method for detecting nonnormality that we consider here, called "the Lilliefors test for normality," was developed by H. W. Lilliefors in the late 1960s. Although it can be used with large samples, it is most helpful when samples are relatively small. The test basically compares the observed relative cumulative frequency distribution of the sample to that of the standard normal distribution. This is done by graphing the observed distribution on a Lilliefors graph. Figure 13.1 gives the Lilliefors graphs needed to test

> H_0: data are from a normal distribution
>
> H_1: data are not from a normal distribution

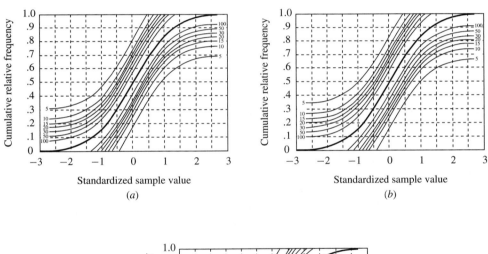

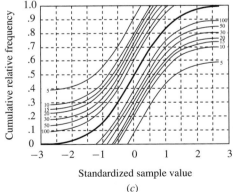

(c)

▨ FIGURE 13.1

(a) 90% Lilliefors bounds for normal samples ($\alpha = .1$); (b) 95% Lilliefors bounds for normal samples ($\alpha = .05$); (c) 99% Lilliefors bounds for normal samples ($\alpha = .01$).(Copyright 1982 by the American Statistical Association. Reprinted with permission.)

▨ **TABLE 13.1**

Column 1 gives the new growth in centimeters of 20 yews, column 2 shows the standardized values, and column 3 is the relative cumulative frequency distribution

Observation	Standardized observation	Relative cumulative frequency
1.1	−1.62	.05
1.3	−1.48	.10
1.4	−1.41	.15
1.5	−1.34	.20
1.9	−1.06	.25
2.5	−.63	.30
2.6	−.56	.35
3.2	−.13	.40
3.5	.08	.45
3.7	.22	.50
3.7	.22	.50
3.9	.36	.60
4.1	.50	.65
4.2	.57	.70
4.2	.57	.70
4.4	.72	.80
4.6	.86	.85
4.8	1.00	.90
4.9	1.07	.95
6.2	1.99	1.00

for various significance levels. The heavy curve in the center of the graph is the cumulative distribution for the standard normal curve. Curves to either side represent the Lilliefors bounds for the sample sizes indicated. If the observed relative cumulative frequency falls outside the bounds given for the specified sample size, then H_0 is rejected and it is concluded that the data are not from a normal distribution. The use of this technique is illustrated in Example 13.1.1.

EXAMPLE 13.1.1. Let X denote the new growth (cm) over a 2-week period of 20 yews grown under identical conditions. The data obtained are shown in Table 13.1. For these data, $\bar{x} = 3.39$ and $s = 1.41$. Since we are to compare the observed relative cumulative frequency distribution to that of the *standard* normal distribution, we first "standardize" these observations by subtracting $\bar{x}$ and dividing by s. The standardized observations are then ordered from smallest to largest and the relative cumulative frequency for each observation is found. The results of these calculations are shown in Table 13.1. To use these data to test

H_0: data are from a normal distribution

H_1: data are not from a normal distribution

at the $\alpha = .05$ level, we graph the observed relative cumulative frequency on the Lilliefors graph of Figure 13.1b. The result is given in Figure 13.2. Since the graph of the observed relative cumulative frequency does not fall outside the bands labeled 20, the size of our

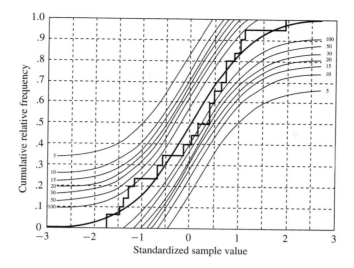

▨ **FIGURE 13.2**

Test for normality of new growth of yews at the $\alpha = .05$ level.

sample, we are unable to reject H_0. We have no evidence that the data are drawn from a nonnormal distribution.

There are several analytic tests available for testing the assumption of normality. Most commercial computer packages include at least one such test.

The natural question to ask is, What do you do if it appears that the normality assumption is not valid? Studies have shown that the use of the normal theory statistics in this case leads to tests that are approximate. In many cases, the approximations are excellent; in others, they are so bad as to be unacceptable. In any case, using normal theory statistics in situations in which the normal theory assumptions are violated leads to results that are suspect. There are two possible courses of action. First, we can try to transform the data so that the normal theory assumptions are met. Some methods for doing so are presented in [5], [7], [16]. Second, we can develop a body of statistical methods that presupposes little about the distribution of the sampled population. Such methods are called *distribution-free*.

In the next six sections we present some of these methods. In particular, we include techniques paralleling those presented earlier. In this way, you have a viable alternative to many normal theory procedures.

Distribution-free statistical procedures have several appealing characteristics. In particular, the derivation of the test statistic in most cases depends only on counting methods, such as those presented in Chapters 2 and 3. Thus the logic behind each test usually is easy to follow. Distribution-free tests often require little computation and can be performed quickly. When sample sizes are small ($n \leq 10$), violations of the normal theory assumptions are hard to detect, but they can have disastrous effects. However, for these small samples, distribution-free tests compare very well with normal theory tests even when all the normal theory assumptions are met. If they are not met, the distribution-free procedure is usually superior. Thus, unless all classical assumptions have been met, for small samples the wiser choice is a distribution-free test. One further advantage of distribution-free techniques should be pointed out. Many distribution-free methods involve analyzing the ranks of the observations, rather than the observations themselves. Thus these techniques are particularly useful with data that consist of ranks rather than measurements or counts.

■ EXERCISES 13.1

1. A new process for producing small precision parts is being studied. The process consists of mixing fine metal powder with a plastic binder, injecting the mixture into a mold, and then removing the binder with a solvent. These data are obtained on parts which should have a 1-inch diameter and whose standard deviation should not exceed .0025 inch.

1.0030	.9997	.9990	1.0054	.9991
1.0041	.9988	1.0026	1.0032	.9943
1.0021	1.0028	1.0002	.9984	.9999

For these data $\bar{x} = 1.00084$ and $s = .00283$.

(a) Use the Lilliefors graph of Figure 13.3 to show that these data do not allow us to reject the normality assumption at the $\alpha = .05$ level.

(b) Test

$$H_0: \mu = 1$$

$$H_1: \mu \neq 1$$

at the $\alpha = .05$ level.

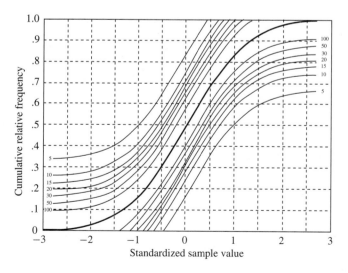

■ FIGURE 13.3

95% Lilliefors bounds for normal samples.

(c) Test

$$H_0: \sigma = .0025$$

$$H_1: \sigma > .0025$$

at the $\alpha = .05$ level.

2. Indoor natatoriums or swimming pools are noted for their poor acoustical properties. The goal is to design a pool in such a way that the average time that it takes a low-frequency sound to die is at most 1.3 seconds with a standard deviation of at most .6 second. Computer simulations of a preliminary design are conducted to see whether these standards are exceeded. These data are obtained on the time required for a low-frequency sound to die. (R. Hughes and M. Johnson, "Acoustic Design in Natatoriums," *The Sound Engineering Magazine,* April 1983, pp. 34–36.)

1.8	3.7	5.0	5.3	6.1	.5
2.8	5.6	5.9	2.7	3.8	5.9
4.6	.3	2.5	1.3	4.4	4.6
5.3	4.3	3.9	2.1	2.3	7.1
6.6	7.9	3.6	2.7	3.3	3.3

For these data $\bar{x} = 3.97$ and $s = 1.89$.

(a) Use the Lilliefors graph of Figure 13.4 to show that these data do not allow us to reject the normality assumption at the $\alpha = .01$ level.

(b) Test

$$H_0: \mu = 1.3$$

$$H_1: \mu > 1.3$$

at the $\alpha = .01$ level.

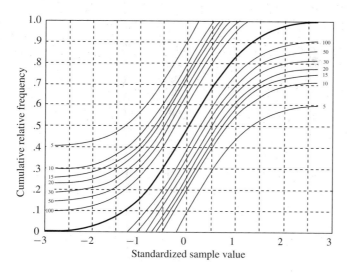

FIGURE 13.4

99% Lilliefors bounds for normal samples.

(c) Test

$$H_0: \ \sigma = .6$$

$$H_1: \ \sigma > .6$$

at the $\alpha = .01$ level. Does it appear that the design specifications are being met?

3. Incompatibility is always a problem when working with computers. A new digital sampling frequency converter is being tested. It takes the sampling frequency from 30 to 52 kHz, word lengths of 14 to 18 bits, and arbitrary formats and converts it to the output sampling frequency. The conversion error is thought to have a standard deviation of less than 150 picoseconds. These data are obtained on the sampling error made in 20 tests of the device. (K. Pohlmann, "The Compatibility Solution," *The Sound Engineering Magazine,* April 1983, pp. 12–14.)

133.2	−11.5	−126.1	17.9	139.4
−81.7	314.8	147.1	−70.4	104.3
56.9	44.4	1.9	−4.7	96.1
−57.3	−43.8	−95.5	−1.2	9.9

For these data $\bar{x} = 28.69$ and $s = 104.93$.

(a) Use the Lilliefors graph of Figure 13.5 to show that these data do not allow us to reject the normality assumption at the $\alpha = .1$ level.

(b) Test

$$H_0: \ \mu = 0$$

$$H_1: \ \mu \neq 0$$

at the $\alpha = .1$ level.

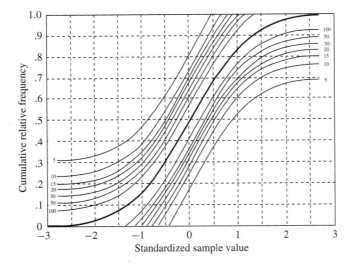

FIGURE 13.5

90% Lilliefors bounds for normal samples.

(c) Test

$$H_0: \sigma = 150$$

$$H_1: \sigma < 150$$

at the $\alpha = .1$ level. Does the converter appear to be as accurate as claimed?

13.2

TESTS OF LOCATION: ONE SAMPLE

In normal theory procedures, the usual measure of the center of location of the distribution of a random variable is its mean. In most distribution-free tests, the center of location is measured by the median of the random variable. The *median* of a random variable X is defined to be the number M such that

$$P[X < M] \leq \tfrac{1}{2} \quad \text{and} \quad P[X \leq M] \geq \tfrac{1}{2}$$

Note that if X is continuous, then

$$P[X < M] = P[X \leq M] = \tfrac{1}{2}$$

That is, for a continuous random variable, the median is the point M such that 50% of the time X lies below M and 50% of the time above M.

We discuss two tests for the median of a continuous random variable. The first, called the *sign test,* is based on the binomial distribution. It assumes only that the random variable under study is continuous.

Sign Test for Median

Assume the X is a continuous random variable with median M. Let $X_1, X_2, \ldots, X_n$ denote a random sample of size n from the distribution of X. If we let M_0 denote the hypothesized value of the median, tests of hypotheses can take any of the usual three forms:

$H_0: M \leq M_0$	$H_0: M \geq M_0$	$H_0: M = M_0$
$H_1: M > M_0$	$H_1: M < M_0$	$H_1: M \neq M_0$
Right-tailed test	Left-tailed test	Two-tailed test

Note that if H_0 is true ($M = M_0$), then each of the continuous random variables X_1, $X_2, \ldots, X_n$ has probability $\tfrac{1}{2}$ of lying below M_0, probability $\tfrac{1}{2}$ of lying above M_0, and probability 0 of assuming the value M_0. This implies that each of the differences $X_1 - M_0, X_2 - M_0, \ldots, X_n - M_0$ has probability $\tfrac{1}{2}$ of being negative, probability $\tfrac{1}{2}$ of being positive, and probability 0 of assuming the value 0. Let N and N' denote the number of negative and positive signs obtained, respectively. If H_0 is true, each of these random variables has a binomial distribution with parameters n and $\tfrac{1}{2}$ and

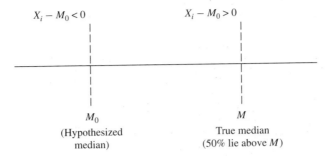

$$X_i - M_0 < 0 \qquad\qquad X_i - M_0 > 0$$

M_0
(Hypothesized
median)

M
True median
(50% lie above M)

▨   **FIGURE 13.6**

Relationship between M and M_0 (right-tailed test: H_1: $M > M_0$).

expected value $n \cdot \frac{1}{2}$. That is, if H_0 is true, we expect half the signs to be positive and half to be negative.

Now consider the diagram of the relationship between M and M_0 for a right-tailed test, shown in Figure 13.6. Clearly, if H_1 is true, then we should observe more positive signs and fewer negative signs than expected. In this case, we use N, the number of negative signs observed, as our test statistic. We reject $H_0(M \leq M_0)$ in favor of $H_1(M > M_0)$ if the observed value of N is too small to have occurred by chance under the assumption that H_0 is true. For a left-tailed test, the situation is reversed. In this case, the test statistic is N', the number of positive signs observed. Once again, H_0 is rejected in favor of H_1 if the observed value of the test statistic is too small to have occurred by chance. The test statistic for a two-tailed test is the smaller of N and N', with rejection of H_0 occurring for small values of this statistic.

We use the sign test for the median in Example 13.2.1.

EXAMPLE 13.2.1. A study of growth based on data gathered from 1971 to 1974 indicates that the median height of men in the 18- to 24-year-old group was 69.7 inches. It is felt that as a result of improvements in health care and nutrition, the median height among young men in this age group is currently larger than 69.7. We wish to test

$$H_0: \ M \leq 69.7 \qquad H_1: \ M > 69.7$$

Since the test is right-tailed, the test statistic is N, the number of negative differences obtained when the hypothesized median (69.7) is subtracted from each observation. These data result:

70.2 (+)	65.8 (−)	78.0 (+)	74.4 (+)
71.4 (+)	67.3 (−)	72.6 (+)	67.5 (−)
69.8 (+)	71.4 (+)	69.9 (+)	70.5 (+)
67.2 (−)	72.1 (+)	73.5 (+)	70.9 (+)
70.1 (+)	73.2 (+)	65.2 (−)	76.0 (+)

Five negative signs are observed. The P value of the test is given by

$$P = P\left[N \leq 5 \,|\, p = \tfrac{1}{2}\right] = .0207$$

(Use the binomial table, Table I of Appendix B, with $n = 20$ and $p = \frac{1}{2}$.) Since this value is small, we reject H_0 and conclude that the median height has increased over the former figure of 69.7 inches.

Several points should be made about the sign test for median. The rationale behind the test is quite logical. It requires very little computation and therefore is quick and easy to apply. It presupposes very little about the distribution of the population from which the sampling is done, requiring only that it be continuous. If, in fact, the distribution is also normal, then the mean and the median are the same. In this case, the sign test is testing the same hypothesis as that tested previously by using the one-sample T test (Chapter 6).

Now we discuss the Wilcoxon signed-rank test for the median. This test, developed by F. Wilcoxon in 1945, tests the null hypothesis that a continuous distribution is symmetric about a hypothesized median M_0.

Wilcoxon Signed-Rank Test

Let $X_1, X_2, X_3, \ldots, X_n$ be a random sample of size n from a continuous distribution. Consider the set of differences $X_1 - M_0, X_2 - M_0, \ldots, X_n - M_0$, where M_0 is the hypothesized median of the distribution from which the sample is drawn. If the null hypothesis is true, then these differences are drawn from a distribution that is symmetric about zero. To conduct the test, we first consider the set of n absolute differences $|X_i - M_0|$ and order them from smallest to largest. We then rank them from 1 to n, with the smallest absolute difference receiving the rank of 1. Each rank R_i is assigned the algebraic sign of the difference score that generated the rank. If the null hypothesis is true and the differences are symmetric about zero, then each rank is just as likely to be assigned a positive sign as a negative sign.

Consider the statistics

$$W_+ = \sum_{\substack{\text{all} \\ \text{positive} \\ \text{ranks}}} R_i \quad \text{and} \quad |W_-| = \left| \sum_{\substack{\text{all} \\ \text{negative} \\ \text{ranks}}} R_i \right|$$

If H_0 is true, each of these should be about the same size. If the true population median is actually larger than the hypothesized median, then we will obtain too many positive differences and too many positive ranks, W_+ will be larger than expected, and $|W_-|$ will be smaller than expected. If the true median is smaller than the hypothesized value, then the situation is reversed. Thus we can use as our test statistic W, the smaller of W_+ and $|W_-|$. The distribution of this statistic has been tabulated for various values of α and n. One such table is Table XI of Appendix B. The table allows us to conduct one-sided tests at α levels of .05, .025, .01, and .005. Two-sided tests can be conducted at the .10, .05, .02, or .01 level. The null hypothesis is always rejected for values of W that are too small to have occurred by chance. Thus we reject H_0 at the α level selected if the observed value of W falls on or below the critical point listed in Table XI.

We show how to use the Wilcoxon signed-rank test in Example 13.2.2.

EXAMPLE 13.2.2. The current median survival time of patients with acute myelogenous leukemia who achieve complete remission from conventional treatment is 21 months. A new procedure is being studied. It is hoped that the median survival time will be improved.

These survival times are noted for 10 patients who received the new treatment:

24.1   25.8   20.5   20.9   27.3
21.5   20.1   28.9   19.2   26.3

To test for symmetry about 21, first we form the set of 10 differences by subtracting 21 from each observed survival time:

X_i	24.1	21.5	25.8	20.1	20.5	28.9	20.9	19.2	27.3	26.3
$X_i - 21$	3.1	.5	4.8	−.9	−.5	7.9	−.1	−1.8	6.3	5.3

Now we order the absolute values of these differences from smallest to largest, rank them from 1 to 10, and assign to each rank the algebraic sign of the difference that generated the rank. Note that because of the continuity assumption, no ties should occur. However, in practice, ties do occur. For example, the absolute difference of .5 is obtained twice. When this happens, all tied scores are assigned the average group rank. This idea is illustrated here:

$|X_i - 21|$	.1	.5	.5	.9	1.8	3.1	4.8	5.3	6.3	7.9
Rank R_i	1	2.5	2.5	4	5	6	7	8	9	10
Signed rank	−1	−2.5	2.5	−4	−5	6	7	8	9	10

The observed values of W_+ and $|W_-|$ are

$$W_+ = \sum_{\substack{\text{all} \\ \text{positive} \\ \text{ranks}}} R_i = 2.5 + 6 + 7 + 8 + 9 + 10 = 42.5$$

and

$$|W_-| = \left| \sum_{\substack{\text{all} \\ \text{negative} \\ \text{ranks}}} R_i \right| = |-1 + (-2.5) + (-4) + (-5)| = 12.5$$

Our test statistic is W, the smaller of the two. Since we are conducting a one-sided test, we enter Table XI with $n = 10$. We see that $P[W \le 11] = .05$. Since the observed value of the test statistic is 12.5, $P = P[W \le 12.5]$ exceeds .05. Thus we do not have sufficient evidence based on this sample that the new procedure has increased the median survival time.

Several things are notable concerning the Wilcoxon signed-rank test. It, like the sign test, assumes that the distribution from which the sampling is done is continuous. If the distribution is also symmetric, then the test is a test for both the median and the mean of the distribution, since in this case these two parameters are identical. Occasionally from past experience we know that a population is symmetric, but more often we do not. When the latter is the case, the sign test is preferred as a test for location. If there is evidence that the distribution is normal, then the Wilcoxon signed-rank test is testing the same hypothesis as that tested by the one-sample T test in normal theory statistics.

▦ EXERCISES 13.2

1. Recent studies of private practices that handle no Medicaid patients indicate that the median length of a patient visit is 22 minutes. It is thought that the median visit length in practices with a large Medicaid load is smaller than this figure. These data are obtained on 20 randomly selected patient visits for one such practice:

Length of patient visit, minutes

21.6	13.4	20.4	16.4
23.5	26.8	24.8	19.3
23.4	9.4	16.8	21.9
24.9	15.6	20.1	16.2
18.7	18.1	19.1	18.9

Based on the sign test, is there sufficient evidence to conclude that for this practice the median length of a patient visit is less than 22 minutes? Explain your answer on the basis of the expected number of positive signs under H_0 and the P value of the test.

2. A study is conducted of nutrition among patients with respiratory failure who require ventilatory support. One variable considered is the creatinine height index, which is a measure of the patient's protein level. An index value less than 6 is considered indicative of a serious protein deficiency. If the median index value among this type of patient is shown to lie below 6, then a new dietary program will be put into effect to correct the problem. These values are obtained from a random sample of 15 patients:

5.7	4.2	4.7	4.6
5.3	5.4	6.8	4.9
4.9	5.8	4.1	5.5
6.4	5.1	4.7	

Based on the sign test, is there evidence that the median index reading is below 6? Explain your answer based on the expected number of positive signs under H_0 and the P value of the test.

3. Well-developed pasture soils should contain indigenous mycorrhizal fungi, which greatly stimulate the growth of clover and rye grass. The median number of spores per gram of soil in good pastureland is 9. In eroded areas, the mycorrhizal infectivity is thought to be highly reduced. Do these data, obtained from 20 eroded areas, tend to support this contention? Explain on the basis of the P value of the sign test.

.01	.12	.28	.54	2.7
.02	.15	.30	.92	2.7
.06	.16	.32	1.52	8.24
.08	.24	.48	1.64	9.3

4. A study is made of alarm calling in ground squirrels. One variable considered is the maximal audible range of a warning call. The median maximal audible range is thought to be more than 87 meters. Do these data support this contention? Explain your answer based on the expected number of negative signs under H_0 and the P value of the test.

Maximal audible range, meters

90.8	79.4	94.4	96.7
91.9	94.3	95.1	84.5
85.2	89.7	82.0	88.2
88.6	95.6	89.4	87.3
98.5	87.1	82.1	86.7

5. Note that $W_+ + |W_-| = 1 + 2 + 3 + \cdots + n$. From high school algebra it is known that this sum is given by $n(n + 1)/2$. This fact can be used as a check on the accuracy of your ranking and computation of the values of W_+ and $|W_-|$ when the Wilcoxon test is utilized. Verify this result for the data of Example 13.2.2, in which $n = 10$.

6. If the null hypothesis is that the distribution from which we are sampling is symmetric about the hypothesized median M_0, then the expected value of W_+ is given by

$$E[W_+] = \frac{n(n + 1)}{4}$$

Find the expected value of W_+ for Example 13.2.2 $(n = 10)$.

7. Whirligig beetles aggregate in the daytime into dense, single-species and multi-species groups, called *rafts,* of hundreds of individuals. The median distance between rafts is thought to be less than .8 km. Use the Wilcoxon signed-rank test to test this hypothesized value, based on these data. Assume symmetry.

.71	.65	.51	.32	.21
.13	.21	1.10	.71	1.63
.16	1.00	1.11	.40	

8. Preliminary studies on black widows indicate that the median time spent on the ground when the spider touches down to attach a fiber during web building is less than 16 seconds. To verify this finding, spiders engaged in active web building are observed. These data result (assume symmetry):

Time on ground, seconds				
18.9	9.3	10.8	20.0	11.9
11.7	19.8	11.1	15.5	9.8
15.9	13.1	23.7	10.4	11.9
25.2	13.5	8.9	12.5	19.9
21.3	8.5	17.5	18.9	13.4

If the true median is 16 seconds, what is the expected value of W_+? (See Exercise 6.) What is the observed value of W_+? Do the data tend to support the contention that the median time spent on the ground is less than 16 seconds? Explain your answer based on the P value of the Wilcoxon test.

9. The median age of onset of diabetes is thought to be 45 years. Assume that the distribution of the variable age of onset is symmetric. We wish to test

$$H_0: M = 45 \qquad H_1: M \neq 45$$

at the $\alpha = .05$ level, using the Wilcoxon signed-rank test based on a sample of size 30. These data result from a study of 30 randomly selected diabetics:

35.5	30.5	40.1	59.8	47.3
44.5	48.9	36.8	52.4	36.6
39.8	42.1	39.3	26.2	55.6
33.3	40.3	65.4	60.9	45.1
51.4	46.8	42.6	45.6	52.2
51.3	38.0	42.8	27.1	43.5

Can H_0 be rejected? To what type of error are we now subject?

10. In 1970 it was reported that the median cost of an initial office visit to a physician was \$14.23. Although the cost for such a visit is certainly higher in current dollars, with inflation taken into account there may not have been a real rise in price relative to the economy as a whole. These data represent the current cost of an initial office visit, adjusted to 1970 dollars. Assuming symmetry, do the data indicate that the median cost is now higher than the 1970 median? Explain your answer on the basis of the P value of the Wilcoxon test.

Current cost, 1970 dollars				
16.14	15.71	16.23	17.44	16.88
15.79	15.10	15.82	15.89	16.99
14.08	16.30	14.88	14.02	14.22
17.22	14.39	16.04	14.56	15.32
16.18	15.26	16.73	16.03	13.94

11. *Normal approximation to W_+.* For large values of n, W_+ and $|W_-|$ are each approximately normally distributed with mean $n(n + 1)/4$ and variance

$$\frac{n(n + 1)(2n + 1)}{24}$$

This fact can be used to approximate P values for values of n not listed in Table XI of Appendix B. We need only standardize W_+ or $|W_-|$ and approximate P, using the standard normal table.
(a) For a sample of size 70, find $P[W_+ \leq 1000]$.
(b) For a sample of size 80, find $P[|W_-| \leq 1500]$.

13.3

TESTS OF LOCATION: PAIRED DATA

We consider now two tests for location that use paired observations. The first, the sign test for median difference, is an extension of the sign test just presented.

Sign Test for Median Difference

Let X and Y be continuous random variables. Let (X_1, Y_1), (X_2, Y_2), . . . , (X_n, Y_n) be a random sample of size n from the distribution of (X, Y). Consider the set of n continuous differences $X_1 - Y_1, X_2 - Y_2, \ldots, X_n - Y_n$. The null hypothesis is that the median difference is zero. That is, we are testing

$$H_0: \ M_{X-Y} = 0$$

If H_0 is true, each of the differences $X_i - Y_i$ has probability $\frac{1}{2}$ of being positive, probability $\frac{1}{2}$ of being negative, and probability 0 of assuming the value 0. Let N and N' denote the number of negative and positive signs obtained, respectively. If H_0 is true, then each of these random variables is binomially distributed with parameters n and $\frac{1}{2}$. Thus if H_0 is true, we expect half the observed differences to be positive and half to be negative. If the median difference is actually positive, then we should obtain too many positive signs and too few negative signs. If the actual median difference is negative, then the situation is reversed. Thus we may use as our test statistic the smaller of N and N'. We reject H_0 in favor of the appropriate alternative if the observed value of the test statistic is too small to have occurred by chance under the assumption that H_0 is true.

The use of this test is illustrated in Example 13.3.1.

EXAMPLE 13.3.1. In a study of the use of Captopril with diuretic-treated hypertensive patients, a 6.25-mg dose is used. Each patient's systolic blood pressure is noted before she or he receives the drug (X) and again 70 minutes after the drug is administered (Y). To determine whether the drug is effective in reducing blood pressure in these patients, we test

$$H_0: M_{X-Y} \leq 0 \qquad H_1: M_{X-Y} > 0$$

If H_1 is true, we expect very few negative differences. The test statistic is therefore N, the number of negative signs obtained. These data result:

X (before)	Y (after)	Sign of $X - Y$
175	140	+
179	143	+
165	135	+
170	133	+
160	162	−
180	150	+
177	182	−
178	139	+
173	140	+
176	141	+

The observed value of N is 2. The P value for the test is given by

$$P = P\left[N \leq 2 \,|\, p = \tfrac{1}{2}\right] = .0547$$

(Use Table I of Appendix B with $n = 10$ and $p = \tfrac{1}{2}$.) Since this probability is fairly small, we reject H_0 and conclude that Captopril is effective in reducing systolic blood pressure in diuretic-treated hypertensive patients.

Note that the sign test for median difference assumes only that both X and Y are continuous. If each is also normal, then $X - Y$ is normal. In this case, the median difference is equal to the mean difference, which, in turn, is equal to the difference in the population means. That is,

$$M_{X-Y} = \mu_{X-Y} = \mu_X - \mu_Y$$

Thus if X and Y are normal, then testing the null hypothesis $H_0: M_{X-Y} = 0$ is equivalent to testing the null hypothesis of equal population means. This is the same hypothesis as that tested by the paired T test in normal theory statistics.

The next test that we consider for use with paired data is the Wilcoxon signed-rank test for matched observations. This test is conducted in exactly the same manner as the signed-rank test for the median illustrated in Section 13.2.

Wilcoxon Signed-Rank Test: Paired Data

Let X and Y be continuous random variables. Let (X_1, Y_1), (X_2, Y_2), . . . , (X_n, Y_n) be a random sample of size n from the distribution of (X, Y). Consider the set of continuous differences $X_1 - Y_1$, $X_2 - Y_2$, . . . , $X_n - Y_n$. The null hypothesis is that these differences are drawn from a population that is symmetric about zero. The test is performed by ordering the absolute values of these differences from smallest to largest and ranking them from 1 to n (assigning tied scores the average group rank). Then each rank is assigned the sign of the difference that generated the rank, and the value is computed of

$$W_+ = \sum_{\substack{\text{all} \\ \text{positive} \\ \text{ranks}}} R_i \quad \text{and} \quad |W_-| = \left| \sum_{\substack{\text{all} \\ \text{negative} \\ \text{ranks}}} R_i \right|$$

The test statistic is W, the smaller of W_+ and $|W_-|$. Hypothesis H_0 is rejected in favor of the appropriate alternative for values of W that are too small to have occurred by chance, based on Table XI of Appendix B.

Example 13.3.2 illustrates the use of Wilcoxon's procedure with paired data.

EXAMPLE 13.3.2. The accidental incorporation of polybrominated biphenyl (PBB) compounds into high-protein dairy pellets led to the contamination of dairy herds in some midwestern states. A study is conducted to determine whether cooking reduces the PBB level in meat from contaminated animals. The experiment is conducted by measuring the PBB level in raw roast sirloin tip (X), cooking the roast, and then measuring the PBB level in the cooked meat (Y). If cooking reduces the PBB level, then we expect very few negative differences when subtraction is done in the order $X - Y$. Our test statistic is therefore $|W_-|$. We conclude that cooking effectively reduces the PBB level if the observed value of this statistic is too *small* to have occurred by chance. These data (in ppm) result (assume symmetry):

X (raw)	Y (cooked)	$X - Y$ (difference)
.19	.15	.04
.20	.10	.10
.01	.02	−.01
.16	.18	−.02
.15	.10	.05
.27	.04	.23
.08	.01	.07
.23	.15	.08
.07	.04	.03
.10	.10	0

We now order the absolute values of the differences smallest to largest and rank them from 1 to 10. In assigning signs to the ranks, there is one problem. What algebraic sign is associated with the difference 0, which is neither positive nor negative? Theoretically, because of the continuity of both X and Y, a zero difference should not occur. However, in practice, as a result of difficulties in measurement, a zero difference does arise occasionally. There are various suggestions as to how to handle the problem. We take a conservative approach. Since the null hypothesis is that the population of differences is symmetric about 0, a zero difference tends to support H_0. Thus logically we should assign to the 0 difference the sign least conducive to the rejection of H_0. In this case, we assign a negative sign, since this will increase the size of $|W_-|$ and make it harder to reject H_0. The results of the signed ranking are as follows:

$\lvert X_i - Y_i \rvert$	0	.01	.02	.03	.04	.05	.07	.08	.10	.23
Rank R_i	1	2	3	4	5	6	7	8	9	10
Signed rank	-1	-2	-3	4	5	6	7	8	9	10

The observed value of $|W_-|$ is

$$|W_-| = \left| \sum_{\substack{\text{all} \\ \text{negative} \\ \text{ranks}}} R_i \right| = |-1 + (-2) + (-3)| = 6$$

From Table XI of Appendix B, the P value of the test ($P[|W_-| \le 6]$) lies between .01 (critical point, 5) and .025 (critical point, 8). Since this value is small, we reject H_0 and conclude that cooking does tend to reduce the PBB level in contaminated meat.

Again, it is important to note the relationship between this test and others previously presented. If the population of differences is known to be symmetric, then you are testing the null hypothesis that the median difference is zero. This is the same hypothesis as that tested by the sign test. If you do not know that the population is symmetric and wish to test a hypothesis about the median, then the sign test is preferable to the Wilcoxon test. If there is evidence that the population of differences is normally distributed, then you are testing H_0: $\mu_X = \mu_Y$, the same hypothesis as that tested by the paired T test in normal theory statistics.

▪ EXERCISES 13.3

1. A 20-week physical conditioning program for women is conducted. One variable studied is the maximal oxygen uptake of the subject. This is measured while she is using a treadmill both before (X) and after (Y) the training period. It is hoped that the training will increase the value of this variable for most subjects.
   (a) The research hypothesis is H_1: $M_{X-Y} < 0$. What is the test statistic for detecting this situation?
   (b) These data result:

Maximal oxygen uptake, liters/minute		
Subject	Before (X)	After (Y)
1	1.98	2.26
2	1.57	1.83
3	1.89	2.31
4	1.42	1.79
5	1.73	1.65
6	1.95	2.26
7	1.69	2.10
8	1.92	2.15
9	1.96	1.54
10	1.94	1.87

Use the sign test to test

$$H_0: M_{X-Y} \geq 0 \qquad H_1: M_{X-Y} < 0$$

Can we conclude that the training tends to increase the maximal oxygen uptake? Explain on the basis of the P value of the test.

2. A study of hand reaction time among Indian hockey players is conducted. The purpose is to compare visual with auditory reaction time. Visual reaction time is measured by noting the time needed to respond to a light signal; auditory reaction time is the time needed to respond to the click of an electric switch. These times are noted for 15 subjects:

Reaction time, milliseconds			Reaction time, milliseconds		
Subject	Visual	Auditory	Subject	Visual	Auditory
1	165.75	162.32	9	195.76	207.34
2	207.57	211.84	10	182.82	198.44
3	240.21	202.65	11	164.37	177.82
4	180.50	166.14	12	232.54	142.28
5	205.89	239.14	13	197.55	187.09
6	192.96	201.51	14	196.58	164.42
7	233.16	184.88	15	216.09	161.39
8	215.86	170.48			

Is there evidence, based on the sign test, that the visual reaction time tends to be slower than the auditory reaction time? Explain on the basis of the P value of the test.

3. A study is run to determine the effects of removing a renal blockage in patients whose renal function is impaired because of advanced metastatic malignancy of nonurologic cause. The arterial blood pressure of each patient is measured before (X) and after (Y) surgery. These data are found:

Arterial blood pressure, mmHg		
Patient	Before (X)	After (Y)
1	150	90
2	132	102
3	130	80
4	116	82
5	107	90
6	100	94
7	101	84
8	96	93
9	90	89
10	78	85

Based on the sign test, can you conclude that the surgery tends to lower arterial blood pressure? Explain on the basis of the P value of the test.

4. A study of the effects of physical training on postcoronary patients included measurements on maximum oxygen uptake, which was determined for each patient before training began (X). After 6 months of bicycle exercise 3 times per week,

each person's oxygen uptake was determined again (Y). These data result (assume symmetry):

Maximum oxygen uptake, ml/(kg)(min)

Patient	Before (X)	After (Y)
1	46.98	40.96
2	23.98	26.21
3	48.25	57.25
4	41.24	38.83
5	42.90	52.17
6	42.45	54.02
7	23.00	24.58
8	30.39	51.51
9	33.80	31.62
10	47.41	54.83

Based on the Wilcoxon signed-rank test, can you conclude at the $\alpha = .05$ level that exercise tends to increase the maximum oxygen uptake in these patients?

5. A study of the courtship behavior of domesticated zebra finches is run to determine the effect of beak color in the female on the number of song patterns sung by the male during courtship. It is thought that the red beak, a sign of maturity, will elicit more patterns than the black beak, which is found in juvenile birds. Each of 10 mature males is presented separately with a live red-beaked and live black-beaked female bird. The male's behavior is observed in each case. The measured variable is the mean number of song patterns over three 10-minute observation periods with each female:

Mean number of song patterns

Bird number	Red beak (X)	Black beak (Y)
1	11.24	2.19
2	12.21	1.69
3	11.7	9.84
4	14.09	13.98
5	15.7	12.66
6	16.9	7.9
7	17.08	14.78
8	11.17	15.66
9	15.18	11.06
10	14.72	20.08

(a) Assume symmetry and use the Wilcoxon signed-rank test to test

$$H_0: \ M_{X-Y} \leq 0 \qquad H_1: \ M_{X-Y} > 0$$

at the $\alpha = .05$ level.

(b) If we do not assume symmetry, then the hypothesis

$$H_0: \ M_{X-Y} \leq 0 \qquad H_1: \ M_{X-Y} > 0$$

is best tested by the sign test. If the sign test is used, can H_0 be rejected at the $\alpha = .05$ level?

6. In a study of mild hypertension among patients aged 21 to 29 years, two groups are used. An experimental group receives chlorthalidone plus reserpine; a second group

receives a placebo. The total cholesterol level for each patient is determined at the outset of the study and again at the end of 1 year of treatment. The following data result:

Total cholesterol level (mg/dl)

Chlorthalidone and reserpine		Placebo	
Before treatment (X)	After treatment (Y)	Before treatment (X)	After treatment (Y)
192.3	172.1	180.5	182.3
178.6	164.1	170.1	170.9
185.7	171.4	174.1	170.2
175.3	152.9	180.4	178.3
183.9	163.9	175.4	175.8
182.6	170.7	188.4	186.1
180.9	165.3	182.8	185.1
184.2	164.2	181.0	177.6

Assuming symmetry, use Wilcoxon's signed-rank test to test

$$H_0: M_{X-Y} \le 0 \qquad H_1: M_{X-Y} > 0$$

at the $\alpha = .05$ level for each group.

13.4

TESTS OF LOCATION: UNMATCHED DATA

In this section we discuss a distribution-free test that can be used to compare the locations of two continuous populations based on independent samples of sizes m and n drawn from those populations. The test is called the *Wilcoxon rank-sum test.*

Wilcoxon Rank-Sum Test

Let X and Y be continuous random variables. Let $X_1, X_2, \ldots, X_m$ and $Y_1, Y_2, \ldots, Y_n$ be independent random samples of sizes m and n from the distribution of X and Y, respectively. Assume that $m \le n$. That is, assume that the X's represent the smaller sample. The null hypothesis is that the X and Y populations are identical. We wish to test this hypothesis with a test that is especially likely to reject H_0 if the populations differ in location. The $m + n$ observations are pooled to form a single sample. These observations are linearly ordered and ranked from 1 to $m + n$, retaining their group identity. Tied scores receive the average group rank, as in previous Wilcoxon tests.

The test statistic is W_m, the sum of the ranks associated with the observations that originally constituted the *smaller* sample (X values). The logic behind this choice of test statistic is as follows. If the X population is located below the Y population, then the smaller ranks will tend to be associated with the X values. This will produce a small value for W_m. If the reverse is true (the X population is located above the Y population), then the larger ranks will be found among the X values, producing a large value of W_m.

Thus we should reject H_0 if the observed value of W_m is too small or too large to have occurred by chance. Table XII of Appendix B gives the probabilities for selected values of m and n. We show how to use this table in Example 13.4.1.

EXAMPLE 13.4.1. In a study of smoking and its effects on sleep patterns, one variable is the time that it takes to fall asleep. A random sample of size 12 is drawn from the population of smokers; an independent sample of size 15 is drawn from the population of non-smokers. These data result:

Time to sleep, minutes			
Smokers (S)		Nonsmokers (N)	
69.3	52.7	28.6	30.6
56.0	34.4	25.1	31.8
22.1	60.2	26.4	41.6
47.6	43.8	34.9	21.1
53.2		29.8	36.0
48.1		28.4	37.9
23.2		38.5	13.9
13.8		30.2	

Do these data indicate that smokers tend to take longer to fall asleep than nonsmokers?

To answer this question, we pool the two samples, order the observations from smallest to largest, retaining their group identity, and rank them from 1 to 27:

Observation	13.8	13.9	21.1	22.1	23.2	25.1	26.4	28.4	28.6
Group	S	N	N	S	S	N	N	N	N
Rank	1	2	3	4	5	6	7	8	9

Observation	29.8	30.2	30.6	31.8	34.4	34.9	36.0	37.9	38.5
Group	N	N	N	N	S	N	N	N	N
Rank	10	11	12	13	14	15	16	17	18

Observation	41.6	43.8	47.6	48.1	52.7	53.2	56.0	60.2	69.3
Group	N	S	S	S	S	S	S	S	S
Rank	19	20	21	22	23	24	25	26	27

Since the sample from the population of smokers ($m = 12$) is smaller than that of non-smokers ($n = 15$), the test statistic W_m is the sum of the ranks associated with the smokers. Since we suspect that smokers take longer to fall asleep than nonsmokers, we reject the null hypothesis of no difference between the two groups if the observed value of W_m is too large to have occurred by chance. For these data

$$W_m = 1 + 4 + 5 + 14 + 20 + 21 + 22 + 23 + 24 + 25 + 26 + 27$$
$$= 212$$

We now turn to Table XII in Appendix B, entering with $m = 12$ and $n = m + 3 = 15$. The critical point for an $\alpha = .05$, right-tailed test is 202. Since $212 > 202$, we reject H_0 and conclude that smokers do tend to take longer to fall asleep than nonsmokers.

If both the X and Y populations are assumed normal, then the Wilcoxon rank-sum test tests the same hypothesis as the pooled T test in normal theory statistics.

Several other distribution-free tests are equivalent to the Wilcoxon rank-sum test. The best known alternative is the Mann-Whitney test. This test also depends on linearly ordering the X and Y observations. The test statistic in this case is U, the number of times that an X value precedes a Y value. If the X population is located below the Y population, then U will be large; if the reverse is true, U will be small. The probability distribution for U also has been tabulated for selected sample sizes. Since the test is equivalent to the Wilcoxon test, there is no need to present both here.

EXERCISES 13.4

1. Nerve growth factor (NGF) is a protein that has been shown to play a role in the development and maintenance of peripheral sympathetic neurons. One approach to the study of NGF is to deprive the animal of NGF and study the effect of this deprivation on various cell types. In this study, the effect on the total protein content in the dorsal root ganglia of rats is considered. Two groups of rats are compared: those born to NGF-deficient females (*in utero*) and those born to normal females but nursed by NGF-deficient females (in milk). These data result:

Total protein content, milligrams of protein per dorsal root ganglion			
In utero (U)		**In milk (M)**	
.12	.09	.19	.20
.19	.13	.21	.22
.17	.21	.21	
.20		.23	

   Do these data indicate at the $\alpha = .05$ level that the total protein content tends to be smaller among rats deprived of NGF *in utero* than among those deprived of the growth factor in milk? What is the P value for the test?

2. Polychlorinated biphenyls (PCBs) are worldwide environmental contaminants of industrial origin that are related to DDT. They are being phased out in the United States, but they will remain in the environment for many years. An experiment is run to study the effects of PCB on the reproductive ability of screech owls. The purpose is to compare the shell thickness of eggs produced by birds exposed to PCB with that of birds not exposed to the contaminant. It is thought that shells of the former group will be thinner than those of the latter. Do these data support this research hypothesis? Explain.

Shell thickness, mm			
Exposed to PCB (E)		**Free of PCB (F)**	
.21	.226	.22	.27
.223	.215	.265	.18
.25	.24	.217	.187
.19	.136	.20	.256
.20		.23	

3. In a study of characteristics of patients experiencing myocardial infarction, the cardiac volume of those whose duration of pain is less than 8 hours is compared with

that of patients whose pain lasted 8 hours or more. These data result:

Cardiac volume, ml			
Less than 8 h (<)		8 h or more (≥)	
793.4	760.5	979.1	940.7
906.5	856.6	797.0	1009.9
604.1	899.1	961.8	1330.3
646.8	806.8	1100.6	909.3
688.1	968.1	843.6	812.4
		739.4	850.0
		1335.8	818.9

Do these data support the research hypothesis that the cardiac volume of those who experience pain for less than 8 hours tends to be smaller than that of those who experience pain for 8 hours or more with myocardial infarction?

4. Sickle-cell anemia is a disease associated with impaired urinary potassium excretion. A study is run to compare the responses of subjects with normal hemoglobin and sickle-cell disease to an oral potassium chloride (KCl) load (.75 meq/kg body weight). Before patients receive the KCl load, no differences in urine pH are detected. These data are obtained at the end of the study. Do they indicate that there is a difference in the way that these groups respond to an oral KCl load relative to the variable urine pH?

Urine pH			
Normal (N)		Sickle cell (S)	
6.6	5.9	5.7	5.2
6.1	5.4	5.6	5.6
6.2	5.7	5.3	5.9
5.8	4.7	5.4	6.0
		4.8	

5. *Normal approximation to W_m.* For large samples, W_m is approximately normally distributed with mean $\mu = m(m + n + 1)/2$ and variance $\sigma^2 = mn(m + n + 1)/12$. These facts can be used to test hypotheses that call for the use of the Wilcoxon procedure for sample sizes not listed in Table XII of Appendix B. We need only standardize W_m and use the standard normal table (Table III of Appendix B) to approximate the P value of the test.

(a) Let $m = 30$ and $n = 60$. Find $P[W_m \leq 1350]$.

(b) Let $m = 40$ and $n = 50$. Find $P[W_m \geq 2000]$.

13.5

KRUSKAL-WALLIS k-SAMPLE TEST FOR LOCATION: UNMATCHED DATA

The idea of using rank sums for comparing two populations based on independent random samples drawn from the populations can be extended to more than two populations. The resulting test was developed by W. H. Kruskal and W. A. Wallis in 1952.

Kruskal-Wallis k-Sample Test

Assume that independent random samples of sizes $n_1, n_2, n_3, \ldots, n_k$ are drawn from k continuous populations, respectively. We wish to test the null hypothesis that these populations are identical with a test that is especially sensitive to differences in location. To do so, the $n_1 + n_2 + n_3 + \cdots + n_k = N$ observations are pooled and ordered from smallest to largest. Then they are ranked from 1 to N, with tied scores receiving the average group rank, as in the Wilcoxon procedures.

Let R_i, $i = 1, 2, \ldots, k$, denote the sum of the ranks associated with the observations drawn from the ith population. If the null hypothesis of no difference among populations is true, then the higher ranks should scatter randomly across the k samples; if one or more populations is located above the others, then the higher ranks should cluster in the samples drawn from those populations. Thus, if H_0 is true, the average rank associated with each group should be moderate in size; otherwise, one or more of these mean ranks should be inflated. The Kruskal-Wallis statistic is given by

$$H = \frac{12}{N(N+1)} \sum_{i=1}^{k} n_i \left(\bar{R}_i - \frac{N+1}{2} \right)^2$$

where $\bar{R}_i = R_i / n_i$, the average rank of the observations drawn from the ith population. Using the methods of Chapters 2 and 4, we can show that if the null hypothesis is true, then $E[\bar{R}_i] = (N+1)/2$. Thus, the Kruskal-Wallis statistic essentially compares the observed average ranks for the k samples with those expected under H_0. If there is a wide discrepancy, then H will be inflated. This implies that H_0 should be rejected for large values of H. It has been found that if H_0 is true, H follows an approximate chi-squared distribution with $k - 1$ degrees of freedom. Therefore, P values for the test are found in Table VIII of Appendix B. As in other cases, there is a form for H that is arithmetically equivalent, but computationally easier to handle. This form is

$$H = \frac{12}{N(N+1)} \sum_{i=1}^{k} \frac{R_i^2}{n_i} - 3(N+1)$$

This is the form that we use in practice.

EXAMPLE 13.5.1. To determine the effect of hemodialysis on the size of the liver, three populations are studied: normal controls, nondialyzed uremic patients, and patients on dialysis. Random samples are obtained from each population, and liver scans are used to determine the area of the liver (in square centimeters) for each subject. These data result (the rank of each observation is given in parentheses):

I (normal controls)		II (nondialyzed patients)		III (dialyzed patients)	
206.9 (14)	143.8 (2)	194.6 (11)	143.0 (1)	288.0 (21)	249.0 (19)
150.0 (5)	192.6 (10)	145.6 (3)	170.0 (6)	269.2 (20)	346.1 (23)
197.3 (12)		174.9 (8)		288.3 (22)	216.6 (16)
173.2 (7)		187.5 (9)		357.5 (24)	202.6 (13)
147.2 (4)		223.4 (17)		229.2 (18)	213.5 (15)

The rank sums are

$$R_1 = 14 + 5 + 12 + \cdots + 10 = 54$$
$$R_2 = 11 + 3 + 8 + \cdots + 6 = 55$$
$$R_3 = 21 + 20 + 22 + \cdots + 15 = 191$$

Note that $n_1 = n_2 = 7$, $n_3 = 10$, and $N = 24$. The observed value of the Kruskal-Wallis statistic for these data is

$$H = \frac{12}{N(N+1)} \sum_{i=1}^{3} \frac{R_i^2}{n_i} - 3(N+1)$$

$$= \frac{12}{24(25)} \left(\frac{54^2}{7} + \frac{55^2}{7} + \frac{191^2}{10} \right) - 3(25) = 14.94$$

The number of degrees of freedom associated with the chi-squared statistic is $k - 1 = 2$. From Table VIII

$$P[X_2^2 \geq 14.94] < .005$$

Since this P value is small, we may conclude that differences in liver size do exist among the three populations.

The Kruskal-Wallis test does assume continuous populations. However, the test can be safely applied to data that originally consist of ranks. If the sampled populations are normal with equal variances, then the hypothesis being tested is the same as that of the one-way classification, completely random design in analysis of variance.

▨ EXERCISES 13.5

1. Vitamin A deficiency is a well-recognized public health problem in many areas. Inadequate dietary intake of vitamin A is the most important factor responsible for this deficiency. A chief source of vitamin A is β carotene, which is derived from vegetables. It has been shown that adding green leafy vegetables to the diet results in an increase in serum vitamin A concentrations. A study is run to determine whether adding fat to the diet has any benefits. A group of 30 children, each of whose serum vitamin A concentration is less than 20 mg vitamin A/100 ml blood serum, is randomly split into three subgroups. Each group receives 40 g spinach daily, but the fat in the diet varies. At the end of the experiment, these data on the serum vitamin A concentration are obtained:

I (no added fat)	II (5 g fat added)	III (10 g fat added)
18.1	29.1	26.6
16.5	15.8	16.1
21.0	20.4	18.8
18.7	23.5	25.0
7.4	18.5	21.8
12.4	21.3	15.4
16.1	23.1	19.9
17.9	23.8	15.5
	20.1	21.1
	11.9	25.5

(a) Compute the rank sum for each group.

(b) Test the null hypothesis that the fat content of the diet has no effect on serum A concentration.

2. Urease is an enzyme known to produce ammonia in the gastrointestinal tract. Ammonia is known to be detrimental to patients with liver disease. A study is conducted to compare the urease concentration in the gastric juices in five populations: normal controls, I; patients with extrahepatic portal vein obstruction, II; patients with amoebic liver abscess, III; patients with viral hepatitis, IV; and patients with idiopathic portal hypertension, V. These data (in milligrams per milliliter) are obtained:

I	II	III	IV	V
261.1	221.9	201.4	600.9	160.6
186.2	188.7	146.1	301.2	135.0
239.1	167.6	96.8	607.9	455.1
243.3	224.9	173.9	283.3	402.3
296.8	178.8	280.8	193.3	457.9
270.5	147.9	100.3	159.4	559.6

Based on these data and the Kruskal-Wallis test, can you claim that these populations differ with respect to the gastric urease concentration?

3. Poisonings may occur owing to extensive contact with pesticide residue on crops. Pesticide absorption through the skin varies with the anatomic region of the body. The palm of the hand is especially sensitive. A study is run to compare the exposure time of the right hand in five different types of agricultural workers. The data are collected by filming the workers for a 17-minute period and determining, for each, how long the right hand is in contact with the crop. These data result:

Tobacco harvesters	Cotton scouts	Peach thinners	Blueberry pickers	Sweet corn packers
14.4	11.7	15.8	16.1	14.3
12.9	13.8	16.2	16.0	14.5
12.0	14.2	15.9	15.9	14.8
13.9	10.3	16.7	16.4	14.9
13.3	7.0	16.4	16.6	14.0

Based on the Kruskal-Wallis test, can you claim that the exposure time of the right hand differs among these groups of workers? Explain your answer based on the P value of the test.

4. Since the liver is the major site of drug metabolism, it is expected that patients with liver disease may have defects in the elimination of drugs metabolized by the liver. One such drug is phenylbutazone. A study is conducted of the response of the system to this drug. Three groups are studied: normal controls, patients with cirrhosis of the liver, and patients with chronic active hepatitis. Each subject is given orally 19 mg phenylbutazone/kg body weight. Based on blood analysis, the time of peak plasma concentration (in hours) is determined for each. These

data result:

Normal	Cirrhosis	Hepatitis
4.0	22.6	16.6
30.6	14.4	12.1
26.8	26.3	7.2
37.9	13.8	6.6
13.7	17.4	12.5
49.0		15.1
		6.7
		20.0

Based on the Kruskal-Wallis test, can you conclude that the three populations differ with respect to the time of peak plasma concentration of phenylbutazone? Explain your answer on the basis of the P value of the test.

5. The supraorbital nasal glands (salt glands) have an important function in marine birds. These glands help to excrete sodium chloride when environmental conditions force the bird to consume more salt than normal. A study is conducted to determine the role of these glands in the excretion of lead, a common environmental pollutant. Three groups of ducks are studied: normal controls, I; ducks force-fed with a dose of commercial lead shot, II; and ducks fed with lead shot and $CaNa_2EDTA$, III. These data are found on the lead concentration (in micrograms of lead per gram of tissue) in the nasal glands:

I	II	III
1.4	11.1	5.0
1.0	10.3	8.2
.9	10.2	4.9
.7	9.7	3.2
.5	7.7	4.4
1.2	10.1	3.1
3.4	11.6	5.1
1.3	13.3	2.9

Use the Kruskal-Wallis test to determine whether differences in the lead concentration in the nasal glands exist among the three populations.

13.6

FRIEDMAN k-SAMPLE TEST FOR LOCATION: MATCHED DATA

In this section we present a distribution-free test for k identical populations when the observations from the k populations are matched. The test, developed by M. Friedman in 1937, is especially sensitive to differences in location.

Friedman Test

Assume that we are interested in comparing the effects of k treatments. It is felt that there is a variable which, although not of direct interest, might interfere with our ability to detect real differences among the k treatments. We want to control this extraneous variable by blocking. That is, we split the experimental units into b groups, or "blocks," each of size k, with members within a block being as nearly alike as possible relative to the extraneous variable. Then we randomly assign the k treatments to units within each block. To test the null hypothesis of identical treatment effects, we rank the observations within each block from 1 to k (smallest to largest), giving tied scores the average group rank. Next we compute R_i, $i = 1, 2, \ldots, k$, the sum of the ranks associated with each of the k treatments. If H_0 is true, each of these rank sums should be moderate in size; otherwise, there should be substantial differences among them. It can be shown that the expected value of each rank sum under H_0 is $b(k + 1)/2$.

The *Friedman statistic S* is designed to compare the observed rank sums with this expected value:

$$S = \sum_{i=1}^{k} \left[R_i - \frac{b(k + 1)}{2} \right]^2$$

Note that if H_0 is true, each of the differences $R_i - b(k + 1)/2$ should be small, yielding a small value of S; otherwise, S will be inflated. The probability distribution for S has been tabulated for a limited number of choices for k (number of treatments) and b (number of blocks). However, it has been found that the statistic

$$\boxed{\frac{12S}{bk(k + 1)}}$$

follows an approximate chi-squared distribution with $k - 1$ degrees of freedom if H_0 is true. Thus this statistic serves as our test statistic with rejection of H_0 occurring for large values of the statistic. The P values are read from Table VIII of Appendix B.

We illustrate the use of the Friedman test in Example 13.6.1.

EXAMPLE 13.6.1. Recent studies have shown that even microliter amounts of crude oil, when applied to the surface of fertile eggs of several avian species, may result in damage to the embryo. In addition to a high aromatic hydrocarbon content, certain crude oils contain high concentrations of nickel and vanadium. The effects of these elements on the embryonic development of mallards are studied. Since ducks from various clutches (nests) have different genetic backgrounds, this factor is controlled by blocking. Six clutches are used in the experiment. Four eggs are randomly selected from each clutch and assigned at random to one of four treatments:

    I. No crude oil applied (control)
   II. Treated with 1 μL crude oil
  III. Treated with 1 μL crude oil with 700 ppm vanadium
  IV. Treated with 1 μL crude oil with 700 ppm nickel

The eggs are allowed to develop for 18 days, at which time the weight, in grams, of each egg is determined. These data result (the rank of each observation *within its block* is given in parentheses):

	Treatment			
Block (clutch)	I	II	III	IV
1	16.77 (4)	14.34 (2)	16.08 (3)	14.29 (1)
2	15.61 (4)	11.92 (1)	13.22 (2)	13.95 (3)
3	14.46 (4)	14.45 (3)	11.72 (1)	13.59 (2)
4	13.08 (3)	16.11 (4)	10.18 (1)	12.22 (2)
5	14.47 (4)	12.85 (1)	13.52 (3)	13.22 (2)
6	12.01 (2)	16.13 (4)	12.68 (3)	10.73 (1)

The treatment rank sums are

$$R_1 = 4 + 4 + 4 + 3 + 4 + 2 = 21$$

$$R_2 = 2 + 1 + 3 + 4 + 1 + 4 = 15$$

$$R_3 = 3 + 2 + 1 + 1 + 3 + 3 = 13$$

$$R_4 = 1 + 3 + 2 + 2 + 2 + 1 = 11$$

Note that if H_0 is true, these rank sums should all be close to the expected value of

$$\frac{b(k + 1)}{2} = \frac{6(4 + 1)}{2} = 15$$

There does seem to be some deviation from this value. Is the deviation enough to conclude that there are differences among the four treatments? To answer, we compute the value of the Friedman statistic S and use it to find the value of the test statistic

$$X_{k-1}^2 = \frac{12S}{bk(k + 1)}$$

For these data,

$$S = \sum_{i=1}^{k} \left[R_i - \frac{b(k + 1)}{2} \right]^2$$

$$= \sum_{i=1}^{4} \left[R_i - \frac{6(4 + 1)}{2} \right]^2$$

$$= (21 - 15)^2 + (15 - 15)^2 + (13 - 15)^2 + (11 - 15)^2$$

$$= 36 + 0 + 4 + 16 = 56$$

The observed value of the $X_{k-1}^2 = X_3^2$ statistic is

$$\frac{12S}{bk(k + 1)} = \frac{12(56)}{6(4)(5)} = 5.6$$

From Table VIII in Appendix B, we see that the P value for this test is between .25 (critical point, 4.11) and .1 (critical point, 6.25). Since this is large, we cannot conclude that there are differences among the treatments.

The Friedman test does assume continuous populations. However, it can be used to analyze data that originally consist of ranks. It is the distribution-free analog of the normal theory randomized complete block design.

■ EXERCISES 13.6

1. During the last few years, an increasing number of cases of suspected penta-chlorophenol (PCP) poisoning of farm animals have been brought to the attention of veterinarians. A study is conducted to consider the effects of varying amounts of PCP on the total weight gain (in kilograms) in pigs. Litter mates are used as blocks to control the effects of natural differences among animals of different parentage. These treatments are used:

  I. Fed lactose (controls)
  II. Fed lactose and 5 mg purified PCP/kg body weight
  III. Fed lactose and 10 mg purified PCP/kg body weight
  IV. Fed lactose and 15 mg purified PCP/kg body weight

These data are obtained on the total weight gained by the end of the experimental period:

Block (litter)	Treatment			
	I	II	III	IV
1	8.9	6.6	5.6	4.2
2	7.2	6.9	7.3	6.9
3	3.1	6.2	7.2	4.1
4	7.1	8.3	6.3	5.8
5	6.7	6.4	5.9	9.4
6	5.3	6.7	8.0	7.9
7	2.4	5.5	6.1	3.1
8	5.7	9.2	9.6	4.2

If the PCP level does not affect total weight gain, each rank sum should lie close to what value? Use the Friedman test to compare the effects of these four treatments on total weight gain.

2. A study is conducted to compare the mercury concentration in the brain, muscle, and eye tissues of trout exposed to a sublethal dose (.3 toxic unit) of methyl mercury. Twelve trout are used in the experiment; each is considered a block. These data on the concentration (in micrograms of mercury per gram of tissue) result:

Block (trout)	Tissue			Block (trout)	Tissue		
	Brain	Muscle	Eye		Brain	Muscle	Eye
1	1.65	.98	.49	7	1.22	1.24	.43
2	1.37	1.17	.40	8	1.66	1.01	.57
3	1.48	1.05	.44	9	1.49	.86	.87
4	1.40	1.45	.55	10	1.67	1.13	.52
5	1.61	.96	.43	11	1.31	1.18	.46
6	1.59	1.00	.39	12	1.55	1.17	.45

If there are no differences in the mercury concentrations in these three tissue types, each rank sum should be close to what value? Use the Friedman test to compare the effects of a .3-toxic-unit dose of methyl mercury on the mercury concentration in the brain, muscle, and eye tissues of trout.

3. A laboratory administrator is considering purchasing a machine to analyze blood samples. Five such machines are on the market. After trial use, each of eight medical technicians is asked to rank the machines in order of preference, with a rank of 1 being assigned to the machine most preferred. These data result:

Block (technician)	Machine				
	I	II	III	IV	V
1	1	3	4	2	5
2	4	5	1	2	3
3	4	1	3	5	2
4	4	1	5	2	3
5	1	3	2	5	4
6	1	2	3	4	5
7	5	1	3	2	4
8	5	1	4	3	2

If there is no clear preference, each of the rank sums should be close to what value? Use the Friedman test to determine whether technicians perceive differences among the machines.

13.7

CORRELATION

In Chapter 11 we discuss the problem of measuring the degree of linear association between two random variables X and Y. This is done by means of the Pearson product-moment coefficient of correlation. Now we introduce a measure of linear association that is particularly useful when either the data consist of ranks or the data set is small enough to be ranked easily. The method was introduced in 1904 by C. Spearman.

Spearman's Rank Correlation Coefficient

Consider a set $(x_1, y_1), (x_2, y_2), (x_3, y_3), \ldots, (x_n, y_n)$ of n paired observations on the random variables X and Y. To estimate the correlation between X and Y, we first rank the observations on X from 1 to n, smallest to largest. We then do the same for the observations on Y. We thus generate a set of n paired ranks, which we denote by $(r_{x_1}, r_{y_1}), (r_{x_2}, r_{y_2}), (r_{x_3}, r_{y_3}), \ldots, (r_{x_n}, r_{y_n})$. Again, we assign tied scores the average group rank. The estimated correlation between X and Y is found by calculating the Pearson coefficient for the set of paired ranks. That is, we define the *Spearman rank correlation coefficient* r_s by

$$r_s = \frac{n \sum r_x r_y - \sum r_x \sum r_y}{\sqrt{\left[n \sum r_x^2 - \left(\sum r_x\right)^2\right]\left[n \sum r_y^2 - \left(\sum r_y\right)^2\right]}}$$

This procedure yields results that are slightly different from those of the Pearson method. However, for large sample sizes, there is close agreement. Furthermore, if there are *no ties*, the Spearman coefficient is given by

$$r_s = 1 - \frac{6 \sum d_i^2}{n(n^2 - 1)}$$

where $d_i = r_{x_i} - r_{y_i}$, the difference between the X and Y ranks. Thus if there are no ties, the Spearman coefficient is easier to compute than the Pearson. The interpretations of the two are the same. Namely, values near 1 indicate a strong positive correlation; large values of X tend to be associated with large values of Y. Values near -1 indicate a strong negative correlation; large values of X tend to be associated with small values of Y. Values near 0 indicate no linear association. It is suggested that the Spearman procedure not be used if there are a large number of ties.

We illustrate the Spearman procedure in Example 13.7.1.

EXAMPLE 13.7.1. A study is run to determine the linear association between an individual's blood nicotine concentration and the nicotine yield of the cigarette smoked. These data are obtained (ranks are in parentheses):

X (blood nicotine concentration, nmol/liter)	Y (nicotine content per cigarette, mg)
185.7 (2)	1.51 (8)
197.3 (5)	.96 (3)
204.2 (8)	1.21 (6)
199.9 (7)	1.66 (10)
199.1 (6)	1.11 (4)
192.8 (3)	.84 (2)
207.4 (9)	1.14 (5)
183.0 (1)	1.28 (7)
234.1 (10)	1.53 (9)
196.5 (4)	.76 (1)

For these data,

$$\sum r_x = \sum r_y = 55 \quad \sum r_x^2 = \sum r_y^2 = 385$$

$$\sum r_x r_y = 2(8) + 5(3) + 8(6) + \cdots + 4(1) = 325$$

Computing r_s directly, we obtain

$$r_s = \frac{n \sum r_x r_y - \sum r_x \sum r_y}{\sqrt{\left[n \sum r_x^2 - \left(\sum r_x\right)^2\right]\left[n \sum r_y^2 - \left(\sum r_y\right)^2\right]}}$$

$$= \frac{10(325) - 55(55)}{\sqrt{[10(385) - 55^2][10(385) - 55^2]}}$$

$$= .27$$

Since there are no ties, r_s can be computed by the shortcut formula:

$$r_s = 1 - \frac{6 \sum d_i^2}{n(n^2 - 1)}$$

$$= 1 - \frac{6[(2 - 8)^2 + (5 - 3)^2 + (8 - 6)^2 + \cdots + (4 - 1)^2]}{10(10^2 - 1)}$$

$$= 1 - \frac{6(120)}{10(99)} = .27$$

Since the Spearman coefficient of correlation does not differ greatly from the Pearson coefficient, we may approximate the coefficient of determination r^2 by r_s^2. In this case, $r_s^2 = .07$. Thus approximately 7% of the variation in the blood nicotine concentration can be attributed to a linear association with the nicotine yield of the cigarette smoked. Since this value is small, we interpret r_s as indicating a weak positive correlation between X and Y.

EXERCISES 13.7

1. Continuous infusion of a drug at a constant rate is supposed to maintain its serum concentration at a constant and predictable level. This does appear to be the case within an individual patient. However, there is a problem in that the same drug dosage does not necessarily produce the same serum concentration in different patients. To study this phenomenon in patients treated with ampicillin for severe purulent meningitis, 24 patients are subjected to a constant-rate infusion of the drug. It is felt that there is a linear relationship between the serum ampicillin concentration and the patient's rate of creatinine clearance. These data are obtained:

x (creatinine clearance, ml/min)	y (serum ampicillin concentration, mg/liter)	x (creatinine clearance, ml/min)	y (serum ampicillin concentration, mg/liter)
69.0	60.0	112.6	12.8
70.0	38.5	116.5	35.0
81.0	92.0	120.2	13.3
85.0	19.2	120.0	59.6
85.1	41.0	122.5	47.8
84.0	69.2	130.1	24.6
95.0	42.7	135.0	18.0
96.1	78.1	132.3	48.5
100.0	50.0	155.7	21.2
107.0	20.0	170.0	23.0
107.5	28.3	121.0	7.4
110.0	15.0	125.0	10.0

(a) Rank each of the sets of observations from 1 to 24.

(b) Find $\sum r_x, \sum r_y, \sum r_x^2, \sum r_y^2$, and $\sum r_x r_y$. Use these values to find r_s from its definition.

(c) Since there are no ties, the shortcut formula can be used. Verify your answer to part b by computing r_s from this formula.

(d) The estimated correlation for the Pearson coefficient is $-.49$. Compare this value to that of Spearman.

(e) Does there appear to be a strong linear association between X and Y? Explain your answer on the basis of the estimated value of r_s^2.

2. Patients with osteoporosis, a disease of the bone that produces a decrease in bone mass, are studied. The patients are treated with human parathyroid hormone fragment. It is hoped that a strong linear relationship exists between the calcium accretion rate during treatment and the final bone volume, so that this variable can be utilized in the future to predict final bone volume. These data result:

x (calcium accretion rate, mmol/24 h)	y (final trabecular bone volume, %)	x (calcium accretion rate, mmol/24 h)	y (final trabecular bone volume, %)
2.5	8.0	15.0	14.9
3.0	12.1	15.2	9.7
4.0	9.1	17.0	15.0
4.6	10.0	20.5	17.0
6.1	11.0	24.6	12.2
7.5	5.2	28.3	47.2
11.0	10.1	30.0	31.4
12.3	18.0		

Find r_s. Does there appear to be a strong positive correlation between X and Y? Explain on the basis of the approximate value of r_s^2.

3. One characteristic of vision is "smooth pursuit" eye movements, or the capacity of the eyes to track objects moving slowly across visual fields. A study is run to explore the relationship between the maximum velocity reached by the eyes during smooth pursuit and blood alcohol content. Twelve subjects are used. The maximum smooth-pursuit velocity is determined for each. Then the subjects are asked to drink either whiskey and water or gin and tonic until they consider themselves unfit to drive. At this point, the maximum velocity of smooth pursuit is measured again, and the subject's blood alcohol content is determined. These data result:

x (blood alcohol content, mg/dl)	y (smooth-pursuit velocity, % decrease)	x (blood alcohol content, mg/dl)	y (smooth-pursuit velocity, % decrease)
20	2	85	19
45	11	86	30
68	30	108	38
68	50	110	10
70	4	120	51
75	6	150	60

Find r_s and interpret this value in a practical sense.

4. To tag baboons for future study, researchers must immobilize the animals temporarily. One drug used for this purpose is phencyclidine hydrochloride. A study is conducted to determine (1) the relationship between the dose administered and the time to complete immobilization and (2) the relationship between the dose administered and the elapsed time from complete immobilization until large movements are seen. These data result:

x (dose, mg drug/kg body weight)	y (time to immobilization, min)	z (time to recovery, min)
1.21	7.6	100.2
1.36	8.2	100.1
1.78	8.7	100.5
1.10	7.9	90.4
1.57	8.0	97.7
1.49	7.4	87.8
1.59	7.7	79.5
1.02	8.5	119.8

(a) Find and interpret the Spearman coefficient of correlation between X and Y.
(b) Find and interpret the Spearman coefficient of correlation between X and Z.

13.8
BARTLETT'S TEST FOR EQUALITY OF VARIANCES

As indicated in Chapter 10, one of the assumptions underlying the F test for equality of means in a one-way classification problem is that population variances are equal. We protect against the violation of this assumption by using equal sample sizes whenever possible. However, if sample sizes vary widely, it is advisable to test

$$H_0:\ \sigma_1^2 = \sigma_2^2 = \cdots = \sigma_k^2$$
$$H_1:\ \sigma_i^2 \neq \sigma_j^2 \qquad \text{for some } i \text{ and } j \text{ (at least two variances differ)}$$

If H_0 is not rejected, we compare means via the F test described in Chapter 10; if H_0 is rejected, the Kruskal-Wallis test given in Section 13.5 is applicable.

The most frequently used test for testing the null hypothesis of equal variances is called *Bartlett's test*. The statistic used in this test can be shown to follow an approximate chi-squared distribution with $k - 1$ degrees of freedom when sampling is done from normal populations.

To conduct Bartlett's test we compute the sample variances $S_1^2, S_2^2, \ldots, S_k^2$ for each of the k samples. We also compute the error mean square, the pooled estimate of σ^2 under the assumption that H_0 is true. In this context, it is convenient to compute MS_E directly from the individual sample variances by means of the formula

$$MS_E = S_p^2 = \sum_{i=1}^{k} \frac{(n_i - 1)S_i^2}{N - k}$$

We next form the statistic Q defined by

$$Q = (N - k) \log_{10} S_p^2 - \sum_{i=1}^{k} (n_i - 1) \log_{10} S_i^2$$

The observed value of this statistic is large when the sample variances S_i^2, $i = 1$, $2, \ldots, k$, are quite different; it is near zero when these sample variances are close in value. The Bartlett statistic is defined by

$$B = \frac{2.3026 Q}{h}$$

where

$$h = 1 + \frac{1}{3(k - 1)} \left(\sum_{i=1}^{k} \frac{1}{n_i - 1} - \frac{1}{N - k} \right)$$

An example should demonstrate the use of Bartlett's test.

EXAMPLE 13.8.1. Let us return to the problem described in Example 10.1.1 in which a study is run to compare the effectiveness of three comprehensive programs for the treatment of mild to moderate acne. These data on the percentage improvement in the number of acne lesions noted per patient at the end of 16 weeks are obtained:

Treatment					
I		**II**		**III**	
48.6	50.8	68.0	71.9	67.5	61.4
49.4	47.1	67.0	71.5	62.5	67.4
50.1	52.5	70.1	69.9	64.2	65.4
49.8	49.0	64.5	68.9	62.5	63.2
50.6	46.7	68.0	67.8	63.9	61.2
		68.3	68.9	64.8	60.5
				62.3	

Since sample sizes are different, the safe line of attack is to test for equal variances and let the results of the test determine whether the data should be analyzed via an F test or by using the Kruskal-Wallis test. For these data

$$n_1 = 10 \qquad n_2 = 12 \qquad n_3 = 13 \qquad N = 35$$

$$s_1^2 = 3.000 \qquad s_2^2 = 4.002 \qquad s_3^2 = 4.938 \qquad k = 3$$

These sample variances are used to compute MS_E as follows:

$$MS_E = S_p^2 = \sum_{i=1}^{3} \frac{(n_i - 1)S_i^2}{N - k}$$

$$= \frac{9(3.000) + 11(4.002) + 12(4.938)}{35 - 3}$$

$$= 4.071$$

The statistic Q is given by

$$Q = (N - k) \log_{10} S_p^2 - \sum_{i=1}^{3} (n_i - 1) \log_{10} S_i^2$$

The logarithms are found using a handheld calculator and are given by

$$\log_{10} S_p^2 = \log_{10}(4.071) = .6097$$

$$\log_{10} S_1^2 = \log_{10}(3.000) = .4771$$

$$\log_{10} S_2^2 = \log_{10}(4.002) = .6023$$

$$\log_{10} S_3^2 = \log_{10}(4.938) = .6936$$

The observed value of Q is

$$Q = (35 - 3)(.6097) - [(9)(.4771) + 11(.6023) + 12(.6936)]$$

$$= .268$$

The Bartlett statistic is given by

$$B = \frac{2.3026 Q}{h}$$

where

$$h = 1 + \frac{1}{3(k-1)} \left(\sum_{i=1}^{k} \frac{1}{n_i - 1} - \frac{1}{N - k} \right)$$

In this case

$$h = 1 + \frac{1}{3(2)} \left(\frac{1}{9} + \frac{1}{11} + \frac{1}{12} - \frac{1}{32} \right)$$

$$= 1.0424$$

and the observed value of the Bartlett statistic is

$$B = \frac{2.3026(.268)}{1.0424} = .5919$$

Since $k = 3$, the P value is found based on the $X_{k-1}^2 = X_2^2$ distribution. From the chi-squared table, we see that

$$P = P[X_2^2 \geq .5919] > .25$$

Since this P value is large, we are unable to reject H_0. We do not have evidence that the three population variances are unequal. In this case, it is reasonable to compare means via the one-way analysis-of-variance F tests as was done in Chapter 10.

▮ EXERCISES 13.8

1. Following a major accidental spill from a chemical manufacturing plant near a river, a study was conducted to determine whether certain species of fish caught from the river differ in terms of the amounts of the chemical absorbed. If differences are found, regulations on human consumption may be recommended. Samples from catches of three major species were measured in parts per million. The

resulting data are given below.

Species		
A	B	C
18.1	29.1	26.6
16.5	15.8	16.1
21.0	20.4	18.8
18.7	23.5	25.0
7.4	18.5	21.8
12.4	21.3	15.4
16.1	23.1	19.9
17.9	23.8	15.5
	20.1	21.1
	11.9	25.5

(a) Use Bartlett's test to test $H_0: \sigma_1^2 = \sigma_2^2 = \sigma_3^2$.

(b) Based on the results of this test, test for equality of location by using either the F test or the Kruskal-Wallis test.

2. Use the data of Exercise 3 of Section 10.1 to test $H_0: \sigma_1^2 = \sigma_2^2 = \sigma_3^2 = \sigma_4^2 = \sigma_5^2$. Was the earlier analysis appropriate?

▨ 13.9

NORMAL APPROXIMATIONS

We saw in Section 4.5 that for large values of n, the Poisson density can be used to approximate the binomial. The normal curve can be utilized to approximate probabilities associated with either variable. The theoretical justification for either approximation procedure is based on the Central Limit Theorem, which is presented in Chapter 6. The argument given here is based strictly on intuition and empirical evidence.

To see how binomial probabilities can be reasonably approximated, we consider a series of binomial variables. In particular, consider four binomial variables, each with probability of success .4 and with values of n of 5, 10, 15, and 20. The densities for these variables, obtained from Table I of Appendix B, together with a rough sketch for each, are given in Figure 13.7a to d.

The point to note from these diagrams is made in Figure 13.7d. Namely, it is not hard to imagine a smooth bell curve that closely fits the block diagram shown. This suggests that binomial probabilities represented by one or more blocks in the diagram can be approximated reasonably well by a carefully selected area under an appropriately chosen normal curve. Which of the infinitely many normal curves is appropriate? Common sense indicates that the normal variable selected should have the same mean and variance as the binomial variable that it approximates. Theorem 13.9.1, offered without formal proof, summarizes these ideas.

THEOREM 13.9.1. Normal approximation to the binomial distribution. Let X be binomial with parameters n and p. For large n, X is approximately normal with mean np and variance $np(1 - p)$.

x	$f(x)$
0	.0778
1	.2592
2	.3456
3	.2304
4	.0768
5	.0102

$n = 5$
$p = .4$

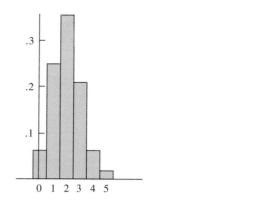

(a)

x	$f(x)$
0	.0060
1	.0404
2	.1209
3	.2150
4	.2508
5	.2007
6	.1114
7	.0425
8	.0106
9	.0016
10	.0001

$n = 10$
$p = .4$

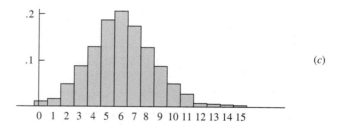

(b)

x	$f(x)$	x	$f(x)$
0	.0005	8	.1181
1	.0047	9	.0612
2	.0219	10	.0245
3	.0634	11	.0074
4	.1268	12	.0016
5	.1859	13	.0003
6	.2066	14	~0
7	.1771	15	~0

$n = 15$
$p = .4$

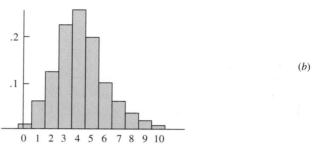

(c)

x	$f(x)$	x	$f(x)$
0	~0	11	.0710
1	.0005	12	.0355
2	.0031	13	.0145
3	.0124	14	.0049
4	.0350	15	.0013
5	.0746	16	.0003
6	.1244	17	~0
7	.1659	18	~0
8	.1797	19	~0
9	.1597	20	~0
10	.1172		

$n = 20$
$p = .4$

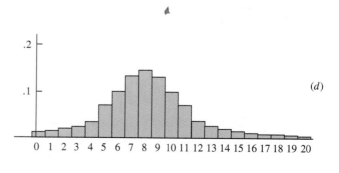

(d)

FIGURE 13.7

Density for X binomial: (a) $n = 5$, $p = .4$; (b) $n = 10$, $p = .4$; (c) $n = 15$, $p = .4$; (d) $n = 20$, $p = .4$.

Admittedly, Theorem 13.9.1 is a bit vague in the sense that the word *large* is not well defined. In the strictest mathematical sense, *large* means as n approaches infinity. For all practical purposes, the approximation is acceptable for values of n and p such that either $p \leq .5$ and $np > 5$ or $p > .5$ and $n(1 - p) > 5$.

EXAMPLE 13.9.1. A study is performed to investigate the connection between maternal smoking during pregnancy and birth defects in children. Of the mothers studied, 40% smoke and 60% do not. When the babies were born, 20 were found to have some sort of birth defect. Let X denote the number of children whose mother smoked while pregnant. If there is no relationship between maternal smoking and birth defects, then X is binomial with $n = 20$ and $p = .4$. What is the probability that 12 or more of the affected children had mothers who smoked?

To answer this question, we need to find $P[X \geq 12]$ under the assumption that X is binomial with $n = 20$ and $p = .4$. This probability can be read from Table I of Appendix B.

$$P[X \geq 12] = 1 - P[X \leq 11]$$
$$= 1 - .9435$$
$$= .0565$$

Note that since $p = .4 \leq .5$ and $np = (20)(.4) = 8 > 5$, the normal approximation should give a result quite close to .0565. Graphically, we are dealing with a normal random variable Y with mean $np = 20(.4) = 8$ and variance $np(1 - p) = 20(.4)(.6) = 4.8$. The exact probability of .0565 is given by the sum of the areas of the blocks centered at 12, 13, 14, 15, 16, 17, 18, 19, and 20, as shown in Figure 13.8. The approximate probability is given by the area under the normal curve above 11.5. That is,

$$P[X \geq 12] \doteq P[Y \geq 11.5]$$

The number .5 is called the *half-unit correction* for continuity. It was subtracted from 12 in the approximation because otherwise half of the area of the block centered at 12 would have been inadvertently ignored, leading to an unnecessary error in the calculation.

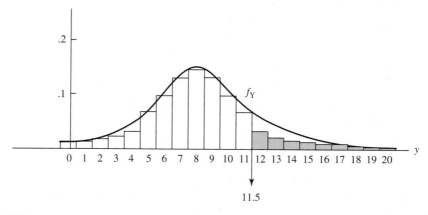

FIGURE 13.8

$P[X \geq 12] = $ area of shaded blocks $\doteq$ area under curve beyond 11.5.

From this point on, the calculation is routine.

$$P[X \geq 12] \doteq P[Y \geq 11.5]$$

$$= P\left[\frac{Y - 8}{\sqrt{4.8}} \geq \frac{11.5 - 8}{\sqrt{4.8}}\right]$$

$$= P[Z \geq 1.59]$$

$$= 1 - P[Z \leq 1.59]$$

$$= 1 - .9441 = .0559$$

Note that even with n as small as 20, the approximated value of .0559 compares quite favorably with the exact value of .0565. In practice, of course, one would not approximate a probability that could be found directly from a binomial table. This was done here only for comparative purposes.

The normal approximation to the Poisson distribution is handled similarly to the binomial. Its theoretical basis is also the Central Limit Theorem. It is reasonably accurate for large values of the Poisson parameter λs, and it employs the half-unit correction factor to adjust for the fact that a discrete distribution is being approximated by a continuous curve. The procedure is based on Theorem 13.9.2.

THEOREM 13.9.2. Normal approximation to the Poisson distribution. Let X be Poisson with parameter λs. Then for large values of λs, X is approximately normal with mean λs and variance λs.

EXAMPLE 13.9.2. A healthy adult male has on the average 5,400,000 red cells per cubic millimeter of blood. A drop of size 1/10,000 cubic millimeter is examined. What is the probability that the number of red cells X will lie between 500 and 580?

Variable X is Poisson with parameter

$$\lambda s = 5,400,000 \frac{1}{10,000} = 540$$

By Theorem 13.9.2, X is approximately normal with mean and variance each equal to 540. Thus, using the half-unit correction factor, we get

$$P[500 \leq X \leq 580] \doteq P[499.5 \leq Y \leq 580.5]$$

$$= P\left[\frac{499.5 - 540}{\sqrt{540}} \leq Z \leq \frac{580.5 - 540}{\sqrt{540}}\right]$$

$$= P[-1.74 \leq Z \leq 1.74]$$

$$= .9591 - .0409 = .9182$$

▇ EXERCISES 13.9

1. Let X be binomial with $n = 20$ and $p = .3$. Use the normal approximation to the binomial to approximate each of the following. Then compare your results with the values obtained from Table I of Appendix B.

(a) $P[X \leq 3]$
(b) $P[3 \leq X \leq 6]$
(c) $P[X \geq 4]$
(d) $P[X = 4]$

2. It is reported that 10% of all human beings have some sort of allergy. One hundred individuals are randomly selected and interviewed. Find the probability that at least 12 will have some sort of allergy. Find the probability that at most eight will have an allergy.

3. The probability of death resulting from the use of contraceptive pills is 3/100,000. Of 1,000,000 women using this form of birth control, how many deaths are expected to be attributable to this use? What is the probability that there will be at most 25 such deaths? What is the probability that the number of deaths owing to this cause is between 25 and 35, inclusive?

4. A laboratory test for heroin in blood samples has a record of 92% accuracy. If 72 samples are analyzed in a month, what is the probability that
   (a) 60 or fewer are accurately evaluated
   (b) Fewer than 60 are accurately evaluated
   (c) Exactly 60 are accurately evaluated

5. One out of every 400 babies born in a large metropolitan hospital is afflicted with the genetic disease phenylketonuria (PKU). Of the next 2000 babies born in this hospital, what is the probability that at least one will have PKU?

6. Assume that male and female rat pups are equally likely to be born to breeding females in the laboratories of a large laboratory animal supply company. What is the probability that of 1000 animals born, 445 or more will be female?

7. Let X be Poisson with parameter $\lambda s = 100$. Use the normal approximation to find the following:
   (a) $P[X \geq 95]$ (c) $P[90 \leq X \leq 110]$
   (b) $P[X \leq 80]$ (d) $P[X = 99]$

8. The average number of jets either arriving at or departing from O'Hare airport is one every 40 seconds. What is the probability that at least 75 such flights will occur during a randomly selected hour? What is the probability that fewer than 100 such flights will take place in an hour?

9. A medium contains 20 killer paramecia (see Exercise 4.5.7). What is the probability that in a $2\frac{1}{2}$-hour period none of these will emit a killer particle? What is the probability that between 5 and 10, inclusive, of these will each emit at least one killer particle? (Killer particles are emitted at a rate of 1 every 5 hours.)

13.10

A SMALL SAMPLE TEST ON PROPORTIONS

In Chapter 8 a method was presented to test H_0: $p = p_0$. This test was derived under the assumption that sample sizes are large enough for the Central Limit Theorem to come into play. If this hypothesis is to be tested and the available data set is small, the binomial distribution can be used to calculate P values. The test statistic used is X, the number of observations in the sample with the trait.

> **EXAMPLE 13.10.1.** A new drug is being developed for use in the treatment of skin cancer. It is hoped that it will be effective on a majority of those patients on whom it is used. The company developing the drug wants to get statistical evidence to support such a claim. Let p denote the proportion of patients for whom the drug will be effective. Since we make whatever is to be supported or detected the alternative hypothesis, the alternative here is that $p > .5$. This automatically implies that the null hypothesis is the negation of H_1, namely, that $p \leq .5$. Thus the two hypotheses involved are
>
> $$H_0:\ p \leq .5$$
> $$H_1:\ p > .5$$

To test H_0 a random sample of 20 patients is selected and the drug is used on each. The test statistic that we shall use is X, the number of patients for whom the drug is effective. If the null hypothesis is true, then X is binomial with $n = 20$, $p = .5$, and $E[X] = np = 10$. Thus if H_0 is true, we would expect the drug to be effective on about 10 patients; if H_1 is true and the effectiveness rate is actually higher than .5, then we would expect to see more than 10 persons helped by the drug. Suppose that when the experiment is conducted, we observe 14 patients for whom the drug is effective. Is this number enough larger than 10 to allow us to reject H_0? To decide, we calculate the P value of the test. In this case

$$P = P[X \geq 14 \,|\, p = .5]$$

From the binomial table, we see that

$$P[X \geq 14 \,|\, p = .5] = 1 - P[X \leq 13 \,|\, p = .5]$$
$$= 1 - .9423$$
$$= .0577$$

Since this P value is small, we reject H_0 and conclude that for a majority of people the drug is effective.

EXERCISES 13.10

1. A public health official feels that more than 70% of the children under age 3 who are treated at a certain clinic get less than the recommended daily allowance of vitamin A. To substantiate this claim, he will take a random sample of 15 children and determine the average vitamin A dosage for each. The test statistic is X, the number receiving less than the recommended daily average of .6 mg. The hypothesis being tested is

$$H_0:\ p \leq .7$$
$$H_1:\ p > .7$$

where p is the proportion receiving less than the recommended daily average.
   (a) If the null value is correct and $p = .7$, what is $E[X]$?
   (b) If when the test is run 12 children appear to be receiving less than the daily minimum, will H_0 be rejected? Explain based on the P value of the test.

2. A new method for grafting oranges has been devised. It is felt that the proportion of grafts that fail to take, p, will be reduced from the current rate of .2. To verify this claim, the new method is used on 20 randomly selected trees, and the number of grafts which fail to take, X, is the test statistic.

(a) Set up the appropriate null and alternative hypotheses for running the test.

(b) If H_0 is true, how many failures would you expect to see?

(c) When the test was run, there were no failures. What practical conclusion should be drawn? Explain based on the P value of the test.

3. A chemical spill occurred in the Xavier River, and wildlife biologists are concerned about toxic accumulation of the chemical in tissues of fish downstream. Previous measurements have shown that only 20% of the fish contain more than 1.5 mg of the chemical per kilogram of body weight. A sample of 16 fish is to be collected following the spill. The statistic to be used to detect the effects of the spill is X, the number of fish that exceed the 1.5-mg limit.

(a) Set up the appropriate null and alternative hypotheses for detecting a situation in which the proportion p of fish that exceeds the accepted limit of 1.5 mg per kilogram of body weight has become larger than 20%.

(b) If H_0 is true, how many of the 16 fish sampled would you expect to exceed the limit?

(c) If the observed value of X is too large to have occurred by chance, H_0 should be rejected. Suppose that of 16 fish examined, 5 are found to exceed the 1.5-mg level. Should H_0 be rejected? Explain by computing the P value of the test.

4. In this problem you will see the interrelationships that exist between α, β, power, and sample size. In each case we predetermine a set of values that lead to the rejection of H_0. That is, we predetermine a critical region. By so doing we preset α. As you move from parts a to d, α will be kept stable as n is allowed to increase. You are asked to think about the effect that this has on power.

A new surgical procedure is to be tested. The current procedure is effective with 50% of the patients on whom it is tried. If the new procedure can be shown to be 60% effective, then it will be put into widespread use. Thus we want to test

$$H_0:\ p = .5$$
$$H_1:\ p = .6$$

The test statistic is X, the number of patients for whom the new procedure is effective. Thus if H_0 is true, X is binomial with parameters n and $p = .5$, $E[X] = n(.5)$, and Var $X = n(.5)(.5)$; if H_1 is true, X is binomial with parameters n and $p = .6$, $E[X] = n(.6)$, and Var $X = n(.6)(.4)$.

(a) For a sample of size 10, we reject H_0 if and only if X is in the set $\{8, 9, 10\}$. That is, the critical region is $\{8, 9, 10\}$. Find α for this test. Find the power of the test. That is, find the probability that $X = 8$, $X = 9$, or $X = 10$ if $p = .6$. With a sample this small, is there a good chance of being able to detect an effectiveness rate of .6 while maintaining an α level of approximately .05?

(b) For a sample of size 15, we use a critical region of $\{11, 12, 13, 14, 15\}$. What is the value of α for this test? What is the power if $p = .6$? Is this sample large enough to expect to detect a p of .6 while maintaining an α level of approximately .05?

(c) If n is increased to 20, what critical region should be chosen to obtain an α level of approximately .05? What is the power for this test if $p = .6$?

(d) It should be clear that to distinguish between $p = .5$ and $p = .6$ with $\alpha \doteq .05$, we must use a sample larger than 20. Use the normal approximation to the binomial distribution to show that for a sample of size 100, $P[X \geq 59] \doteq .05$. Show that when $p = .6$, the power for this test is over .50. That is, find $P[X \geq 59]$ if X is binomial with $n = 100$ and $p = .6$. (Use the normal approximation to the binomial distribution explained in Section 13.9 to find P.)

Summation Notation and Rules for Expectation and Variance

SUMMATION NOTATION

In many statistical procedures it is necessary to manipulate sets of numerical observations. A shorthand notation has been developed to help simplify these operations. The notation uses the Greek letter sigma (Σ) to indicate addition. The use of this notation is illustrated below.

EXAMPLE A.1. Consider the following set of observations:

$$x_1 = 4 \qquad x_3 = 2 \qquad x_5 = -3$$
$$x_2 = 1 \qquad x_4 = 5$$

$$\sum_{i=1}^{5} x_i = x_1 + x_2 + x_3 + x_4 + x_5 \qquad \text{(add the } x\text{'s)}$$
$$= 4 + 1 + 2 + 5 + (-3) = 9$$

$$\sum_{i=1}^{5} x_i^2 = x_1^2 + x_2^2 + x_3^2 + x_4^2 + x_5^2 \qquad \text{(add the}$$
$$= 4^2 + 1^2 + 2^2 + 5^2 + (-3)^2 \qquad \text{squares of } x\text{'s)}$$
$$= 16 + 1 + 4 + 25 + 9 = 55$$

$$\sum_{i=1}^{5} 2x_i = 2x_1 + 2x_2 + 2x_3 + 2x_4 + 2x_5 \qquad \text{(multiply each } x\text{)}$$
$$= 2(4) + 2(1) + 2(2) + 2(5) + 2(-3) \qquad \text{by 2, then add)}$$
$$= 8 + 2 + 4 + 10 + (-6) = 18$$

$$\sum_{i=1}^{5} (x_i - 1) = (4 - 1) + (1 - 1) + (2 - 1) \qquad \text{(subtract 1 from each}$$
$$+ (5 - 1) + (-3 - 1) \qquad \text{observation, then add)}$$
$$= 3 + 0 + 1 + 4 - 4 = 4$$

$$\sum_{i=1}^{3} x_i = x_1 + x_2 + x_3 \qquad \text{(add first}$$
$$= 4 + 1 + 2 = 7 \qquad \text{three observations)}$$

$$\sum_{i=3}^{5} x_i^3 = x_3^3 + x_4^3 + x_5^3 \qquad \text{(add cubes of}$$
$$= 2^3 + 5^3 + (-3)^3 \qquad \text{last three observations)}$$
$$= 8 + 125 - 27 = 106$$

In most statistical applications, all the observations are used in the computations. When this is true, the limits of summation and the subscripts may be omitted. In this case, we could write $\sum x = 9$, $\sum x^2 = 55$, $\sum 2x = 18$, and $\sum (x - 1) = 4$. The limits of summation and the subscripts cannot be dropped in the last two calculations.

PRACTICE 1. Consider this set of observations:

$$y_1 = 3 \qquad y_3 = 1 \qquad y_5 = 2$$

$$y_2 = 6 \qquad y_4 = -1 \qquad y_6 = -4$$

Find $\sum y$, $\sum y^2$, $\sum 3y$, $\sum (y + 2)$, $\sum_{i=1}^{3} y_i$, $\sum_{i=3}^{6} y_i^2$, $\sum_{i=2}^{5} 2y_i$. (Answers are given at the end of Appendix A.)

RULES FOR SUMMATION. The following rules allow us to simplify complex expressions so they can be evaluated quickly:

RULE 1 $\qquad\qquad\qquad \sum_{i=1}^{n} c = nc \qquad\qquad\qquad$ (*c* is any real number)

RULE 2 $\qquad\qquad\qquad \sum_{i=1}^{n} cx_i = c \sum_{i=1}^{n} x_i \qquad\qquad$ (constants can be factored out of summation expressions)

RULE 3 $\qquad \sum_{i=1}^{n} (x_i + y_i) = \sum_{i=1}^{n} x_i + \sum_{i=1}^{n} y_i \qquad$ (sums can be split and evaluated separately)

EXAMPLE A.2. Consider these two data sets:

$$x_1 = 2 \qquad\qquad y_1 = 2$$
$$x_2 = 3 \qquad\qquad y_2 = -1$$
$$x_3 = 5 \qquad\qquad y_3 = 4$$
$$x_4 = 2 \qquad\qquad y_4 = 6$$
$$\sum_{i=1}^{4} x_i = 12 \qquad \sum_{i=1}^{4} y_i = 11$$

Consider the expression

$$\sum_{i=1}^{4} (2x_i - 3y_i + 3)$$

The rules for summation can be used to simplify this expression as follows:

$$\sum_{i=1}^{4} (2x_i - 3y_i + 3) = \sum_{i=1}^{4} 2x_i + \sum_{i=1}^{4} (-3)y_i + \sum_{i=1}^{4} 3 \qquad \text{(rule 3)}$$

$$= 2 \sum_{i=1}^{4} x_i - 3 \sum_{i=1}^{4} y_i + \sum_{i=1}^{4} 3 \qquad \text{(rule 2)}$$

$$= 2(12) - 3(11) + 4(3)$$

$$= 24 - 33 + 12 = 3$$

(rule 1 and substitution)

PRACTICE 2. Consider these two data sets:

$$x_1 = 1 \qquad y_1 = -2$$

$$x_2 = 4 \qquad y_2 = 4$$

$$x_3 = -3 \qquad y_3 = 5$$

Find $\sum x$, $\sum y$, $\sum x^2$, $\sum y^2$, $\sum (2x + y)$, $\sum (3x - 2y)$, $\sum (3x + 2y - 1)$, and $\sum (x + 3y + 4)$.

RULES FOR EXPECTATION AND VARIANCE

There are three rules for expectation and three rules for variance that are useful in proving some of the statistical results that are stated in the text. These rules are given and illustrated here. Our first application of the rules will be in proving that $E[\bar{X}] = \mu$ and Var $\bar{X} = \sigma^2/n$.

RULES FOR EXPECTATION. Let X and Y be random variables, and let c be any real number.

1. $E[c] = c$ (The expected value of any constant is that constant.)
2. $E[cX] = cE[X]$ (Constants can be factored from expectations.)
3. $E[X + Y] = E[X] + E[Y]$ (The expected value of a sum is equal to the sum of the expected values.)

EXAMPLE A.3. Let X and Y be random variables such that $E[X] = 3$ and $E[Y] = -2$. Then

$$E[X + Y] = E[X] + E[Y] = 3 + (-2) = 1$$

$$E[2X + Y] = E[2X] + E[Y]$$

$$= 2E[X] + E[Y]$$

$$= 2(3) + (-2) = 4$$

$$E[X - 3Y + 1] = E[X] + E[-3Y] + E[1]$$

$$= E[X] + (-3)E[Y] + E[1]$$

$$= 3 + (-3)(-2) + 1$$

$$= 10$$

RULES FOR VARIANCE. Let X and Y be random variables and c any real number. Then

1. Var $c = 0$.
2. Var $cX = c^2$ Var X.
3. If X and Y are independent, then $\text{Var}(X + Y) = \text{Var } X + \text{Var } Y$. (Two variables are independent if the value assumed by one has no influence on the value assumed by the other.)

EXAMPLE A.4. Let X and Y be independent with $\mu_X = 2$, $\mu_Y = 6$, $\sigma_X^2 = 9$, and $\sigma_Y^2 = 3$. Then

$$E[2X - 3Y - 6] = 2E[X] - 3E[Y] - 6$$
$$= 2(2) - 3(6) - 6$$
$$= -20$$

$$\text{Var}[2X - 3Y - 6] = \text{Var } 2X + \text{Var}[-3Y] + \text{Var}[-6]$$
$$= 4 \text{ Var } X + 9 \text{ Var } Y + 0$$
$$= 4(9) + 9(3)$$
$$= 63$$

To say that $X_1, X_2, \ldots, X_n$ is a random sample from the distribution of X means that each of these random variables has exactly the same mean and variance as X as well as the same shape. If X is normally distributed with mean 10 and variance 16, then each of the random variables $X_1, X_2, \ldots, X_n$ is also normally distributed with mean 10 and variance 16. Furthermore, the term *random sample* implies that these random variables are independent. With these ideas in mind it is possible to use the rules for expectation and variance to verify the claims concerning $\bar{X}$ made in Section 6.2.

EXAMPLE A.5. Assume that $\bar{X}$ is the sample mean based on a random sample of size n drawn from a distribution with mean μ and variance σ^2. Since $X = (X_1 + X_2 + \cdots + X_n)/n$,

$$E[\bar{X}] = E\left[\frac{X_1 + X_2 + \cdots + X_n}{n}\right]$$

By rule 2 for expectation, the constant $1/n$ can be factored to yield

$$E[\bar{X}] = \left(\frac{1}{n}\right) E[X_1 + X_2 + \cdots + X_n]$$

Rule 3 for expectation allows us to rewrite the expression as

$$E[\bar{X}] = \left(\frac{1}{n}\right) \{E[X_1] + E[X_2] + \cdots + E[X_n]\}$$

However, $E[X]$ and μ are interchangeable symbols for the average value of X. Since each of the random variables $X_1, X_2, \ldots, X_n$ has the same average value as X, we can replace $E[X_1], E[X_2], \ldots, E[X_n]$ each by μ. We can conclude that

$$E[\bar{X}] = \frac{1}{n} \underbrace{(\mu + \mu + \cdots + \mu)}_{n \text{ terms}}$$

$$= \frac{1}{n}(n\mu)$$

$$= \mu$$

as claimed in Section 6.2. Now consider Var $\bar{X}$.

$$\text{Var } \bar{X} = \text{Var}\left[\frac{1}{n}(X_1 + X_2 + \cdots + X_n)\right]$$

$$= \left(\frac{1}{n}\right)^2 \text{Var}(X_1 + X_2 + \cdots + X_n)$$

$$= \left(\frac{1}{n}\right)^2 (\sigma^2 + \sigma^2 + \cdots + \sigma^2)$$

$$= \left(\frac{1}{n}\right)^2 n\sigma^2 = \frac{\sigma^2}{n}$$

Note that since σ^2 is a constant, as n increases in size, σ^2/n becomes smaller. Thus, for large n, Var $\bar{X}$ is rather small. This means that for large n, most observed sample means will lie close to μ as desired.

PRACTICE 3. Let X and Y be independent such that $\mu_X = 2$, $\mu_Y = 6$, $\sigma_X^2 = 9$, $\sigma_Y^2 = 16$. Find the numerical values of parts a through f.

(*a*) σ_X, σ_Y
(*b*) $E[X^2]$, $E[Y^2]$
(*c*) $E[X + 2Y]$, $\text{Var}[X + 2Y]$
(*d*) $E[3X - 2Y - 2]$, $\text{Var}[3X - 2Y - 2]$
(*e*) $E[(X - 2)/3]$, $\text{Var}[(X - 2)/3]$
(*f*) $E[(Y - 6)/4]$, $\text{Var}[(Y - 6)/4]$
(*g*) The results of parts *e* and *f* are not coincidental. Try to generalize the pattern observed there.

PRACTICE 4. If 5 is systematically added to each observed value of some random variable X to form a new variable Y, what is the relationship between the mean of X and the mean of Y? Between the variance of X and the variance of Y? Between the standard deviation of X and the standard deviation of Y?

PRACTICE 5. If each observed value of X is systematically multiplied by 10 to form a new variable Y, what is the relationship between the mean of X and the mean of Y? Between the variance of X and the variance of Y? Between the standard deviation of X and the standard deviation of Y?

PRACTICE 6. Use the rules of expectation and the rules of variance to prove Theorem 5.3.1. Assume that $(X - \mu)/\sigma$ is normal.

Answers to Practice Problems

1. 7, 67, 21, 19, 10, 22, 16
2. 2, 7, 26, 45, 11, −8, 17, 35

Statistical Tables

TABLE I

Cumulative binomial distribution

$$F_X(t) = P[X \leq t] = \sum_{x \leq t} \binom{n}{x} p^x (1-p)^{n-x}$$

							p					
n	t	0.1	0.2	0.25	0.3	0.4	0.5	0.6	0.7	0.75	0.8	0.9
5	0	0.5905	0.3277	0.2373	0.1681	0.0778	0.0312	0.0102	0.0024	0.0010	0.0003	0.0000
	1	0.9185	0.7373	0.6328	0.5282	0.3370	0.1875	0.0870	0.0308	0.0156	0.0067	0.0005
	2	0.9914	0.9421	0.8965	0.8369	0.6826	0.5000	0.3174	0.1631	0.1035	0.0579	0.0086
	3	0.9995	0.9933	0.9844	0.9692	0.9130	0.8125	0.6630	0.4718	0.3672	0.2627	0.0815
	4	1.0000	0.9997	0.9990	0.9976	0.9898	0.9688	0.9222	0.8319	0.7627	0.6723	0.4095
	5	1.0000	1.0000	1.0000	1.0000	1.0000	1.0000	1.0000	1.0000	1.0000	1.0000	1.0000
6	0	0.5314	0.2621	0.1780	0.1176	0.0467	0.0156	0.0041	0.0007	0.0002	0.0001	0.0000
	1	0.8857	0.6554	0.5339	0.4202	0.2333	0.1094	0.0410	0.0109	0.0046	0.0016	0.0001
	2	0.9841	0.9011	0.8306	0.7443	0.5443	0.3437	0.1792	0.0705	0.0376	0.0170	0.0013
	3	0.9987	0.9830	0.9624	0.9295	0.8208	0.6562	0.4557	0.2557	0.1694	0.0989	0.0159
	4	0.9999	0.9984	0.9954	0.9891	0.9590	0.8906	0.7667	0.5798	0.4661	0.3446	0.1143
	5	1.0000	0.9999	0.9998	0.9993	0.9959	0.9844	0.9533	0.8824	0.8220	0.7379	0.4686
	6	1.0000	1.0000	1.0000	1.0000	1.0000	1.0000	1.0000	1.0000	1.0000	1.0000	1.0000
7	0	0.4783	0.2097	0.1335	0.0824	0.0280	0.0078	0.0016	0.0002	0.0001	0.0000	0.0000
	1	0.8503	0.5767	0.4449	0.3294	0.1586	0.0625	0.0188	0.0038	0.0013	0.0004	0.0000
	2	0.9743	0.8520	0.7564	0.6471	0.4199	0.2266	0.0963	0.0288	0.0129	0.0047	0.0002
	3	0.9973	0.9667	0.9294	0.8740	0.7102	0.5000	0.2898	0.1260	0.0706	0.0333	0.0027
	4	0.9998	0.9953	0.9871	0.9712	0.9037	0.7734	0.5801	0.3529	0.2436	0.1480	0.0257
	5	1.0000	0.9996	0.9987	0.9962	0.9812	0.9375	0.8414	0.6706	0.5551	0.4233	0.1497
	6	1.0000	1.0000	0.9999	0.9998	0.9984	0.9922	0.9720	0.9176	0.8665	0.7903	0.5217
	7	1.0000	1.0000	1.0000	1.0000	1.0000	1.0000	1.0000	1.0000	1.0000	1.0000	1.0000
8	0	0.4305	0.1678	0.1001	0.0576	0.0168	0.0039	0.0007	0.0001	0.0000	0.0000	0.0000
	1	0.8131	0.5033	0.3671	0.2553	0.1064	0.0352	0.0085	0.0013	0.0004	0.0001	0.0000
	2	0.9619	0.7969	0.6785	0.5518	0.3154	0.1445	0.0498	0.0113	0.0042	0.0012	0.0000
	3	0.9950	0.9437	0.8862	0.8059	0.5941	0.3633	0.1737	0.0580	0.0273	0.0104	0.0004
	4	0.9996	0.9896	0.9727	0.9420	0.8263	0.6367	0.4059	0.1941	0.1138	0.0563	0.0050
	5	1.0000	0.9988	0.9958	0.9887	0.9502	0.8555	0.6846	0.4482	0.3215	0.2031	0.0381

TABLE I

(*Continued*)

n	t	0.1	0.2	0.25	0.3	0.4	0.5	0.6	0.7	0.75	0.8	0.9
							p					
	6	1.0000	0.9999	0.9996	0.9987	0.9915	0.9648	0.8936	0.7447	0.6329	0.4967	0.1869
	7	1.0000	1.0000	1.0000	0.9999	0.9993	0.9961	0.9832	0.9424	0.8999	0.8322	0.5695
	8	1.0000	1.0000	1.0000	1.0000	1.0000	1.0000	1.0000	1.0000	1.0000	1.0000	1.0000
9	0	0.3874	0.1342	0.0751	0.0404	0.0101	0.0020	0.0003	0.0000	0.0000	0.0000	0.0000
	1	0.7748	0.4362	0.3003	0.1960	0.0705	0.0195	0.0038	0.0004	0.0001	0.0000	0.0000
	2	0.9470	0.7382	0.6007	0.4628	0.2318	0.0898	0.0250	0.0043	0.0013	0.0003	0.0000
	3	0.9917	0.9144	0.8343	0.7297	0.4826	0.2539	0.0994	0.0253	0.0100	0.0031	0.0001
	4	0.9991	0.9804	0.9511	0.9012	0.7334	0.5000	0.2666	0.0988	0.0489	0.0196	0.0009
	5	0.9999	0.9969	0.9900	0.9747	0.9006	0.7461	0.5174	0.2703	0.1657	0.0856	0.0083
	6	1.0000	0.9997	0.9987	0.9957	0.9750	0.9102	0.7682	0.5372	0.3993	0.2618	0.0530
	7	1.0000	1.0000	0.9999	0.9996	0.9962	0.9805	0.9295	0.8040	0.6997	0.5638	0.2252
	8	1.0000	1.0000	1.0000	1.0000	0.9997	0.9980	0.9899	0.9596	0.9249	0.8658	0.6126
	9	1.0000	1.0000	1.0000	1.0000	1.0000	1.0000	1.0000	1.0000	1.0000	1.0000	1.0000
10	0	0.3487	0.1074	0.0563	0.0282	0.0060	0.0010	0.0001	0.0000	0.0000	0.0000	0.0000
	1	0.7361	0.3758	0.2440	0.1493	0.0464	0.0107	0.0017	0.0001	0.0000	0.0000	0.0000
	2	0.9298	0.6778	0.5256	0.3828	0.1673	0.0547	0.0123	0.0016	0.0004	0.0001	0.0000
	3	0.9872	0.8791	0.7759	0.6496	0.3823	0.1719	0.0548	0.0106	0.0035	0.0009	0.0000
	4	0.9984	0.9672	0.9219	0.8497	0.6331	0.3770	0.1662	0.0473	0.0197	0.0064	0.0001
	5	0.9999	0.9936	0.9803	0.9527	0.8338	0.6230	0.3669	0.1503	0.0781	0.0328	0.0016
	6	1.0000	0.9991	0.9965	0.9894	0.9452	0.8281	0.6177	0.3504	0.2241	0.1209	0.0128
	7	1.0000	0.9999	0.9996	0.9984	0.9877	0.9453	0.8327	0.6172	0.4744	0.3222	0.0702
	8	1.0000	1.0000	1.0000	0.9999	0.9983	0.9893	0.9536	0.8507	0.7560	0.6242	0.2639
	9	1.0000	1.0000	1.0000	1.0000	0.9999	0.9990	0.9940	0.9718	0.9437	0.8926	0.6513
	10	1.0000	1.0000	1.0000	1.0000	1.0000	1.0000	1.0000	1.0000	1.0000	1.0000	1.0000
11	0	0.3138	0.0859	0.0422	0.0198	0.0036	0.0005	0.0000	0.0000	0.0000	0.0000	0.0000
	1	0.6974	0.3221	0.1971	0.1130	0.0302	0.0059	0.0007	0.0000	0.0000	0.0000	0.0000
	2	0.9104	0.6174	0.4552	0.3127	0.1189	0.0327	0.0059	0.0006	0.0001	0.0000	0.0000
	3	0.9815	0.8389	0.7133	0.5696	0.2963	0.1133	0.0293	0.0043	0.0012	0.0002	0.0000
	4	0.9972	0.9496	0.8854	0.7897	0.5328	0.2744	0.0994	0.0216	0.0076	0.0020	0.0000
	5	0.9997	0.9883	0.9657	0.9218	0.7535	0.5000	0.2465	0.0782	0.0343	0.0117	0.0003
	6	1.0000	0.9980	0.9924	0.9784	0.9006	0.7256	0.4672	0.2103	0.1146	0.0504	0.0028
	7	1.0000	0.9998	0.9988	0.9957	0.9707	0.8867	0.7037	0.4304	0.2867	0.1611	0.0185
	8	1.0000	1.0000	0.9999	0.9994	0.9941	0.9673	0.8811	0.6873	0.5448	0.3826	0.0896
	9	1.0000	1.0000	1.0000	1.0000	0.9993	0.9941	0.9698	0.8870	0.8029	0.6779	0.3026
	10	1.0000	1.0000	1.0000	1.0000	1.0000	0.9995	0.9964	0.9802	0.9578	0.9141	0.6862
	11	1.0000	1.0000	1.0000	1.0000	1.0000	1.0000	1.0000	1.0000	1.0000	1.0000	1.0000
12	0	0.2824	0.0687	0.0317	0.0138	0.0022	0.0002	0.0000	0.0000	0.0000	0.0000	0.0000
	1	0.6590	0.2749	0.1584	0.0850	0.0196	0.0032	0.0003	0.0000	0.0000	0.0000	0.0000
	2	0.8891	0.5583	0.3907	0.2528	0.0834	0.0193	0.0028	0.0002	0.0000	0.0000	0.0000
	3	0.9744	0.7946	0.6488	0.4925	0.2253	0.0730	0.0153	0.0017	0.0004	0.0001	0.0000
	4	0.9957	0.9274	0.8424	0.7237	0.4382	0.1938	0.0573	0.0095	0.0028	0.0006	0.0000
	5	0.9995	0.9806	0.9456	0.8822	0.6652	0.3872	0.1582	0.0386	0.0143	0.0039	0.0001
	6	0.9999	0.9961	0.9857	0.9614	0.8418	0.6128	0.3348	0.1178	0.0544	0.0194	0.0005
	7	1.0000	0.9994	0.9972	0.9905	0.9427	0.8062	0.5618	0.2763	0.1576	0.0726	0.0043
	8	1.0000	0.9999	0.9996	0.9983	0.9847	0.9270	0.7747	0.5075	0.3512	0.2054	0.0256
	9	1.0000	1.0000	1.0000	0.9998	0.9972	0.9807	0.9166	0.7472	0.6093	0.4417	0.1109
	10	1.0000	1.0000	1.0000	1.0000	0.9997	0.9968	0.9804	0.9150	0.8416	0.7251	0.3410

TABLE I

(Continued)

n	t	0.1	0.2	0.25	0.3	0.4	0.5	0.6	0.7	0.75	0.8	0.9
							p					
	11	1.0000	1.0000	1.0000	1.0000	1.0000	0.9998	0.9978	0.9862	0.9683	0.9313	0.7176
	12	1.0000	1.0000	1.0000	1.0000	1.0000	1.0000	1.0000	1.0000	1.0000	1.0000	1.0000
13	0	0.2542	0.0550	0.0238	0.0097	0.0013	0.0001	0.0000	0.0000	0.0000	0.0000	0.0000
	1	0.6213	0.2336	0.1267	0.0637	0.0126	0.0017	0.0001	0.0000	0.0000	0.0000	0.0000
	2	0.8661	0.5017	0.3326	0.2025	0.0579	0.0112	0.0013	0.0001	0.0000	0.0000	0.0000
	3	0.9658	0.7473	0.5843	0.4206	0.1686	0.0461	0.0078	0.0007	0.0001	0.0000	0.0000
	4	0.9935	0.9009	0.7940	0.6543	0.3530	0.1334	0.0321	0.0040	0.0010	0.0002	0.0000
	5	0.9991	0.9700	0.9198	0.8346	0.5744	0.2905	0.0977	0.0182	0.0056	0.0012	0.0000
	6	0.9999	0.9930	0.9757	0.9376	0.7712	0.5000	0.2288	0.0624	0.0243	0.0070	0.0001
	7	1.0000	0.9988	0.9944	0.9818	0.9023	0.7095	0.4256	0.1654	0.0802	0.0300	0.0009
	8	1.0000	0.9998	0.9990	0.9960	0.9679	0.8666	0.6470	0.3457	0.2060	0.0991	0.0065
	9	1.0000	1.0000	0.9999	0.9993	0.9922	0.9539	0.8314	0.5794	0.4157	0.2527	0.0342
	10	1.0000	1.0000	1.0000	0.9999	0.9987	0.9888	0.9421	0.7975	0.6674	0.4983	0.1339
	11	1.0000	1.0000	1.0000	1.0000	0.9999	0.9983	0.9874	0.9363	0.8733	0.7664	0.3787
	12	1.0000	1.0000	1.0000	1.0000	1.0000	0.9999	0.9987	0.9903	0.9762	0.9450	0.7458
	13	1.0000	1.0000	1.0000	1.0000	1.0000	1.0000	1.0000	1.0000	1.0000	1.0000	1.0000
14	0	0.2288	0.0440	0.0178	0.0068	0.0008	0.0001	0.0000	0.0000	0.0000	0.0000	0.0000
	1	0.5846	0.1979	0.1010	0.0475	0.0081	0.0009	0.0001	0.0000	0.0000	0.0000	0.0000
	2	0.8416	0.4481	0.2811	0.1608	0.0398	0.0065	0.0006	0.0000	0.0000	0.0000	0.0000
	3	0.9559	0.6982	0.5213	0.3552	0.1243	0.0287	0.0039	0.0002	0.0000	0.0000	0.0000
	4	0.9908	0.8702	0.7415	0.5842	0.2793	0.0898	0.0175	0.0017	0.0003	0.0000	0.0000
	5	0.9985	0.9561	0.8883	0.7805	0.4859	0.2120	0.0583	0.0083	0.0022	0.0004	0.0000
	6	0.9998	0.9884	0.9617	0.9067	0.6925	0.3953	0.1501	0.0315	0.0103	0.0024	0.0000
	7	1.0000	0.9976	0.9897	0.9685	0.8499	0.6047	0.3075	0.0933	0.0383	0.0116	0.0002
	8	1.0000	0.9996	0.9978	0.9917	0.9417	0.7880	0.5141	0.2195	0.1117	0.0439	0.0015
	9	1.0000	1.0000	0.9997	0.9983	0.9825	0.9102	0.7207	0.4158	0.2585	0.1298	0.0092
	10	1.0000	1.0000	1.0000	0.9998	0.9961	0.9713	0.8757	0.6448	0.4787	0.3018	0.0441
	11	1.0000	1.0000	1.0000	1.0000	0.9994	0.9935	0.9602	0.8392	0.7189	0.5519	0.1584
	12	1.0000	1.0000	1.0000	1.0000	0.9999	0.9991	0.9919	0.9525	0.8990	0.8021	0.4154
	13	1.0000	1.0000	1.0000	1.0000	1.0000	0.9999	0.9992	0.9932	0.9822	0.9560	0.7712
	14	1.0000	1.0000	1.0000	1.0000	1.0000	1.0000	1.0000	1.0000	1.0000	1.0000	1.0000
15	0	0.2059	0.0352	0.0134	0.0047	0.0005	0.0000	0.0000	0.0000	0.0000	0.0000	0.0000
	1	0.5490	0.1671	0.0802	0.0353	0.0052	0.0005	0.0000	0.0000	0.0000	0.0000	0.0000
	2	0.8159	0.3980	0.2361	0.1268	0.0271	0.0037	0.0003	0.0000	0.0000	0.0000	0.0000
	3	0.9444	0.6482	0.4613	0.2969	0.0905	0.0176	0.0019	0.0001	0.0000	0.0000	0.0000
	4	0.9873	0.8358	0.6865	0.5155	0.2173	0.0592	0.0093	0.0007	0.0001	0.0000	0.0000
	5	0.9978	0.9389	0.8516	0.7216	0.4032	0.1509	0.0338	0.0037	0.0008	0.0001	0.0000
	6	0.9997	0.9819	0.9434	0.8689	0.6098	0.3036	0.0950	0.0152	0.0042	0.0008	0.0000
	7	1.0000	0.9958	0.9827	0.9500	0.7869	0.5000	0.2131	0.0500	0.0173	0.0042	0.0000
	8	1.0000	0.9992	0.9958	0.9848	0.9050	0.6964	0.3902	0.1311	0.0566	0.0181	0.0003
	9	1.0000	0.9999	0.9992	0.9963	0.9662	0.8491	0.5968	0.2784	0.1484	0.0611	0.0022
	10	1.0000	1.0000	0.9999	0.9993	0.9907	0.9408	0.7827	0.4845	0.3135	0.1642	0.0127
	11	1.0000	1.0000	1.0000	0.9999	0.9981	0.9824	0.9095	0.7031	0.5387	0.3518	0.0556
	12	1.0000	1.0000	1.0000	1.0000	0.9997	0.9963	0.9729	0.8732	0.7639	0.6020	0.1841
	13	1.0000	1.0000	1.0000	1.0000	1.0000	0.9995	0.9948	0.9647	0.9198	0.8329	0.4510
	14	1.0000	1.0000	1.0000	1.0000	1.0000	1.0000	0.9995	0.9953	0.9866	0.9648	0.7941
	15	1.0000	1.0000	1.0000	1.0000	1.0000	1.0000	1.0000	1.0000	1.0000	1.0000	1.0000

▨ **TABLE I**
(*Continued*)

n	t	0.1	0.2	0.25	0.3	0.4	0.5	0.6	0.7	0.75	0.8	0.9
16	0	0.1853	0.0281	0.0100	0.0033	0.0003	0.0000	0.0000	0.0000	0.0000	0.0000	0.0000
	1	0.5147	0.1407	0.0635	0.0261	0.0033	0.0003	0.0000	0.0000	0.0000	0.0000	0.0000
	2	0.7892	0.3518	0.1971	0.0994	0.0183	0.0021	0.0001	0.0000	0.0000	0.0000	0.0000
	3	0.9316	0.5981	0.4050	0.2459	0.0651	0.0106	0.0009	0.0000	0.0000	0.0000	0.0000
	4	0.9830	0.7982	0.6302	0.4499	0.1666	0.0384	0.0049	0.0003	0.0000	0.0000	0.0000
	5	0.9967	0.9183	0.8103	0.6598	0.3288	0.1051	0.0191	0.0016	0.0003	0.0000	0.0000
	6	0.9995	0.9733	0.9204	0.8247	0.5272	0.2272	0.0583	0.0071	0.0016	0.0002	0.0000
	7	0.9999	0.9930	0.9729	0.9256	0.7161	0.4018	0.1423	0.0257	0.0075	0.0015	0.0000
	8	1.0000	0.9985	0.9925	0.9743	0.8577	0.5982	0.2839	0.0744	0.0271	0.0070	0.0001
	9	1.0000	0.9998	0.9984	0.9929	0.9417	0.7728	0.4728	0.1753	0.0796	0.0267	0.0005
	10	1.0000	1.0000	0.9997	0.9984	0.9809	0.8949	0.6712	0.3402	0.1897	0.0817	0.0033
	11	1.0000	1.0000	1.0000	0.9997	0.9951	0.9616	0.8334	0.5501	0.3698	0.2018	0.0170
	12	1.0000	1.0000	1.0000	1.0000	0.9991	0.9894	0.9349	0.7541	0.5950	0.4019	0.0684
	13	1.0000	1.0000	1.0000	1.0000	0.9999	0.9979	0.9817	0.9006	0.8029	0.6482	0.2108
	14	1.0000	1.0000	1.0000	1.0000	1.0000	0.9997	0.9967	0.9739	0.9365	0.8593	0.4853
	15	1.0000	1.0000	1.0000	1.0000	1.0000	1.0000	0.9997	0.9967	0.9900	0.9719	0.8147
	16	1.0000	1.0000	1.0000	1.0000	1.0000	1.0000	1.0000	1.0000	1.0000	1.0000	1.0000
17	0	0.1668	0.0225	0.0075	0.0023	0.0002	0.0000	0.0000	0.0000	0.0000	0.0000	0.0000
	1	0.4818	0.1182	0.0501	0.0193	0.0021	0.0001	0.0000	0.0000	0.0000	0.0000	0.0000
	2	0.7618	0.3096	0.1637	0.0774	0.0123	0.0012	0.0001	0.0000	0.0000	0.0000	0.0000
	3	0.9174	0.5489	0.3530	0.2019	0.0464	0.0064	0.0005	0.0000	0.0000	0.0000	0.0000
	4	0.9779	0.7582	0.5739	0.3887	0.1260	0.0245	0.0025	0.0001	0.0000	0.0000	0.0000
	5	0.9953	0.8943	0.7653	0.5968	0.2639	0.0717	0.0106	0.0007	0.0001	0.0000	0.0000
	6	0.9992	0.9623	0.8929	0.7752	0.4478	0.1662	0.0348	0.0032	0.0006	0.0001	0.0000
	7	0.9999	0.9891	0.9598	0.8954	0.6405	0.3145	0.0919	0.0127	0.0031	0.0005	0.0000
	8	1.0000	0.9974	0.9876	0.9597	0.8011	0.5000	0.1989	0.0403	0.0124	0.0026	0.0000
	9	1.0000	0.9995	0.9969	0.9873	0.9081	0.6855	0.3595	0.1046	0.0402	0.0109	0.0001
	10	1.0000	0.9999	0.9994	0.9968	0.9652	0.8338	0.5522	0.2248	0.1071	0.0377	0.0008
	11	1.0000	1.0000	0.9999	0.9993	0.9894	0.9283	0.7361	0.4032	0.2347	0.1057	0.0047
	12	1.0000	1.0000	1.0000	0.9999	0.9975	0.9755	0.8740	0.6113	0.4261	0.2418	0.0221
	13	1.0000	1.0000	1.0000	1.0000	0.9995	0.9936	0.9536	0.7981	0.6470	0.4511	0.0826
	14	1.0000	1.0000	1.0000	1.0000	0.9999	0.9988	0.9877	0.9226	0.8363	0.6904	0.2382
	15	1.0000	1.0000	1.0000	1.0000	1.0000	0.9999	0.9979	0.9807	0.9499	0.8818	0.5182
	16	1.0000	1.0000	1.0000	1.0000	1.0000	1.0000	0.9998	0.9977	0.9925	0.9775	0.8332
	17	1.0000	1.0000	1.0000	1.0000	1.0000	1.0000	1.0000	1.0000	1.0000	1.0000	1.0000
18	0	0.1501	0.0180	0.0056	0.0016	0.0001	0.0000	0.0000	0.0000	0.0000	0.0000	0.0000
	1	0.4503	0.0991	0.0395	0.0142	0.0013	0.0001	0.0000	0.0000	0.0000	0.0000	0.0000
	2	0.7338	0.2713	0.1353	0.0600	0.0082	0.0007	0.0000	0.0000	0.0000	0.0000	0.0000
	3	0.9018	0.5010	0.3057	0.1646	0.0328	0.0038	0.0002	0.0000	0.0000	0.0000	0.0000
	4	0.9718	0.7164	0.5187	0.3327	0.0942	0.0154	0.0013	0.0000	0.0000	0.0000	0.0000
	5	0.9936	0.8671	0.7175	0.5344	0.2088	0.0481	0.0058	0.0003	0.0000	0.0000	0.0000
	6	0.9988	0.9487	0.8610	0.7217	0.3743	0.1189	0.0203	0.0014	0.0002	0.0000	0.0000
	7	0.9998	0.9837	0.9431	0.8593	0.5634	0.2403	0.0576	0.0061	0.0012	0.0002	0.0000
	8	1.0000	0.9957	0.9807	0.9404	0.7368	0.4073	0.1347	0.0210	0.0054	0.0009	0.0000
	9	1.0000	0.9991	0.9946	0.9790	0.8653	0.5927	0.2632	0.0596	0.0193	0.0043	0.0000
	10	1.0000	0.9998	0.9988	0.9939	0.9424	0.7597	0.4366	0.1407	0.0569	0.0163	0.0002
	11	1.0000	1.0000	0.9998	0.9986	0.9797	0.8811	0.6257	0.2783	0.1390	0.0513	0.0012
	12	1.0000	1.0000	1.0000	0.9997	0.9942	0.9519	0.7912	0.4656	0.2825	0.1329	0.0064

TABLE I

(*Concluded*)

n	t	0.1	0.2	0.25	0.3	0.4	0.5	0.6	0.7	0.75	0.8	0.9
	13	1.0000	1.0000	1.0000	1.0000	0.9987	0.9846	0.9058	0.6673	0.4813	0.2836	0.0282
	14	1.0000	1.0000	1.0000	1.0000	0.9998	0.9962	0.9672	0.8354	0.6943	0.4990	0.0982
	15	1.0000	1.0000	1.0000	1.0000	1.0000	0.9993	0.9918	0.9400	0.8647	0.7287	0.2662
	16	1.0000	1.0000	1.0000	1.0000	1.0000	0.9999	0.9987	0.9858	0.9605	0.9009	0.5497
	17	1.0000	1.0000	1.0000	1.0000	1.0000	1.0000	0.9999	0.9984	0.9944	0.9820	0.8499
	18	1.0000	1.0000	1.0000	1.0000	1.0000	1.0000	1.0000	1.0000	1.0000	1.0000	1.0000
19	0	0.1351	0.0144	0.0042	0.0011	0.0001	0.0000	0.0000	0.0000	0.0000	0.0000	0.0000
	1	0.4203	0.0829	0.0310	0.0104	0.0008	0.0000	0.0000	0.0000	0.0000	0.0000	0.0000
	2	0.7054	0.2369	0.1113	0.0462	0.0055	0.0004	0.0000	0.0000	0.0000	0.0000	0.0000
	3	0.8850	0.4551	0.2631	0.1332	0.0230	0.0022	0.0001	0.0000	0.0000	0.0000	0.0000
	4	0.9648	0.6733	0.4654	0.2822	0.0696	0.0096	0.0006	0.0000	0.0000	0.0000	0.0000
	5	0.9914	0.8369	0.6678	0.4739	0.1629	0.0318	0.0031	0.0001	0.0000	0.0000	0.0000
	6	0.9983	0.9324	0.8251	0.6655	0.3081	0.0835	0.0116	0.0006	0.0001	0.0000	0.0000
	7	0.9997	0.9767	0.9225	0.8180	0.4878	0.1796	0.0352	0.0028	0.0005	0.0000	0.0000
	8	1.0000	0.9933	0.9713	0.9161	0.6675	0.3238	0.0885	0.0105	0.0023	0.0003	0.0000
	9	1.0000	0.9984	0.9911	0.9674	0.8139	0.5000	0.0861	0.0326	0.0089	0.0016	0.0000
	10	1.0000	0.9997	0.9977	0.9895	0.9115	0.6762	0.3325	0.0839	0.0287	0.0067	0.0000
	11	1.0000	1.0000	0.9995	0.9972	0.9648	0.8204	0.5122	0.1820	0.0775	0.0233	0.0003
	12	1.0000	1.0000	0.9999	0.9994	0.9884	0.9165	0.6919	0.3345	0.1749	0.0676	0.0017
	13	1.0000	1.0000	1.0000	0.9999	0.9969	0.9682	0.8371	0.5261	0.3322	0.1631	0.0086
	14	1.0000	1.0000	1.0000	1.0000	0.9994	0.9904	0.9304	0.7178	0.5346	0.3267	0.0352
	15	1.0000	1.0000	1.0000	1.0000	0.9999	0.9978	0.9770	0.8668	0.7369	0.5449	0.1150
	16	1.0000	1.0000	1.0000	1.0000	1.0000	0.9996	0.9945	0.9538	0.8887	0.7631	0.2946
	17	1.0000	1.0000	1.0000	1.0000	1.0000	1.0000	0.9992	0.9896	0.9690	0.9171	0.5797
	18	1.0000	1.0000	1.0000	1.0000	1.0000	1.0000	0.9999	0.9989	0.9958	0.9856	0.8649
	19	1.0000	1.0000	1.0000	1.0000	1.0000	1.0000	1.0000	1.0000	1.0000	1.0000	1.0000
20	0	0.1216	0.0115	0.0032	0.0008	0.0000	0.0000	0.0000	0.0000	0.0000	0.0000	0.0000
	1	0.3917	0.0692	0.0243	0.0076	0.0005	0.0000	0.0000	0.0000	0.0000	0.0000	0.0000
	2	0.6769	0.2061	0.0913	0.0355	0.0036	0.0002	0.0000	0.0000	0.0000	0.0000	0.0000
	3	0.8670	0.4114	0.2252	0.1071	0.0160	0.0013	0.0000	0.0000	0.0000	0.0000	0.0000
	4	0.9568	0.6296	0.4148	0.2375	0.0510	0.0059	0.0003	0.0000	0.0000	0.0000	0.0000
	5	0.9887	0.8042	0.6172	0.4164	0.1256	0.0207	0.0016	0.0000	0.0000	0.0000	0.0000
	6	0.9976	0.9133	0.7858	0.6080	0.2500	0.0577	0.0065	0.0003	0.0000	0.0000	0.0000
	7	0.9996	0.9679	0.8982	0.7723	0.4159	0.1316	0.0210	0.0013	0.0002	0.0000	0.0000
	8	0.9999	0.9900	0.9591	0.8867	0.5956	0.2517	0.0565	0.0051	0.0009	0.0001	0.0000
	9	1.0000	0.9974	0.9861	0.9520	0.7553	0.4119	0.1275	0.0171	0.0039	0.0006	0.0000
	10	1.0000	0.9994	0.9961	0.9829	0.8725	0.5881	0.2447	0.0480	0.0139	0.0026	0.0000
	11	1.0000	0.9999	0.9991	0.9949	0.9435	0.7483	0.4044	0.1133	0.0409	0.0100	0.0001
	12	1.0000	1.0000	0.9998	0.9987	0.9790	0.8684	0.5841	0.2277	0.1018	0.0321	0.0004
	13	1.0000	1.0000	1.0000	0.9997	0.9935	0.9423	0.7500	0.3920	0.2142	0.0867	0.0024
	14	1.0000	1.0000	1.0000	1.0000	0.9984	0.9793	0.8744	0.5836	0.3828	0.1958	0.0113
	15	1.0000	1.0000	1.0000	1.0000	0.9997	0.9941	0.9490	0.7625	0.5852	0.3704	0.0432
	16	1.0000	1.0000	1.0000	1.0000	1.0000	0.9987	0.9840	0.8929	0.7748	0.5886	0.1330
	17	1.0000	1.0000	1.0000	1.0000	1.0000	0.9998	0.9964	0.9645	0.9087	0.7939	0.3231
	18	1.0000	1.0000	1.0000	1.0000	1.0000	1.0000	0.9995	0.9924	0.9757	0.9308	0.6083
	19	1.0000	1.0000	1.0000	1.0000	1.0000	1.0000	1.0000	0.9992	0.9968	0.9885	0.8784
	20	1.0000	1.0000	1.0000	1.0000	1.0000	1.0000	1.0000	1.0000	1.0000	1.0000	1.0000

TABLE II
Poisson distribution function

$$F_X(t) = P[X \le t] = \sum_{x \le t} e^{-\lambda s}(\lambda s)^x/x!$$

t	0.5	1.0	2.0	3.0	4.0	5.0	6.0	7.0	8.0	9.0	10.0	11.0	12.0	13.0	14.0	15.0
0	0.607	0.368	0.135	0.050	0.018	0.007	0.002	0.001	0.000	0.000	0.000	0.000	0.000	0.000	0.000	0.000
1	0.910	0.736	0.406	0.199	0.092	0.040	0.017	0.007	0.003	0.001	0.000	0.000	0.000	0.000	0.000	0.000
2	0.986	0.920	0.677	0.423	0.238	0.125	0.062	0.030	0.014	0.006	0.003	0.001	0.001	0.000	0.000	0.000
3	0.998	0.981	0.857	0.647	0.433	0.265	0.151	0.082	0.042	0.021	0.010	0.005	0.002	0.001	0.000	0.000
4	1.000	0.996	0.947	0.815	0.629	0.440	0.285	0.173	0.100	0.055	0.029	0.015	0.008	0.004	0.002	0.001
5	1.000	0.999	0.983	0.916	0.785	0.616	0.446	0.301	0.191	0.116	0.067	0.038	0.020	0.011	0.006	0.003
6	1.000	1.000	0.995	0.966	0.889	0.762	0.606	0.450	0.313	0.207	0.130	0.079	0.046	0.026	0.014	0.008
7	1.000	1.000	0.999	0.988	0.949	0.867	0.744	0.599	0.453	0.324	0.220	0.143	0.090	0.054	0.032	0.018
8	1.000	1.000	1.000	0.996	0.979	0.932	0.847	0.729	0.593	0.456	0.333	0.232	0.155	0.100	0.062	0.037
9	1.000	1.000	1.000	0.999	0.992	0.968	0.916	0.830	0.717	0.587	0.458	0.341	0.242	0.166	0.109	0.070
10	1.000	1.000	1.000	1.000	0.997	0.986	0.957	0.901	0.816	0.706	0.583	0.460	0.347	0.252	0.176	0.118
11	1.000	1.000	1.000	1.000	0.999	0.995	0.980	0.947	0.888	0.803	0.697	0.579	0.462	0.353	0.260	0.185
12	1.000	1.000	1.000	1.000	1.000	0.998	0.991	0.973	0.936	0.876	0.792	0.689	0.576	0.463	0.358	0.268
13	1.000	1.000	1.000	1.000	1.000	0.999	0.996	0.987	0.966	0.926	0.864	0.781	0.682	0.573	0.464	0.363
14	1.000	1.000	1.000	1.000	1.000	1.000	0.999	0.994	0.983	0.959	0.917	0.854	0.772	0.675	0.570	0.466
15	1.000	1.000	1.000	1.000	1.000	1.000	0.999	0.998	0.992	0.978	0.951	0.907	0.844	0.764	0.669	0.568
16	1.000	1.000	1.000	1.000	1.000	1.000	1.000	0.999	0.996	0.989	0.973	0.944	0.899	0.835	0.756	0.664
17	1.000	1.000	1.000	1.000	1.000	1.000	1.000	1.000	0.998	0.995	0.986	0.968	0.937	0.890	0.827	0.749
18	1.000	1.000	1.000	1.000	1.000	1.000	1.000	1.000	0.999	0.998	0.993	0.982	0.963	0.930	0.883	0.819
19	1.000	1.000	1.000	1.000	1.000	1.000	1.000	1.000	1.000	0.999	0.997	0.991	0.979	0.957	0.923	0.875
20	1.000	1.000	1.000	1.000	1.000	1.000	1.000	1.000	1.000	1.000	0.998	0.995	0.988	0.975	0.952	0.917
21											0.999	0.998	0.994	0.986	0.971	0.947
22											1.000	0.999	0.997	0.992	0.983	0.967
23											1.000	1.000	0.999	0.996	0.991	0.981
24											1.000	1.000	0.999	0.998	0.995	0.989
25											1.000	1.000	1.000	0.999	0.997	0.994
26											1.000	1.000	1.000	1.000	0.999	0.997
27											1.000	1.000	1.000	1.000	0.999	0.998
28											1.000	1.000	1.000	1.000	1.000	0.999
29											1.000	1.000	1.000	1.000	1.000	1.000

TABLE III
Cumulative distribution: Standard normal

$$F_Z(z) = P[Z \le z]$$

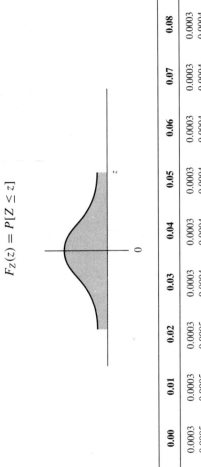

z	0.00	0.01	0.02	0.03	0.04	0.05	0.06	0.07	0.08	0.09
−3.4	0.0003	0.0003	0.0003	0.0003	0.0003	0.0003	0.0003	0.0003	0.0003	0.0002
−3.3	0.0005	0.0005	0.0005	0.0004	0.0004	0.0004	0.0004	0.0004	0.0004	0.0003
−3.2	0.0007	0.0007	0.0006	0.0006	0.0006	0.0006	0.0006	0.0005	0.0005	0.0005
−3.1	0.0010	0.0009	0.0009	0.0009	0.0008	0.0008	0.0008	0.0008	0.0007	0.0007
−3.0	0.0013	0.0013	0.0013	0.0012	0.0012	0.0011	0.0011	0.0011	0.0010	0.0010
−2.9	0.0019	0.0018	0.0018	0.0017	0.0016	0.0016	0.0015	0.0015	0.0014	0.0014
−2.8	0.0026	0.0025	0.0024	0.0023	0.0023	0.0022	0.0021	0.0021	0.0020	0.0019
−2.7	0.0035	0.0034	0.0033	0.0032	0.0031	0.0030	0.0029	0.0028	0.0027	0.0026
−2.6	0.0047	0.0045	0.0044	0.0043	0.0041	0.0040	0.0039	0.0038	0.0037	0.0036
−2.5	0.0062	0.0060	0.0059	0.0057	0.0055	0.0054	0.0052	0.0051	0.0049	0.0048
−2.4	0.0082	0.0080	0.0078	0.0075	0.0073	0.0071	0.0069	0.0068	0.0066	0.0064
−2.3	0.0107	0.0104	0.0102	0.0099	0.0096	0.0094	0.0091	0.0089	0.0087	0.0084
−2.2	0.0139	0.0136	0.0132	0.0129	0.0125	0.0122	0.0119	0.0116	0.0113	0.0110
−2.1	0.0179	0.0174	0.0170	0.0166	0.0162	0.0158	0.0154	0.0150	0.0146	0.0143
−2.0	0.0228	0.0222	0.0217	0.0212	0.0207	0.0202	0.0197	0.0192	0.0188	0.0183
−1.9	0.0287	0.0281	0.0274	0.0268	0.0262	0.0256	0.0250	0.0244	0.0239	0.0233
−1.8	0.0359	0.0351	0.0344	0.0336	0.0329	0.0322	0.0314	0.0307	0.0301	0.0294
−1.7	0.0446	0.0436	0.0427	0.0418	0.0409	0.0401	0.0392	0.0384	0.0375	0.0367
−1.6	0.0548	0.0537	0.0526	0.0516	0.0505	0.0495	0.0485	0.0475	0.0465	0.0455
−1.5	0.0668	0.0655	0.0643	0.0630	0.0618	0.0606	0.0594	0.0582	0.0571	0.0559
−1.4	0.0808	0.0793	0.0778	0.0764	0.0749	0.0735	0.0721	0.0708	0.0694	0.0681
−1.3	0.0968	0.0951	0.0934	0.0918	0.0901	0.0885	0.0869	0.0853	0.0838	0.0823
−1.2	0.1151	0.1131	0.1112	0.1093	0.1075	0.1056	0.1038	0.1020	0.1003	0.0985
−1.1	0.1357	0.1335	0.1314	0.1292	0.1271	0.1251	0.1230	0.1210	0.1190	0.1170
−1.0	0.1587	0.1562	0.1539	0.1515	0.1492	0.1469	0.1446	0.1423	0.1401	0.1379
−0.9	0.1841	0.1814	0.1788	0.1762	0.1736	0.1711	0.1685	0.1660	0.1635	0.1611
−0.8	0.2119	0.2090	0.2061	0.2033	0.2005	0.1977	0.1949	0.1921	0.1894	0.1867

z										
-0.7	0.2148	0.2177	0.2206	0.2236	0.2266	0.2296	0.2327	0.2358	0.2389	0.2420
-0.6	0.2451	0.2483	0.2514	0.2546	0.2578	0.2611	0.2643	0.2676	0.2709	0.2743
-0.5	0.2776	0.2810	0.2843	0.2877	0.2912	0.2946	0.2981	0.3015	0.3050	0.3085
-0.4	0.3121	0.3156	0.3192	0.3228	0.3264	0.3300	0.3336	0.3372	0.3409	0.3446
-0.3	0.3483	0.3520	0.3557	0.3594	0.3632	0.3669	0.3707	0.3745	0.3783	0.3821
-0.2	0.3859	0.3897	0.3936	0.3974	0.4013	0.4052	0.4090	0.4129	0.4168	0.4207
-0.1	0.4247	0.4286	0.4325	0.4364	0.4404	0.4443	0.4483	0.4522	0.4562	0.4602
-0.0	0.4641	0.4681	0.4721	0.4761	0.4801	0.4840	0.4880	0.4920	0.4960	0.5000
0.0	0.5359	0.5319	0.5279	0.5239	0.5199	0.5160	0.5120	0.5080	0.5040	0.5000
0.1	0.5753	0.5714	0.5675	0.5636	0.5596	0.5557	0.5517	0.5478	0.5438	0.5398
0.2	0.6141	0.6103	0.6064	0.6026	0.5987	0.5948	0.5910	0.5871	0.5832	0.5793
0.3	0.6517	0.6480	0.6443	0.6406	0.6368	0.6331	0.6293	0.6255	0.6217	0.6179
0.4	0.6879	0.6844	0.6808	0.6772	0.6736	0.6700	0.6664	0.6628	0.6591	0.6554
0.5	0.7224	0.7190	0.7157	0.7123	0.7088	0.7054	0.7019	0.6985	0.6950	0.6915
0.6	0.7549	0.7517	0.7486	0.7454	0.7422	0.7389	0.7357	0.7324	0.7291	0.7257
0.7	0.7852	0.7823	0.7794	0.7764	0.7734	0.7704	0.7673	0.7642	0.7611	0.7580
0.8	0.8133	0.8106	0.8078	0.8051	0.8023	0.7995	0.7967	0.7939	0.7910	0.7881
0.9	0.8389	0.8365	0.8340	0.8315	0.8289	0.8264	0.8238	0.8212	0.8186	0.8159
1.0	0.8621	0.8599	0.8577	0.8554	0.8531	0.8508	0.8485	0.8461	0.8438	0.8413
1.1	0.8830	0.8810	0.8790	0.8770	0.8749	0.8729	0.8708	0.8686	0.8665	0.8643
1.2	0.9015	0.8997	0.8980	0.8962	0.8944	0.8925	0.8907	0.8888	0.8869	0.8849
1.3	0.9177	0.9162	0.9147	0.9131	0.9115	0.9099	0.9082	0.9066	0.9049	0.9032
1.4	0.9319	0.9306	0.9292	0.9279	0.9265	0.9251	0.9236	0.9222	0.9207	0.9192
1.5	0.9441	0.9429	0.9418	0.9406	0.9394	0.9382	0.9370	0.9357	0.9345	0.9332
1.6	0.9545	0.9535	0.9525	0.9515	0.9505	0.9495	0.9484	0.9474	0.9463	0.9452
1.7	0.9633	0.9625	0.9616	0.9608	0.9599	0.9591	0.9582	0.9573	0.9564	0.9554
1.8	0.9706	0.9699	0.9693	0.9686	0.9678	0.9671	0.9664	0.9656	0.9649	0.9641
1.9	0.9767	0.9761	0.9756	0.9750	0.9744	0.9738	0.9732	0.9726	0.9719	0.9713
2.0	0.9817	0.9812	0.9808	0.9803	0.9798	0.9793	0.9788	0.9783	0.9778	0.9772
2.1	0.9857	0.9854	0.9850	0.9846	0.9842	0.9838	0.9834	0.9830	0.9826	0.9821
2.2	0.9890	0.9887	0.9884	0.9881	0.9878	0.9875	0.9871	0.9868	0.9864	0.9861
2.3	0.9916	0.9913	0.9911	0.9909	0.9906	0.9904	0.9901	0.9898	0.9896	0.9893
2.4	0.9936	0.9934	0.9932	0.9931	0.9929	0.9927	0.9925	0.9922	0.9920	0.9918
2.5	0.9952	0.9951	0.9949	0.9948	0.9946	0.9945	0.9943	0.9941	0.9940	0.9938
2.6	0.9964	0.9963	0.9962	0.9961	0.9960	0.9959	0.9957	0.9956	0.9955	0.9953
2.7	0.9974	0.9973	0.9972	0.9971	0.9970	0.9969	0.9968	0.9967	0.9966	0.9965
2.8	0.9981	0.9980	0.9979	0.9979	0.9978	0.9977	0.9977	0.9976	0.9975	0.9974
2.9	0.9986	0.9986	0.9985	0.9985	0.9984	0.9984	0.9983	0.9982	0.9982	0.9981
3.0	0.9990	0.9990	0.9989	0.9989	0.9989	0.9988	0.9988	0.9987	0.9987	0.9987
3.1	0.9993	0.9993	0.9992	0.9992	0.9992	0.9992	0.9991	0.9991	0.9991	0.9990
3.2	0.9995	0.9995	0.9995	0.9994	0.9994	0.9994	0.9994	0.9994	0.9993	0.9993
3.3	0.9997	0.9996	0.9996	0.9996	0.9996	0.9996	0.9996	0.9995	0.9995	0.9995
3.4	0.9998	0.9997	0.9997	0.9997	0.9997	0.9997	0.9997	0.9997	0.9997	0.9997

TABLE IV

Random digits

Line/Col.	(1)	(2)	(3)	(4)	(5)	(6)	(7)	(8)	(9)	(10)	(11)	(12)	(13)	(14)
1	10480	15011	01536	02011	81647	91646	69179	14194	62590	36207	20969	99570	91291	90700
2	22368	46573	25595	85393	30995	89198	27982	53402	93965	34095	52666	19174	39615	99505
3	24130	48360	22527	97265	76393	64809	15179	24830	49340	32081	30680	19655	63348	58629
4	42167	93093	06243	61680	07856	16376	39440	53537	71341	57004	00849	74917	97758	16379
5	37570	39975	81837	16656	06121	91782	60468	81305	49684	60672	14110	06927	01263	54613
6	77921	06907	11008	42751	27756	53498	18602	70659	90655	15053	21916	81825	44394	42880
7	99562	72905	56420	69994	98872	31016	71194	18738	44013	48840	63213	21069	10634	12952
8	96301	91977	05463	07972	18876	20922	94595	56869	69014	60045	18425	84903	42508	32307
9	89579	14342	63661	10281	17453	18103	57740	84378	25331	12566	58678	44947	05585	56941
10	85475	36857	43342	53988	53060	59533	38867	62300	08158	17983	16439	11458	18593	64952
11	28918	69578	88231	33276	70997	79936	56865	05859	90106	31595	01547	85590	91610	78188
12	63553	40961	48235	03427	49626	69445	18663	72695	52180	20847	12234	90511	33703	90322
13	09429	93969	52636	92737	88974	33488	36320	17617	30015	08272	84115	27156	30613	74952
14	10365	61129	87529	85689	48237	52267	67689	93394	01511	26358	85104	20285	29975	89868
15	07119	97336	71048	08178	77233	13916	47564	81056	97735	85977	29372	74461	28551	90707
16	51085	12765	51821	51259	77452	16308	60756	92144	49442	53900	70960	63990	75601	40719
17	02368	21382	52404	60268	89368	19885	55322	44819	01188	65255	64835	44919	05944	55157
18	01011	54092	33362	94904	31273	04146	18594	29852	71585	85030	51132	01915	92747	64951
19	52162	53916	46369	58586	23216	14513	83149	98736	23495	64350	94738	17752	35156	35749
20	07056	97628	33787	09998	42698	06691	76988	13602	51851	46104	88916	19509	25625	58104
21	48663	91245	85828	14346	09172	30168	90229	04734	59193	22178	30421	61666	99904	32812
22	54164	58492	22421	74103	47070	25306	76468	26384	58151	06646	21524	15227	96909	44592
23	32639	32363	05597	24200	13363	38005	94342	28728	35806	06912	17012	64161	18296	22851
24	29334	27001	87637	87308	58731	00256	45834	15398	46557	41135	10367	07684	36188	18510
25	02488	33062	28834	07351	19731	92420	60952	61280	50001	67658	32586	86679	50720	94953
26	81525	72295	04839	96423	24878	82651	66566	14778	76797	14780	13300	87074	79666	95725
27	29676	20591	68086	26432	46901	20849	89768	81536	86645	12659	92259	57102	80428	25280
28	00742	57392	39064	66432	84673	40027	32832	61362	98947	96067	64760	64584	96096	98253
29	05366	04213	25669	26422	44407	44048	37937	63904	45766	66134	75470	66520	34693	90449
30	91921	26418	64117	94305	26766	25940	39972	22209	71500	64568	91402	42416	07844	69618
31	00582	04711	87917	77341	42206	35126	74087	99547	81817	42607	43808	76655	62028	76630
32	00725	69884	62797	56170	86324	88072	76222	36086	84637	93161	76038	65855	77919	88006
33	69011	65797	95876	55293	18988	27354	26575	08625	40801	59920	29841	80150	12777	48501
34	25976	57948	29888	88604	67917	48708	18912	82271	65424	69774	33611	54262	85963	03547
35	09763	83473	73577	12908	30883	18317	28290	35797	05998	41688	34952	37888	38917	88050
36	91567	42595	27958	30134	04024	86385	29880	99730	55536	84855	29080	09250	79656	73211
37	17955	56349	90999	49127	20044	59931	06115	20542	18059	02008	73708	83517	36103	42791
38	46503	18584	18845	49618	02304	51038	20655	58727	28168	15475	56942	53389	20562	87338
39	92157	89634	94824	78171	84610	82834	09922	25417	44137	48413	25555	21246	35509	20468
40	14577	62765	35605	81263	39667	47358	56873	56307	61607	49518	89656	20103	77490	18062
41	98427	07523	33362	64270	01638	92477	66969	98420	04880	45585	46565	04102	46880	45709
42	34914	63976	88720	82765	34476	17032	87589	40836	32427	70002	70663	88863	77775	69348
43	70060	28277	39475	46473	23219	53416	94970	25832	69975	94884	19661	72828	00102	66794
44	53976	54914	06990	67245	68350	82948	11398	42878	80287	88267	47363	46634	06541	97809
45	76072	29515	40980	07391	58745	25774	22987	80059	39911	96189	41151	14222	60697	59583
46	90725	52210	83974	29992	65831	38857	50490	83765	55657	14361	31720	57375	56228	41546
47	64364	67412	33339	31926	14883	24413	59744	92351	97473	89286	35931	04110	23726	51900
48	08962	00358	31662	25388	61642	34072	81249	35648	56891	69352	48373	45578	78547	81788
49	95012	68379	93526	70765	10593	04542	76463	54328	02349	17247	28865	14777	62730	92277
50	15664	10493	20492	38391	91132	21999	59516	81652	27195	48223	46751	22923	32261	85653

Reprinted with permission from W. H. Beyer (ed.), *CRC Handbook of Tables for Probability and Statistics*, 2d ed., 1968, p. 480. Copyright CRC Press, Boca Raton, Florida.

TABLE V
Mean diameter at breast height for a stand of loblolly pines

Tree	Square	MDBH	Tree	Square	MDBH	Tree	Square	MDBH
1	1	5.86	51	14	6.97	101	29	5.17
2	1	6.02	52	14	5.87	102	29	6.56
3	1	6.27	53	14	5.75	103	29	5.69
4	1	6.25	54	15	6.35	104	29	6.20
5	1	7.76	55	15	5.59	105	29	6.65
6	2	6.09	56	15	7.19	106	29	6.73
7	2	5.23	57	16	5.39	107	30	6.73
8	2	6.97	58	16	5.05	108	30	6.88
9	2	6.04	59	17	5.78	109	30	5.90
10	3	7.65	60	17	6.34	110	31	6.33
11	3	5.51	61	17	6.10	111	31	6.24
12	4	5.15	62	17	7.25	112	31	7.39
13	4	7.07	63	18	6.63	113	31	5.66
14	4	5.80	64	18	7.50	114	31	5.85
15	4	6.17	65	18	5.79	115	31	7.46
16	4	5.92	66	18	5.99	116	32	6.87
17	5	5.62	67	19	5.86	117	32	5.45
18	5	5.66	68	19	5.37	118	33	6.13
19	5	6.80	69	19	4.92	119	33	4.88
20	6	7.03	70	19	6.24	120	33	5.92
21	6	5.88	71	19	6.14	121	33	4.46
22	6	6.62	72	20	5.70	122	34	6.07
23	6	7.01	73	20	6.54	123	34	6.25
24	6	5.19	74	20	8.29	124	34	5.09
25	7	6.15	75	21	6.55	125	35	5.74
26	7	6.51	76	21	4.97	126	35	5.83
27	8	6.01	77	21	6.29	127	35	5.22
28	8	7.82	78	21	6.67	128	35	6.59
29	8	6.47	79	21	5.49	129	36	5.70
30	8	6.54	80	22	5.24	130	36	7.29
31	8	6.13	81	22	7.11	131	37	6.66
32	9	6.66	82	22	6.26	132	37	6.18
33	9	6.92	83	23	5.33	133	37	5.02
34	9	7.21	84	23	6.19	134	37	5.23
35	9	6.62	85	24	5.77	135	37	5.77
36	10	6.96	86	24	5.60	136	38	6.11
37	10	6.71	87	24	6.20	137	38	5.74
38	10	6.47	88	24	5.95	138	39	7.86
39	11	6.29	89	24	6.87	139	39	5.50
40	11	5.88	90	24	6.56	140	40	6.71
41	12	6.89	91	25	5.74	141	40	5.89
42	12	6.53	92	25	6.27	142	40	6.56
43	12	6.32	93	25	6.16	143	40	5.28
44	13	5.42	94	25	6.63	144	40	7.00
45	13	6.70	95	26	7.07	145	41	6.24
46	13	7.19	96	26	6.92	146	41	6.37
47	13	7.08	97	26	6.47	147	41	6.42
48	13	6.23	98	27	6.63	148	42	5.53
49	14	5.41	99	27	6.34	149	42	7.07
50	14	7.54	100	28	7.11	150	42	6.74

TABLE V

(Continued)

Tree	Square	MDBH	Tree	Square	MDBH	Tree	Square	MDBH
151	42	6.74	201	55	6.57	251	71	6.17
152	42	4.72	202	56	6.83	252	71	6.60
153	42	5.17	203	56	7.02	253	71	7.67
154	43	7.37	204	57	6.03	254	71	7.13
155	43	6.10	205	57	6.54	255	72	6.95
156	44	5.93	206	57	6.11	256	72	5.14
157	44	6.96	207	58	6.33	257	73	6.17
158	44	5.52	208	58	5.88	258	73	6.13
159	45	7.06	209	58	6.37	259	74	7.16
160	45	7.25	210	59	5.46	260	74	7.49
161	45	6.53	211	59	6.57	261	74	6.52
162	46	6.51	212	59	6.25	262	75	6.24
163	46	6.03	213	60	7.23	263	75	7.29
164	46	6.10	214	60	5.21	264	75	6.64
165	46	6.52	215	60	5.04	265	76	6.35
166	47	7.20	216	60	6.16	266	76	6.62
167	47	5.91	217	60	5.70	267	77	6.00
168	47	6.51	218	61	5.80	268	77	6.49
169	48	7.48	219	61	5.15	269	77	6.52
170	48	6.73	220	61	6.79	270	77	6.16
171	49	6.16	221	62	5.80	271	77	6.34
172	49	4.76	222	62	7.60	272	78	5.61
173	49	6.70	223	62	6.35	273	78	6.80
174	49	5.83	224	62	6.01	274	78	6.64
175	49	6.60	225	63	7.16	275	79	6.54
176	50	8.07	226	63	6.55	276	79	6.46
177	50	5.66	227	63	5.69	277	79	6.54
178	50	6.12	228	63	5.46	278	79	5.86
179	50	6.27	229	63	6.01	279	80	6.12
180	51	6.66	230	64	6.47	280	80	5.85
181	51	5.99	231	64	5.56	281	80	5.84
182	51	5.51	232	64	5.37	282	81	4.86
183	51	6.98	233	64	6.26	283	84	6.41
184	52	6.13	234	65	6.51	284	84	6.52
185	52	7.11	235	65	6.40	285	81	6.30
186	52	5.47	236	65	6.97	286	81	6.85
187	52	5.18	237	66	5.56	287	82	6.36
188	53	6.30	238	66	6.20	288	82	6.95
189	53	5.11	239	66	6.26	289	83	7.00
190	53	7.32	240	67	6.13	290	83	5.91
191	53	7.20	241	68	7.00	291	83	6.88
192	54	5.41	242	68	5.70	292	84	7.03
193	54	6.43	243	68	6.56	293	84	6.06
194	54	5.79	244	69	7.49	294	84	5.20
195	54	6.24	245	69	6.91	295	84	5.54
196	55	6.45	246	69	5.97	296	85	6.78
197	55	4.95	247	69	5.23	297	85	5.98
198	55	6.88	248	70	6.46	298	85	5.49
199	55	6.22	249	70	5.11	299	86	5.48
200	55	4.61	250	70	6.47	300	86	6.73

TABLE V

(*Continued*)

Tree	Square	MDBH	Tree	Square	MDBH	Tree	Square	MDBH
301	87	5.33	351	99	6.15	401	120	6.40
302	87	6.26	352	100	7.16	402	120	5.76
303	87	4.25	353	100	5.37	403	120	5.15
304	87	6.36	354	101	7.84	404	121	7.34
305	87	5.54	355	101	5.94	405	121	5.22
306	88	6.60	356	101	6.59	406	121	6.92
307	88	5.91	357	102	7.04	407	122	6.77
308	88	6.44	358	102	7.05	408	122	6.53
309	88	6.41	359	103	5.61	409	123	6.15
310	89	6.42	360	103	5.82	410	123	5.98
311	89	6.03	361	103	5.52	411	123	7.38
312	89	6.17	362	104	6.62	412	124	4.99
313	90	6.85	363	104	5.70	413	124	5.11
314	90	5.55	364	105	6.84	414	125	6.60
315	90	5.73	365	105	7.10	415	125	6.15
316	91	6.07	366	105	5.82	416	125	6.44
317	91	4.57	367	106	6.35	417	126	6.56
318	91	5.45	368	106	6.64	418	126	5.60
319	91	5.77	369	107	6.13	419	127	6.82
320	91	5.42	370	107	7.07	420	128	6.35
321	92	7.24	371	108	5.79	421	128	6.44
322	92	5.36	372	108	6.99	422	128	5.86
323	93	6.99	373	108	5.45	423	129	6.87
324	93	6.65	374	109	6.22	424	129	8.32
325	93	6.22	375	109	7.61	425	130	5.99
326	93	7.57	376	109	6.95	426	130	6.28
327	94	5.61	377	109	6.29	427	131	7.61
328	94	6.07	378	109	6.10	428	132	6.32
329	94	7.29	379	110	6.10	429	132	6.56
330	95	4.98	380	110	7.91	430	132	8.37
331	95	5.96	381	110	6.95	431	132	7.63
332	95	6.88	382	111	7.44	432	133	5.53
333	95	6.49	383	112	5.66	433	133	6.97
334	95	6.57	384	112	6.70	434	134	6.80
335	95	6.12	385	113	6.84	435	134	6.07
336	96	5.52	386	113	6.52	436	134	5.76
337	96	6.05	387	113	6.19	437	134	6.60
338	96	5.62	388	114	5.63	438	135	6.52
339	96	5.78	389	114	4.37	439	135	6.57
340	97	6.11	390	115	6.27	440	136	6.16
341	97	5.80	391	115	8.48	441	136	6.57
342	97	6.27	392	115	5.52	442	136	7.11
343	97	6.09	393	116	6.68	443	137	5.88
344	98	5.38	394	117	6.68	444	137	5.26
345	98	6.03	395	117	5.70	445	138	6.36
346	98	6.27	396	118	6.21	446	138	5.90
347	99	6.07	397	118	6.48	447	138	5.91
348	99	6.79	398	118	6.05	448	139	6.89
349	99	7.12	399	119	6.16	449	139	5.03
350	99	6.70	400	119	5.66	450	140	6.61

TABLE V
(Concluded)

Tree	Square	MDBH	Tree	Square	MDBH	Tree	Square	MDBH
451	140	6.79	503	160	6.50	555	179	6.30
452	140	5.88	504	160	6.40	556	180	6.42
453	141	6.89	505	160	7.29	557	180	6.70
454	141	6.09	506	160	5.89	558	181	5.42
455	142	6.12	507	160	7.08	559	181	6.90
456	142	7.06	508	161	6.59	560	181	7.20
457	142	7.19	509	161	5.92	561	182	6.97
458	143	5.78	510	161	7.48	562	182	6.24
459	143	6.50	511	162	6.70	563	183	7.05
460	143	6.55	512	162	5.95	564	183	6.26
461	143	5.71	513	163	6.38	565	184	5.91
462	144	5.55	514	163	5.65	566	184	6.27
463	144	5.97	515	164	6.15	567	184	5.60
464	145	6.23	516	164	6.83	568	185	5.95
465	146	5.72	517	164	5.30	569	185	5.21
466	146	5.90	518	165	7.89	570	186	6.38
467	146	6.26	519	166	5.41	571	186	5.42
468	147	6.28	520	166	5.73	572	186	5.86
469	147	4.46	521	166	5.94	573	186	6.11
470	148	5.81	522	167	6.45	574	187	6.45
471	148	6.22	523	167	4.99	575	187	5.89
472	149	6.25	524	168	5.80	576	188	6.51
473	149	5.58	525	168	7.39	577	188	7.31
474	149	5.69	526	169	5.92	578	189	6.46
475	150	5.17	527	169	5.89	579	189	5.21
476	150	6.11	528	170	5.49	580	190	6.64
477	150	6.16	529	170	7.11	581	191	5.35
478	151	6.14	530	171	6.47	582	191	6.35
479	151	5.60	531	171	6.26	583	191	6.05
480	152	5.34	532	171	6.76	584	192	6.30
481	152	6.19	533	172	6.62	585	193	7.29
482	152	6.53	534	172	5.64	586	194	6.53
483	152	6.10	535	172	5.67	587	194	6.29
484	153	4.81	536	172	5.89	588	195	6.21
485	153	6.28	537	173	7.26	589	195	6.21
486	154	6.56	538	173	5.36	590	195	6.49
487	154	6.81	539	174	5.49	591	196	5.68
488	154	5.73	540	174	5.40	592	196	7.53
489	154	5.62	541	174	4.90	593	197	6.05
490	155	5.62	542	175	5.96	594	198	5.47
491	155	6.60	543	175	6.69	595	198	6.78
492	155	6.39	544	175	6.94	596	199	6.61
493	156	6.82	545	175	5.75	597	199	4.73
494	156	5.99	546	176	5.63	598	200	5.41
495	157	5.80	547	176	8.02	599	200	6.21
496	157	6.12	548	177	7.83	600	200	7.01
497	157	7.18	549	177	7.60			
498	158	6.30	550	177	5.82			
499	158	5.37	551	178	4.98			
500	158	5.48	552	178	6.01			
501	159	5.92	553	178	7.08			
502	159	6.05	554	179	6.80			

MDBH	
Mean	**Std. Dev.**
6.2536	0.6949

TABLE VI
Cumulative *T* distribution

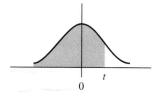

$$F(t) = P[T \le t]$$

ν	.40 .60	.25 .75	.10 .90	.05 .95	.025 .975	.01 .99	.005 .995	.001 .999	.0005 (Area to right) .9995 (Area to left)
1	0.325	1.000	3.078	6.314	12.706	31.821	63.657	318.317	636.607
2	0.289	0.816	1.886	2.920	4.303	6.965	9.925	22.327	31.598
3	0.277	0.765	1.638	2.353	3.182	4.541	5.841	10.215	12.924
4	0.271	0.741	1.533	2.132	2.776	3.747	4.604	7.173	8.610
5	0.267	0.727	1.476	2.015	2.571	3.365	4.032	5.893	6.869
6	0.265	0.718	1.440	1.943	2.447	3.143	3.707	5.208	5.959
7	0.263	0.711	1.415	1.895	2.365	2.998	3.499	4.785	5.408
8	0.262	0.706	1.397	1.860	2.306	2.896	3.355	4.501	5.041
9	0.261	0.703	1.383	1.833	2.262	2.821	3.250	4.297	4.781
10	0.260	0.700	1.372	1.812	2.228	2.764	3.169	4.144	4.587
11	0.260	0.697	1.363	1.796	2.201	2.718	3.106	4.025	4.437
12	0.259	0.695	1.356	1.782	2.179	2.681	3.055	3.930	4.318
13	0.259	0.694	1.350	1.771	2.160	2.650	3.012	3.852	4.221
14	0.258	0.692	1.345	1.761	2.145	2.624	2.977	3.787	4.140
15	0.258	0.691	1.341	1.753	2.131	2.602	2.947	3.733	4.073
16	0.258	0.690	1.337	1.746	2.120	2.583	2.921	3.686	4.015
17	0.257	0.689	1.333	1.740	2.110	2.567	2.898	3.646	3.965
18	0.257	0.688	1.330	1.734	2.101	2.552	2.878	3.611	3.922
19	0.257	0.688	1.328	1.729	2.093	2.539	2.861	3.579	3.883
20	0.257	0.687	1.325	1.725	2.086	2.528	2.845	3.552	3.850
21	0.257	0.686	1.323	1.721	2.080	2.518	2.831	3.527	3.819
22	0.256	0.686	1.321	1.717	2.074	2.508	2.819	3.505	3.792
23	0.256	0.685	1.319	1.714	2.069	2.500	2.807	3.485	3.768
24	0.256	0.685	1.318	1.711	2.064	2.492	2.797	3.467	3.745
25	0.256	0.684	1.316	1.708	2.060	2.485	2.787	3.450	3.725
26	0.256	0.684	1.315	1.706	2.056	2.479	2.779	3.435	3.707
27	0.256	0.684	1.314	1.703	2.052	2.473	2.771	3.421	3.690
28	0.256	0.683	1.313	1.701	2.048	2.467	2.763	3.408	3.674
29	0.256	0.683	1.311	1.699	2.045	2.462	2.756	3.396	3.659
30	0.256	0.683	1.310	1.697	2.042	2.457	2.750	3.385	3.646
31	0.256	0.682	1.309	1.696	2.040	2.453	2.744	3.375	3.633
32	0.255	0.682	1.309	1.694	2.037	2.449	2.738	3.365	3.622
33	0.255	0.682	1.308	1.692	2.035	2.445	2.733	3.356	3.611
34	0.255	0.682	1.307	1.691	2.032	2.441	2.728	3.348	3.601
35	0.255	0.682	1.306	1.690	2.030	2.438	2.724	3.340	3.591

TABLE VI

(Continued)

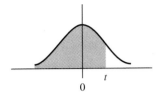

$$F(t) = P[T \leq t]$$

v	.40 .60	.25 .75	.10 .90	.05 .95	.025 .975	.01 .99	.005 .995	.001 .999	.0005 (Area to right) .9995 (Area to left)
36	0.255	0.681	1.306	1.688	2.028	2.434	2.719	3.333	3.582
37	0.255	0.681	1.305	1.687	2.026	2.431	2.715	3.326	3.574
38	0.255	0.681	1.304	1.686	2.024	2.429	2.712	3.319	3.566
39	0.255	0.681	1.304	1.685	2.023	2.426	2.708	3.313	3.558
40	0.255	0.681	1.303	1.684	2.021	2.423	2.704	3.307	3.551
41	0.255	0.681	1.303	1.683	2.020	2.421	2.701	3.301	3.544
42	0.255	0.680	1.302	1.682	2.018	2.418	2.698	3.296	3.538
43	0.255	0.680	1.302	1.681	2.017	2.416	2.695	3.291	3.532
44	0.255	0.680	1.301	1.680	2.015	2.414	2.692	3.286	3.526
45	0.255	0.680	1.301	1.679	2.014	2.412	2.690	3.281	3.520
46	0.255	0.680	1.300	1.679	2.013	2.410	2.687	3.277	3.515
47	0.255	0.680	1.300	1.678	2.012	2.408	2.685	3.273	3.510
48	0.255	0.680	1.299	1.677	2.011	2.407	2.682	3.269	3.505
49	0.255	0.680	1.299	1.677	2.010	2.405	2.680	3.265	3.500
50	0.255	0.679	1.299	1.676	2.009	2.403	2.678	3.261	3.496
51	0.255	0.679	1.298	1.675	2.008	2.402	2.676	3.258	3.492
52	0.255	0.679	1.298	1.675	2.007	2.400	2.674	3.255	3.488
53	0.255	0.679	1.298	1.674	2.006	2.399	2.672	3.251	3.484
54	0.255	0.679	1.297	1.674	2.005	2.397	2.670	3.248	3.480
55	0.255	0.679	1.297	1.673	2.004	2.396	2.668	3.245	3.476
56	0.255	0.679	1.297	1.673	2.003	2.395	2.667	3.242	3.473
57	0.255	0.679	1.297	1.672	2.002	2.394	2.665	3.239	3.470
58	0.255	0.679	1.296	1.672	2.002	2.392	2.663	3.237	3.466
59	0.254	0.679	1.296	1.671	2.001	2.391	2.662	3.234	3.463
60	0.254	0.679	1.296	1.671	2.000	2.390	2.660	3.232	3.460
61	0.254	0.679	1.296	1.670	2.000	2.389	2.659	3.229	3.457
62	0.254	0.678	1.295	1.670	1.999	2.388	2.658	3.227	3.455
63	0.254	0.678	1.295	1.669	1.998	2.387	2.656	3.225	3.452
64	0.254	0.678	1.295	1.669	1.998	2.386	2.655	3.223	3.449
65	0.254	0.678	1.295	1.669	1.997	2.385	2.654	3.221	3.447

TABLE VI
(*Concluded*)

ν	.40 .60	.25 .75	.10 .90	.05 .95	.025 .975	.01 .99	.005 .995	.001 .999	.0005 (Area to right) .9995 (Area to left)
66	0.254	0.678	1.295	1.668	1.997	2.384	2.652	3.218	3.444
67	0.254	0.678	1.294	1.668	1.996	2.383	2.651	3.217	3.442
68	0.254	0.678	1.294	1.668	1.995	2.382	2.650	3.215	3.440
69	0.254	0.678	1.294	1.667	1.995	2.382	2.649	3.213	3.437
70	0.254	0.678	1.294	1.667	1.994	2.381	2.648	3.211	3.435
71	0.254	0.678	1.294	1.667	1.994	2.380	2.647	3.209	3.433
72	0.254	0.678	1.293	1.666	1.993	2.379	2.646	3.207	3.431
73	0.254	0.678	1.293	1.666	1.993	2.379	2.645	3.206	3.429
74	0.254	0.678	1.293	1.666	1.993	2.378	2.644	3.204	3.427
75	0.254	0.678	1.293	1.665	1.992	2.377	2.643	3.203	3.425
76	0.254	0.678	1.293	1.665	1.992	2.376	2.642	3.201	3.423
77	0.254	0.678	1.293	1.665	1.991	2.376	2.641	3.200	3.422
78	0.254	0.678	1.292	1.665	1.991	2.375	2.640	3.198	3.420
79	0.254	0.678	1.292	1.664	1.990	2.375	2.640	3.197	3.418
80	0.254	0.678	1.292	1.664	1.990	2.374	2.639	3.195	3.416
81	0.254	0.678	1.292	1.664	1.990	2.373	2.638	3.194	3.415
82	0.254	0.677	1.292	1.664	1.989	2.373	2.637	3.193	3.413
83	0.254	0.677	1.292	1.663	1.989	2.372	2.636	3.191	3.412
84	0.254	0.677	1.292	1.663	1.989	2.372	2.636	3.190	3.410
85	0.254	0.677	1.292	1.663	1.988	2.371	2.635	3.189	3.409
86	0.254	0.677	1.291	1.663	1.988	2.371	2.634	3.188	3.407
87	0.254	0.677	1.291	1.663	1.988	2.370	2.634	3.187	3.406
88	0.254	0.677	1.291	1.662	1.987	2.369	2.633	3.186	3.405
89	0.254	0.677	1.291	1.662	1.987	2.369	2.632	3.184	3.403
90	0.254	0.677	1.291	1.662	1.987	2.369	2.632	3.183	3.402
91	0.254	0.677	1.291	1.662	1.986	2.368	2.631	3.182	3.401
92	0.254	0.677	1.291	1.662	1.986	2.368	2.630	3.181	3.400
93	0.254	0.677	1.291	1.661	1.986	2.367	2.630	3.180	3.398
94	0.254	0.677	1.291	1.661	1.986	2.367	2.629	3.179	3.397
95	0.254	0.677	1.291	1.661	1.985	2.366	2.629	3.178	3.396
96	0.254	0.677	1.290	1.661	1.985	2.366	2.628	3.177	3.395
97	0.254	0.677	1.290	1.661	1.985	2.365	2.627	3.176	3.394
98	0.254	0.677	1.290	1.661	1.984	2.365	2.627	3.176	3.393
99	0.254	0.677	1.290	1.660	1.984	2.365	2.626	3.175	3.392
100	0.254	0.677	1.290	1.660	1.984	2.364	2.626	3.174	3.391
∞	0.253	0.674	1.282	1.645	1.960	2.326	2.576	3.090	3.291

TABLE VII
Sample size for testing the mean

Level of t test

Value of Δ = $\frac{\mu-\mu_0}{\sigma}$	Single-sided α = 0.005 / Double-sided α = 0.01					Single-sided α = 0.01 / Double-sided α = 0.02					Single-sided α = 0.025 / Double-sided α = 0.05					Single-sided α = 0.05 / Double-sided α = 0.1				
β =	0.01	0.05	0.1	0.2	0.5	0.01	0.05	0.1	0.2	0.5	0.01	0.05	0.1	0.2	0.5	0.01	0.05	0.1	0.2	0.5
0.05																				
0.10																				122
0.15																				70
0.20															99				101	45
0.25					110					139				128	64			139	71	32
0.30				134	78				115	90			119	90	45		122	97	52	24
0.35			125	99	58			109	85	63		109	88	67	34		90	72	40	19
0.40		115	97	77	45		101	85	66	47	117	84	68	51	26	101	70	55	33	15
0.45		92	77	62	37	110	81	68	53	37	93	67	54	41	21	80	55	44	27	13
0.50	100	75	63	51	30	90	66	55	43	30	76	54	44	34	18	65	45	36	22	11
0.55	83	63	53	42	26	75	55	46	36	25	63	45	37	28	15	54	38	30	19	9
0.60	71	53	45	36	22	63	47	39	31	21	53	38	32	24	13	46	32	26	17	8
0.65	61	46	39	31	20	55	41	34	27	18	46	33	27	21	12	39	28	22	15	8
0.70	53	40	34	28	17	47	35	30	24	16	40	29	24	19	10	34	24	19	13	8
0.75	47	36	30	25	16	42	31	27	21	14	35	26	21	16	9	30	21	17	12	7
0.80	41	32	27	22	14	37	28	24	19	13	31	22	19	15	9	27	19	15	11	6
0.85	37	29	24	20	13	33	25	21	17	12	28	21	17	13	8	24	17	14	11	6
0.90	34	26	22	18	12	29	23	19	16	11	25	19	16	12	7	21	15	13	10	5
0.95	31	24	20	17	11	27	21	18	14	10	23	17	14	11	7	19	14	11	9	5
1.00	28	22	19	16	10	25	19	16	13	9	21	16	13	10	6	18	13	11	8	5

Value of $\Delta = \dfrac{\mu - \mu_0}{\sigma}$																			
1.1	24	19	16	14	9	21	16	14	12	8	18	13	11	9	6	15	11	9	7
1.2	21	16	14	12	8	18	14	12	10	7	15	12	10	8	5	13	10	8	6
1.3	18	15	13	11	8	16	13	11	9	6	14	10	9	7		11	8	7	6
1.4	16	13	12	10	7	14	11	10	9	6	12	9	8	7		10	8	7	5
1.5	15	12	11	9	7	13	10	9	8	6	11	8	7	6		9	7	6	
1.6	13	11	10	8	6	12	10	9	7	5	10	8	7	6		8	6	6	
1.7	12	10	9	8	6	11	9	8	7		9	7	6	5		8	6	5	
1.8	12	10	9	8	6	10	8	7	7		8	7	6			7	6		
1.9	11	9	8	7	6	10	8	7	6		8	6	6			7	5		
2.0	10	8	8	7	5	9	7	7	6		7	6	5			6			
2.1	10	8	7	7		8	7	6	6		7	6				6			
2.2	9	8	7	6		8	7	6	5		7	6				6			
2.3	9	7	7	6		8	6	6			6	5				5			
2.4	8	7	7	6		7	6	6			6								
2.5	8	7	6	6		7	6	6			6								
3.0	7	6	6	5		6	5	5			5								
3.5	6	5	5			5													
4.0	6																		

Reprinted with permission from W. H. Beyer (ed.), *CRC Handbook of Tables for Probability and Statistics*, 2d ed., 1968, p. 282. Copyright CRC Press, Boca Raton, Florida.

TABLE VIII
Cumulative chi-squared distribution

$$F(\chi^2) = P[X^2 \le \chi^2]$$

γ \ F	.005	.010	.025	.050	.100	.250	.500	.750	.900	.950	.975	.990	.995
1	.0000393	.000157	.000982	.00393	.0158	.102	.455	1.32	2.71	3.84	5.02	6.63	7.88
2	.0100	.0201	.0506	.103	.211	.575	1.39	2.77	4.61	5.99	7.38	9.21	10.6
3	.0717	.115	.216	.352	.584	1.21	2.37	4.11	6.25	7.81	9.35	11.3	12.8
4	.207	.297	.484	.711	1.06	1.92	3.36	5.39	7.78	9.49	11.1	13.3	14.9
5	.412	.554	.831	1.15	1.61	2.67	4.35	6.63	9.24	11.1	12.8	15.1	16.7
6	.676	.872	1.24	1.64	2.20	3.45	5.35	7.84	10.6	12.6	14.4	16.8	18.5
7	.989	1.24	1.69	2.17	2.83	4.25	6.35	9.04	12.0	14.1	16.0	18.5	20.3
8	1.34	1.65	2.18	2.73	3.49	5.07	7.34	10.2	13.4	15.5	17.5	20.1	22.0
9	1.73	2.09	2.70	3.33	4.17	5.90	8.34	11.4	14.7	16.9	19.0	21.7	23.6
10	2.16	2.56	3.25	3.94	4.87	6.74	9.34	12.5	16.0	18.3	20.5	23.2	25.2
11	2.60	3.05	3.82	4.57	5.58	7.58	10.3	13.7	17.3	19.7	21.9	24.7	26.8
12	3.07	3.57	4.40	5.23	6.30	8.44	11.3	14.8	18.5	21.0	23.3	26.2	28.3
13	3.57	4.11	5.01	5.89	7.04	9.30	12.3	16.0	19.8	22.4	24.7	27.7	29.8
14	4.07	4.66	5.63	6.57	7.79	10.2	13.3	17.1	21.1	23.7	26.1	29.1	31.3
15	4.60	5.23	6.26	7.26	8.55	11.0	14.3	18.2	22.3	25.0	27.5	30.6	32.8

16	5.14	5.81	6.91	7.96	9.31	11.9	15.3	19.4	23.5	26.3	28.8	32.0	34.3
17	5.70	6.41	7.56	8.67	10.1	12.8	16.3	20.5	24.8	27.6	30.2	33.4	35.7
18	6.26	7.01	8.23	9.39	10.9	13.7	17.3	21.6	26.0	28.9	31.5	34.8	37.2
19	6.84	7.63	8.91	10.1	11.7	14.6	18.3	22.7	27.2	30.1	32.9	36.2	38.6
20	7.43	8.26	9.59	10.9	12.4	15.5	19.3	23.8	28.4	31.4	34.2	37.6	40.0
21	8.03	8.90	10.3	11.6	13.2	16.3	20.3	24.9	29.6	32.7	35.5	38.9	41.4
22	8.64	9.54	11.0	12.3	14.0	17.2	21.3	26.0	30.8	33.9	36.8	40.3	42.8
23	9.26	10.2	11.7	13.1	14.8	18.1	22.3	27.1	32.0	35.2	38.1	41.6	44.2
24	9.89	10.9	12.4	13.8	15.7	19.0	23.3	28.2	33.2	36.4	39.4	43.0	45.6
25	10.5	11.5	13.1	14.6	16.5	19.9	24.3	29.3	34.4	37.7	40.6	44.3	46.9
26	11.2	12.2	13.8	15.4	17.3	20.8	25.3	30.4	35.6	38.9	41.9	45.6	48.3
27	11.8	12.9	14.6	16.2	18.1	21.7	26.3	31.5	36.7	40.1	43.2	47.0	49.6
28	12.5	13.6	15.3	16.9	18.9	22.7	27.3	32.6	37.9	41.3	44.5	48.3	51.0
29	13.1	14.3	16.0	17.7	19.8	23.6	28.3	33.7	39.1	42.6	45.7	49.6	52.3
30	13.8	15.0	16.8	18.5	20.6	24.5	29.3	34.8	40.3	43.8	47.0	50.9	53.7

Reprinted with permission from W. H. Beyer (ed.), *CRC Handbook of Tables for Probability and Statistics*, 2d ed., 1968, p. 294. Copyright CRC Press, Inc., Boca Raton, Florida.

TABLE IX
Cumulative F distribution

$$P[F_{\gamma_1,\gamma_2} \le f] = .90$$

γ_2 \ γ_1	1	2	3	4	5	6	7	8	9	10	12	15	20	24	30	40	60	120	∞
1	39.86	49.50	53.59	55.83	57.24	58.20	58.91	59.44	59.86	60.19	60.71	61.22	61.74	62.00	62.26	62.53	62.79	63.06	63.33
2	8.53	9.00	9.16	9.24	9.29	9.33	9.35	9.37	9.38	9.39	9.41	9.42	9.44	9.45	9.46	9.47	9.47	9.48	9.49
3	5.54	5.46	5.39	5.34	5.31	5.28	5.27	5.25	5.24	5.23	5.22	5.20	5.18	5.18	5.17	5.16	5.15	5.14	5.13
4	4.54	4.32	4.19	4.11	4.05	4.01	3.98	3.95	3.94	3.92	3.90	3.87	3.84	3.83	3.82	3.80	3.79	3.78	3.76
5	4.06	3.78	3.62	3.52	3.45	3.40	3.37	3.34	3.32	3.30	3.27	3.24	3.21	3.19	3.17	3.16	3.14	3.12	3.10
6	3.78	3.46	3.29	3.18	3.11	3.05	3.01	2.98	2.96	2.94	2.90	2.87	2.84	2.82	2.80	2.78	2.76	2.74	2.72
7	3.59	3.26	3.07	2.96	2.88	2.83	2.78	2.75	2.72	2.70	2.67	2.63	2.59	2.58	2.56	2.54	2.51	2.49	2.47
8	3.46	3.11	2.92	2.81	2.73	2.67	2.62	2.59	2.56	2.54	2.50	2.46	2.42	2.40	2.38	2.36	2.34	2.32	2.29
9	3.36	3.01	2.81	2.69	2.61	2.55	2.51	2.47	2.44	2.42	2.38	2.34	2.30	2.28	2.25	2.23	2.21	2.18	2.16
10	3.29	2.92	2.73	2.61	2.52	2.46	2.41	2.38	2.35	2.32	2.28	2.24	2.20	2.18	2.16	2.13	2.11	2.08	2.06
11	3.23	2.86	2.66	2.54	2.45	2.39	2.34	2.30	2.27	2.25	2.21	2.17	2.12	2.10	2.08	2.05	2.03	2.00	1.97
12	3.18	2.81	2.61	2.48	2.39	2.33	2.28	2.24	2.21	2.19	2.15	2.10	2.06	2.04	2.01	1.99	1.96	1.93	1.90
13	3.14	2.76	2.56	2.43	2.35	2.28	2.23	2.20	2.16	2.14	2.10	2.05	2.01	1.98	1.96	1.93	1.90	1.88	1.85
14	3.10	2.73	2.52	2.39	2.31	2.24	2.19	2.15	2.12	2.10	2.05	2.01	1.96	1.94	1.91	1.89	1.86	1.83	1.80
15	3.07	2.70	2.49	2.36	2.27	2.21	2.16	2.12	2.09	2.06	2.02	1.97	1.92	1.90	1.87	1.85	1.82	1.79	1.76
16	3.05	2.67	2.46	2.33	2.24	2.18	2.13	2.09	2.06	2.03	1.99	1.94	1.89	1.87	1.84	1.81	1.78	1.75	1.72
17	3.03	2.64	2.44	2.31	2.22	2.15	2.10	2.06	2.03	2.00	1.96	1.91	1.86	1.84	1.81	1.78	1.75	1.72	1.69
18	3.01	2.62	2.42	2.29	2.20	2.13	2.08	2.04	2.00	1.98	1.93	1.89	1.84	1.81	1.78	1.75	1.72	1.69	1.66
19	2.99	2.61	2.40	2.27	2.18	2.11	2.06	2.02	1.98	1.96	1.91	1.86	1.81	1.79	1.76	1.73	1.70	1.67	1.63
20	2.97	2.59	2.38	2.25	2.16	2.09	2.04	2.00	1.96	1.94	1.89	1.84	1.79	1.77	1.74	1.71	1.68	1.64	1.61
21	2.96	2.57	2.36	2.23	2.14	2.08	2.02	1.98	1.95	1.92	1.87	1.83	1.78	1.75	1.72	1.69	1.66	1.62	1.59
22	2.95	2.56	2.35	2.22	2.13	2.06	2.01	1.97	1.93	1.90	1.86	1.81	1.76	1.73	1.70	1.67	1.64	1.60	1.57
23	2.94	2.55	2.34	2.21	2.11	2.05	1.99	1.95	1.92	1.89	1.84	1.80	1.74	1.72	1.69	1.66	1.62	1.59	1.55
24	2.93	2.54	2.33	2.19	2.10	2.04	1.98	1.94	1.91	1.88	1.83	1.78	1.73	1.70	1.67	1.64	1.61	1.57	1.53
25	2.92	2.53	2.32	2.18	2.09	2.02	1.97	1.93	1.89	1.87	1.82	1.77	1.72	1.69	1.66	1.63	1.59	1.56	1.52
26	2.91	2.52	2.31	2.17	2.08	2.01	1.96	1.92	1.88	1.86	1.81	1.76	1.71	1.68	1.65	1.61	1.58	1.54	1.50
27	2.90	2.51	2.30	2.17	2.07	2.00	1.95	1.91	1.87	1.85	1.80	1.75	1.70	1.67	1.64	1.60	1.57	1.53	1.49
28	2.89	2.50	2.29	2.16	2.06	2.00	1.94	1.90	1.87	1.84	1.79	1.74	1.69	1.66	1.63	1.59	1.56	1.52	1.48
29	2.89	2.50	2.28	2.15	2.06	1.99	1.93	1.89	1.86	1.83	1.78	1.73	1.68	1.65	1.62	1.58	1.55	1.51	1.47
30	2.88	2.49	2.28	2.14	2.05	1.98	1.93	1.88	1.85	1.82	1.77	1.72	1.67	1.64	1.61	1.57	1.54	1.50	1.46
40	2.84	2.44	2.23	2.09	2.00	1.93	1.87	1.83	1.79	1.76	1.71	1.66	1.61	1.57	1.54	1.51	1.47	1.42	1.38
60	2.79	2.39	2.18	2.04	1.95	1.87	1.82	1.77	1.74	1.71	1.66	1.60	1.54	1.51	1.48	1.44	1.40	1.35	1.29
120	2.75	2.35	2.13	1.99	1.90	1.82	1.77	1.72	1.68	1.65	1.60	1.55	1.48	1.45	1.41	1.37	1.32	1.26	1.19
∞	2.71	2.30	2.08	1.94	1.85	1.77	1.72	1.67	1.63	1.60	1.55	1.49	1.42	1.38	1.34	1.30	1.24	1.17	1.00

$$P[F_{\gamma_1,\gamma_2} \leq f] = .95$$

γ_2 \ γ_1	1	2	3	4	5	6	7	8	9	10	12	15	20	24	30	40	60	120	8
1	161.4	199.5	215.7	224.6	230.2	234.0	236.8	238.9	240.5	241.9	243.9	245.9	248.0	249.1	250.1	251.1	252.2	253.3	254.3
2	18.51	19.00	19.16	19.25	19.30	19.33	19.35	19.37	19.38	19.40	19.41	19.43	19.45	19.45	19.46	19.47	19.48	19.49	19.50
3	10.13	9.55	9.28	9.12	9.01	8.94	8.89	8.85	8.81	8.79	8.74	8.70	8.66	8.64	8.62	8.59	8.57	8.55	8.53
4	7.71	6.94	6.59	6.39	6.26	6.16	6.09	6.04	6.00	5.96	5.91	5.86	5.80	5.77	5.75	5.72	5.69	5.66	5.63
5	6.61	5.79	5.41	5.19	5.05	4.95	4.88	4.82	4.77	4.74	4.68	4.62	4.56	4.53	4.50	4.46	4.43	4.40	4.36
6	5.99	5.14	4.76	4.53	4.39	4.28	4.21	4.15	4.10	4.06	4.00	3.94	3.87	3.84	3.81	3.77	3.74	3.70	3.67
7	5.59	4.74	4.35	4.12	3.97	3.87	3.79	3.73	3.68	3.64	3.57	3.51	3.44	3.41	3.38	3.34	3.30	3.27	3.23
8	5.32	4.46	4.07	3.84	3.69	3.58	3.50	3.44	3.39	3.35	3.28	3.22	3.15	3.12	3.08	3.04	3.01	2.97	2.93
9	5.12	4.26	3.86	3.63	3.48	3.37	3.29	3.23	3.18	3.14	3.07	3.01	2.94	2.90	2.86	2.83	2.79	2.75	2.71
10	4.96	4.10	3.71	3.48	3.33	3.22	3.14	3.07	3.02	2.98	2.91	2.85	2.77	2.74	2.70	2.66	2.62	2.58	2.54
11	4.84	3.98	3.59	3.36	3.20	3.09	3.01	2.95	2.90	2.85	2.79	2.72	2.65	2.61	2.57	2.53	2.49	2.45	2.40
12	4.75	3.89	3.49	3.26	3.11	3.00	2.91	2.85	2.80	2.75	2.69	2.62	2.54	2.51	2.47	2.43	2.38	2.34	2.30
13	4.67	3.81	3.41	3.18	3.03	2.92	2.83	2.77	2.71	2.67	2.60	2.53	2.46	2.42	2.38	2.34	2.30	2.25	2.21
14	4.60	3.74	3.34	3.11	2.96	2.85	2.76	2.70	2.65	2.60	2.53	2.46	2.39	2.35	2.31	2.27	2.22	2.18	2.13
15	4.54	3.68	3.29	3.06	2.90	2.79	2.71	2.64	2.59	2.54	2.48	2.40	2.33	2.29	2.25	2.20	2.16	2.11	2.07
16	4.49	3.63	3.24	3.01	2.85	2.74	2.66	2.59	2.54	2.49	2.42	2.35	2.28	2.24	2.19	2.15	2.11	2.06	2.01
17	4.45	3.59	3.20	2.96	2.81	2.70	2.61	2.55	2.49	2.45	2.38	2.31	2.23	2.19	2.15	2.10	2.06	2.01	1.96
18	4.41	3.55	3.16	2.93	2.77	2.66	2.58	2.51	2.46	2.41	2.34	2.27	2.19	2.15	2.11	2.06	2.02	1.97	1.92
19	4.38	3.52	3.13	2.90	2.74	2.63	2.54	2.48	2.42	2.38	2.31	2.23	2.16	2.11	2.07	2.03	1.98	1.93	1.88
20	4.35	3.49	3.10	2.87	2.71	2.60	2.51	2.45	2.39	2.35	2.28	2.20	2.12	2.08	2.04	1.99	1.95	1.90	1.84
21	4.32	3.47	3.07	2.84	2.68	2.57	2.49	2.42	2.37	2.32	2.25	2.18	2.10	2.05	2.01	1.96	1.92	1.87	1.81
22	4.30	3.44	3.05	2.82	2.66	2.55	2.46	2.40	2.34	2.30	2.23	2.15	2.07	2.03	1.98	1.94	1.89	1.84	1.78
23	4.28	3.42	3.03	2.80	2.64	2.53	2.44	2.37	2.32	2.27	2.20	2.13	2.05	2.01	1.96	1.91	1.86	1.81	1.76
24	4.26	3.40	3.01	2.78	2.62	2.51	2.42	2.36	2.30	2.25	2.18	2.11	2.03	1.98	1.94	1.89	1.84	1.79	1.73
25	4.24	3.39	2.99	2.76	2.60	2.49	2.40	2.34	2.28	2.24	2.16	2.09	2.01	1.96	1.92	1.87	1.82	1.77	1.71
26	4.23	3.37	2.98	2.74	2.59	2.47	2.39	2.32	2.27	2.22	2.15	2.07	1.99	1.95	1.90	1.85	1.80	1.75	1.69
27	4.21	3.35	2.96	2.73	2.57	2.46	2.37	2.31	2.25	2.20	2.13	2.06	1.97	1.93	1.88	1.84	1.79	1.73	1.67
28	4.20	3.34	2.95	2.71	2.56	2.45	2.36	2.29	2.24	2.19	2.12	2.04	1.96	1.91	1.87	1.82	1.77	1.71	1.65
29	4.18	3.33	2.93	2.70	2.55	2.43	2.35	2.28	2.22	2.18	2.10	2.03	1.94	1.90	1.85	1.81	1.75	1.70	1.64
30	4.17	3.32	2.92	2.69	2.53	2.42	2.33	2.27	2.21	2.16	2.09	2.01	1.93	1.89	1.84	1.79	1.74	1.68	1.62
40	4.08	3.23	2.84	2.61	2.45	2.34	2.25	2.18	2.12	2.08	2.00	1.92	1.84	1.79	1.74	1.69	1.64	1.58	1.51
60	4.00	3.15	2.76	2.53	2.37	2.25	2.17	2.10	2.04	1.99	1.92	1.84	1.75	1.70	1.65	1.59	1.53	1.47	1.39
120	3.92	3.07	2.68	2.45	2.29	2.17	2.09	2.02	1.96	1.91	1.83	1.75	1.66	1.61	1.55	1.50	1.43	1.35	1.25
8	3.84	3.00	2.60	2.37	2.21	2.10	2.01	1.94	1.88	1.83	1.75	1.67	1.57	1.52	1.46	1.39	1.32	1.22	1.00

TABLE IX
(Continued)

$$P[F_{\gamma_1, \gamma_2} \leq f] = .975$$

γ_2 \ γ_1	1	2	3	4	5	6	7	8	9	10	12	15	20	24	30	40	60	120	∞
1	647.8	799.5	864.2	899.6	921.8	937.1	948.2	956.7	963.3	968.6	976.7	984.9	993.1	997.2	1001	1006	1010	1014	1018
2	38.51	39.00	39.17	39.25	39.30	39.33	39.36	39.37	39.39	39.40	39.41	39.43	39.45	39.46	39.46	39.47	39.48	39.49	39.50
3	17.44	16.04	15.44	15.10	14.88	14.73	14.62	14.54	14.47	14.42	14.34	14.25	14.17	14.12	14.08	14.04	13.99	13.95	13.90
4	12.22	10.65	9.98	9.60	9.36	9.20	9.07	8.98	8.90	8.84	8.75	8.66	8.56	8.51	8.46	8.41	8.36	8.31	8.26
5	10.01	8.43	7.76	7.39	7.15	6.98	6.85	6.76	6.68	6.62	6.52	6.43	6.33	6.28	6.23	6.18	6.12	6.07	6.02
6	8.81	7.26	6.60	6.23	5.99	5.82	5.70	5.60	5.52	5.46	5.37	5.27	5.17	5.12	5.07	5.01	4.96	4.90	4.85
7	8.07	6.54	5.89	5.52	5.29	5.12	4.99	4.90	4.82	4.76	4.67	4.57	4.47	4.42	4.36	4.31	4.25	4.20	4.14
8	7.57	6.06	5.42	5.05	4.82	4.65	4.53	4.43	4.36	4.30	4.20	4.10	4.00	3.95	3.89	3.84	3.78	3.73	3.67
9	7.21	5.71	5.08	4.72	4.48	4.32	4.20	4.10	4.03	3.96	3.87	3.77	3.67	3.61	3.56	3.51	3.45	3.39	3.33
10	6.94	5.46	4.83	4.47	4.24	4.07	3.95	3.85	3.78	3.72	3.62	3.52	3.42	3.37	3.31	3.26	3.20	3.14	3.08
11	6.72	5.26	4.63	4.28	4.04	3.88	3.76	3.66	3.59	3.53	3.43	3.33	3.23	3.17	3.12	3.06	3.00	2.94	2.88
12	6.55	5.10	4.47	4.12	3.89	3.73	3.61	3.51	3.44	3.37	3.28	3.18	3.07	3.02	2.96	2.91	2.85	2.79	2.72
13	6.41	4.97	4.35	4.00	3.77	3.60	3.48	3.39	3.31	3.25	3.15	3.05	2.95	2.89	2.84	2.78	2.72	2.66	2.60
14	6.30	4.86	4.24	3.89	3.66	3.50	3.38	3.29	3.21	3.15	3.05	2.95	2.84	2.79	2.73	2.67	2.61	2.55	2.49
15	6.20	4.77	4.15	3.80	3.58	3.41	3.29	3.20	3.12	3.06	2.96	2.86	2.76	2.70	2.64	2.59	2.52	2.46	2.40
16	6.12	4.69	4.08	3.73	3.50	3.34	3.22	3.12	3.05	2.99	2.89	2.79	2.68	2.63	2.57	2.51	2.45	2.38	2.32
17	6.04	4.62	4.01	3.66	3.44	3.28	3.16	3.06	2.98	2.92	2.82	2.72	2.62	2.56	2.50	2.44	2.38	2.32	2.25
18	5.98	4.56	3.95	3.61	3.38	3.22	3.10	3.01	2.93	2.87	2.77	2.67	2.56	2.50	2.44	2.38	2.32	2.26	2.19
19	5.92	4.51	3.90	3.56	3.33	3.17	3.05	2.96	2.88	2.82	2.72	2.62	2.51	2.45	2.39	2.33	2.27	2.20	2.13
20	5.87	4.46	3.86	3.51	3.29	3.13	3.01	2.91	2.84	2.77	2.68	2.57	2.46	2.41	2.35	2.29	2.22	2.16	2.09
21	5.83	4.42	3.82	3.48	3.25	3.09	2.97	2.87	2.80	2.73	2.64	2.53	2.42	2.37	2.31	2.25	2.18	2.11	2.04
22	5.79	4.38	3.78	3.44	3.22	3.05	2.93	2.84	2.76	2.70	2.60	2.50	2.39	2.33	2.27	2.21	2.14	2.08	2.00
23	5.75	4.35	3.75	3.41	3.18	3.02	2.90	2.81	2.73	2.67	2.57	2.47	2.36	2.30	2.24	2.18	2.11	2.04	1.97
24	5.72	4.32	3.72	3.38	3.15	2.99	2.87	2.78	2.70	2.64	2.54	2.44	2.33	2.27	2.21	2.15	2.08	2.01	1.94
25	5.69	4.29	3.69	3.35	3.13	2.97	2.85	2.75	2.68	2.61	2.51	2.41	2.30	2.24	2.18	2.12	2.05	1.98	1.91
26	5.66	4.27	3.67	3.33	3.10	2.94	2.82	2.73	2.65	2.59	2.49	2.39	2.28	2.22	2.16	2.09	2.03	1.95	1.88
27	5.63	4.24	3.65	3.31	3.08	2.92	2.80	2.71	2.63	2.57	2.47	2.36	2.25	2.19	2.13	2.07	2.00	1.93	1.85
28	5.61	4.22	3.63	3.29	3.06	2.90	2.78	2.69	2.61	2.55	2.45	2.34	2.23	2.17	2.11	2.05	1.98	1.91	1.83
29	5.59	4.20	3.61	3.27	3.04	2.88	2.76	2.67	2.59	2.53	2.43	2.32	2.21	2.15	2.09	2.03	1.96	1.89	1.81
30	5.57	4.18	3.59	3.25	3.03	2.87	2.75	2.65	2.57	2.51	2.41	2.31	2.20	2.14	2.07	2.01	1.94	1.87	1.79
40	5.42	4.05	3.46	3.13	2.90	2.74	2.62	2.53	2.45	2.39	2.29	2.18	2.07	2.01	1.94	1.88	1.80	1.72	1.64
60	5.29	3.93	3.34	3.01	2.79	2.63	2.51	2.41	2.33	2.27	2.17	2.06	1.94	1.88	1.82	1.74	1.67	1.58	1.48
120	5.15	3.80	3.23	2.89	2.67	2.52	2.39	2.30	2.22	2.16	2.05	1.94	1.82	1.76	1.69	1.61	1.53	1.43	1.31
∞	5.02	3.69	3.12	2.79	2.57	2.41	2.29	2.19	2.11	2.05	1.94	1.83	1.71	1.64	1.57	1.48	1.39	1.27	1.00

$$P[F_{\gamma_1,\gamma_2} \leq f] = .99$$

γ_2 \ γ_1	1	2	3	4	5	6	7	8	9	10	12	15	20	24	30	40	60	120	∞
1	4052	4999.5	5403	5625	5764	5859	5928	5982	6022	6056	6106	6157	6209	6235	6261	6287	6313	6339	6366
2	98.50	99.00	99.17	99.25	99.30	99.33	99.36	99.37	99.39	99.40	99.42	99.43	99.45	99.46	99.47	99.47	99.48	99.49	99.50
3	34.12	30.82	29.46	28.71	28.24	27.91	27.67	27.49	27.35	27.23	27.05	26.87	26.69	26.60	26.50	26.41	26.32	26.22	26.13
4	21.20	18.00	16.69	15.98	15.52	15.21	14.98	14.80	14.66	14.55	14.37	14.20	14.02	13.93	13.84	13.75	13.65	13.56	13.46
5	16.26	13.27	12.06	11.39	10.97	10.67	10.46	10.29	10.16	10.05	9.89	9.72	9.55	9.47	9.38	9.29	9.20	9.11	9.02
6	13.75	10.92	9.78	9.15	8.75	8.47	8.26	8.10	7.98	7.87	7.72	7.56	7.40	7.31	7.23	7.14	7.06	6.97	6.88
7	12.25	9.55	8.45	7.85	7.46	7.19	6.99	6.84	6.72	6.62	6.47	6.31	6.16	6.07	5.99	5.91	5.82	5.74	5.65
8	11.26	8.65	7.59	7.01	6.63	6.37	6.18	6.03	5.91	5.81	5.67	5.52	5.36	5.28	5.20	5.12	5.03	4.95	4.86
9	10.56	8.02	6.99	6.42	6.06	5.80	5.61	5.47	5.35	5.26	5.11	4.96	4.81	4.73	4.65	4.57	4.48	4.40	4.31
10	10.04	7.56	6.55	5.99	5.64	5.39	5.20	5.06	4.94	4.85	4.71	4.56	4.41	4.33	4.25	4.17	4.08	4.00	3.91
11	9.65	7.21	6.22	5.67	5.32	5.07	4.89	4.74	4.63	4.54	4.40	4.25	4.10	4.02	3.94	3.86	3.78	3.69	3.60
12	9.33	6.93	5.95	5.41	5.06	4.82	4.64	4.50	4.39	4.30	4.16	4.01	3.86	3.78	3.70	3.62	3.54	3.45	3.36
13	9.07	6.70	5.74	5.21	4.86	4.62	4.44	4.30	4.19	4.10	3.96	3.82	3.66	3.59	3.51	3.43	3.34	3.25	3.17
14	8.86	6.51	5.56	5.04	4.69	4.46	4.28	4.14	4.03	3.94	3.80	3.66	3.51	3.43	3.35	3.27	3.18	3.09	3.00
15	8.68	6.36	5.42	4.89	4.56	4.32	4.14	4.00	3.89	3.80	3.67	3.52	3.37	3.29	3.21	3.13	3.05	2.96	2.87
16	8.53	6.23	5.29	4.77	4.44	4.20	4.03	3.89	3.78	3.69	3.55	3.41	3.26	3.18	3.10	3.02	2.93	2.84	2.75
17	8.40	6.11	5.18	4.67	4.34	4.10	3.93	3.79	3.68	3.59	3.46	3.31	3.16	3.08	3.00	2.92	2.83	2.75	2.65
18	8.29	6.01	5.09	4.58	4.25	4.01	3.84	3.71	3.60	3.51	3.37	3.23	3.08	3.00	2.92	2.84	2.75	2.66	2.57
19	8.18	5.93	5.01	4.50	4.17	3.94	3.77	3.63	3.52	3.43	3.30	3.15	3.00	2.92	2.84	2.76	2.67	2.58	2.49
20	8.10	5.85	4.94	4.43	4.10	3.87	3.70	3.56	3.46	3.37	3.23	3.09	2.94	2.86	2.78	2.69	2.61	2.52	2.42
21	8.02	5.78	4.87	4.37	4.04	3.81	3.64	3.51	3.40	3.31	3.17	3.03	2.88	2.80	2.72	2.64	2.55	2.46	2.36
22	7.95	5.72	4.82	4.31	3.99	3.76	3.59	3.45	3.35	3.26	3.12	2.98	2.83	2.75	2.67	2.58	2.50	2.40	2.31
23	7.88	5.66	4.76	4.26	3.94	3.71	3.54	3.41	3.30	3.21	3.07	2.93	2.78	2.70	2.62	2.54	2.45	2.35	2.26
24	7.82	5.61	4.72	4.22	3.90	3.67	3.50	3.36	3.26	3.17	3.03	2.89	2.74	2.66	2.58	2.49	2.40	2.31	2.21
25	7.77	5.57	4.68	4.18	3.85	3.63	3.46	3.32	3.22	3.13	2.99	2.85	2.70	2.62	2.54	2.45	2.36	2.27	2.17
26	7.72	5.53	4.64	4.14	3.82	3.59	3.42	3.29	3.18	3.09	2.96	2.81	2.66	2.58	2.50	2.42	2.33	2.23	2.13
27	7.68	5.49	4.60	4.11	3.78	3.56	3.39	3.26	3.15	3.06	2.93	2.78	2.63	2.55	2.47	2.38	2.29	2.20	2.10
28	7.64	5.45	4.57	4.07	3.75	3.53	3.36	3.23	3.12	3.03	2.90	2.75	2.60	2.52	2.44	2.35	2.26	2.17	2.06
29	7.60	5.42	4.54	4.04	3.73	3.50	3.33	3.20	3.09	3.00	2.87	2.73	2.57	2.49	2.41	2.33	2.23	2.14	2.03
30	7.56	5.39	4.51	4.02	3.70	3.47	3.30	3.17	3.07	2.98	2.84	2.70	2.55	2.47	2.39	2.30	2.21	2.11	2.01
40	7.31	5.18	4.31	3.83	3.51	3.29	3.12	2.99	2.89	2.80	2.66	2.52	2.37	2.29	2.20	2.11	2.02	1.92	1.80
60	7.08	4.98	4.13	3.65	3.34	3.12	2.95	2.82	2.72	2.63	2.50	2.35	2.20	2.12	2.03	1.94	1.84	1.73	1.60
120	6.85	4.79	3.95	3.48	3.17	2.96	2.79	2.66	2.56	2.47	2.34	2.19	2.03	1.95	1.86	1.76	1.66	1.53	1.38
∞	6.63	4.61	3.78	3.32	3.02	2.80	2.64	2.51	2.41	2.32	2.18	2.04	1.88	1.79	1.70	1.59	1.47	1.32	1.00

Reprinted with permission from W. H. Beyer (ed.), *CRC Handbook of Tables for Probability and Statistics*, 2d ed., 1968, pp. 306–308. Copyright CRC Press, Boca Raton, Florida.

TABLE X

Duncan's tables

Least significant studentized ranges r_p $\alpha = 0.05$ P						Least significant studentized ranges r_p $\alpha = 0.01$ P					
r	2	3	4	5	6	r	2	3	4	5	6
1	17.97	17.97	17.97	17.97	17.97	1	90.03	90.03	90.03	90.03	90.03
2	6.085	6.085	6.085	6.085	6.085	2	14.04	14.04	14.04	14.04	14.04
3	4.501	4.516	4.516	4.516	4.516	3	8.261	8.321	8.321	8.321	8.321
4	3.927	4.013	4.033	4.033	4.033	4	6.512	6.677	6.740	6.756	6.756
5	3.635	3.749	3.797	3.814	3.814	5	5.702	5.893	5.898	6.040	6.065
6	3.461	3.587	3.649	3.680	3.694	6	5.243	5.439	5.549	5.614	5.655
7	3.344	3.477	3.548	3.588	3.611	7	4.949	5.145	5.260	5.334	5.383
8	3.261	3.399	3.475	3.521	3.549	8	4.746	4.939	5.057	5.135	5.189
9	3.199	3.339	3.420	3.470	3.502	9	4.596	4.787	4.906	4.986	5.043
10	3.151	3.293	3.376	3.430	3.465	10	4.482	4.671	4.790	4.871	4.931
11	3.113	3.256	3.342	3.397	3.435	11	4.392	4.579	4.697	4.780	4.841
12	3.082	3.225	3.313	3.370	3.410	12	4.320	4.504	4.622	4.706	4.767
13	3.055	3.200	3.289	3.348	3.389	13	4.260	4.442	4.560	4.644	4.706
14	3.033	3.178	3.268	3.329	3.372	14	4.210	4.391	4.508	4.591	4.654
15	3.014	3.160	3.250	3.312	3.356	15	4.168	4.347	4.463	4.547	4.610
16	2.998	3.144	3.235	3.298	3.343	16	4.131	4.309	4.425	4.509	4.572
17	2.984	3.130	3.222	3.285	3.331	17	4.099	4.275	4.391	4.475	4.539
18	2.971	3.118	3.210	3.274	3.321	18	4.071	4.246	4.362	4.445	4.509
19	2.960	3.107	3.199	3.264	3.311	19	4.046	4.220	4.335	4.419	4.483
20	2.950	3.097	3.190	3.255	3.303	20	4.024	4.197	4.312	4.395	4.459
24	2.919	3.066	3.160	3.226	3.276	24	3.956	4.126	4.239	4.322	4.386
30	2.888	3.035	3.131	3.199	3.250	30	3.889	4.506	4.168	4.250	4.314
40	2.858	3.006	3.102	3.171	3.224	40	3.825	3.988	4.098	4.180	4.244
60	2.829	2.976	3.073	3.143	3.198	60	3.762	3.922	4.031	4.111	4.174
120	2.800	2.947	3.045	3.116	3.172	120	3.702	3.858	3.965	4.044	4.107
∞	2.772	2.918	3.017	3.089	3.146	∞	3.643	3.796	3.900	3.978	4.040

Abridgment of H. L. Harter's "Critical Values for Duncan's New Multiple Range Test," *Biometrics,* vol. 16, no. 4 (1960). With permission from the Biometric Society.

TABLE XI
Wilcoxon signed-rank test

One-sided	Two-sided	$n = 5$	$n = 6$	$n = 7$	$n = 8$	$n = 9$	$n = 10$
$P = .05$	$P = .10$	1	2	4	6	8	11
$P = .025$	$P = .05$		1	2	4	6	8
$P = .01$	$P = .02$			0	2	3	5
$P = .005$	$P = .01$				0	2	3

One-sided	Two-sided	$n = 11$	$n = 12$	$n = 13$	$n = 14$	$n = 15$	$n = 16$
$P = .05$	$P = .10$	14	17	21	26	30	36
$P = .025$	$P = .05$	11	14	17	21	25	30
$P = .01$	$P = .02$	7	10	13	16	20	24
$P = .005$	$P = .01$	5	7	10	13	16	19

One-sided	Two-sided	$n = 17$	$n = 18$	$n = 19$	$n = 20$	$n = 21$	$n = 22$
$P = .05$	$P = .10$	41	47	54	60	68	75
$P = .025$	$P = .05$	35	40	46	52	59	66
$P = .01$	$P = .02$	28	33	38	43	49	56
$P = .005$	$P = .01$	23	28	32	37	43	49

One-sided	Two-sided	$n = 23$	$n = 24$	$n = 25$	$n = 26$	$n = 27$	$n = 28$
$P = .05$	$P = .10$	83	92	101	110	120	130
$P = .025$	$P = .05$	73	81	90	98	107	117
$P = .01$	$P = .02$	62	69	77	85	93	102
$P = .005$	$P = .01$	55	61	68	76	84	92

One-sided	Two-sided	$n = 29$	$n = 30$	$n = 31$	$n = 32$	$n = 33$	$n = 34$
$P = .05$	$P = .10$	141	152	163	175	188	201
$P = .025$	$P = .05$	127	137	148	159	171	183
$P = .01$	$P = .02$	111	120	130	141	151	162
$P = .005$	$P = .01$	100	109	118	128	138	149

One-sided	Two-sided	$n = 35$	$n = 36$	$n = 37$	$n = 38$	$n = 39$	
$P = .05$	$P = .10$	214	228	242	256	271	
$P = .025$	$P = .05$	195	208	222	235	250	
$P = .01$	$P = .02$	174	186	198	211	224	
$P = .005$	$P = .01$	160	171	183	195	208	

One-sided	Two-sided	$n = 40$	$n = 41$	$n = 42$	$n = 43$	$n = 44$	$n = 45$
$P = .05$	$P = .10$	287	303	319	336	353	371
$P = .025$	$P = .05$	264	279	295	311	327	344
$P = .01$	$P = .02$	238	252	267	281	297	313
$P = .005$	$P = .01$	221	234	248	262	277	292

One-sided	Two-sided	$n = 46$	$n = 47$	$n = 48$	$n = 49$	$n = 50$	
$P = .05$	$P = .10$	389	408	427	446	466	
$P = .025$	$P = .05$	361	379	397	415	434	
$P = .01$	$P = .02$	329	345	362	380	398	
$P = .005$	$P = .01$	307	323	339	356	373	

Reprinted with permission from W. H. Beyer (ed.), *CRC Handbook of Tables for Probability and Statistics*, 2d ed., 1968, p. 400. Copyright CRC Press, Boca Raton, Florida.

TABLE XII

Wilcoxon rank-sum test

$m = 3(1)25$ and $n = m(1)m + 25$
$P = .05$ one-sided; $P = .10$ two-sided

n	$m = 3$	$m = 4$	$m = 5$	$m = 6$	$m = 7$	$m = 8$	$m = 9$	$m = 10$	$m = 11$	$m = 12$	$m = 13$	$m = 14$
$n = m$	6,15	12,24	19,36	28,50	39,66	52,84	66,105	83,127	101,152	121,179	143,208	167,239
$n = m + 1$	7,17	13,27	20,40	30,54	41,71	54,90	69,111	86,134	105,159	125,187	148,216	172,248
$n = m + 2$	7,20	14,30	22,43	32,58	43,76	57,95	72,117	89,141	109,166	129,195	152,225	177,257
$n = m + 3$	8,22	15,33	24,46	33,63	46,80	60,100	75,123	93,147	112,174	134,202	157,233	182,266
$n = m + 4$	9,24	16,36	25,50	35,67	48,85	62,106	78,129	96,154	116,181	138,210	162,241	187,275
$n = m + 5$	9,27	17,39	26,54	37,71	50,90	65,111	81,135	100,160	120,188	142,218	166,250	192,284
$n = m + 6$	10,29	18,42	27,58	39,75	52,95	67,117	84,141	103,167	124,195	147,225	171,258	197,293
$n = m + 7$	11,31	19,45	29,61	41,79	54,100	70,122	87,147	107,173	128,202	151,233	176,266	203,301
$n = m + 8$	11,34	20,48	30,65	42,84	57,104	73,127	90,153	110,180	132,209	155,241	181,274	208,310
$n = m + 9$	12,36	21,51	32,68	44,88	59,109	75,133	93,159	114,186	136,216	159,249	185,283	213,319
$n = m + 10$	13,38	22,54	33,72	46,92	61,114	78,138	96,165	117,193	139,224	164,256	190,291	218,328
$n = m + 11$	13,41	23,57	34,76	48,96	63,119	80,144	100,170	120,200	143,231	168,264	195,299	223,337
$n = m + 12$	14,43	24,60	36,79	50,100	65,124	83,149	103,176	124,206	147,238	172,272	199,308	228,346
$n = m + 13$	15,45	25,63	37,83	52,104	68,128	86,154	106,182	127,213	151,245	177,279	204,316	234,354
$n = m + 14$	15,48	26,66	39,86	53,109	70,133	88,160	109,188	131,219	155,252	181,287	209,324	239,363
$n = m + 15$	16,50	27,69	40,90	55,113	72,138	91,165	112,194	134,226	159,259	185,295	214,332	244,372
$n = m + 16$	17,52	28,72	42,93	57,117	74,143	94,170	115,200	138,232	163,266	190,302	218,341	249,381
$n = m + 17$	17,55	29,75	43,97	59,121	77,147	96,176	118,206	141,239	167,273	194,310	223,349	254,390
$n = m + 18$	18,57	30,78	44,101	61,125	79,152	99,181	121,212	145,245	171,280	198,318	228,357	260,398
$n = m + 19$	19,59	31,81	46,104	62,130	81,157	102,186	124,218	148,252	175,287	203,325	233,365	265,407
$n = m + 20$	19,62	32,84	47,108	64,134	83,162	104,192	127,224	152,258	178,295	207,333	237,374	270,416
$n = m + 21$	20,64	33,87	49,111	66,138	86,166	107,197	130,230	155,265	182,302	211,341	242,382	275,425
$n = m + 22$	21,66	34,90	50,115	68,142	88,171	109,203	133,236	159,271	186,309	216,348	247,390	280,434
$n = m + 23$	21,69	35,93	52,118	70,146	90,176	112,208	136,242	162,278	190,316	220,356	252,398	285,443
$n = m + 24$	22,71	37,95	53,122	72,150	92,181	115,213	139,248	166,284	194,323	224,364	257,406	291,451
$n = m + 25$	23,73	38,98	54,126	73,155	94,186	117,219	142,254	169,291	198,330	229,371	261,415	296,460

$$m = 3(1)25 \text{ and } n = m(1)m + 25$$
$$P = .05 \text{ one-sided}; \ P = .10 \text{ two-sided}$$

n	$m = 15$	$m = 16$	$m = 17$	$m = 18$	$m = 19$	$m = 20$	$m = 21$	$m = 22$	$m = 23$	$m = 24$	$m = 25$
$n = m$	192,273	220,308	249,346	280,386	314,427	349,471	386,517	424,566	465,616	508,668	552,723
$n = m + 1$	198,282	226,318	256,356	287,397	321,439	356,484	394,530	433,579	474,630	517,683	562,738
$n = m + 2$	203,292	232,328	262,367	294,408	328,451	364,496	402,543	442,592	483,644	527,697	572,753
$n = m + 3$	209,301	238,338	268,378	301,419	336,462	372,508	410,556	450,606	492,658	536,712	582,768
$n = m + 4$	215,310	244,348	275,388	308,430	343,474	380,520	418,569	459,619	501,672	546,726	592,783
$n = m + 5$	220,320	250,358	281,399	315,441	350,486	387,533	427,581	468,632	511,685	555,741	602,798
$n = m + 6$	226,329	256,368	288,409	322,452	358,497	395,545	435,594	476,646	520,699	565,755	612,813
$n = m + 7$	231,339	262,378	294,420	329,463	365,509	403,557	443,607	485,659	529,713	574,770	622,828
$n = m + 8$	237,348	268,388	301,430	336,474	372,521	411,569	451,620	494,672	538,727	584,784	632,843
$n = m + 9$	242,358	274,398	307,441	342,486	380,532	419,581	459,633	502,686	547,741	594,798	642,858
$n = m + 10$	248,367	280,408	314,451	349,497	387,544	426,594	468,645	511,699	556,755	603,813	652,873
$n = m + 11$	254,376	286,418	320,462	356,508	394,556	434,606	476,658	520,712	565,769	613,827	662,888
$n = m + 12$	259,386	292,428	327,472	363,519	402,567	442,618	484,671	528,726	574,783	622,842	672,903
$n = m + 13$	265,395	298,438	333,483	370,530	409,579	450,630	492,684	537,739	584,796	632,856	682,918
$n = m + 14$	270,405	304,448	340,493	377,541	416,591	458,642	501,696	546,752	593,810	642,870	692,933
$n = m + 15$	276,414	310,458	346,504	384,552	424,602	465,655	509,709	554,766	602,824	651,885	702,948
$n = m + 16$	282,423	316,468	353,514	391,563	431,614	473,667	517,722	563,779	611,838	661,899	712,963
$n = m + 17$	287,433	322,478	359,525	398,574	438,626	481,679	526,734	572,792	620,852	670,914	723,977
$n = m + 18$	293,442	328,488	366,535	405,585	446,637	489,691	534,747	581,805	629,866	680,928	733,992
$n = m + 19$	299,451	334,498	372,546	412,596	453,649	487,703	542,760	589,819	639,879	690,942	743,1007
$n = m + 20$	304,461	340,508	379,556	419,607	461,660	505,715	550,773	598,832	648,893	699,957	753,1022
$n = m + 21$	310,470	347,517	385,568	426,618	468,672	512,728	559,785	607,845	657,907	709,971	763,1037
$n = m + 22$	315,480	353,527	392,577	433,629	475,684	520,740	567,798	615,859	666,921	718,986	773,1052
$n = m + 23$	321,489	359,537	398,588	439,641	483,695	528,752	575,811	624,872	675,935	728,1000	783,1067
$n = m + 24$	327,498	365,547	405,598	446,652	490,707	536,764	583,824	633,885	684,949	738,1014	793,1082
$n = m + 25$	332,508	371,557	411,609	453,663	498,718	544,776	592,836	642,898	694,962	747,1029	803,1097

TABLE XII
(Continued)

$$m = 3(1)25 \text{ and } n = m(1)m + 25$$
$$P = .025 \text{ one-sided}; P = .05 \text{ two-sided}$$

n	m = 3	m = 4	m = 5	m = 6	m = 7	m = 8	m = 9	m = 10	m = 11	m = 12	m = 13	m = 14
n = m	5,16	11,25	18,37	26,52	37,68	49,87	63,108	79,131	96,157	116,184	137,214	160,246
n = m + 1	6,18	12,28	19,41	28,56	39,73	51,93	66,114	82,138	100,164	120,192	141,223	165,255
n = m + 2	6,21	12,32	20,45	29,61	41,78	54,98	68,121	85,145	103,172	124,200	146,231	170,264
n = m + 3	7,23	13,35	21,49	31,65	43,83	56,104	71,127	88,152	107,179	128,208	150,240	174,274
n = m + 4	7,26	14,38	22,53	32,70	45,88	58,110	74,133	91,159	110,187	131,217	154,249	179,283
n = m + 5	8,28	15,41	24,56	34,74	46,94	61,115	77,139	94,166	114,194	135,225	159,257	184,292
n = m + 6	8,31	16,44	25,60	36,78	48,99	63,121	79,146	97,173	118,201	139,233	163,266	189,301
n = m + 7	9,33	17,47	26,64	37,83	50,104	65,127	82,152	101,179	121,209	143,241	168,274	194,310
n = m + 8	10,35	17,51	27,68	39,87	52,109	68,132	85,158	104,186	125,216	147,249	172,283	198,320
n = m + 9	10,38	18,54	29,71	41,91	54,114	70,138	88,164	107,193	128,224	151,257	176,292	203,329
n = m + 10	11,40	19,57	30,75	42,96	56,119	72,144	90,171	110,200	132,231	155,265	181,300	208,338
n = m + 11	11,43	20,60	31,79	44,100	58,124	75,149	93,177	113,207	135,239	159,273	185,309	213,347
n = m + 12	12,45	21,63	32,83	45,105	60,129	77,155	96,183	117,213	139,246	163,281	190,317	218,356
n = m + 13	12,48	22,66	33,87	47,109	62,134	80,160	99,189	120,220	143,253	167,289	194,326	222,366
n = m + 14	13,50	23,69	35,90	49,113	64,139	82,166	101,196	123,227	146,261	171,297	198,335	227,375
n = m + 15	13,53	24,72	36,94	50,118	66,144	84,172	104,202	126,234	150,268	175,305	203,343	232,384
n = m + 16	14,55	24,76	37,98	52,122	68,149	87,177	107,208	129,241	153,276	179,313	207,352	237,393
n = m + 17	14,58	25,79	38,102	53,127	70,154	89,183	110,214	132,248	157,283	183,321	212,360	242,402
n = m + 18	15,60	26,82	40,105	55,131	72,159	92,188	113,220	136,254	161,290	187,329	216,369	247,411
n = m + 19	15,63	27,85	41,109	57,135	74,164	94,194	115,227	139,261	164,298	191,337	221,377	252,420
n = m + 20	16,65	28,88	42,113	58,140	76,169	96,200	118,233	142,268	168,305	195,345	225,386	256,430
n = m + 21	16,68	29,91	43,117	60,144	78,174	99,205	121,239	145,275	171,313	199,353	229,395	261,439
n = m + 22	17,70	30,94	45,120	61,149	80,179	101,211	124,245	148,282	175,320	203,361	234,403	266,448
n = m + 23	17,73	31,97	46,124	63,153	82,184	103,217	127,251	152,288	179,327	207,369	238,412	271,457
n = m + 24	18,75	31,101	47,128	65,157	84,189	106,222	129,258	155,295	182,335	211,377	243,420	276,466
n = m + 25	18,78	32,104	48,132	66,162	86,194	108,228	132,264	158,302	186,342	216,384	247,429	281,475

$$m = 3(1)25 \text{ and } n = m(1)m + 25$$
$$P = .025 \text{ one-sided}; \quad P = .05 \text{ two-sided}$$

n	$m = 15$	$m = 16$	$m = 17$	$m = 18$	$m = 19$	$m = 20$	$m = 21$	$m = 22$	$m = 23$	$m = 24$	$m = 25$
$n = m$	185,280	212,316	240,355	271,395	303,438	337,483	373,530	411,579	451,630	493,683	536,739
$n = m + 1$	190,290	217,327	246,366	277,407	310,450	345,495	381,543	419,593	460,644	502,698	546,754
$n = m + 2$	195,300	223,337	252,377	284,418	317,462	352,508	389,556	428,606	468,659	511,713	555,770
$n = m + 3$	201,309	229,347	258,388	290,430	324,474	359,521	397,569	436,620	477,673	520,728	565,785
$n = m + 4$	206,319	234,358	264,399	297,441	331,486	367,533	404,583	444,634	486,687	529,743	574,801
$n = m + 5$	211,329	240,368	271,409	303,453	338,498	374,546	412,596	452,648	494,702	538,758	584,816
$n = m + 6$	216,339	245,379	277,420	310,464	345,510	381,559	420,609	460,662	503,716	547,773	593,832
$n = m + 7$	221,349	251,389	283,431	316,476	351,523	389,571	428,622	469,675	512,730	556,788	603,847
$n = m + 8$	227,358	257,399	289,442	323,487	358,535	396,584	436,635	477,689	520,745	565,803	612,863
$n = m + 9$	232,368	262,410	295,453	329,499	365,547	403,597	443,649	485,703	529,759	575,817	622,878
$n = m + 10$	237,378	268,420	301,464	336,510	372,559	411,609	451,662	493,717	538,773	584,832	632,893
$n = m + 11$	242,388	274,430	307,475	342,522	379,571	418,622	459,675	502,730	546,788	593,847	641,909
$n = m + 12$	248,397	279,441	313,486	349,533	386,583	426,634	467,688	510,744	555,802	602,862	651,924
$n = m + 13$	253,407	285,451	319,497	355,545	393,595	433,647	475,701	518,758	564,816	611,877	660,940
$n = m + 14$	258,417	291,461	325,508	362,556	400,607	440,660	482,715	526,772	572,831	620,892	670,955
$n = m + 15$	263,427	296,472	331,519	368,568	407,619	448,672	490,728	535,785	581,845	629,907	679,971
$n = m + 16$	269,436	302,482	338,529	375,579	414,631	455,685	498,741	543,799	590,859	638,922	689,986
$n = m + 17$	274,446	308,492	344,540	381,591	421,643	463,697	506,754	551,813	599,873	648,936	699,1001
$n = m + 18$	279,456	314,502	350,551	388,602	428,655	470,710	514,767	560,826	607,888	657,951	708,1017
$n = m + 19$	284,466	319,513	356,562	395,613	435,667	477,723	522,780	568,840	616,902	666,966	718,1032
$n = m + 20$	290,475	325,523	362,573	401,625	442,679	485,735	530,793	576,854	625,916	675,981	727,1048
$n = m + 21$	295,485	331,533	368,584	408,636	449,691	492,748	537,807	584,868	633,931	684,996	737,1063
$n = m + 22$	300,495	336,544	374,595	414,648	456,703	500,760	545,820	593,881	642,945	693,1011	747,1078
$n = m + 23$	306,504	342,554	380,606	421,659	463,715	507,773	553,833	601,895	651,959	703,1025	756,1094
$n = m + 24$	311,514	348,564	387,616	427,671	470,727	515,785	561,846	609,909	660,973	712,1040	766,1109
$n = m + 25$	316,524	353,575	393,627	434,682	477,739	522,798	569,859	618,922	668,988	721,1055	775,1125

TABLE XIII

Blood pressure data

Patient	Sex	Systolic pressure	Diastolic pressure	Patient	Sex	Systolic pressure	Diastolic pressure
1	M	112	80	61	F	142	80
2	F	112	80	62	F	120	80
3	M	130	76	63	M	136	86
4	M	157	86	64	M	142	80
5	F	152	80	65	F	95	80
6	F	130	80	66	M	110	80
7	M	140	90	67	F	118	80
8	M	120	74	68	M	97	75
9	F	100	82	69	M	120	84
10	M	118	100	70	F	110	60
11	F	120	90	71	M	110	80
12	M	122	72	72	F	118	88
13	F	130	80	73	M	117	76
14	M	96	65	74	M	100	78
15	F	90	56	75	F	152	88
16	M	102	70	76	M	112	80
17	F	115	80	77	F	160	88
18	M	130	80	78	M	110	75
19	M	136	94	79	M	128	85
20	F	130	80	80	F	118	90
21	M	122	80	81	M	140	100
22	M	118	84	82	F	90	58
23	M	108	76	83	M	110	70
24	M	110	86	84	F	102	60
25	F	140	88	85	M	140	90
26	M	130	80	86	F	110	80
27	F	120	80	87	M	116	74
28	M	120	76	88	M	118	81
29	M	125	80	89	F	140	85
30	F	130	80	90	M	106	70
31	M	120	80	91	F	110	72
32	M	110	84	92	M	120	75
33	M	115	70	93	F	110	80
34	F	120	100	94	M	120	80
35	M	142	94	95	M	116	80
36	F	120	85	96	F	122	95
37	M	102	64	97	M	130	90
38	M	110	78	98	M	110	70
39	F	118	80	99	F	150	80
40	M	120	80	100	M	122	80
41	F	120	78	101	M	108	58
42	M	126	76	102	F	132	88
43	M	144	100	103	M	110	70
44	F	140	95	104	M	122	82
45	M	116	80	105	F	140	100
46	M	108	80	106	M	138	96
47	F	136	98	107	M	127	90
48	M	135	85	108	F	130	80
49	M	114	76	109	M	130	80
50	F	150	90	110	M	110	70
51	F	110	50	111	F	130	90
52	M	120	70	112	M	130	82
53	M	120	80	113	M	160	105
54	F	122	80	114	F	132	80
55	M	120	80	115	M	120	80
56	M	165	70	116	M	123	73
57	M	120	80	117	F	110	80
58	F	136	90	118	M	112	80
59	M	140	70	119	F	118	72
60	M	110	66	120	M	140	78

R E F E R E N C E S

1. Beyer, William, ed.: *Handbook of Tables for Probability and Statistics,* 2d ed., CRC Press, Boca Raton, Fla., 1968.
2. Bradley, James V.: *Distribution Free Statistical Tests,* Prentice-Hall, Englewood Cliffs, N.J., 1968.
3. Conover, W. J.: *Practical Non-parametric Statistics,* Wiley, New York, 1971.
4. Daniel, W.: *Applied Nonparametric Statistics,* PWS-Kent, Boston, 1990.
5. Hoaglin, D., F. Mosteller, and J. Tukey: *Understanding Robust and Exploratory Data Analysis,* Wiley, New York, 1983.
6. Iman, R.: "Graphs for Use with the Lilliefors Test for Normal and Exponential Distributions," *The American Statistician,* vol. 36, no. 2, 1982.
7. Koopmans, Lambert: *An Introduction to Contemporary Statistics,* PWS-Kent, Boston, 1985.
8. Larson, Harold: *Introduction to Probability Theory and Statistical Inference,* Wiley, New York, 1982.
9. LeOntnor, M., and T. Bishop: *Experimental Design and Analysis,* Valley Book Company, Blacksburg, Va., 1986.
10. Lentner, M., J. Arnold, and K. Hinkelmann: "How to Use the Ratio of MS (Blocks) and MS (Error) Correctly," *American Statistician,* vol. 43, no. 2, 1989, pp. 100–108.
11. Milton, J. S., and J. Arnold: *Introduction to Probability and Statistics: Principles and Applications for Engineering and the Computing Sciences,* McGraw-Hill, New York, 1990.
12. Myers, R.: *Classical and Modern Regression with Applications,* PWS-Kent, Boston, 1990.
13. Myers, R., and J. S. Milton: *A First Course in the Theory of Linear Statistical Models,* PWS-Kent, Boston, 1991.
14. *SAS User's Guide,* Version 5, SAS Institute Inc., Raleigh, N.C., 1985.
15. Snedecor, G. W., and William Cochran: *Statistical Methods,* 6th ed., Iowa State University Press, Ames, 1967.
16. Tukey, John: *Exploratory Data Analysis,* Addison-Wesley, Reading, Mass., 1977.

Answers to
Odd Numbered Problems

Exercises 1.1

1. (a)

Category	Frequency	Relative frequency	Percentage
MI	7	7/24 = .2917	29.17
MR	3	3/24 = .1250	12.5
PI	14	14/24 = .5833	58.33

3. Diagnosis

Sex	MI	MR	PI	Distribution of sex
F	4	1	10	15
	.1667	.0417	.4167	.625
	16.67%	4.17%	41.67%	62.5%
M	3	2	4	9
	.125	.0833	.1667	.375
	12.5%	8.33%	16.67%	37.5%
Distribution of diagnosis	7	3	14	24
	.2917	.125	.5833	
	29.17%	12.5%	58.33%	

5. (a) Headache

Sex	V	T	C	Distribution of sex
F	66	30	34	130
	.3729	.1695	.1921	.7345
	37.29%	16.95%	19.21%	73.45%
M	17	16	14	47
	.0960	.0904	.0791	.2655
	9.60%	9.04%	7.9%	26.55%
Distribution of diagnosis	83	46	48	177
	.4689	.2599	.2712	
	46.89%	25.99%	27.12%	

Cell frequencies are divided by 177.

(b)

Sex	V	T	C		
F	66	30	34	‖	130
	.5077	.2308	.2615	‖	
	50.77%	23.08%	26.15%	‖	
				‖	
M	17	16	14	‖	
	.3617	.3404	.2979	‖	47
	36.17%	34.04%	29.79%	‖	

Cell frequencies for females are divided by 130; those for males are divided by 47.

7. (a) species 2; 46.15% of this species participated in the grooming activity versus 38.46% of the other species
  (b) 42.31%
  (c) yes; the percentages stated in part *a* do seem to be rather different, indicating that species 2 seems to participate in grooming substantially more often than does species 1

Exercises 1.2

1. (a)
```
 4 | 05
 5 | 123
 6 | 122678
 7 | 011189
 8 | 124
 9 | 018
10 | 0
11 | 1
```
  (b) The data suggest a bell shape.
  (c) yes; almost all of these data points lie below the "normal" range of 1.0 to 2.9

3. (a)
```
12 | 12
12 | 5678
13 | 0123344
13 | 5678
14 | 01
14 | 6
```
  (b) no
  (c) average is somewhere in the "low" thirteens; maybe around 13.3; no, all of these readings are well above the standard protective level of 1 mg/ml

5. (a)

Acoustic	Visual
08 |	07 | 01123
08 | 6	07 | 578
09 |	08 | 01
09 | 9	08 | 9
10 | 0123	09 | 0
11 | 34	09 | 579
11 | 57	10 | 012334
12 | 0	10 |
12 | 6	

  (b) no; both diagrams appear to be symmetric
  (c) yes; latency for visual appears to be U-shaped
  (d) visual; more data points are clustered away from the center

7.

Home 1	Home 2
1|88	
2|035899	
3|0114555569	3|6
4|0112227	4|89
5|011269	5|45677
6|1245	6|2334579
7|126	7|128
8|79	8|01339
	9|2

They are similar in shape but not in location. Patients at home 2 tend on the average to be older than those at home 1.

9. (a)

Sterile	Nonsterile
0|	0|23
0|99	0|6679
1|0001	1|11344
1|578	1|5689
2|	2|0
2|5688	2|
3|004	
3|5	

"Nonsterile" forms a rough bell. "Sterile" seems to be more widely dispresed. "Nonsterile" seems to have a lower center of location.

(b)

Sterile	Nonsterile
|0|23	
99|0|6679	
1000|1|11344	
875|1|5689	
|2|0	
8865|2|	
400|3|	
5|3|	

Radishes seem to grow better in sterile soil. However, their growth seems to be more consistent in nonsterile soil.

Exercises 1.3

1. (a) 12,130; 737   **(b)** 11,393   **(c)** 6   **(d)** 1898.833   **(e)** 1899   **(f)** 736.5

(g)

Class	Boundaries	Frequency	Relative frequency	Cumulative frequency	Relative cumulative frequency
1	736.5 to 2635.5	8	0.178	8	0.178
2	2635.5 to 4534.5	9	0.200	17	0.378
3	4534.5 to 6433.5	9	0.200	26	0.578
4	6433.5 to 8332.5	12	0.267	38	0.845
5	8332.5 to 10231.5	5	0.111	43	0.956
6	10231.5 to 12130.5	2	0.044	45	1.000

3. (a)

Class	Boundaries	Frequency	Relative frequency	Cumulative frequency	Relative cumulative frequency
1	1499.5 to 2320.5	9	0.375	9	0.375
2	2320.5 to 3141.5	1	0.042	10	0.417
3	3141.5 to 3962.5	10	0.417	20	0.834
4	3962.5 to 4783.5	0	0.000	20	0.834
5	4783.5 to 5604.5	4	0.167	24	1.000

5. (b) .616

7. (a)
```
0|578
1|01223455677888999
2|00123333444556778
3|0011245678
4|05
5|0
```

(b) yes; the distribution might be skewed right

(c)

Class	Boundaries	Frequency	Relative frequency	Cumulative frequency	Relative cumulative frequency
1	.45 to 1.25	7	.14	7	.14
2	1.25 to 2.05	15	.30	27	.44
3	2.05 to 2.85	15	.30	37	.74
4	2.85 to 3.65	8	.16	45	.90
5	3.65 to 4.45	3	.06	48	.96
6	4.45 to 5.25	2	.04	50	1.00

9. (a) no; the text procedure calls for 6 classes to be used for the burned data, whereas SAS uses 7

(b) .4

(c) .4; no; yes, a future observation of .400 would fall on this boundary

(d) burned: .1085 to .5125; unburned: .0095 to .3755; no

11.

Experimental	Control
	08
	08	8
	09	0
	09	68
	10	012
	10	5699
	11	012222
	11	556789
	12	012334
	12	8
0	13		
98887765	13		
44322	14		
9877655	14		
4211110	15		
65	15		

There is a major difference in location. The double stem-and-leaf graphed back-to-back gives a better picture of the distribution than do the separately graphed histograms.

Exercises 1.4

1. set I: $\bar{x} = 2.1$, $\tilde{x} = 2$
set II: $\bar{x} = 3.5$, $\tilde{x} = 3.5$

3. (a) robins: $\bar{x} = 100.48$, $\tilde{x} = 75.0$
doves: $\bar{x} = 224.66$, $\tilde{x} = 170$

   (b) $\bar{x} = 184.02$, $\tilde{x} = 168.35$
       The median is least affected by the presence of an outlier.
5. $\bar{x} = .72$, $\tilde{x} = .71$
7. $\bar{x} = 1.1$

Exercises 1.5

1. set I: range $= 4$, $s = 1.5$, $s^2 = 2.11$
   set II: range $= 6$, $s = 2.2$, $s^2 = 4.94$
3. **(a)** robin: $s = 62.54$, $s^2 = 3911.446$ **(b)** $s = 119.62$; no
       dove: $s = 234.52$, $s^2 = 55000.499$ $s^2 = 14308.124$
   (c) robin: 90.25; dove: 220.6   **(d)** 216.35; yes   **(e)** robin: 255.0; dove: 1186.1
   (f) 367.8; no
5. $s = .98$, $s^2 = .954$, range $= 4.5$, iqr $= 1.3$
7. **(a)** 0|1   **(b)** site I: $\bar{x} = 20.0$, $\tilde{x} = 19.0$ **(c)** site I: $s = 10.1$, $s^2 = 102.13$
       0|9   site II: $\bar{x} = 16.6$, $\tilde{x} = 17.5$ site II: $s = 6.1$, $s^2 = 37.44$
       1|0234 $\tilde{x} = .71$, $s^2 = .1956$, iqr $= .22$
       1|55789
       2|001234
       2|5
9. **(a)** Any number that is a fair amount larger than the largest value or smaller than the small-
       est value will change the range but have little effect on the median. For example, 5
       would work.
   (b) Any value that is close to the average value would work.

Exercises 1.6

1. **(a)** 0|2   **(b)** $\bar{x} = 11$, $q_1 = 9$, $q_3 = 13$, iqr $= 4$, $f_1 = 3$, $f_3 = 19$,
       0|67889 $F_1 = -3$, $F_3 = 25$, $a_1 = 6$, $a_3 = 16$
       1|00111122334   **(c)** The values 2 and 20 are each mild outliers.
       1|556
       2|0
3. $\tilde{x} = 2.72$, $q_1 = 1.32$, $q_3 = 5.25$, iqr $= 3.93$, $f_1 = 4.57$, $f_3 = 11.145$; no outliers
5. **(a)** A: $\tilde{x} = 130$, $q_1 = 119.5$, $q_3 = 139.0$, iqr $= 19.5$, $f_1 = 90.25$, $f_3 = 168.25$,
           $F_1 = 61.0$, $F_3 = 197.5$
       outliers: 12.5;, 170,200
       $a_1 = 105$, $a_3 = 156$
       R: $\tilde{x} = 253$, $q_1 = 238$, $q_3 = 271$, iqr $= 33$, $f_1 = 188.5$, $f_3 = 320.5$, $F_1 = 139.0$,
           $F_3 = 370.0$
       outlier: 561
       $a_1 = 221$, $a_3 = 283$
   (b) $\bar{x} = 128.07$, $s^2 = 1282.681$ **(c)** $\bar{x} = 133.95$, $s^2 = 503.83$
   (d) 516 is an outlier; no
7. **(a)** 1: 7.7; 2: 5.5   **(b)** group 2   **(c)** group 1
   (d) group 1; no, it might be an error in data entry or a botched experimental point
   (e) yes

Exercises 1.7

1. (a)

Class	Midpoint	Cumulative frequency
1	7	1
2	12	3
3	17	8
4	22	11

(b) $\bar{x} \doteq 16.5$, $s^2 \doteq 22.27$, $s \doteq 4.7$, $\tilde{x} \doteq 17.5$

3. (a) Men   Women

Class	Midpoint	Cumulative frequency	Class	Midpoint	Cumulative frequency
1	7	1	1	7	0
2	12	5	2	12	2
3	17	12	3	17	12
4	22	35	4	22	19
5	27	51	5	27	22
6	32	58	6	32	27
7	37	68	7	37	29

(b) men: $\bar{x} \doteq 25.1$, $s^2 = 52.26$, $s \doteq 7.2$, $\tilde{x} \doteq 24.4$
women: $\bar{x} = 22.9$, $s^2 \doteq 51.91$, $s \doteq 7.2$, $\tilde{x} \doteq 21.6$

Exercises 2.1

1. relative frequency/personal   **3.** relative frequency; $\frac{5}{150}$ **5.** classical; $\frac{1}{4}$

7. relative frequency; $\frac{8}{100}$ **9.** classical; $\frac{1}{5}$

11. (a) .800

(b) 5% of the time there is a reaction in the first 5.9 minutes so 95% of the time there is no reaction; therefore, $p \doteq .95$

(c) .15

13. high; due to the seriousness of the consequences of the stick, a 1 in 20 chance seems to be rather high

Exercises 2.2

1.

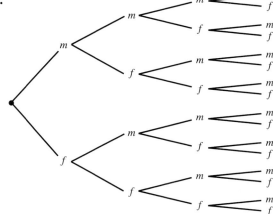

$\frac{1}{2}$; $\frac{6}{16}$; $\frac{4}{16}$; 0

3. (a)

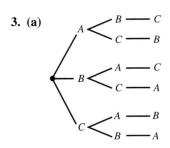

(b) $\frac{1}{3}$

5. (a)

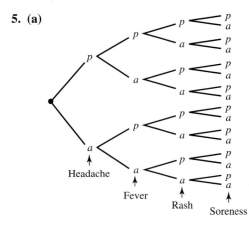

Headache

Fever

Rash

Soreness

(b) pppp, pppa, papp, papa, appp, appa, aapp, aapa

(c) pppp, ppap, appp, apap

(d) pppp, appp

(e) ppaa, paap, paaa, apaa, aaap, aaaa

7. (a)

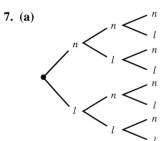

(b) The paths are equally likely if, on each test, the cell count is just as likely to be normal as low; no

9. (a)

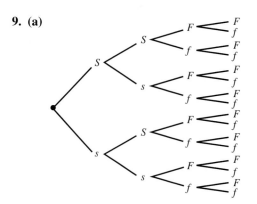

(b) (i) $\frac{1}{16}$ **(ii)** $\frac{9}{16}$ **(iii)** $\frac{4}{16}$ **(iv)** $\frac{12}{16}$

11. (a) tall, yellow, round
(b)

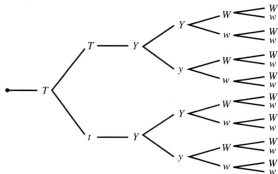

(c) each is tall and yellow; some are wrinkled and some are round
(d) 1   **(e)** $\frac{4}{16}$ **(f)** 0

13. (a)

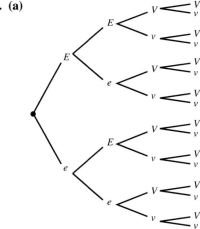

(b) 4   **(c)** 12   **(d)** $\frac{12}{16}, \frac{1}{6}, \frac{15}{16}$

Exercises 2.3

1. permutation   **3.** combination   **5.** normal-high-high-normal-low; nnhhl; permutation
7. tutu = tagged-untagged-tagged-untagged
   tuut = tagged-untagged-untagged-tagged
9. combination; pppwwwwp; pwpwpwwp; permutation

Exercises 2.4

1. $20 \cdot 15 = 300$ **3.** $5 \cdot 24 \cdot 23 \cdot 22 \cdot 21 = 1{,}275{,}120$
5. (a) $1 \cdot 4 \cdot 2 = 8$ **(b)** $1 \cdot 2 \cdot 2 = 4$ **(c)** $\frac{4}{64}$

(d)

$* = no\ repetition$

7. $1 \cdot 1 \cdot 4 = 4$

9. $64 \cdot 64 \cdot 64 = 262,144$; $64 \cdot 63 \cdot 62 = 249,984$; $262,144 - 249,984 = 12,160$ (number with repetition); $P[\text{repetition}] = \dfrac{12,160}{262,144}$

$61 \cdot 60 \cdot 59 = 215,940 =$ number with no repetition and codes an amino acid;

$P[\text{no repetition and codes an amino acid}] = \dfrac{215,940}{262,144}$

11. (a) $7! = 5040$

(b) $2 \cdot 1 \cdot 5! = 240$ ways to have A and B in positions one and two; $P[A$ and B in positions one and two$] = \dfrac{240}{5040} = .0476$

(c) yes; the probability that this would occur by chance is small $(.0476)$

13. (a) 16   **(b)** 5

15. (a) $n, n-1, n-2, \ldots, n-r+1$ **(c)** $_{10}P_4 = 10 \cdot 9 \cdot 8 \cdot 7$ **(d)** $_nP_n = n!$

(e) $_{10}P_3 = 10 \cdot 9 \cdot 8 = 720$

Exercises 2.5

1. $\dfrac{3!}{2!\,1!} = 3$ **3.** $\dfrac{14!}{4!\,10!} = 1001$

5. $\dfrac{8!}{4!\,2!\,2!} = 420$ (the rest periods alternate with the activity period and the observation ends with a rest period)

$\dfrac{7!}{4!\,2!\,1!} = 105$ ways to have the long activity periods consecutive; $\dfrac{105}{420}$

7. $\dfrac{10!}{3!\,2!\,4!\,1!} = 12,600$; $\dfrac{9!}{3!\,2!\,4!} = 1,260$ ways to have stop at the end; $12,600 - 1,260 =$

$11,340$ ways to have the stop elsewhere; $P[\text{stop not at the end}] = \dfrac{11,340}{12,600}$

Exercises 2.6

1. (a) 15   **(b)** 56   **(c)** 1   **(d)** 1

3. $\dfrac{\binom{7}{7}\binom{8}{0}}{\binom{15}{7}} = \dfrac{1}{6435}$; $\dfrac{\binom{7}{5}\binom{8}{2}}{\binom{15}{7}} = \dfrac{588}{6435}$ **5.** $\dfrac{\binom{4}{2}\binom{6}{1}}{\binom{10}{3}} = \dfrac{36}{120}$

7. $\dfrac{\binom{5}{0}\binom{95}{15}}{\binom{100}{15}} = .4357, \quad \dfrac{\binom{5}{0}\binom{95}{14}}{\binom{100}{15}} = .4034$

$P[\text{at most } 1] = .4357 + .4034 = .8391$

9. $\binom{50}{15} \doteq 2{,}250{,}000{,}000{,}000$

Exercises 3.1

1. (a) have leukemia and the white cell count is high
   (b) have leukemia or the white cell count is high
   (c) have leukemia but the white cell count is not high
   (d) does not have leukemia and the white cell count is not high
3. (a) The child has received both vaccines.

(b) 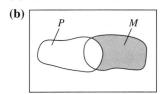   **(c)**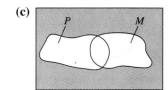

(d) 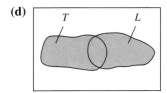   **(e)**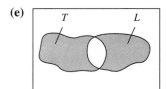

5. b, c, d, f, g, h   **7.** .65   **9.** .10
11. (a) .27   **(b)** .67   **(c)** .18   **(d)** .82
13. S or $\varnothing = S$. Hence $P[S \text{ or } \varnothing] = P[S]$. Since S and $\varnothing$ are mutually exclusive, $P[S] = P[S \text{ or } \varnothing] = P[S] + P[\varnothing]$ by Axiom 3. By Axiom 1, $P[S] = 1$. Hence

$$1 = 1 + P[\varnothing]$$

Solve for $P[\varnothing]$ to obtain $P[\varnothing] = 0$.
15. (a) $B = A$ or (B but not A). Since A and B but not A are mutually exclusive, $P[B] = P[A] + P[B \text{ but not } A]$ by Axiom 3. By Axiom 2

$$P[B \text{ but not } A] \geq 0$$

Add $P[A]$ to each side of the above inequality to obtain

$$P[A] + P[B \text{ but not } A] \geq P[A]$$

Substitution yields

$$P[B] \geq P[A]$$

(b) Note that since C is an event, C is contained in S. By part a $P[C] \leq P[S]$. Since by Axiom 1 $P[S] = 1$, we have $P[C] \leq 1$.

Exercises 3.2

1.
(a) .12   **(b)** .02   **(c)** .06   **(d)** .88

3.

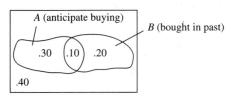

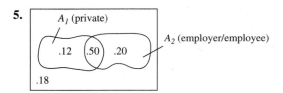

(a) .60   **(b)** .20
(c) .40(5000)(100) = 200,000

5.

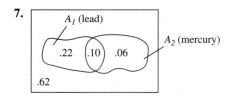

.82; .20

7.

$P[A_1 \text{ or } A_2] = P[A_1] + P[A_2] - P[\text{both}]$
$.38 = .32 + P[A_2] - .10$
$P[A_2] = .16$

.16; .22

Exercises 3.3

1. (a) $\frac{6}{16}$ **(b)** $\frac{2}{8}$ **(c)** $\frac{1}{2}$ **(d)** $\frac{1}{2}$

3. (a) A_1: 65 or older
   A_2: mild heart failure

   $P[A_1 \text{ or } A_2] = P[A_1] + P[A_2] - P[A_1 \text{ and } A_2]$
   $.104 = .10 + .01 - P[A_1 \text{ and } A_2]$
   $P[A_1 \text{ and } A_2] = .006$

(b)

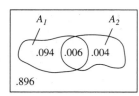

(c) $\dfrac{.006}{.094} = .0638$ **(d)** $\dfrac{.004}{.900} = .0044$

5.

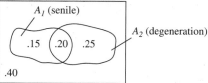

$\dfrac{.20}{.45} = .4444$; $\dfrac{.25}{.65} = .3846$

7.

A_1 (low sugar)

A_2 (convulsions)

.33 (.07) .18

.42

$.42$; $\dfrac{.07}{.40} = .175$

9.

A_1 (HIV)

A_2 (herpes)

.0005 (.0005) .0095

.9895

$.0095 + .9895 = .999$; $\dfrac{.9895}{.99} = .9995$

Exercises 3.4

1. $\alpha = P[\text{test} + \,|\, \text{true} -] = \frac{12}{142}$ $\beta = P[\text{test} - \,|\, \text{true} +] = \frac{4}{58}$

3. $\alpha \doteq \frac{7}{402}$; $\beta \doteq \frac{19}{98}$

5. $\frac{130}{142}$; high because specificity is the probability of getting a correct test result among true negative subjects

7.

		True state		
		−	+	
Test	+	13	92	105
result	−	62	8	70
		75	100	175

$\alpha \doteq \frac{3}{75}$

9. (a) $\alpha \doteq \frac{1000}{99969} \doteq .01$; specificity $= 1 - \alpha \doteq .99$

    (b) $\beta \doteq \frac{1}{31}$; sensitivity $= 1 - \beta = \frac{30}{31}$

11. $\frac{130}{134}$

13. $\alpha \doteq \frac{83}{115}$; $\frac{116}{199}$; no, the positive predictive value is only about .58

15. (a)

		TB Present		
		yes	no	
abuse	yes	11	296	307
drugs	no	35	1650	1685
		46	1946	1992

(b) $\dfrac{\frac{11}{307}}{\frac{35}{1685}} = 1.725$

Exercises 3.5

1. A_1, B_1: not independent, not mutually exclusive
   A_2, B_2: not independent, not mutually exclusive
   A_3, B_3: independent, not mutually exclusive
   A_4, B_4: not independent, mutually exclusive
   A_5, B_5: not independent, not mutually exclusive
   A_6, B_6: not independent, not mutually exclusive
   A_7, B_7: independent, not mutually exclusive

3. $P[\text{high BOD}] \cdot P[\text{high acidity}] = .35(.10) = .035$

Since this product is not equal to .04, the probability that both events occur, the events are not independent.

$P[\text{high acid} \mid \text{high BOD}] = \frac{.04}{.35} = \frac{4}{35}$

5. $P[\text{both ok}] = (.99)^2 = .9801$

7. (a) .0112 (pppp)   .0048 (appp)   **(b)** .1   **(c)** .16   **(d)** .756
      .0448 (pppa)   .0192 (appa)
      .1008 (ppap)   .0432 (apap)
      .4032 (ppaa)   .1728 (apaa)
      .0028 (papp)   .0012 (aapp)
      .0112 (papa)   .0048 (aapa)
      .0252 (paap)   .0108 (aaap)
      .1008 (paaa)   .0432 (aaaa)

9. (a)

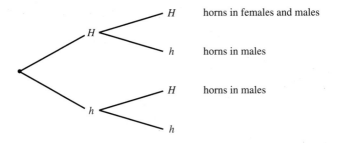

H	horns in females and males
h	horns in males
H	horns in males
h	

(b) $P[\text{male and horns}] = \frac{1}{2} \cdot \frac{3}{4} = \frac{3}{8}$; $P[\text{female and horns}] = \frac{1}{2} \cdot \frac{1}{4} = \frac{1}{8}$
(c) $P[\text{horns}] = P[\text{male and horns}] + P[\text{female and horns}] = \frac{4}{8}$;
   $P[\text{horns}|\text{male}] = \frac{3}{4} \neq P[\text{horns}]$

11. (a) $P[AB^-] = P[AB]P[RH^-] = (.04)(.15) = .006$
  (b) $P[AB^-] = (.04)(.15) = .006$
  (c) yes; the probability of AB^- blood is the same regardless of race
  (d) no; for whites $P[A^-] = (.40)(.15) = .06$ but for blacks $P[A^-] = (.27)(.15) = .0405$
13. $P[\text{at least one false positive}] = 1 - P[\text{no false positive}]$
$$= 1 - (.95)^{10}$$
$$= .4013$$

Exercises 3.6

1. $P[- \ -] = .15; P[+ \ +] = .37$
 $P[\text{mother is } - \ - \text{ and father is } + \ +] = .15(.37) = .0555$
 $P[\text{erythroblastosis}] = .0360 + .0555 = .0915$
3. $P[\text{male and survive}] = P[\text{survive} \mid \text{male}] \, P[\text{male}]$
$$= (.35) \, (.52)$$
$$= .182$$
5. $P[\text{diabetes and unaware}] = P[\text{unaware} \mid \text{diabetes}]P[\text{diabetes}]$
$$= (.50)(.02)$$
$$= .01$$
7. $P[\text{error and observable}] = P[\text{observable} \mid \text{error}]P[\text{error}]$
$$= .35(.4)$$
$$= .14$$
9. (a) $P[\text{yes}] = P[\text{yes and } A] + P[\text{yes and } B]$
$$= P[\text{yes} \mid A]P[A] + P[\text{yes} \mid B]P[B]$$
  Solve for $P[\text{yes} \mid B]$ to obtain
$$P[\text{yes} \mid B] = \frac{P[\text{yes}] - P[\text{yes} \mid A]P[A]}{P[B]}$$
 (b) $P[\text{fraud}] = P[\text{yes} \mid B] = \dfrac{.60 - .5(.5)}{.5} = .70$

Exercises 3.7

1. (a) B = black
  D = die

 (b) $P[B \mid D] = \dfrac{P[D \text{ and } B]}{P[D]} = \dfrac{.000064}{.000064 + .000153} \doteq .295$
 (c) $P[B \mid D] = \dfrac{P[D \mid B]P[B]}{P[D \mid B]P[B] + P[D \mid B']P[B']}$
$$= \frac{.00064(.10)}{.00064(.10) + .00017(.90)} = .295$$

3. $P[B \text{ alone} \mid \text{remission}] =$

$$\frac{P[\text{remission} \mid B]P[B]}{P[\text{remission} \mid B]P[B] + P[\text{remission} \mid A]P[A] + P[\text{remission} \mid C]P[C]}$$

$$= \frac{\frac{3}{4}\left(\frac{1}{3}\right)}{\frac{3}{4}\left(\frac{1}{3}\right) + \frac{1}{2}\left(\frac{1}{3}\right) + \frac{6}{10}\left(\frac{1}{3}\right)}$$

$$= \frac{\frac{1}{4}}{\left(\frac{1}{4}\right) + \left(\frac{1}{6}\right) + \left(\frac{2}{10}\right)} \doteq .4054$$

5. (a) $P[\text{true} + \mid \text{test} +] = \dfrac{P[\text{test} + \mid \text{true}+]P[\text{true}+]}{P[\text{test} + \mid \text{true} +]P[\text{true} +] + P[\text{test} + \mid \text{true} -]P[\text{true} -]}$

$$= \frac{.95(.10)}{.95(.10) + 0(.90)}$$

$$= 1$$

(b) $\dfrac{.95(.10)}{.95(.10) + .50(.90)} = .1743$

(c) decreases from 1 to .1743 (difference $= .8257$)

(d) $\dfrac{1(.10)}{1(.10) + .05(.90)} \doteq .6896$

(e) $\dfrac{.5(.10)}{.5(.10) + .05(.90)} \doteq .5263$

(f) decreases from .6896 to .5263 (difference $= .1633$)

Exercises 4.1

1. discrete   **3.** continuous   **5.** discrete   **7.** continuous   **9.** continuous
11. discrete   **13.** continuous

Exercises 4.2

1. (a) .09; $P[X = 5]$ **(b)** .41; $P[X \le 2] = P[\text{at most 2 persons will seek treatment unnecessarily on a randomly selected day}]$ **(c)** .11   **(d)** .19

3. (a)

x	0	1	2	3	4
$f(x)$	$(.1)^4$	$4(.1)^3(.9)^1$	$6(.1)^2(.9)^2$	$4(.1)(.9)^3$	$.9^4$

or

x	0	1	2	3	4
$f(x)$	.0001	.0036	.0486	.2916	.6561

(b) .0037; $P[X \le 1] = P[\text{at most 1 patient will obtain relief}]$
(c) yes; $P[\text{no one will get relief}] = f(0) = .0001$; it would be very unusual for this even to occur

5. $E[X] = \mu = .2$

7. (a) 8.75   **(b)** 67.25   **(c)** 13.32   **(d)** .36

(e) $E[(X - \mu)^2] = E[(X - .2)^2]$
$$= (-2.2)^2(.1) + (-1.2)^2(.2) + (-.2)^2(.3) + (.8)^2(.2) + (1.8)^2(.2)$$
$$= 1.56$$

(f) $E[(X - \mu)^2] = E[(X - 3)^2]$
$$= (-2)^2(.1) + (-1)^2(.15) + (0)^2(.5) + (1)^2(.15) + (2)^2(.1)$$
$$= 1.1$$

9. (b) $E[X^2] - (E[X])^2 = 8.75 - (2.75)^2 = 1.1875$
(c) $67.25 - (8.15)^2 = .8275$

11. (a)

x	0	1	2	3
f(x)	$(.05)^3$	$3(.95)(.05)^2$	$3(.95)^2(.05)$	$(.95)^3$

or

x	0	1	2	3
f(x)	.000125	.007125	.135375	.857375

(b) $E[X]$ = average number of patients desensitized = 2.85
(c) $\mu = E[X] = 2.85$
(d) $E[X^2] = 8.265$
(e) $\sigma^2 =$ Var $X = .1425$; $\sigma = \sqrt{.1425} \doteq .3775$

13. (a) 0   1   2

$$P[|X - 1| \leq 2] = P[|X - 1| \leq 4\sigma] \geq 1 - \frac{1}{4^2} = \frac{15}{16}$$

The probability that X will lie above 2 or below 0 is at most $\frac{1}{16}$. Since rainfall cannot be negative, $P[X > 2]$ is at most $\frac{1}{16}$.
(b) Since 2 lies 7.5σ away from the mean, $P[X \geq 2] \leq \frac{1}{(7.5)^2} = \frac{4}{225}$

Exercises 4.3

1. (a)

x	6	7	8	9	10
f(x)	.05	.15	.75	.90	1.00

(b) .75   **(c)** $P[X > 7] = 1 - P[X \leq 7] = .85$
(d) $P[7 \leq X \leq 9] = P[X \leq 9] - P[X \leq 6] = .90 - .05 = .85$

3. (a)

x	0	1	2	3
f(x)	.15	.40	.90	1.00

(b) $P[X \leq 1] = .40$ **(c)** $P[X \geq 2] = 1 - P[X \leq 1] = .60$

5. (a) .6, .9, .1, .6
(b)

x	0	1	2	3	4	5	6
f(x)	.1	.1	.1	.3	.2	.1	.1

(c) 3.1   **(d)** 2.89   **(e)** $\sqrt{2.89}$; AIDS cases

Exercises 4.4

1. (a) binomial; $n = 5$; $p = .006$
(b) binomial; $n = 5$; $p = .001$
(c) binomial; $n = 10$; $p = .9$
(d) not binomial; p changes due to sampling without replacement from a small group of objects
(e) approximately binomial; $n = 8$; $p \doteq .05$
(f) not binomial; the number of trials is not fixed

3. (b) $f(x) = \dfrac{10!}{x!\,(10-x)!}(.01)^x(.99)^{10-x}$ $\qquad x = 0, 1, 2, \ldots, 10$

(c) $E[X] = 10(.01) = .1$ $\qquad$ **(d)** no; trials would not be independent

 Var $X = 10(.01)(.99) = .099$

 $\sigma = \sqrt{.099}$

5. (a) $\dfrac{4!}{x!\,(4-x)!}(.2)^x(.8)^{4-x}$ $\qquad x = 0, 1, 2, 3, 4$ $\qquad$ **(b)** $f(0) = \dfrac{4!}{0!\,4!}(.2)^0(.8)^4 = .4096$

(c) $f(1) = \dfrac{4!}{1!\,3!}(.2)^1(.8)^3 = .4096,$ so $P[X \le 1] = .4096 + .4096 = .8192$; $n = 4$ is

 not listed in the table

7. (a) .6331 $\qquad$ **(b)** .3823 $\qquad$ **(c)** .2508 $\qquad$ **(d)** .3669 $\qquad$ **(e)** .0548 $\qquad$ **(f)** .7779

 **(g)** .6054 $\qquad$ **(h)** .6665 $\qquad$ **(i)** .3546

9. $E[X] = 20(.6) = 12;$ $P[X \le 9] = .1275$

Exercises 4.5

1. (a) 10 $\qquad$ **(b)** $f(x) = \dfrac{e^{-10}10^x}{x!}$ $\qquad x = 0, 1, 2, \ldots$ $\qquad$ **(c)** .029 $\qquad$ **(d)** .933 $\qquad$ **(e)** .782

 **(f)** .125

3. $\lambda = 2;$ $s = 3;$ $\lambda s = 6;$ $P[X \le 4] = .285;$ $E[X] = 6$

 $P[X \ge 12] = 1 - P[X \le 11] = 1 - .98 = .02$

5. $\lambda = 5;$ $s = \frac{16}{20} = .8;$ $\lambda s = 4;$ $P[X = 0] = .018$

 $P[X \ge 9] = 1 - P[X \le 8] = 1 - .979 = .021$

7. $\lambda = 1;$ $s = .5;$ $\lambda s = .5;$ $P[X = 0] = .607$

 $P[X \ge 1] = 1 - .607 = .393$

9.

x	3	4	5	6	7	8	9	10
Binomial	.8670	.9568	.9887	.9976	.9996	.9999	1.000	1.000
Poisson	.857	.947	.983	.995	.999	1.000	1.000	1.000

11. $n = 2,000,000;$ $p = \dfrac{5}{1,000,000};$ $np = \lambda s = 10$

 $P[X \ge 1] = 1 - P[X = 0] \doteq 1.000$

13. $E[X] = (150)(.10) = 15;$ $P[X = 10] = P[X \le 10] - P[X \le 9] \doteq .118 - .07 = .048$

Exercises 5.1

1. (c) $P[\text{at most .2 cc should be prescribed}] = P[Z \le .2]$

 **(d)** $P[\text{at most .1 cc should be prescribed}] = P[Z \le .1]$

 **(e)** $P[\text{between .1 and .2 cc should be prescribed}] = P[.1 \le Z \le .2]$

 **(f)** subtract answer for part d from answer for part c

 **(g)** μ should be close to .2

 **(h)** $f(.2) = \frac{200}{9} \cdot \frac{2}{10} = \frac{40}{9};$ $P[X \le .2] = \frac{1}{2}\left(\frac{2}{10}\right)\frac{40}{9} = \frac{4}{9}$

 **(i)** $f(.1) = \frac{200}{9} \cdot \frac{1}{10} = \frac{20}{9};$ $P[X \le .1] = \frac{1}{2}\left(\frac{1}{10}\right)\frac{20}{9} = \frac{1}{9}$

 **(j)** $\frac{4}{9} - \frac{1}{9} = \frac{3}{9}$

3. (b) $\frac{9}{16}$ **(c)** 0 (X is continuous)

5. (c) $P[X > 3] = 2 \cdot \frac{1}{5} = \frac{2}{5}$ **(d)** 2.5 minutes

Exercises 5.2

1. (a) I and II
  (b) $P[\text{pacemaker lasts between 2 and 4 years}] = P[2 \leq X \leq 4]$
  (c) $P[\text{pacemaker lasts at least 8 years}] = P[X \geq 8]; 1 - F(8)$
  (d) $F(4)$
3. (a) I, II, and III   **(b)** $1 - F(18)$; III, IV, and V   **(c)** $F(36) - F(27)$; IV

Exercises 5.3

1. (a) $f(x) = \dfrac{1}{2\sqrt{2\pi}} e^{-1/2(x-5/2)^2}$ $-\infty < x < \infty$ **(b)** 5 ± 2 (3 and 7)

3. (a) .0643   **(b)** .9147   **(c)** .9147   **(d)** .9222   **(e)** .0239   **(f)** .8451
  (g) 0   **(h)** -1.645 **(i)** .67   **(j)** 1.28   **(k)** $-.84$ **(l)** 1.96   **(m)** 2.575

5. (a) $z = \dfrac{100 - 153}{25} = -2.12; P[Z \leq -2.12] = .0170$

  (b) $z = \dfrac{180 - 153}{25} = 1.08; P[Z \geq 1.08] = .1401$

  (c) $z = -2.12$ and $z = \dfrac{175 - 153}{25} = .88; P[-2.12 \leq Z \leq .88] = .7936$

  (d) $z = \dfrac{128 - 153}{25} = -1$ and $z = \dfrac{178 - 153}{25} = 1; P[-1 \leq Z \leq 1] = .6827$

  (e) $\dfrac{x_0 - 153}{25} = -1.28; x_0 = 153 + 25(-1.28) = 121$

  (f) $\dfrac{x_0 - 153}{25} = -1.555; x_0 = 153 + 25(1.555) = 191.875$

7. (a) $P[X \leq 120] = P\left[Z \leq \dfrac{120 - 106}{8}\right] = P[Z \leq 1.75] = .9599$
  (b) $P[90 \leq X \leq 120] = P[-2 \leq Z \leq 1.75] = .9599 - .0228 = .9371$ or 93.71%
  (c) $P[106 \leq X \leq 110] = P[0 \leq Z \leq .5] = .6915 - .5 = .1915$
  (d) $P[X \geq 121] = P[Z \geq 1.875] = 1 - .9699 = .0301$
  (e) $\dfrac{x_0 - 106}{8} = -.67; x_0 = 106 - 8(.67) = 100.64$

9. (a) $f(x) = \dfrac{1}{.2\sqrt{2\pi}} e^{-1/2(x-1.5/.2)^2}$ $-\infty < x < \infty$

  $P[-1.1 \leq X \leq 1.9] = P[-2 < Z < 2] = .9544$

  (b) $P[X < .9] = P\left[Z < \dfrac{.9 - 1.5}{.2}\right] = P[Z < -3] = .0013$

  (c) $P[X > 2] = P[Z > 2.5] = .0062$; yes, this is an unusual event

Exercises 5.4

1. $\mu = 20.3$ and $\sigma = 1.4$; 18.9 to 21.7 is within one standard deviation of μ; this occurs with probability about .68; it is not unusual
3. $\mu = .25$ and $\sigma = .11$; .03 to .47 is within two standard deviations of μ; this occurs with probability about .95
5. (a) male under 21: 140 to 180   (c) Age 20 and 125 is unusually low.
       male 21 to 29: 140 to 260   Age 20 and 200 is unusually high.
       male 30 or over: 160 to 280

Exercises 6.2

1. $\bar{x} = 408.3$ 3. shorter
7. (a) Var $\bar{X} = \dfrac{\sigma^2}{n} = \dfrac{.4829}{10} = .04829$ (c) standard error $= \sqrt{.04829} = .21975$

9. $E[\bar{X}] = \mu = 13$; Var $\bar{X} = \dfrac{\sigma^2}{n} = \dfrac{9}{16}$; standard error $= \dfrac{3}{4}$

11. (a)

x	0	1
$f(x_i)$	1/2	1/2

$E[X_i] = 0\left(\frac{1}{2}\right) + 1\left(\frac{1}{2}\right) = \frac{1}{2}$

$E[X_i^2] = 0^2\left(\frac{1}{2}\right) + 1^2\left(\frac{1}{2}\right) = \frac{1}{2}$

Var $X_i = E[X_i^2] - (E[X_i])^2 = \frac{1}{2} - \frac{1}{4} = \frac{1}{4}$

(b) $\sum X_i =$ number of heads so $\dfrac{\sum X_i}{n} =$ proportion of heads

(c) $\bar{X}$ is approximately normally distributed with mean $\frac{1}{2}$ and variance $\left(\frac{1}{4}\right)$ 30
(d) standard normal

Exercises 6.3

1. (a) 0|4   There is a rough bell shape.
       0|7877
       1|1400011000
       1|7655
       2|2

(b) $\bar{x} = 11.533$; $s = 4.210$; $s^2 = 17.7258$
3. (a) 1.753   (b) 2.131   (c) -1.753 (d) -2.131 (e) .01   (f) .10
   (g) .90   (h) 2.131   (i) 2.947
5. $\bar{x} \pm 1.96(s/\sqrt{n})$ or $9.5 \pm 1.96(.5/\sqrt{1000})$; $9.5 \pm .031$; $(9.469, 9.531)$

7. $\bar{x} \pm 1.699 \left(\dfrac{s}{\sqrt{n}}\right)$ or $41.2 \pm 1.699 \left(\dfrac{2.1}{\sqrt{30}}\right)$; $41.2 \pm .65$; $(40.55, 41.85)$; longer; no;
   the entire interval is above 35%

9. $\bar{x} \pm 3.355 \left(\dfrac{s}{\sqrt{n}}\right)$ or $5.66 \pm 3.355 \left(\dfrac{.49}{\sqrt{9}}\right)$; $(5.11, 6.21)$

11. $\bar{x} \pm 2.131 \left(\dfrac{s}{\sqrt{n}}\right)$ or $11.533 \pm 1.729 \left(\dfrac{4.210}{\sqrt{20}}\right)$; $(11.146; 11.920)$

Exercises 6.4

1. (a) H_0: $\mu \geq .08$, H_1: $\mu < .08$

(b) You believe that the average percentage of metal in household waste has been reduced when, in fact, it has not.

(c) You are unable to show that the average percentage of metal in household waste has been reduced when, in fact, it *has* been reduced.

3. (a) $H_0: \mu \geq 9$, $H_1: \mu < 9$

   (b) Type I: You believe that the DDT level is lower than it actually is. Therefore, controls might not be enforced or strengthened as carefully as needed.

   Type II: You are unable to show that the DDT level has been reduced when, in fact, it has. Controls that are already working could be made even more stringent.

5. Type I: You obtain a "false positive" result. The patient believes that he or she has the AIDS virus when, in fact, this is not true.

   Type II: The virus is present but it is not detected. This is a "false negative" test result.

   Probably Type II is more serious.

7. $H_1: \mu < 8$, $H_0: \mu \geq 8$

   Type I: It is thought that acid rain is stunting the growth of dogwood saplings, but this is not true.

Exercises 6.5

1. $P = P[T_A > 3]$; $.001 < P < .005$; reject H_0

3. $P = P[T_{15} < -1.5] + [T_{15} > 1.5]$; $.10 < P < .20$; fail to reject H_0

5. (a) $H_0: \mu \leq .035\%$, $H_1: \mu > .035\%$

   (b) $\dfrac{\bar{x} - \mu_0}{s/\sqrt{n}} = \dfrac{.09 - .035}{.25/\sqrt{144}} = 2.64$; $P = P[T_{143} > 2.64]$; using row ∞,

   $.001 < P < .005$

7. $H_1 = \mu > 25$; $\dfrac{\bar{x} - \mu_0}{s/\sqrt{n}} = \dfrac{27 - 25}{18/\sqrt{80}} = .99$; $P = P[T_{79} > .99]$; $.10 < P < .25$

   These data do not support the research claim. If the claim is made, the probability of error is between .10 and .25.

9. yes; yes; no

   In Exercises 1 and 2, P is less than .05. In Exercise 3, P exceeds .05.

11. (a) $H_0: \mu = 2.5$, $H_1: \mu \neq 2.5$

    (b) $\bar{x} = 2.66$; $\dfrac{\bar{x} - \mu_0}{s/\sqrt{n}} = \dfrac{2.66 - 2.50}{.2/\sqrt{10}} = 2.53$; $s = .20$

    $P = P[T_9 < -2.53] + P[T_9 > 2.53]$; $.05 < P < .10$

    Reject H_0 at the $\alpha = .10$ level because $P < .10$. A Type I error is possible.

13. $H_0: \mu \geq 1.3$, $H_1: \mu < 1.3$; $\bar{x} = .8$; $s = .8$; $\dfrac{\bar{x} - \mu_0}{s/\sqrt{n}} = \dfrac{.8 - 1.3}{.8/\sqrt{20}} = -2.80$

    $P = P[T_{19} < -2.80]$; $.005 < P < .01$; since $P < .01$, H_0 can be rejected at $\alpha = .01$ level.

Exercises 6.6

1. $n = \dfrac{z^2 s^2}{d^2} = \dfrac{(2.576)^2 (.066)}{(.1)^2} = 43.796 \doteq 44$

3. $s = 1.43$; $n = \dfrac{(1.96)^2 (1.43)^2}{(.5)^2} \doteq 32$

5. $s = 2.3$; $\Delta = \frac{2}{2.3} = .9$; $\alpha = .05$; $\beta = .05$; $n = 15$ (one-sided test)

Exercises 7.1

1. (a) .01   **(b)** .25   **(c)** .05   **(d)** 19.0   **(e)** 2.09   **(f)** $\chi_1^2 = 3.33$; $\chi_2^2 = 16.9$

3. (a) $\bar{x} = 3840.2$ **(b)** $s^2 = 1261.69$

(c) $\bar{x} \pm 1.86 \left(\dfrac{s}{\sqrt{n}} \right)$ or $3840.2 \pm 1.86(35.5/\sqrt{9})$; $(3818.2, 3862.2)$

(d) $L_1 = \dfrac{8(1261.69)}{15.5} = 651.19$

$L_2 = \dfrac{8(1261.69)}{2.73} = 3697.26$; $(651.19, 3697.26)$; $(\sqrt{651.19}, \sqrt{3697.26})$

5. (a) $\chi_{.05}^2 \doteq \frac{1}{2}\left[1.645 + \sqrt{2(79) - 1}\right]^2 = 100.46$

$\chi_{.90}^2 \doteq \frac{1}{2}\left[-1.28 + \sqrt{2(79) - 1}\right]^2 = 63.28$

(b) $\chi_{.025}^2 \doteq \frac{1}{2}\left[-1.96 + \sqrt{2(99) - 1}\right]^2 = 72.91$

$\chi_{.975}^2 \doteq \frac{1}{2}\left[1.96 + \sqrt{2(99) - 1}\right]^2 = 127.93$

(c) $\chi_{.005}^2 \doteq \frac{1}{2}\left[-2.575 + \sqrt{2(74) - 1}\right]^2 = 45.59$

$\chi_{.995}^2 \doteq \frac{1}{2}\left[2.575 + \sqrt{2(74) - 1}\right]^2 = 108.04$

7. (a) $\bar{x} \pm 1.671 \left(\dfrac{s}{\sqrt{n}} \right)$ or $3400 \pm 1.671 \left(\dfrac{100}{\sqrt{61}} \right)$; $(3378.6, 3421.4)$

(b) $\chi_{.05}^2 = \frac{1}{2}\left[-1.645 + \sqrt{2(60) - 1}\right]^2 = 42.91$; $\chi_{.95}^2 = \frac{1}{2}\left[1.645 + \sqrt{2(60) - 1}\right]^2$

$= 78.80$

$L_1 = \dfrac{60(100)^2}{78.80} = 7614.21$; $L_2 = \dfrac{60(100)^2}{42.91} = 13982.75$

$\sqrt{L_1} = 87.3$; $\sqrt{L_2} = 118.2$

Exercises 7.2

1. (a) $\bar{x} = 12.11$, $s = 1.48$, $s^2 = 2.186$

(b) $\dfrac{\bar{x} - \mu_0}{\dfrac{s}{\sqrt{n}}} = \dfrac{12.11 - 13}{\dfrac{1.48}{\sqrt{12}}} = -2.08$; $P = P[T_{11} < 2.08]$; yes, $.025 < P < .05$

(c) $\dfrac{(n-1)s^2}{\sigma_0^2} = \dfrac{11(2.186)}{2.25} = 10.69$; $P = P[X_{11}^2 < 10.69]$; no, $.50 < P < .75$

3. (a) $\dfrac{\bar{x} - \mu_0}{\sigma_0^2} = \dfrac{6.3 - 6.5}{\dfrac{1.7}{\sqrt{25}}} = -.588$; $P = P[T_{24} < -.588]$; no, $.25 < P < .40$ and

therefore $P > .05$

(b) $\dfrac{(n-1)s^2}{\sigma_0^2} = \dfrac{24(1.7)^2}{(1.2)^2} = 48.17$; $P = P[X_{24}^2 > 48.17]$; yes, $P < .005$ and

therefore $P < .05$

Exercises 8.1

1. $\hat{p} = \frac{32}{36} = .889$ 3. $\hat{p} = \frac{11}{15} = .733$

7. (a) $E[X_i] = 0(1 - p) + 1(p) = p;\ E[X_i^2] = 0^2(1 - p) + 1^2(p) = p;$
   $\text{Var } X_i = E[X_i^2] - (E[X_i])^2 = p - p^2 = p(1 - p)$
   (d) standard normal

Exercises 8.2

1. $.027 \pm 1.96\sqrt{\dfrac{.027(.973)}{150}}$ or $(.001,\ .053)$; shorter

3. (a) $\hat{p} = \dfrac{125}{200} = .625$ (b) $.625 \pm 1.645\sqrt{\dfrac{.625(.375)}{200}}$ or $(.569,\ .681)$
   (c) no; the values 60–68% are contained in the interval

5. $\hat{p} = .3;\ .3 \pm 1.645\sqrt{\dfrac{.3(.7)}{1000}}$ or $(.276,\ .324)$; $.276$ (2 billion) $= 552$ million,
   $.324$ (2 billion) $= 648$ million

7. $.84 \pm 1.96\sqrt{\dfrac{.84(.16)}{191}}$ or $(.788,\ .892)$

Exercises 8.3

1. $.08 \pm 2.33\sqrt{\dfrac{.08(.92)}{13573}}$ or $(.075,\ .085)$ 3. $n \doteq \dfrac{(1.88)^2}{4(.03)^2} \doteq 982$

5. $\hat{p} = .84;\ n \doteq \dfrac{(1.88)^2(.84)(.16)}{(.03)^2} \doteq 528$

7. (a) $g'(p) = 1 - 2p$
   (b) $1 - 2p = 0$
   $2p = 1$
   $p = \frac{1}{2}$
   (c) $g''(p) = -2$; a negative second derivative implies downward concavity and therefore
   a maximum

Exercises 8.4

1. (a) $H_0\colon p \le \frac{1}{2},\ H_1\colon p > \frac{1}{2}$
   (b) $\hat{p} = \dfrac{270}{500} = .54;\ \dfrac{\hat{p} - p_0}{\sqrt{\dfrac{p_0(1 - p_0)}{n}}} = \dfrac{.54 - .50}{\sqrt{\dfrac{.50(.50)}{500}}} = 1.79$

   $P = P[Z > 1.79] = .036$; reject H_0 because P is small; subject to a Type I error; the dam
   project might be stopped unnecessarily

3. $\hat{p} = \frac{14}{50} = .28;\ z = \dfrac{.28 - .70}{\sqrt{\dfrac{.7(.3)}{50}}} = -6.48;\ P < .0002$

5. We need z to be at least 1.96 ($z_{.025}$). Therefore, we need

$$\frac{\hat{p} - .7}{\sqrt{\frac{.7(.3)}{50}}} \geq 1.96$$

Solve for $\hat{p}$ to see that $\hat{p}$ must be at least .827. This means that $\frac{x}{50}$ must be at least .827 or x must be at least 50 (.827) = 42.

7. (a) $H_1: p > .85$ **(b)** $\hat{p} = \frac{123}{139} = .885$; maybe, because $\hat{p} > .85$

(c) $z = \dfrac{.885 - .850}{\sqrt{\dfrac{.850(.150)}{139}}} = 1.16$; $P = P[Z > 1.16] = .123$; unable to reject H_0 at the

$\alpha = .10$ level because $P > .10$
(d) The sample size is rather small.

Exercises 8.5

1. $\hat{p}_1 = \frac{29}{742} = .039$; $\hat{p}_2 = \frac{13}{733} = .018$; $\hat{p}_1 - \hat{p}_2 = .021$
3. $\hat{p}_1 - \hat{p}_2 = .40 - .19 = .21$

5. $.316 \pm 1.645\sqrt{\dfrac{.895(.105)}{19} + \dfrac{.579(.421)}{19}}$ or $.316 \pm .219$; $(.097, .535)$; yes, because the

interval contains only positive values

7. $\hat{p}_1 - \hat{p}_2 = .89 - .504 = .386$; $.386 \pm 1.645\sqrt{\dfrac{.89(.11)}{500} + \dfrac{.504(.496)}{500}}$ or

$.386 \pm .043$; $(.343, .429)$

9. $n = \dfrac{(1.96)^2[.039(.961) + .018(.982)]}{(.02)^2} \doteq 530$;

$n = (1.645)^2 \dfrac{[.039(.961) + .018(.982)]}{(.02)^2} \doteq 374$

11. $n = \dfrac{(1.96)^2}{2(.02)^2} \doteq 4802$

Having a prior estimate available allows us to use a smaller sample in the actual study.

Exercises 8.6

1. Type II; Vitamin C might actually be effective but this is not detected so an effective treatment might be missed; no; it has not been proved ineffective; we simply have not shown that it is effective
3. $H_0: p_1 \leq p_2$, $H_1: p_1 > p_2$; $\hat{p}_1 = \frac{38}{101} = .376$; $\hat{p}_2 = \frac{6}{31} = .194$; $\hat{p}_1 - \hat{p}_2 = .182$;

$$\hat{p} = \frac{38 + 6}{132} = .333; \; z = \frac{.182}{\sqrt{.333(.667)\left(\dfrac{1}{101} + \dfrac{1}{31}\right)}} = 1.88$$

$P = P[Z > 1.88] = .0301$; reject H_0 at the $\alpha = .05$ level because $P < .05$

5. H_0: $p_1 - p_2$, H_1: $p_1 - p_2$; $\hat{p}_1 = \frac{162}{2055} = .079$, $\hat{p}_2 = \frac{14}{266} = .053$;

$$\hat{p}_1 - \hat{p}_2 = .026; \quad \hat{p} = \frac{162 + 14}{2055 + 266} = .076$$

$$z = \frac{.026}{\sqrt{.076(.924)\left(\dfrac{1}{2055} + \dfrac{1}{266}\right)}} = 1.51; \quad P = P[Z > 1.51] = .0655; \quad \text{reject at}$$

$a = .10$ but not at $a = .05$

Exercises 9.1

1. $\bar{x}_1 = 3.65$; $\bar{X}_2 = 3.5$; $\widehat{\mu_1 - \mu_2} = .15$

3. $E[\bar{x}_1 - \bar{x}_2] = 15 - 10 = 5$; $\text{Var}(\bar{X}_1 - \bar{X}_2) = \frac{16}{20} + \frac{18}{25} = 1.52$; $\sigma = \sqrt{1.52} = 1.23$; Z

5. $\widehat{\mu_1 - \mu_2} = 5.4 - 6.8 = -1.4$

Exercises 9.2

1. $s_1^2/s_2^2 = (6.34)^2/(3.20)^2 \doteq 3.93$; there is evidence that $\sigma_1^2 \neq \sigma_2^2$

3. $s_2^2/s_1^2 = (11.02)^2/(8.68)^2 = 1.61$; unable to conclude that $\sigma_1^2 \neq \sigma_2^2$

5. **(a)** $b = 2.57$ $a = 1/2.76 \doteq .36$ **(b)** $b = 2.75$ $a = 1/2.91 \doteq .34$
    (c) $b = 2.85$ $a = 1/3.29 \doteq .30$

7. $s^2 = .092$; $s_w^2 = .291$; $s_w^2/s_m^2 = 3.16$; $P = P[F_{7,9} > 3.16]$; $.05 < P < .10$
   Since $P > .05$, H_0 cannot be rejected at the $\alpha = .05$ level.

9. **(a)** yes; yes   **(b)** yes; no   **(c)** $F_{20,10}$; $s_1^2/s_2^2 = 3.00$ **(d)** $F_{20,10}$; $s_1^2/s_2^2 = 2.00$
   (e) No; if the tabled F value is more than 2, then the rule of thumb leads to rejection even
      though the F test might not. If the table F value is 2 or less, then the rule of thumb and
      the F test would both level to rejection.

Exercises 9.3

1. **(a)** $s_P^2 = \dfrac{9(42) + 13(37)}{10 + 14 - 2} = 39.05$ **(b)** $s_P^2 = \dfrac{28 + 30}{2} = 29$

   (c) $s_P^2 = \dfrac{9(20) + 49(40)}{10 + 50 - 2} = 36.896$

3. men: $s^2 = .092$, $\bar{x} = 3.65$
   women: $s^2 = .291$, $\bar{x} = 3.50$
   $\dfrac{.291}{.092} = 3.16 > 2$; by the rule of thumb, pooling is not appropriate

5. $s_1^2/s_2^2 = (10.1)^2/(10)^2 = 1.02 < 2$; pooling is appropriate;

   $$s_P^2 = \frac{(10.1)^2 + (10)^2}{2} = 101.005$$

   $(\bar{x}_1 - \bar{x}_2) \pm 1.746\sqrt{101.005\left(\frac{1}{9} + \frac{1}{9}\right)}$ or 1 ± 8.27; $(-7.27, 9.27)$; cannot conclude that

   there is a difference in average survival time because 0 lies in this interval

7. $s_1^2/s_2^2 = (9.9)^2/(9.5)^2 = 1.09 < 2$; pooling is appropriate;

   $$s_P^2 = \frac{17(9.9)^2 + 4(9.5)^2}{18 + 5 - 2} = 96.53$$

$H_0: \mu \le \mu_2,\ H_1: \mu_1 > \mu_2;\ t = \dfrac{(42.7 - 27.7)}{\sqrt{96.53 \left(\frac{1}{18} + \frac{1}{5}\right)}} = 3.02;\ P = P[T_{21} > 3.02];$

$.001 < P < .005$; reject H_0

9. $s_2^2/s_1^2 = (2)^2/(1.9)^2 = 1.11 < 2$; pooling is appropriate;

$s_P^2 = \dfrac{50(1.9)^2 + 40(2)^2}{90} = 3.78$

$H_0: \mu_1 \ge \mu_2,\ H_1: \mu_1 < \mu_2;\ t = \dfrac{59.1 - 65.2}{\sqrt{3.78\left(\frac{1}{51} + \frac{1}{41}\right)}} = -14.96;$

$P = P[T_{90} < -14.96];\ P < .0005$; reject H_0

11. $s_1^2/s_2^2 = \frac{4}{3.5} = 1.14 < 2$; pooling is appropriate; $s_P^2 = \dfrac{32(4) + 13(3.5)}{45} = 3.856$

$H_0: \mu_1 \ge \mu_2,\ H_1: \mu_1 < \mu_2;\ t = \dfrac{11.3 - 12.6}{\sqrt{3.856\left(\frac{1}{33} + \frac{1}{14}\right)}} = -2.08;$

$P = P[T_{45} < -2.08];\ .01 < P < .025$; reject H_0

Exercises 9.4

1. $t = 1.83$; 67; $.025 < P < .05$; the P value is affected but the conclusion remains the same

3. $s_1^2/s_2^2 = (6.5)^2/(3.6)^2 = 3.26 > 2$; do not pool
$H_0: \mu_1 \ge \mu_2,\ H_1: \mu_1 > \mu_2;\ t = 15.53'\ df = 33.95;\ P < .005$

5. pool; $s_P^2 = \dfrac{3460(8.68)^2 + 2237(11.02)^2}{5697} = 93.44$

$H_0: \mu_1 \le \mu_2,\ H_1: \mu_1 > \mu_2;\ t = 852.76;\ P < .0005$; reject H_0

7. do not pool; $H_0: \mu_1 \le \mu_2,\ H_1: \mu_1 > \mu_2;\ t = 8.73;\ df = 24.03;\ P < .0005$

9. do not pool; $df = 11.06$; $(-8.28, -.00014)$; yes, because 0 does not lie in this interval

11. $s_2^2/s_1^2 = 36/25 \equiv 1.44 < 2$; pooling is appropriate;

$s_P^2 = \dfrac{96319(25) + 81608(36)}{96320 + 81609 - 2} = 30.05;\ (-5.521, -5.419)$

Exercises 9.5

1. $\bar{d} = 12.55$; $s_d = 24.47$; $(-25.92, .82)$; no, because 0 lies in this interval

3. $H_0: \mu_D \le 0,\ H_1: \mu_D > 0;\ t = 2.76;\ .001 < P < .005$; reject H_0

5. $H_0: \mu_D \le 0,\ H_1: \mu_D > 0;\ t = 4.63;\ P.0005$

Exercises 10.1

1. (a) They are of particular interest to the researcher and were not selected randomly.

    (b) $H_0: \mu_1 = \mu_2 = \mu_3 = \mu_4 = \mu_5$

    (c) $T_1. = 591.4$ $T.. = 1835.4$

            $T_2. = 460.4$ $\bar{X}.. = 36.71$

            $T_3. = 364.5$ $\sum\sum x^2 = 79896.22$

            $T_4. = 254.7$

            $T_5. = 164.4$

(d) $SS_{Total} = 12522.36$, $SS_{Tr} = 11274.32$, $SS_E = 1248.04$
(e) $MS_{Tr} = 2818.58$, $MS_E = 27.73$
(f) $F_{4,45} = 101.64$
(g) yes; $P < .01$ ($P \doteq 0$ via TI83)
(h) normality and equal variances

3. ANOVA

Source	DF	SS	MS	F
Treatment	4	3.935	.984	8.07
Error	37	4.497	.122	
Total	41			

$P = P[F_{4,37} > 8.09]$; $P < .01$; conclude that there are differences in the mean sulfur content among these five coal seams

5. ANOVA

Source	DF	SS	MS	F
Treatment	2	7.73	3.865	107.36
Error	29	1.04	.036	
Total	31			

reject H_0: $\mu_1 = \mu_2 = \mu_3$; $P < .01$

Exercises 10.2

1. (a)

$\bar{x}_{2.}$	$\bar{x}_{1.}$	$\bar{x}_{4.}$	$\bar{x}_{3.}$	$\bar{x}_{5.}$
38.7	46.0	50.0	51.3	60.0

(b) $\binom{6}{2} = 15$ (c) $\binom{10}{2} = 45$

3. $\alpha' \leq 1 - (1 - .05)^3 = .1426$; .5367; .9006

5. (a) ANOVA

Source	DF	SS	MS	F
Treatment	2	225.625	112.8125	4.9471
Error	21	478.875	22.8036	
Total	23			

$P = P[F_{2,21} > 4.9471]$; $.01 < P < .025$; reject H_0: $\mu_1 = \mu_2 = \mu_3$

(b) $\dfrac{b}{c} = \dfrac{.15}{3} = .05$

$|\bar{x}_{1.} - \bar{x}_{2.}|$ must exceed $2.080\sqrt{22.8036\left(\frac{1}{8} + \frac{1}{9}\right)} = 4.83$

$|\bar{x}_{1.} - \bar{x}_{3.}|$ must exceed $2.080\sqrt{22.8036\left(\frac{1}{8} + \frac{1}{7}\right)} = 5.14$

$|\bar{x}_{2.} - \bar{x}_{3.}|$ must exceed $2.080\sqrt{22.8036\left(\frac{1}{9} + \frac{1}{7}\right)} = 5.01$

$\bar{x}_{2.}$	$\bar{x}_{3.}$	$\bar{x}_{1.}$
16.33	22.0	23.125

7.

p	2	3
r_p	4.024	4.197
SSR_p	.685	.715

$df = 21$ (use 20)
$MSE = .232$
$n = 8$

$\bar{x}_1$	$\bar{x}_3$	$\bar{x}_2$
$-.9$	0	.2

9.

p	2	3	4
r_p	3.889	4.506	4.168
SSR'_p	.135	.156	.144

$df = 36$ (use 30)
$MSE = .012$
$n = 10$

$\bar{x}_{5.}$	$\bar{x}_{4.}$	$\bar{x}_{2.}$	$\bar{x}_{3.}$
.491	.656	1.604	1.623

11. (a) ANOVA

Source	DF	SS	MS	F
Treatment	2	189.22	94.61	.44
Error	15	3193.06	212.87	
Total	17			

unable to reject H_0: $\mu_1 = \mu_2 = \mu_3$
(b) not applicable

Exercises 10.3

1. ANOVA

Source	DF	SS	MS	F
Treatment	3	586.6	195.53	2.90
Error	76	512.2	67.42	
Total	79	5710.8		

$P = P[F_{3,76} > 2.90]$; $.025 < P < .05$; reject H_0: $\sigma_{Tr}^2 = 0$

Exercises 10.4

1. (a) no interaction; the difference from block 1 to block 2 is 2 for each treatment, and the difference from block 2 to block 3 is -2 for each treatment
   (b) interaction; for treatment A the difference between block 1 and block 2 is 3, whereas this difference is 5 for treatment C
   (c) interaction; for treatment A the difference between block 1 and block 2 is 3, whereas this difference is 2 for treatment B
3. (a) Since $RE > 1$, blocking is effective. The completely randomized design requires twice as many observations as the randomized complete block design to perform as well.
   (b) blocking is effective; requires 10 times as many observations
   (c) blocking is not effective; do not block in the future
   (d) blocking is not effective; do not block in the future
   (e) designs are equivalent

5. (a) $T_{1.} = 1872.3$ $\quad \bar{X}_{1.} = 936.15$ $\quad T_{.1} = 3967.9$ $\quad \bar{X}_{.1} = 991.975$
$T_{2.} = 1618.9$ $\quad \bar{X}_{2.} = 809.45$ $\quad T_{.2} = 3183.5$ $\quad \bar{X}_{.2} = 795.875$
$T_{3.} = 1781.3$ $\quad \bar{X}_{3.} = 890.65$
$T_{4.} = 1878.9$ $\quad \bar{X}_{4.} = 939.45$

$T_{..} = 7151.4$ $\quad \bar{X}_{..} = 893.925$ $\quad \sum\limits_{i=1}^{4}\sum\limits_{j=1}^{2} X_{ij}^2 = 6501860.16$

$N = 8$ $\qquad T_{..}^2/N = 6392815.245$

(b) ANOVA

Source	DF	SS	MS	F
Treatment	3	22004.455	7334.82	2.17
Block	1	76910.42	76910.42	
Error	3	10130.04	3376.68	
Total	7	109044.95		

$P = P[F_{3,3} > 2.17]$; $P > .10$; unable to reject H_0: $\mu_{1.} = \mu_{2.} = \mu_{3.} = \mu_{4.}$

(c) $C = 2(3)/7 = .857$; $RE = .857 + .143(22.78) = 4.11$; blocking appears to be useful

7.

p	2	3	4
r_p	3.956	4.126	4.239
SSR_p	1.697	1.769	1.818

$df = 27$ (use 24)
$MSE = 1.84$
$n = b = 10$

$\bar{x}_{3.}$	$\bar{x}_{4.}$	$\bar{x}_{2.}$	$\bar{x}_{1.}$
19.9	51.1	59.5	89.0

9. *Standard Taping*

$T_1 = 74$ $\qquad \bar{X}_{1.} = 4.625$ $\qquad T_{..} = 159$
$T_2 = 39$ $\qquad \bar{X}_{2.} = 2.4375$ $\qquad N = 48$
$T_3 = 46$ $\qquad \bar{X}_{3.} = 2.875$ $\qquad T^2/N = 526.6875$

$T_{.1} = 7.5$ $\qquad T_{.9} = 15.0$ $\qquad \sum\limits_{i=1}^{3}\sum\limits_{j=1}^{16} X_{ij}^2 = 879.5$

$T_{.2} = 16.5$ $\qquad T_{.10} = 14.5$
$T_{.3} = 11.0$ $\qquad T_{.11} = 2.5$
$T_{.4} = 4.5$ $\qquad T_{.12} = 15.5$
$T_{.5} = 15.0$ $\qquad T_{.13} = 5.5$
$T_{.6} = 7.0$ $\qquad T_{.14} = 14.5$
$T_{.7} = 16.5$ $\qquad T_{.15} = 2.0$
$T_{.8} = 6.0$ $\qquad T_{.16} = 5.5$

ANOVA

Source	DF	SS	MS	F
Treatment	2	42.875	21.4375	3.848
Block	15	142.8125	9.5208	
Error	30	167.125	5.5708	
Total	47	352.8125		

$P = P[F_{2,30} > 3.848]$; $.01 < P < .025$; reject H_0: $\mu_{1.} = \mu_{2.} = \mu_{3.}$

$\binom{3}{2} = 3$ Bonferroni-type paired T tests can be run. If each is run at the $\alpha = .05$ level then

$\alpha' \le 1 - (.95)^3 = .1426$.

$H_0: \mu_1 = \mu_2$, $H_1: \mu_1 \ne \mu_2$; $t = \dfrac{\bar{d}}{\sqrt{S_d/n}} = 2.39$; $P = .03 < .05$ (found via TI83)

Reject H_0 and conclude that flexibility was different before taping than after taping.

$H_0: \mu_1 = \mu_3$, $H_1: \mu_1 \ne \mu_3$; $t = 2.04$; $P = .059 > .05$ (found via TI83)

Unable to reject H_0; cannot detect any difference in flexibility after taping and after running.

$H_0: \mu_2 = \mu_3$, $H_1: \mu_2 \ne \mu_3$; $t = -.607$; $P = .55 > .05$ (found via TI83)

Unable to reject H_0; cannot detect any difference in flexibility after taping and after running.

Reinforced Taping

$T_1 = 77$	$\bar{X}_1 = 4.8125$	$T_{..} = 168.5$
$T_2 = 37$	$\bar{X}_2 = 2.3125$	$N = 48$
$T_3 = 54.5$	$\bar{X}_3 = 3.40625$	$T_{..}^2/N = 591.51$

$T_{.1} = 13.5$ $T_{.9} = -7.0$ $\displaystyle\sum_{i=1}^{3}\sum_{j=1}^{16} X_{ij}^2 = 1075.75$

$T_{.2} = 13.0$ $T_{.10} = 4.0$

$T_{.3} = 12.5$ $T_{.11} = 5.5$

$T_{.4} = 16.0$ $T_{.12} = 22.5$

$T_{.5} = 10.5$ $T_{.13} = 11.0$

$T_{.6} = 9.0$ $T_{.14} = 11.5$

$T_{.7} = 17.0$ $T_{.15} = .5$

$T_{.8} = 19.0$ $T_{.16} = 10.0$

ANOVA

Source	DF	SS	MS	F
Treatment	2	50.256	25.128	4.377
Block	15	261.74	17.449	
Error	30	172.244	5.741	
Total	47	484.24		

$P = P[F_{2,30} > 4.377]$; $.01 < P < .025$; reject $H_0: \mu_1 = \mu_2 = \mu_3$.

$H_0: \mu_1 = \mu_2$, $H_1: \mu_1 \ne \mu_2$; $t = 3.03$; $P = .008 < .05$

Reject H_0 and conclude that there is a difference in flexibility before and after taping.

$H_0: \mu_1 = \mu_3$, $H_1: \mu_1 \ne \mu_3$; $t = 1.63$; $P = .123 > .05$

Unable to detect any difference in flexibility before taping and after running.

$H_0: \mu_2 = \mu_3$, $H_1: \mu_2 \ne \mu_3$; $t = -1.28$; $P = .219 > .05$

Unable to detect any difference in flexibility after taping and after running.

Results for standard and reinforced taping are similar.

Exercises 10.5

1. **(b)** $T_{..}^2/N = (3366)^2/36 = 314,721$; $SS_{\text{Total}} = 12,710.42$

   (c) $SS_{\text{Tr}} = 12,489$; $SS_E = SS_{\text{Total}} - SS_{\text{Tr}} = 221.42$

   (d) $SS_A = 10,842$; $SS_B = 1225$; $SS_{AB} = = SS_{\text{Tr}} - SS_A - SS_B = 422$

(e/f) ANOVA

Source	DF	SS	MS	F
Treatment	5	12,489	2,497.8	338.42
A	2	10,842	5,421	734.48
B	1	1,225	1,225	165.97
AB	2	422	211	28.59
Error	30	221.42	7.3807	
Total	35	12,710.42		

H_0: $(\alpha\beta)_{ij} = 0$ (no interaction)
H_1: $(\alpha\beta)_{ij} \neq 0$ (interaction exists)

Reject H_0 with $P < .01$. Conclude that interaction exists. Therefore, we compare levels of factor A at each level of factor B.

ANOVA

Source	DF	SS	MS	F
Treatment	2	7564	3782	460.097 *P < .01
Error	15	123.3	8.22	
Total	17			

Reject H_0: $\mu_{11.} = \mu_{21.} = \mu_{31.}$ and H_1: $\mu_{i1.} \neq \mu_{k1.}$ for some i and k.

p	2	3	$df = 15$
r_p	4.168	4.347	$MSE = 8.22$
SSR_p	4.879	5.088	$n = 6$

$\bar{x}_{11.}$	$\bar{x}_{21.}$	$\bar{x}_{31.}$
73.0	102.0	123.0

ANOVA

Source	DF	SS	MS	F
Treatment	2	3700	1850	282.82 *P < .01
Error	15	98.12	6.54	
Total	17			

Reject H_0: $\mu_{12.} = \mu_{22.} = \mu_{32.}$ and H_1: $\mu_{i2.} \neq \mu_{k2.}$ for some i and k.

p	2	3	$df = 15$
r_p	4.168	4.347	$MSE = 6.54$
SSR_p	4.35	4.54	$n = 6$

$\bar{x}_{12.}$	$\bar{x}_{22.}$	$\bar{x}_{32.}$
71.0	86.0	106.0

3.   **(b)** $T_{..}^2/N = (859)^2/20 = 36894.05$; $SS_{\text{Total}} = 953.21$

    (c) $SS_{\text{Tr}} = 471.45$; $SS_E = 481.76$

    (d) $SS_A = 151.25$; $SS_B = .2$; $SS_{AB} = 320.0$

    (e) yes; there is a crossover

    (f) **ANOVA**

Source	DF	SS	MS	F
Treatment	3	471.45	157.15	5.22
A	1	151.25	151.25	5.02
B	1	.20	.20	.007
AB	1	320.0	320.0	10.63
Error	16	481.76	30.11	
Total	19	953.21		

H_0: $(\alpha\beta)_{ij} = 0$ (no interaction)
H_1: $(\alpha\beta)_{ij} \neq 0$ (interaction exists)
$P = P[F_{1,16} > 10.63]$; reject H_0 with $P < .01$
H_0: $\mu_{11.} = \mu_{21.}$, H_1: $\mu_{11.} \neq \mu_{21.}$; $f = 9.375$; $.01 < P < .025$; reject H_0
H_0: $\mu_{12.} = \mu_{22.}$, H_1: $\mu_{12.} \neq \mu_{22.}$; $f = 1.34$; $P > .10$; unable to reject H_0

5.   **(a)** **ANOVA**

Source	DF	SS	MS	F
Treatment	5	1,201,750.417	240,350.08	87.96
A	2	102,443.17	51,221.58	18.75
B	1	1,020,250.08	1,020,250.08	373.39
AB	2	79,057.167	39,528.58	14.47
Error	6	16,394.48	2,732.41	
Total	11	1,218,144.9		

$$\sum_{i=1}^{3}\sum_{j=1}^{2}\sum_{k=1}^{2} X_{ijk}^2 = 3,175,929$$

$$T_{...}^2/N = (4847)^2/12 = 1,957,784.083$$

  (b) H_0: $(\alpha\beta)_{ij} = 0$ (no interaction)

    H_1: $(\alpha\beta)_{ij} \neq 0$ (interaction exists); reject H_0 with $P < .01$

    H_0: $\mu_{11.} = \mu_{21.} = \mu_{31.}$ and

    H_1: $\mu_{i1.} \neq \mu_{j1.}$ for some i and j.

    ANOVA

    Reject H_0 with $P = .0276$ (TI83)

    $|X_{i1.} - X_{j1.}|$ must exceed $3.182\sqrt{4989.83\left(\frac{1}{2} + \frac{1}{2}\right)} = (224.77)$

$\bar{x}_{31.}$	$\bar{x}_{11.}$	$\bar{x}_{21.}$
490.5	722.5	873.5

    H_0: $\mu_{12.} = \mu_{22.} = \mu_{32.}$ and H_1: $\mu_{i2.} \neq \mu_{j2.}$ for some i and j.

ANOVA

Source	DF	SS	MS	F
Treatment	2	32,624.33	16,312.17	34.34
Error	3	1,425	475	
Total	5			

Reject H_0 with $P < .01$.

$|X_{i2.} - X_{j2.}|$ must exceed $3.182\sqrt{475\left(\frac{1}{2} + \frac{1}{2}\right)} = 69.35$

$\bar{x}_{32.}$	$\bar{x}_{22.}$	$\bar{x}_{12.}$
56.0	64.5	216.5

7. No interaction is found. Site differences are found. No differences are found among weeks.

Exercises 11.1

1. yes; the scattergram exhibits a linear trend   **3.** questionable

Exercises 11.2

1. $\sum x = 36.2$ $\sum y = 85.6$ $\bar{x} = 2.59$
$\sum x^2 = 105.66$ $\sum xy = 244.8$ $\bar{y} = 6.11$

$$b = \frac{14(244.8) - 36.2(85.6)}{14(105.66) - (36.2)^2} = \frac{328.48}{168.80} = 1.95$$

$a = 6.11 - 1.95(2.59) = 1.06; \mu_{Y|x} = 1.06 + 1.95x;$
$\mu_{Y|x=3.7} = 1.06 + 1.95(3.7) = 8.275; \hat{y} = 8.275$

3. $b = \dfrac{106(75989.6) - 366.1(12623)}{106(2435.63) - 366.1^2} = \dfrac{3433617.3}{124147.57} = 27.66$

$a = 119.08 - 27.66(3.45) = 23.65; \hat{\mu}_{Y|x} = 23.65 + 27.66x;$
$\hat{y} = 23.65 + 27.66(5.5) = 175.78$
no; 16 lies above the values used to generate the regression equation

5. (a) $\sum x = 56.6$ $\sum y = 151.1$ **(b)** $b = 1.996$ $\hat{\mu}_{Y|x} = 1.361 + 1.996x$
      $\sum x^2 = 117.68$ $\sum xy = 311.96$ $a = 1.361$
(c) $\hat{y} = 5.853$

7. (b) $\hat{\mu}_{Y|x} = 7.227 - .03296x$ **(c)** $\hat{\mu}_{Y|x=18} = \hat{y} = 6.634$

Exercises 11.3

1. (b) close to 1
      (c) $\sum x = 15$ $\sum y = 30.1$ $\sum xy = 92.75$
      $\sum x^2 = 47.5$ $\sum y^2 = 183.65$
      (d) $r \doteq .99$; strong positive

3. (b) close to 0; there is little linear trend
      (c) $\sum x = 21$ $\sum y = 38.2$ $\sum xy = 114.46$
      $\sum x^2 = 67.12$ $\sum y^2 = 228.98$
      (d) $r \doteq .015$; weak negative

5. (a) $\sum x = 2405$ $\sum y = 2503$ $\sum xy = 902{,}475$
$\sum x^2 = 900{,}775$ $\sum y^2 = 919{,}489$

(b) $r \doteq .978$

(c) yes; it gives almost the same readings as the manual method and should be easier to use

7. (b) As worry increases, there is a tendency for depression to increase. As satisfaction increases, there is a tendency for depression to decrease. As worry increases, there is a tendency for satisfaction to decrease.

(c) $H_0: \rho = 0$, $H_1: \rho \neq 0$

Exercises 11.4

1. (b) $\sum x = 1776$ $\sum y = 3018$ $\sum xy = 549{,}705$
$\sum x^2 = 322{,}062$ $\sum y^2 = 941{,}056$ $r \doteq .967$

(c) $r^2 \doteq .9351$; 93.51% of the variation in a lifter's best clean-and-jerk lift is associated with body weight

(d) ANOVA

Source	DF	SS	MS	F
Regression	1	28,280	28,280	116.4 *$P < .01$
Error	8	1,943.6	242.95	
Total	9	30,223.6		

$$S_{xy} = \frac{10(549{,}705) - 1776(3018)}{10} = 13708.2$$

$$S_{xx} = \frac{10(322{,}062) - (1776)^2}{10} = 6644.4$$

$$b = \frac{S_{xy}}{S_{xx}} = 2.063$$

$$a = -64.61$$

$$S_{yy} = \frac{10(941{,}056) - (3018)^2}{10} = 30223.6$$

$$\hat{\mu}_{y|x} = -64.61 + 2.063x$$

$$\hat{y} = 347.39 \text{ pounds}$$

5. $r^2 \doteq (.978)^2 = .956$; yes

7. .09; .1296; .0256

Exercises 11.5

1. (a) yes

(b) ANOVA

Source	DF	SS	MS	F
Regression	1	4,269.44	4,269.44	11.26 *$P < .01$
Error	9	3,411.11	379.01	
Total	10	7,680.55		

$\sum x = 548$ $\sum y = 620$ $\sum xy = 28{,}895$ $\bar{x} = 49.818$
$\sum x^2 = 28{,}230$ $\sum y^2 = 42{,}626$ $b = -2.143$
$S_{xy} = -1992.27$ $S_{xx} = 929.64$ $S = \sqrt{379.01} = 19.468$

(c) $a = 163.127$; $b = -2.143$

(d) $163.127 \pm 2.262 \left[\dfrac{19.468\sqrt{28230}}{\sqrt{11(929.64)}} \right]$ or 163.127 ± 73.17; 95% confident that α lies in the interval $(89.957; 236.297)$

$-2.143 \pm 2.262 \left[\dfrac{19.468}{\sqrt{929.64}} \right]$ or -2.143 ± 1.444; 95% confident that β lies in the interval $(-3.587, - .699)$

(e) $\hat{\mu}_{Y|x} = 163.127 - 2.143(35) = 88.122$ days;

$88.122 \pm 2.262(19.468)\sqrt{\dfrac{1}{11} + \dfrac{(35 - 49.818)^2}{929.64}}$ or 88.122 ± 25.186; 95% confident that $\mu_{Y|x=35}$ lies in the interval $(62.936, 113.308)$

(f) 88.122; $88.122 \pm 2.262 \, (19.468) \sqrt{1 + \dfrac{1}{11} + \dfrac{(35 - 49.818)^2}{929.64}}$ or 88.122 ± 50.73; 95% confident that $Y|_{x=35}$ lies in the interval $(37.392, 138.852)$

Exercises 11.6

1. $\hat{\mu}_{Y|x} = \hat{y} = 54.079 + .097(233) + .034(260) + .522(82) - 2.655(80) + 2.559(88)$
$= 141.116$

3. decrease the estimate by 2.655

5. (a) 73% of the variation in porosity is attributed to the linear association with the three regressors

(b) .0018; .018

(c) $- .72(20) = - 14.40$

7. $2^5 - 1 = 31$

Exercises 12.1

1. Table rearranged so that rows are fixed.

Hepatitis			
Vaccinated	**Yes**	**No**	
Yes	11 (41.06)	538 (507.94)	549 (fixed)
No	70 (39.94)	464 (494.06)	534 (fixed)
	81	1002	1083

$\chi_1^2 = 48.24$; $P < .005$; evidence shows that the proportion of those vaccinated with hepatitis is not the same as the proportion with hepatitis among those not vaccinated

3.

Rubella			
Cataracts	**Yes**	**No**	
Yes	14 (10.67)	6 (9.33)	20 (fixed)
No	10 (13.33)	15 (11.67)	25 (fixed)
	24	21	

$\chi_1^2 = 4.018$; $.025 < P < .05$; evidence shows that the proportion of those whose mother had rubella among those with cataracts is different from that among those whose mother did not have rubella

5.

	Allergy present		
Leukemia	Yes	No	
No	5 (10.39)	12 (6.61)	17 (fixed)
Yes	17 (11.61)	2 (7.39)	19 (fixed)
	22	14	36

$\chi_1^2 = 13.62$; $P < .005$; proportion of those with allergies differs between those with and without leukemia

7.

	Age		
Allergic	3 or under	Over 3	
Yes	32 (28.34)	30 (33.66)	62
No	80 (83.66)	103 (99.34)	183
	112	133	245

$\chi_1^2 = 1.16$; $P > .10$; no association is found between age and allergy to eggs; independence

9. $\hat{p}_1 = \dfrac{52}{300} = .173$; $\hat{p}_2 = \dfrac{48}{320} = .150$; $\hat{p} = \dfrac{52 + 48}{620} = .1613$

$$z = \frac{\hat{p} - \hat{p}_2}{\sqrt{\hat{p}(1 - \hat{p})\left(\dfrac{1}{n_1} + \dfrac{1}{n_2}\right)}} = \frac{.173 - .150}{\sqrt{.1613(.8387)\left(\dfrac{1}{300} + \dfrac{1}{320}\right)}} \doteq .778$$

$(.778)^2 = .605$; the difference between Z^2 and χ_1^2 is due to rounding differences

Exercises 12.2

1. Patients: $\hat{p}_A = \dfrac{472}{1301} = .363$ Controls: $\hat{p}_A = \dfrac{2625}{6313} = .415$

$\hat{p}_B = \dfrac{102}{1301} = .078$ $\hat{p}_B = \dfrac{570}{6313} = .090$

$\hat{p}_B = \dfrac{29}{1301} = .022$ $\hat{p}_{AB} = \dfrac{226}{6313} = .036$

The proportions appear to differ for all blood groups except possibly group B.

3. (a) no **(b)** independence **(c)** H_0: fragrance and color are independent
H_1: fragrance and color are not independent

(d)

	Flower color		
Fragrance	White	Pink	Orange	
Yes	12 (40.3)	60 (45.5)	58 (44.2)	130
No	50 (21.7)	10 (24.5)	10 (23.8)	70
	62	70	68	200

$\chi_2^2 = 82.29$; $P < .005$; conclude that color and fragrance are not independent

Given that a flower has a fragrance, there is a 9.23% chance that it is white, a 46.15% chance that it is pink, and a 44.62% chance that it is orange.

5. **(a)** test of homogeneity

(b)

SO$_2$ level	Chloroplast level			
	High	**Normal**	**Low**	
High	3 (5)	4 (8.33)	13 (6.67)	20
Normal	5 (5)	10 (8.33)	5 (6.67)	20
Low	7 (5)	11 (8.33)	2 (6.67)	20
	15	25	20	60

$\chi_4^2 = 14.74$; $.005 < P < .01$; reject H$_0$; conclude that the chloroplast level is affected by the SO$_2$ level

(c) $\hat{p}_H = \frac{13}{20} = .65$; $\hat{p} = \frac{2}{20} = .10$; $\hat{p} = \frac{5}{20} = .25$

It appears that SO$_2$ tends to decrease the chloroplast level.

7.

Location	Species							
	A	**B**	**C**	**D**	**E**	**F**	**G**	
Up	37 (34.70)	12 (11.31)	6 (9.80)	18 (13.58)	7 (5.28)	6 (9.05)	0 (2.26)	86
Down	9 (11.30)	3 (3.69)	7 (3.20)	0 (4.42)	0 (1.72)	6 (2.95)	3 (.74)	28
	46	15	13	18	7	12	3	114

$\chi_6^2 = 28.35$; $P < .005$

These data do not meet the size guidelines given as there is an expected cell frequency less than 1 and several others less than 5. More data are needed for the test to be valid. However, it appears from the data that the plant is probably having an adverse effect on plant life, with a particularly large impact on species D and E.

Exercises 13.1

1. **(a)** unable to reject H$_0$; data do not refute the assumption of normality

    (b) $t = 1.149$; $P > .10$

    Since $P > .05$, H$_0$ cannot be rejected at the $\alpha = .05$ level.

    (c) $\chi_{14}^2 = \dfrac{(.000008)}{(.0025)^2} = 17.94$; $.10 < P < .25$

    Since $P > .05$, H$_0$ cannot be rejected at the $\alpha = .05$ level.

3. **(b)** $t = 1.22$; $10 < P < .25$

    Since $P > .10$, H$_0$ cannot be rejected at the $\alpha = .10$ level.

    (c) $\chi_{19}^2 = \dfrac{20(104.93)^2}{(150)^2} = 9.79$; $.025 < P < .05$

    Since $P < .10$, H$_0$ can be rejected at the $\alpha = .10$ level. yes

Exercises 13.2

1. H$_0$: $M \geq 22$, H$_1$: $M < 22$

    If H$_0$ is true, $E[N'] = 10$; if H$_1$ is true, there should be too few positive signs.

    $N' = 5$; $P = P[N' \leq 5 | p = \frac{1}{2}] = .0207$; reject H$_0$

3. H_0: $M \geq 9$, H_1: $M < 9$

$E[N'] = 10$; $P = P\left[N' \leq 1 | p = \frac{1}{2}\right] \doteq 0.0000$; reject H_0

Yes, because P is extremely small.

5. $W_+ = 42.5$, $|W_-| = 12.5$

$$W_+ + |W_-| = 55 = \frac{10(11)}{2}$$

7.

x_i	0.71	0.13	0.16	0.65	0.21	1.00	0.51
$x_i - 8$	−0.09	−0.67	−0.64	−0.15	−0.59	0.2	−0.29
$|x_i - 8|$	0.09	0.67	0.64	0.15	0.59	0.2	0.29
Rank	1.5	13	12	3	10.5	4	5
Signed rank	−1.5	−13	−12	−3	−10.5	4	−5

x_i	1.1	1.11	0.32	0.71	0.4	0.21	1.63
$x_i - 8$	0.3	0.31	−0.48	−0.09	−0.4	−0.59	0.83
$|x_i - 8|$	0.3	0.31	0.48	0.09	0.4	0.59	0.83
Rank	6	7	9	1.5	8	10.5	14
Signed rank	6	7	−9	−1.5	−8	−10.5	14

H_0: $M \geq .8$, H_1: $M < .8$

If H_1 is true, we expect too many negative signs and too few positive ones. The test statistic is W_+.

$P = P[W_+ \leq 31]$; $P > .05$; unable to reject H_0 at the $\alpha = .05$ level because $31 > 26$

9.

x_i	35.5	44.5	39.8	33.3	51.4	51.3	30.5	48.9	42.1
$x_i - 45$	−9.5	−0.5	−5.5	−11.7	6.4	6.3	−14.5	3.9	−2.9
$|x_i - 45|$	9.5	0.5	5.5	11.7	6.4	6.3	14.5	3.9	2.9
Rank	22	2	13	24	16	15	25	10	9
Signed rank	−22	−2	−13	−24	16	15	−25	10	−9

x_i	40.3	46.8	38	40.1	36.8	39.3	65.4	42.6	42.8
$x_i - 45$	−4.7	1.8	−7	−4.9	−8.2	−5.7	20.4	−2.4	−2.2
$|x_i - 45|$	4.7	1.8	7	4.9	8.2	5.7	20.4	2.4	2.2
Rank	11	5	17	12	20	14	30	8	6
Signed rank	−11	5	−17	−12	−20	−14	30	−8	−6

x_i	59.8	52.4	26.2	60.9	45.6	27.1	47.3	36.6	
$x_i - 45$	14.8	7.4	−18.8	15.9	0.6	−17.9	2.3	−8.4	
$|x_i - 45|$	14.8	7.4	18.8	15.9	0.6	17.9	2.3	8.4	
Rank	26	19	29	27	3	28	7	21	
Signed rank	26	19	−29	27	3	−28	7	−21	

x_i	55.6	45.1	52.2	43.5
$x_i - 45$	10.6	0.1	7.2	−1.5
$|x_i - 45|$	10.6	0.1	7.2	1.5
Rank	23	1	18	4
Signed rank	23	1	18	−4

$W_+ = 200$, $|W_-| = 265$; $P = P[W_+ \leq 200] > .10$ because $200 > 152$; Type II

11. (a) $E[W_+] = \dfrac{70(71)}{4} = 1242.5$; $\text{Var } W_+ = \dfrac{70(71)(141)}{24} = 29198.75$;

$P[W_+ \leq 1000] = P[Z \leq -1.42] = .0778$

(b) $E[|W_-|] = \dfrac{80(81)}{4} = 1620$; $\text{Var } |W_-| = \dfrac{80(81)(161)}{24} = 4347$;

$P[|W_-|] \leq 1500 = P[Z \leq -.58] = .2810$

Exercises 13.3

1. **(a)** number of positive signs

(b) $P = P[N' \leq 3 | p = \frac{1}{2}] = .1719$; unable to reject H_0

3. H_0: $M_{X,Y} \leq 0$, H_1: $M_{X,Y} > 0$; $P = P[N \leq 1 | p = \frac{1}{2}] = .0107$; reject H_0

5. **(a)**

d_i	9.05	10.52	1.86	0.11	3.04	9	2.3	−4.49	4.12	−5.36
$|d_i|$	9.05	10.52	1.86	0.11	3.04	9	2.3	4.49	4.12	5.36
Rank	9	10	2	1	4	8	3	6	5	7
Signed rank	9	10	2	1	4	8	3	−6	5	−7

$W_+ = 42$, $|W_-| = 13$; $P = P[|W_-| \leq 13] > .05$ because $13 > 11$; unable to reject H_0 at the $\alpha = .05$ level

(b) $P = P[N \leq 2 | p = \frac{1}{2}] = .0547$; unable to reject at $\alpha = .05$ because $P > .05$

Exercises 13.4

1.

Observation	0.09	0.12	0.13	0.17	0.19	0.19
Group	U	U	U	U	U	U
Rank	1	2	3	4	5.5	5.5

Observation	0.2	0.2	0.21	0.21	0.21	0.22	0.23
Group	U	M	U	M	M	M	M
Rank	7.5	7.5	10	10	10	12	13

$W_m = 58$; reject if W_m is too large; $P < .025$; reject H_0 and conclude that the total protein content tends to be smaller among rats deprived of NGF in utero than among those deprived of the growth factor in milk

3.

Observation	604.1	646.8	688.1	739.4	760.5	793.5
Group	<	<	<	≥	<	<
Rank	1	2	3	4	5	6

Observation	797.0	806.8	812.4	818.9	843.6	850.0	856.6
Group	≥	<	≥	≥	≥	≥	<
Rank	7	8	9	10	11	12	13

Observation	899.1	906.5	909.3	940.7	961.8	968.1	979.1
Group	<	<	≥	≥	≥	<	≥
Rank	14	15	16	17	18	19	20

Observation	1009.9	1100.6	1330.3	1335.8
Group	≥	≥	≥	≥
Rank	21	22	23	24

W_m = sum of ranks of $<$ group; reject if W_m is too small; $W_m = 86$; reject with $P < .025$ (cutoff point is 91)

5. **(a)** $E[W_m] = \dfrac{30(91)}{2} = 1365$; Var $W_m = \dfrac{30(60)(91)}{12} = 13650$;

$P[W_m \leq 1350] = P[Z \leq -.13] = .4483$

(b) $E[W_m] = \dfrac{40(91)}{2} = 1820$; Var $W_m = \dfrac{40(50)(91)}{12} = 15166.67$;

$P[W_m \geq 2000] = 1 - P[Z \leq 1.46] = .0721$

Exercises 13.5

1. (a) $R_1 = 72.5$ **(b)** $H = \dfrac{12}{28(29)}\left[\dfrac{(72.5)^2}{8} + \dfrac{(170)^2}{10} + \dfrac{(163.5)^2}{10}\right] - 3(29) = 4.92;$
  $R_2 = 170$
  $R_3 = 163.5$ $P = P[X_2^2 \geq 4.92];\ .05 < P < .10$

3. $R_1 = 35$ $H = \dfrac{12}{25(26)}\left[\dfrac{(35)^2}{5} + \dfrac{(23)^2}{5} + \dfrac{(102)^2}{5} + \dfrac{(103)^2}{5} + \dfrac{(62)^2}{5}\right] - 3(26)$

  $R_2 = 23$ $H = 20.256;\ P = P[X_4^2 \geq 20.256];\ P < .005$
  $R_3 = 102$
  $R_4 = 103$
  $R_5 = 62$

5. $R_1 = 39$ $H = \dfrac{12}{24(25)}\left[\dfrac{(39)^2}{8} + \dfrac{(163)^2}{8} + \dfrac{(98)^2}{8}\right] - 3(25)$

  $R_2 = 163$ $H = 19.235;\ P = P[X_2^2 \geq 19.235];\ P < .005$
  $R_3 = 98$

Exercises 13.6

1. $R_1 = 18$ $\dfrac{b(k+1)}{2} = \dfrac{8(5)}{2} = 20$

  $R_2 = 21.5$
  $R_3 = 25$
  $R_4 = 15.5$
  $S = [(18 - 20) + (21.5 - 20) + (25 - 20) + (15.5 - 20)]^2 = 51.5$
  $X_3^2 = \dfrac{12S}{bk(k+1)} = \dfrac{12(51.5)}{8(4)5} = 3.8625;\ P = P[\chi_3^2 \geq 3.8625];\ .25 < P < .50;$
  unable to reject H_0

3. $R_1 = 25$ $\dfrac{b(k+1)}{2} = \dfrac{8(6)}{2} = 24$

  $R_2 = 17$
  $R_3 = 25$
  $R_4 = 25$
  $R_5 = 28$
  $S = 68;\ X_4^2 = \dfrac{12(68)}{40(6)} = 3.4;\ P = P[\chi_4^2 \geq 3.4];\ .25 < P < .50;$ unable to reject H_0

Exercises 13.7

1. (b) $\sum r_x = \sum r_y = 300;\quad \sum r_x^2 = \sum x_y^2 = 4900;\quad \sum r_x r_y = 3196;$

  $r_s = \dfrac{24(3196) - (300)^2}{\sqrt{[24(4900) - (300)^2][24(4900) - (300)^2]}} = -.4817$

(c) $\sum d^2 = 3408;\ r_s = 1 - \dfrac{6(3408)}{24(575)} = -.4817$

(d) the difference is very small
(e) $r_s^2 = .2320;$ weak negative correlation

3. $\sum r_x^2 = \sum r_y^2 = 649.5$; $\sum r_x = \sum r_y = 78$; $\sum r_x r_y = 588.25$; $r_s = .57$

There is a moderate positive correlation between blood alcohol content and smooth pursuit velocity.

Exercises 13.8

1. $n_1 = 8, n_2 = 10, n_3 = 10, N = 28$

$s_1^2 = 18.2124,$ $s_2^2 = 22.3162,$ $s_3^2 = 17.5645,$ $K = 3$

$$s_p^2 = \frac{7(18.2124) + 9(22.3162) + 9(17.5645)}{25} = 19.4565$$

$log\ s_p^2 = 1.2891$ $Q = 25(1.2891) - [7(1.2604) + 9(1.3486) + 9(1.2446)]$

$log\ s_1^2 = 1.2604$ $Q = .0659$

$log\ s_2^2 = 1.3486$

$log\ s_3^2 = 1.2446$

$$h = 1 + \frac{1}{3(2)}\left[\left(\frac{1}{7} + \frac{1}{9} + \frac{1}{9}\right)^{-1/25}\right] = 1.3584$$

$$B = \frac{2.3026(.0659)}{1.3584} = .1117; P = P\left[X_2^2 \ge .1117\right]; P > .90; \text{ do not reject } H_0$$

Exercises 13.9

1. (a) $P[X \le 3] \doteq P\left[Z \le \dfrac{3.5 - 6}{\sqrt{4.2}}\right] = P[Z \le -1.22] = .1112\ (.1071 \text{ binomial})$

(b) $P[3 \le X \le 6] \doteq P\left[\dfrac{2.5 - 6}{\sqrt{4.2}} \le Z \le \dfrac{6.5 - 6}{\sqrt{4.2}}\right] = P[-1.71 \le Z \le .24] = .5512$

   (.5725 binomial)

(c) $P[X \ge 4] = 1 - P[X \le 3] = 1 - P\left[Z \le \dfrac{3.5 - 6}{\sqrt{4.2}}\right] = P[-1.22 \le Z \le -.73];$

   .1215 (.1304 binomial)

3. $E[X] = 30$; Var $X = .99997$

$$P[X \le 25] \doteq P\left[Z \le \frac{25.5 - 30}{29.9991}\right] = P[Z \le -.82] \doteq .2061$$

$$P[25 \le X \le 35] \doteq P\left[\frac{24.5 - 30}{\sqrt{29.9991}} \le Z \le \frac{35.5 - 30}{\sqrt{29.9991}}\right]$$

$$= P[-1.000 \le Z \le 1.00] = .6826$$

5. $E[X] = 5$; Var $X = 4.9875$; $P[X \ge 1] \doteq P\left[Z \ge \dfrac{.5 - 5}{\sqrt{4.9875}}\right] = P[Z \ge -2.01] = .9778$

7. (a) $P[X \ge 95] \doteq P\left[Z \ge \dfrac{94.5 - 100}{10}\right] = P[Z \ge -.55] = .7088$

$$P\left[Z \le \frac{80.5 - 100}{10}\right] = P[Z \le -1.95] = .0256$$

c) $P[90 \le X \le 110] \doteq P\left[\dfrac{89.5 - 100}{10} \le Z \le \dfrac{110.5 - 100}{10}\right]$

$= P[-1.05 \le Z \le 1.05] = .7062$

(d) $P[X = 99] \doteq P\left[\dfrac{98.5 - 100}{10} \le Z \le \dfrac{99.5 - 100}{10}\right] = P[-.15 \le Z \le -.05] = .0397$

9. $\lambda = 1$; $s = .5$; $\lambda s = .5$; $X = $ number of killer particles per paramecia;

$P[X = 0] = .607$ (Poisson table)

$Y = $ number of killers that emit a killer particle; success = emission of a killer particle;

$p = .393$

$E[Y] = 20(.393) = 7.86$; Var $Y = 4.771$

$P[Y = 0] \doteq P\left[\dfrac{-.5 - 7.86}{\sqrt{4.771}} \le Z \le \dfrac{.5 - 7.86}{\sqrt{4.771}}\right] = P[-3.83 \le Z \le 3.37] = .9996$

$P[5 \le Y \le 10] \doteq P\left[\dfrac{4.5 - 7.86}{\sqrt{4.771}} \le Z \le \dfrac{10.5 - 7.86}{\sqrt{4.771}}\right]$

$= P[-1.54 \le Z \le 1.21] = .8251$

Exercises 13.10

1. (a) 10.5   (b) $P = P[X \ge 12 \mid p = .7] = .2969$; unable to reject H_0
3. (a) $H_0: p \le .20$, $H_1: p > .20$
   (b) 3.2
   (c) $P = P[X \ge 5 \mid p = .2] = .2018$; unable to reject H_0